Exploring the Nutrition and Health Benefits of Functional Foods

Hossain Uddin Shekhar
University of Dhaka, Bangladesh

Zakir Hossain Howlader
University of Dhaka, Bangladesh

Yearul Kabir
University of Dhaka, Bangladesh

A volume in the Advances in Environmental Engineering and Green Technologies (AEEGT) Book Series

Medical Information Science Reference
An Imprint of IGI Global

Published in the United States of America by
Medical Information Science Reference (an imprint of IGI Global)
701 E. Chocolate Avenue
Hershey PA, USA 17033
Tel: 717-533-8845
Fax: 717-533-8661
E-mail: cust@igi-global.com
Web site: http://www.igi-global.com

Library of Congress Cataloging-in-Publication Data

Names: Shekhar, Hossain Uddin, 1965- editor. | Howlader, Zakir Hossain, 1968- editor. | Kabir, Yearul, 1958- editor.
Title: Exploring the nutrition and health benefits of functional foods / Hossain Uddin Shekhar, Zakir Hossain Howlader, and Yearul Kabir, editors.
Description: Hershey, PA : Medical Information Science Reference, [2017] | Includes bibliographical references and index.
Identifiers: LCCN 2016017433| ISBN 9781522505914 (h/c) | ISBN 9781522505921 (eISBN)
Subjects: | MESH: Functional Food
Classification: LCC RA784 | NLM QU 145.5 | DDC 613.2--dc23 LC record available at https://lccn.loc.gov/2016017433

This book is published in the IGI Global book series Advances in Environmental Engineering and Green Technologies (AEEGT) (ISSN: 2326-9162; eISSN: 2326-9170)

British Cataloguing in Publication Data
A Cataloguing in Publication record for this book is available from the British Library.

All work contributed to this book is new, previously-unpublished material. The views expressed in this book are those of the authors, but not necessarily of the publisher.

For electronic access to this publication, please contact: eresources@igi-global.com.

Advances in Environmental Engineering and Green Technologies (AEEGT) Book Series

ISSN: 2326-9162
EISSN: 2326-9170

Mission

Growing awareness and an increased focus on environmental issues such as climate change, energy use, and loss of non-renewable resources have brought about a greater need for research that provides potential solutions to these problems. Research in environmental science and engineering continues to play a vital role in uncovering new opportunities for a "green" future.

The **Advances in Environmental Engineering and Green Technologies (AEEGT)** book series is a mouthpiece for research in all aspects of environmental science, earth science, and green initiatives. This series supports the ongoing research in this field through publishing books that discuss topics within environmental engineering or that deal with the interdisciplinary field of green technologies.

Coverage

- Contaminated Site Remediation
- Cleantech
- Industrial Waste Management and Minimization
- Water Supply and Treatment
- Renewable Energy
- Sustainable Communities
- Electric Vehicles
- Biofilters and Biofiltration
- Radioactive Waste Treatment
- Green Transportation

IGI Global is currently accepting manuscripts for publication within this series. To submit a proposal for a volume in this series, please contact our Acquisition Editors at Acquisitions@igi-global.com or visit: http://www.igi-global.com/publish/.

The Advances in Environmental Engineering and Green Technologies (AEEGT) Book Series (ISSN 2326-9162) is published by IGI Global, 701 E. Chocolate Avenue, Hershey, PA 17033-1240, USA, www.igi-global.com. This series is composed of titles available for purchase individually; each title is edited to be contextually exclusive from any other title within the series. For pricing and ordering information please visit http://www.igi-global.com/book-series/advances-environmental-engineering-green-technologies/73679. Postmaster: Send all address changes to above address.

Titles in this Series

For a list of additional titles in this series, please visit: www.igi-global.com

Smart Cities as a Solution for Reducing Urban Waste and Pollution
Goh Bee Hua (National University of Singapore, Singapore)
Information Science Reference • copyright 2016 • 362pp • H/C (ISBN: 9781522503026) • US $190.00 (our price)

Food Science, Production, and Engineering in Contemporary Economies
Andrei Jean-Vasile (Petroleum-Gas University of Ploiesti, Romania)
Information Science Reference • copyright 2016 • 473pp • H/C (ISBN: 9781522503415) • US $240.00 (our price)

Smart Grid as a Solution for Renewable and Efficient Energy
Ayaz Ahmad (COMSATS Institute of Information Technology, Pakistan) and Naveed Ul Hassan (LUMS School of Science & Engineering, Pakistan)
Information Science Reference • copyright 2016 • 415pp • H/C (ISBN: 9781522500728) • US $220.00 (our price)

Biologically-Inspired Energy Harvesting through Wireless Sensor Technologies
Vasaki Ponnusamy (Universiti Tunku Abdul Rahman, Malaysia) Noor Zaman (King Faisal University, Saudi Arabia) Tang Jung Low (Universiti Teknologi Petronas, Malaysia) and Anang Hudaya Muhamad Amin (Multimedia University, Malaysia)
Information Science Reference • copyright 2016 • 318pp • H/C (ISBN: 9781466697928) • US $200.00 (our price)

Handbook of Research on Waste Management Techniques for Sustainability
Ulas Akkucuk (Bogazici University, Turkey)
Information Science Reference • copyright 2016 • 438pp • H/C (ISBN: 9781466697232) • US $240.00 (our price)

Control and Treatment of Landfill Leachate for Sanitary Waste Disposal
Hamidi Abdul Aziz (Universiti Sains Malaysia, Malaysia) and Salem Abu Amr (Universiti Sains Malaysia, Malaysia)
Information Science Reference • copyright 2016 • 459pp • H/C (ISBN: 9781466696105) • US $220.00 (our price)

Toxicity and Waste Management Using Bioremediation
Ashok K. Rathoure (Vardan Environet Guargaon, India) and Vinod K. Dhatwalia (Uttaranchal University, India)
Engineering Science Reference • copyright 2016 • 421pp • H/C (ISBN: 9781466697348) • US $205.00 (our price)

Handbook of Research on Climate Change Impact on Health and Environmental Sustainability
Soumyananda Dinda (Sidho-Kanho-Birsha University, India)
Information Science Reference • copyright 2016 • 711pp • H/C (ISBN: 9781466688148) • US $325.00 (our price)

IGI GLOBAL
DISSEMINATOR OF KNOWLEDGE
www.igi-global.com

701 E. Chocolate Ave., Hershey, PA 17033
Order online at www.igi-global.com or call 717-533-8845 x100
To place a standing order for titles released in this series, contact: cust@igi-global.com
Mon-Fri 8:00 am - 5:00 pm (est) or fax 24 hours a day 717-533-8661

Table of Contents

Detailed Table of Contents

Emerging influence of Cardiovascular Diseases (CVDs) and its impact on the society has raised much awareness for its prevention. Healthy food habits and physical exercise has drawn a lot of attention of the people from scientific as well as common world. The role of food-based bioactive compounds in reducing risk of CVDs has been established with various health benefits apart from the basic nutrition have been reported. The present chapter provides an overview of the role of different foods on cardiovascular health of humans. Biological effects of plant derived food products and their bioactive compounds in the context of relevance to cardiovascular health promotion are discussed in detail. The chapter also covers the effects of the consumption of functional food on the intermediate clinical markers of CVDs including cholesterolemia, hypertension, endothelial function and inflammation. The chapter will enable the better understanding of the current knowledge on the potential health benefits of different functional foods and bioactive compounds on cardiovascular health.

Functional foods containing physiologically-active components, have been reported to confer several health benefits. Longitudinal cohort studies indicate that certain foods and dietary patterns play an important role in primary prevention of numerous disease conditions and this has led to the identification of putative functional foods. Research is necessary to substantiate the potential health benefits of various functional foods for which the diet–health relationships have yet not been scientifically validated. The term 'functional foods' may include health/functional health foods, foods fortified with minerals/vitamins, dietary supplements or even the traditional medicines.

Lentils have been part of human diet from ancient times. This chapter focuses on the nutritional composition, presence of bioactive substances, antioxidants and health rendering properties of lentils. Recent definitions have considered lentils as a prophylactic and therapeutic functional food due to its considerable content of essential macronutrients, namely functional proteins and carbohydrates, and essential micronutrients, as well as bioactive phytochemicals such as phytates and polyphenols. Indeed, the presence of an impressive arsenal of secondary metabolites, minerals and bioactive constituents in lentils have shown to be promising contributors in the management and prevention of several human chronic diseases, attributed to their anticarcinogenic, hypoglycemic, hypocholesterolemic and blood-pressure lowering properties.

Kimchi is a traditional Korean food manufactured by fermenting vegetables with probiotic Lactic Acid Bacteria (LAB). Many bacteria are involved in the fermentation of kimchi, but LAB become dominant while the putrefactive bacteria are suppressed during salting of baechu cabbage and the fermentation. The addition of other subingredients and formation of fermentation byproducts of LAB promote the fermentation process of LAB to eventually lead to eradication of putrefactive and pathogenic bacteria, and also increase the functionalities of kimchi. Accordingly, kimchi can be considered a vegetable probiotic food that contributes health benefits in a similar manner as yogurt as a dairy probiotic food. Further, the major ingredients of kimchi are cruciferous vegetables; and other healthy functional foods such as garlic, ginger, red pepper powder, and so on are added to kimchi as subingredients. As all of these ingredients undergo fermentation by LAB, kimchi is regarded as a source of LAB; and the fermentative byproducts from the functional ingredients significantly boost its functionality. Because kimchi is both tasty and highly functional, it is typically served with steamed rice at every Korean meal. Health functionality of kimchi, based upon our research and that of other, includes anticancer, antiobesity, anticonstipation, colorectal health promotion, probiotic properties, cholesterol reduction, fibrolytic effect, antioxidative and antiaging properties, brain health promotion, immune promotion, and skin health promotion. In this review we describe the health functionalities of kimchi and the probiotic properties of its LAB.

Tea is the second most widely consumed beverage throughout the world, after water. "Tea" is referred to the aromatic beverage prepared by incubating cured leaves of the plant *Camellia sinensis* with hot or boiling water. The origin of tea has remained a mystery and has been associated with legends in the Chinese history. Under experimental conditions in laboratory, tea has been reported to act as an anti-cancer agent in various models of lung, pancreas, liver, breast, fore-stomach, oesophagus, duodenum, colon, and skin cancers induced by chemical carcinogens. Tea also contains a wide range of antioxidants and has been found to possess several others health benefits. This chapter summarizes the history behind its use, various health benefits, and current state of scientific literature and epidemiological evidence of its usefulness.

This chapter per the authors will introduce the reader to Complementary and Alternative Medicine (CAM) and shall discuss herbalism as a subset of CAM. Particular emphasis will be placed on herbal teas or rather infusions and decoctions used in disease therapy. This chapter will enumerate the different types of teas and shall use maps, graphs, and other tools to illustrate location, consumption, use and availability. Furthermore, the authors will highlight potential health benefits, recent studies (in vitro, in vivo) undertaken by research scientists to validate efficacy, and shall call for more research (clinical data management, clinical trials, etc.) and support for ongoing work in this area of expertise. The authors shall place a spotlight on the plant family, Asteraceae, and their herbal plants of interest, Artemisia annua and Brickellia cavanillesii. Extensive studies have been performed to determine the therapeutic potential of Brickellia cavanillesii plant at Ernest E. Smith laboratory, The Institute of Environmental and Human Health (TIEHH), Texas Tech University, Lubbock, USA.

This chapter focuses on the potential health benefits of camel milk including angiotension I-converting enzyme-inhibitory, anti-cancer and antioxidant activities, antidiabetic, antimicrobial and hypoallergenicity effects. The bioactivity of oligosaccharide, conjugated linoleic acid and D-amino acid in camel milk is provided. The proposed mechanisms behind these bioactive components and potential health claims are explained. This chapter also describes camel milk composition, nutritional value, production and population. The current available information in the literature on camel milk is not abundant. More research is needed to give better understanding on functional properties of camel milk.

Pomegranate (Punica granatum L.), the fruit and its peel have been shown to hold tremendous potential for the treatment of various ailments. Incorporation of pomegranate, peel and their extracts, as key functional ingredients in various ethnopharmacological formulations are widely accepted in almost all cultures of the World. In addition to their disease ameliorating features, pomegranate and the peel extracts have gained significant popularity in functional food market as ingredient of choice in foods designed to prevent onset of various non-communicable diseases. Health promoting features of the pomegranate peel and fruit extracts define the scope of this natural reserve in global nutraceutical and functional food industry. On account of their unique phytochemicals profile, plentiful pool of antioxidants, dietary fibers, minerals and natural colors, both the valuable reserves have been remained as highly explored plant material in last two decades. Building levels of interest in this fruit has created a deeper insight among researchers to understand actual potential and pathways of pomegranate biomolecules reactivity in human models. The chapter in hand meticulously deals with pomegranate and its extracts as source of innovative healthy components responsible for averting cardiovascular diseases, inflammatory and non-inflammatory disorders, type 2 diabetes, gastric ulcers, various types of cancers and neurodegenerative disorders.

Yerba mate (Ilex paraguariensis) is a plant original from the subtropical regions of South America, present in Southern Brazil, Northeastern Argentina, Paraguay and Uruguay. It is primarily consumed as a beverage made by steeping the leaves of the plant in hot water. The growing interest in mate products has made it paramount that research on this herbal tea continues, as it has shown extraordinary possibilities not only as a consumer beverage but also in the nutraceutical industry. Yet, there is much to be done: human-based studies to support the properties verified in vitro and in vivo models with animas are scarce.

Rice is a fundamental food in many cultural cuisines around the world, and it is an important cereal crop that feeds more than half of the world's population. The two main categories are white rice and whole grain rice or bow ice. Whole grain rice is not processed very much, so it is high in nutritional value, whereas white rice is processed so that the bran or outer covering is removed, leaving it with less nutritional value. People choose different styles of rice for particular flavors, depending on their culinary needs, the availability, and the potential for healthy benefits as well.

In Asian countries, soybeans have been used as food and food ingredients for centuries and their consumption have been associated with beneficial health effects. In addition to their nutritive value, soybeans have many active chemical compounds, among which isoflavones are the most important. Isoflavones are plant-derived phytoestrogens, chemically comparable in their structure and properties to human estrogens. For isoflavones to become bioavailable, their activation and/or conversion into more active metabolites, such equol from daidzein, must occur. Equol is the isoflavone metabolite with the greatest estrogenic activity and antioxidant capacity. Epidemiological studies have suggested that high intakes of isoflavones reduce the symptoms of menopause as well as the incidence of hormone-dependent and aging-associated diseases such as osteoporosis, cardiovascular disease and cancer. This chapter reviews soy consumption, isoflavone metabolism, and briefly summarizes the results of recent clinical trials on, and meta-analyses of, the effects of isoflavone consumption on human health.

In recent years, the consumer demands for healthier meat and meat products with reduced level of fat, cholesterol, decreased contents of sodium chloride and nitrite, improved composition of fatty acid profile and incorporated health enhancing ingredients are rapidly increasing worldwide and prevent the risk of diseases. This review focuses on strategies to investigate the changes in physical, physicochemical and microbial properties of meat and meat products in dietary processed sulfur fed animals. Overall, this review focuses on sulfur supplementation to pigs, growth performance of pigs and meat quality, enhancing the nutritional and functional values, shelf-life extension, improve sensory quality characteristics and health benefit etc. This review further discusses the current status, consumer acceptance, and market for functional foods from the global viewpoints. Future prospects for functional meat and meat products are also discussed.

Association between food and health is complex. Healthy food can promote and maintain good human health. Healthy food and nutrition is a key regulating factor for boosting the immunity and therapeutic effectiveness of a treatment strategy. Oxidative stress is well involved in the pathogenesis of diverse diseases and aging. Food always considered as good source of nutrients, protein, fat, carbohydrates, vitamins, minerals and antioxidants. Consumed as part of a normal diet, phytochemicals present in food like vitamins (vitamin C & E), minerals (like, zinc, selenium), phytoconstituents (phenolic compounds, flavonoids, carotenoids) confer additional health benefits, by virtue of their antioxidant property. A diet rich that rich in antioxidant molecule reduces the risk of several oxidative stress related diseases. Numerous antioxidant molecules isolated from food showed the curative and health promotion effect. This chapter majorly deals with the role antioxidant/pro-oxidant substances present in different foods on human body.

Non-degradable packaging materials are doing much damage to the environment. So the interest has been developed in biodegradable films and coatings these days. Use of edible films and coatings is eco-friendly technology used for enhancing the shelf life of the fruits and vegetables. The use of antimicrobial compounds in edible coatings of proteins, starch, cellulose derivatives, chitosan, alginate, fruit puree,

Preface

In the last few decades, our understanding of functional foods has increased greatly and people around the world are aware of the concept of functional foods. To them it is more than just a source of simple nutrition. People are starting to realize not only the physiological and nutritional value of these foods, but their health benefits as well. We now have a revolution in the way we understand nutrition and health.

Functional foods are an important part to the diet and play a vital role in health and nutrition. We may have different ways of defining "functional food". However, it is any fresh or processed food which is supposed to have a health-promoting and/or disease-preventing property apart from providing only the basic nutritional function of supplying nutrients. In the general category we have processed food made from functional food ingredients, or fortified with health-promoting additives, like "vitamin-enriched" products, and also fresh foods (e.g., *vegetables*) that have specific health claims attached to them. Fermented foods with live cultures are often also considered to be functional foods with probiotic benefits. The most noteworthy aspects of functional foods are their biological functions that augment several health benefits to consumers due to the functional properties linked with them.

During the past few decades or so, consumption of functional foods has developed as a major health trend among conscious people who want to have a greater control over their health and well being. It is apparent that this life style trend will continue and gain momentum, so there is a continuous need for scientific information on all aspects of functional foods in this evolving sector. Being a part of a regular diet, functional foods are understood to provide a wide range of physiological benefits and potential health benefits. This book on functional foods discusses these and other functional properties of foods available and consumed by people. The book also reviews functional foods for the prevention and treatment of diseases from a multidisciplinary perspective and covers a wide range of topics. Although many topics have been included in this book, we do not claim the coverage to be comprehensive.

The necessity to provide a better understanding together with the need to disseminate the latest developments in this rapidly expanding field, this book, covers a wide range of functional foods, including the source of the functional foods, their history, functionality, chemical, physical and physiological properties, health benefits, mechanisms of antioxidant action, anticancer, antidiabetic properties, as well as clinical and epidemiological evidence. This book discusses the theoretical and practical aspects of functional foods, from the fundamental concepts of biochemistry, nutrition, and physiology to the technologies involved in food processing.

In recent years, the health-promoting effects of foods have evolved into an area of intense research and there is now a wealth of scientific evidence that supports the role of various foods and their components in promoting human health. Recently, a great deal of consideration has been made to anti-carcinogenicity, anti-mutagenicity, anti-oxidative and anti-aging properties of certain foods and such studies have revealed their potential health significance. These studies have also provided an understanding of the relationship between diet and optimal health, particularly with respect to age-related degenerative disease risk reduction such as cancer, heart disease, osteoporosis, diabetes, and stroke. This book offers an assortment of important information on functional foods and provides scientific evidence on therapeutic applications of foods.

Due to potential health benefits of functional foods, consumers around the world have intensified their interest in food selection and preparation as a means of maintaining good health and also for protection against diseases and age related conditions. Such interest and changes in the approach of consumers, together with the continuous advances made in food science and technology, have provided food companies with substantial incentives to produce health-promoting foods and diets with advanced formulations that takes into consideration the needs of the increasingly health conscious consumers who are interested in self-administered health care.

Today more and more people have the firm belief that traditional functional foods can reduce disease risk, maintain health, and thus make their dreams of having a long and healthy life come true. The history of traditional functional foods is based on herbal products which are in use as traditional medicines from time immemorial. This together with health care which is based on natural products has given new worldwide meaning tofunctional foods.

This book provides food scientists and technologists, food process engineers, biochemists, nutritionists, medical doctors, public health professionals, entrepreneurs as well as students and researchers interested in functional foods with comprehensive information on selected functional foods in terms of the physiological effects of foods and food components able to promote good health and prevent or alleviate diseases. Individuals who believe in the need for real foods that combines nutritional and medical benefits and who believe that such foods can be produced, will find this book to be immensely helpful. The information provided in the book would be of enormous help to those who are keen in preserving health through prevention of diseases. Augmented understanding of the role of functional foods will open new possibilities of producing new elements for nutritionally optimized foods that care of both the health and nutrition of a consumer.

This book will also be an invaluable source of information for a detailed understanding of the impact of functional food nutrients on human metabolic pathways. Therefore, researchers and policy makers in life sciences will find this information greatly resourceful for them. We believe a contemporary reference and source book such as this, which describes, distils, and disseminates important and relevant scientific information and advances in this field, is valuable for the flow of such information.

This book consists of a series of chapters focusing on the current state of functional properties of foods in relation to health and diseases. It examines health-promoting and therapeutic properties of functional foods and the resulting benefits to nutritional value and long-term health.

Chapters 1 and 2 describe the contribution of functional foods to the prevention of cardiovascular health of humans and attempts to identify the role of dietary factors while bearing in mind the impact of physiologically active components. The chapter also covers the role of functional foods in the treatment of cardiovascular disorders. The chapters provide a better understanding of the current knowledge on the potential health benefits of different functional foods and bioactive compounds such as dietary fiber, omega-3 fatty acids, antioxidants, photochemical as well as probiotics, prebiotics and synbiotics and its relation to the health of heart and blood vessels.

Chapter 3 provides information on the abilities of functional foods to prevent and manage hypertension by virtue of their capability to influence bio-macromolecules in the cells. The chapter also describes the etiology and pathophysiology of hypertension and the role of functional components of foods such as long chain fatty acids, glucosinolate and polyphenols in the wellbeing of humans in relation to hypertension.

Chapters 4 and 5 focus on the potential health benefits of tea which contains a wide range of antioxidants. These chapters also summarize the history behind the consumption of tea and describe the current research on the mode of operation of the antioxidants as well as epidemiological evidence of health benefits of tea. The functionality and physiological properties of conventional and medicinal herbal tea in terms of their role in anti-aging and chronic diseases such as cancer has also been discussed.

Topics of Chapter 6 cover the functional benefits and risks of consumption of rice on human health. Heath benefits of rice are described in terms of antioxidant properties of rice and the presence of phytochemical such as flavonoids, tocopherol, tocotrienol, anthocyanins and steryl fevulate.

Chapter 7 describes the current research on kimchi, a traditional fermented Korean dish (made from vegetables using an assortment of seasonings and its health benefits) as a vegetable probiotic food. Health promoting effects of kimchi such as lipid lowering, antiatherosclerosis, anithrombotic, antihypertensive, antioxidant, anti-aging, anticancer, antiviral, anti-asthma, obesity preventing, skin care, etc. has been discussed.

Topics of Chapter 8 focus on the nutritional composition, presence of antioxidants and other bioactive substances in relation to the health rendering benefits of lentils. This chapter provides information on the presence of nutrients and bioactive phytochemicals that have prophylactic and therapeutic functional properties in lentils. It also describes the role of lentils in the management and prevention of several human chronic illnesses due to their anti-carcinogenic, hypo-glycemic, hypo-cholesterolemic properties together with their blood-pressure lowering activities.

Chapter 9 focuses on the potential health benefits of camel milk in relation to different bioactive components present in the milk. The presence of bioactive components such as oligosaccharide, conjugated linoleic acid, D and L amino acid have been particularly mentioned and the functional role of the constituents of camel milk on antidiabetic, antimicromial, antioxidant, anticancer, hypoallergenicity and Angiotension Converting Enzyme (ACE) inhibitory activity has been described. The proposed mechanisms behind the activity of these bioactive components and potential health claims are also described.

In Chapter 10, the role of pomegranate (*Punicagranatum* L.) and its extract in the treatment of various ailments is discussed, focusing particularly on antioxidants, phytochemicals and dietary fiber. Since ancient times pomegranates have been turned to for their immense medical benefits responsible for protection against a range of mild infections to several life threatening degenerative disorders. Pomegranate and its extracts as source of bioactive healthy components responsible for averting cardiovascular diseases, inflammatory and non-inflammatory disorders, type 2 diabetes, gastric ulcers, various types of cancers and neurodegenerative disorders have also been described.

Chapter 11 discusses the beneficial health effects of soy and soy products in addition to their nutritive value. The chapter focuses on the relationship between functional bioactive components of soybean, such as isoflavones and equol, and their health benefits. The mode of action and the role of isoflavones on menopause symptoms, bone health, cardiovascular and central nervous system and hormone-dependent cancers have been illustrated in this chapter.

Chapter 12 covers the functional benefits of plant food, Yerba Mate. This chapter is devoted to different functional properties of this plant food. Some of the yerba health benefits are less widely known, at least for those who do not live in a yerba-drinking part of the world. It is used as an antioxidant and antimicrobial agent. It is also used for the improvement of oral health. This chapter elaborates the role yerba mate has in cancer prevention, as a hypo-cholesterolemic agent and as a source of photochemicals. Relationship between bioactive food components and their health benefits has also been discussed.

Chapter 13 discusses some of the important functional foods of the Indian subcontinent. It describes the presence of various chemical and biological functional components and their role in improving human health. The functional constituents of various food commodities consumed by the people of the Indian Subcontinent e.g., cereals, legumes, oilseeds, milk and milk products, herbs and condiments and exotic fruits such as Ber (*Zizpplus*), Jamun (*Syzgium cumini*) has been described in this chapter. Consumption of such food on the corrective and preventive potential of gastrointestinal health, bone health, cardiovascular diseases, various types of cancers, neurodegenerative diseases, ill-effects of obesity, and metabolic syndrome has also been illustrated.

Chapter 14 discusses the unique nutritional and health-promoting bioactive compounds present in traditional African foods that contribute to human health and influence various physiological pathways involved in health promotion. The chapter also outlines the abilities of functional components of traditional African foods to prevent and manage chronic diseases, such as diabetes, hypertension, obesity, cardiovascular diseases, cancer, and others. The chapter also includes the health benefits of traditional African fermented foods.

Chapter 15 mainly focuses on the antioxidant functional components of different foods and identifies the role of antioxidant/pro-oxidant substances present in different foods on health benefits. The chapter also describes the association of health improvement and prevention of disease in relation to consumption of natural foods containing various antioxidant molecules.

Chapter 16 reviews the current literature on the history, composition, classification and functional properties of edible film coating, with regard to controlling microbiological growth and extension of shelf-life of various foods. The chapter also presents the action of microbial films and coatings on food, uses of antimicrobial food agents and additives in edible films with respect to food sensory quality and nutrition. The impact and advantages of edible film coating in terms of food safety and consumer acceptability and health benefits has also been discussed.

Finally, Chapter 17 deals with sulfur supplementation to pigs and its impact on growth performance and meat quality, and ways to enhance nutritional and functional values, extend shelf-life; improve sensory quality characteristics and health benefits etc. This chapter further discusses the current status, consumer acceptance, and market for functional foods from a global viewpoint. Future prospects for functional meat and meat products are also discussed.

Functional foods in nutrition and health benefit is a rapidly advancing area of research and this book discusses the science behind these foods and offers a great deal of information on how they can be used to fight disease and improve overall health. This book will serve as a useful source book in understanding what functional food is, its impact, potential, and how it relates to the well-being of human. The chapters are clear, easy to read, and interesting for anyone who wishes to become more knowledgeable about functional foods. This book is a compilation of various aspects of functionality and health benefits of selected functional foods of the world.

1. Food and Cardiac Health: Protective effects of food on cardiovascular system by *Aditi Jain and Vibha Rani*
2. Functional foods and cardiac health by *Santosh Jain Passi*
3. Functional Food in hypertension by *Anil Kumar Gupta*
4. Health benefits of tea by *Sumonto Mitra and Shashi Khandelwal*
5. Herbal benefits of tea by *Etetor Roland Eshiet and Ernest E. Smith*
6. Health benefits and Risks of Rice by *Zakir Hossain Howlader and Hossain Uddin Shekhar*
7. Health promoting effects of kimchi by *Kim Hyun Ju and Han Eung-Soo*
8. Lentils (*Lens culinaris*, L.): A novel functional food by *"Mo'ez Al-Islam" Ezzat Faris and Amita Attlee*
9. Functional properties of camel milk by *Omar Amin Alhaj*
10. Pomegranate peel and fruit extracts - a novel approach to avert degenerative disorders by *Saeed Akhtar, Tariq Ismail and Muhammad Riaz*
11. Soy and soy products, isoflavones, equol and health by *Baltasar Mayo, Lucia Guadamuro, Ana Belen Florez and Susana Delgado*
12. Yerba Mate: Chemistry, technology and biological properties by *Roberto Buffo*
13. Functional foods of Indian subcontinent by *Jiwan S. Sidhu and Tasleem A. Zafar*
14. Traditional African foods and their potential to contribute to health and nutrition by *John H. Muyonga, Sophie Nansereko, Ilona Steenkamp, Marena Manley and Judith Kanensi Okoth*
15. Food in Health Preservation and Promotion - A Special Focus on the Interplay between Oxidative Stress and Pro-oxidant / Antioxidant by *Saikat Sen and Raja Chakraborty*
16. Antimicrobial edible films and coatings for fruits and vegetables by *Amrita Poonia*
17. Application of the dietary processed Sulphur supplementation for enhancing nutritional and functional properties of meat products by *Chi Ho Lee*

There are several professional books on this subject matter and the choice for any particular one depends on the needs of the users. The 17 chapters in this book represent collections of selected reviews on the role of functional foods in nutrition and health benefits from a multidisciplinary perspective. It not only introduces functional foods, but also shows the investigations and research that led to their creation with modern approaches in the prevention and treatment of chronic diseases such as cardiovascular disease. As functional foods continue to become popular worldwide, a concrete understanding of these functional foods will help food scientists take advantage of them to better maintain and promote health.

Each chapter has been contributed by dedicated professionals from across the globe representing academia, government institutes, and industry. We hope this book would be a valuable information source and reference book for scientists of diverse backgrounds including biologists, biochemists, chemists, dieticians, food scientist, and nutritionists, medical doctors and pharmacologists from universities, research institutes, and food industries. We sincerely hope this book addresses the needs of its readers and advances their understanding and knowledge of functional food. We believe that this book will lead to further stimulation of research and development in this emerging field, and will provide consumers with up-dated information about products that could reduce disease risk and assist them in maintaining a healthy life style. It is a joint effort of many individuals who worked hard to make this book a comprehensive one. This effort signifies significant cooperation and outstanding teamwork.

We express our gratitude to all the contributing authors who accepted our invitation to give their time and effort and share the expertise they have achieved through their hard work and extensive research. We also thank the reviewers for giving their valuable comments leading to improvements in the contents of each chapter. We acknowledge and thank the members of the production team at IGI for their time, effort, advice, and expertise, especially, Ms. Erin O'Dea and Ms. Courtney Tychinski for their guidance and support to this project. They are the ones who made this book possible. It has been a pleasure to work with IGI publisher and the co-operation of the editorial and production staff is highly appreciated. We are grateful to our families and the institution we work for. It would not have been possible for us to publish this book without their endless encouragement and their faith in us.

Yearul Kabir
On behalf of the Editors

Chapter 1
Food and Cardiac Health:
Protective Effects of Food on Cardiovascular System

Aditi Jain
Jaypee Institute of Information Technology, India

Vibha Rani
Jaypee Institute of Information Technology, India

ABSTRACT

Emerging influence of Cardiovascular Diseases (CVDs) and its impact on the society has raised much awareness for its prevention. Healthy food habits and physical exercise has drawn a lot of attention of the people from scientific as well as common world. The role of food-based bioactive compounds in reducing risk of CVDs has been established with various health benefits apart from the basic nutrition have been reported. The present chapter provides an overview of the role of different foods on cardiovascular health of humans. Biological effects of plant derived food products and their bioactive compounds in the context of relevance to cardiovascular health promotion are discussed in detail. The chapter also covers the effects of the consumption of functional food on the intermediate clinical markers of CVDs including cholesterolemia, hypertension, endothelial function and inflammation. The chapter will enable the better understanding of the current knowledge on the potential health benefits of different functional foods and bioactive compounds on cardiovascular health.

INTRODUCTION

Cardiovascular Diseases (CVDs) have a substantial influence on public health from past several decades and it still remain the major cause of mortality and morbidity throughout the globe. CVDs comprise group of different cardiac and vascular complications including hypertension, coronary heart, atherosclerosis, cerebrovascular disease (stroke), peripheral artery disease, rheumatic heart disease, heart failure etc. Major lifestyle causes of CVDs include tobacco intake, physical inactivity and unhealthy diet (World health organization, 2009). Major CVD events arise due to atherosclerosis, a pathophysi-

DOI: 10.4018/978-1-5225-0591-4.ch001

ological complication of innermost layer of arterial wall and such events can be prevented by nutritional supplementation (O'Toole et al. 2008). Different parameters have been studied in this regard and life-style changes have been suggested as the most helpful practices including physical activity and healthy food habits. Healthy diet and food habits show an inverse relationship with onset of vascular diseases as well as affect the longevity. Food provides both the essential nutrients required for basic life processes as well as bioactive compounds that help in disease prevention and health enhancement. Balanced diet including fruits, vegetables, whole grains and other plant foods helps in acquiring the required amounts of nutrients, antioxidants, bioactive compounds and phytochemicals thereby prevents various health related complications. Potential health promoting benefits of the natural bioactive compounds have been studied over time. There is keen interest in assessing the role of food-based bioactive compounds in reducing risk of chronic diseases including Cancer, CVD and diabetes mellitus.

For the reduction of coronary heart diseases, much emphasis is given on reducing the saturated fat, trans fat and cholesterol to lower the low-density lipoprotein-cholesterol (LDL-C) levels. Other pathways involved in the protective effects mediated by different food products with respect to CVDs onset has also been studied extensively. Oxidative stress results in cellular damage by affecting proteins, DNA and lipids, thereby increasing the risk CVDs. Oxidized LDL-C are a major factor that contributes to the cardiac diseases. Antioxidant potential of fruits and vegetables accounts for the most of the health promoting benefits and CVD prevention (Pandey & Rizvi, 2009). Major oxidative stress mediated events that lead to various cardiovascular complications are summarized in the Figure 1. Other factors include preventing vascular inflammation, reducing platelet hyper activity, vasodilation, cardiac hypertrophy etc.

Figure 1. Oxidative stress induced cardiac complications

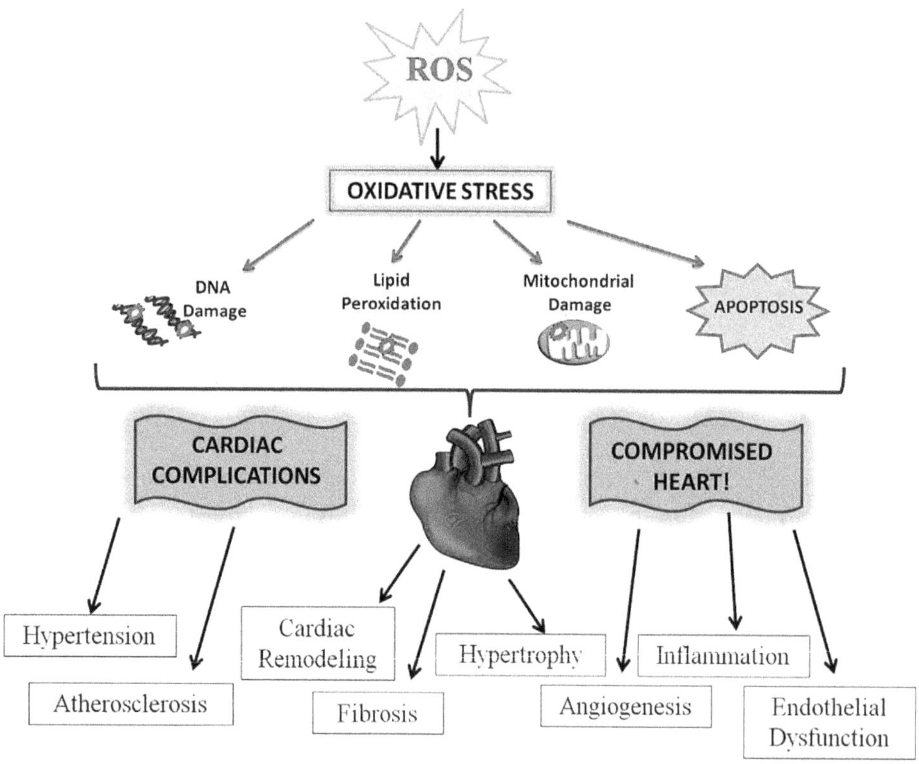

Inflammation is a critical factor in CVDs and its systemic marker, C-reactive protein, plays an important role in disease progression. Inflammation promotes atherosclerosis initiation and progression resulting in severe thrombotic complications of atherosclerosis (Shrivastava et al, 2015). Platelet activation and aggregation play a key role in the pathogenesis of myocardial infarction and ischaemic cardiac complications. Cardiac hypertrophy is a compensatory patholphysiological response of the heart to chronic pressure, and is a critical risk factor for ischemic heart disease, arrhytmia and sudden death. Dietary supplementation can promote the proper platelet function by reducing the hyper-reactivity of platelets and maintain cardiovascular health.

Based on the extensive studies done in the previous decades, a throughout general observation has been made to support the hypothesis that the precise intake of foods and beverages with high amount of flavonoids and polyphenols play an important role in reducing CVD risk by improving vascular function and modulating inflammation (Habauzit & Morand, 2012). There are ample epidemiologic evidences from numerous studies that suggest a strong relationship between the consumption of diets high in fruits and vegetables, legumes, whole grains, fish and cardiovascular disease protection. Phenolic compounds including flavonoids, tannins etc. are present in almost all the plants and vegetables. These compounds have been studied in detail for their protective and beneficial roles in human health.

NATURAL FOODS WITH CARDIOPROTECTIVE BENEFITS

There are increasing facts suggesting the uptake of natural food products as they are enriched in micronutrients including minerals, vitamins and essential fatty acids that are required to sustain the cellular antioxidant levels and other stress response mechanisms (Visioli & Hagen, 2007). It has also been demonstrated in various studies that intake of a healthy balanced diet including whole food is evidently more beneficial as compared to the consumption of processed food. It may be contributed to the fact that isolated compounds either loses their biological activity or may not behave in the similar way as in the whole foods. Hence, the usually present combination of phytochemicals of natural food products is responsible for the various potential preventive effects. Number of food item has been reported to play a significant role in prevention and cure of CVDs. These are discussed in detail in the following section and their different mechanisms are depicted in Figure 2.

Fruits, vegetables, legumes, whole grains and fish are high in fiber and omega 3 (or *n*-3) fatty acids as well as low in saturated fat, trans fat and dietary cholesterol. Whole grains, nuts and green leafy vegetables are the rich source of vitamin E, which is well known for reducing the risk for atherosclerosis and coronary heart diseases. Fruit and vegetables have sufficient amount of antioxidants including phytochemicals, phenolics and carotenoids that protect cellular systems and reduces the risk of various diseases including CVDs. In a very recent UK Women's Cohort Study, it has been eastablished that total fruit intake lowers the risk of CVD mortality, with a 6–7% reduction in risk for each 80 g/day portion consumed. Also, women in the highest intake group of grapes and citrus experienced a significant reduction in risk of CVD and stroke as compared with the non-consumers (Lai et al., 2015).

Garlic, or *Allium sativum* has been used in daily food practices across the worlds from centuries and it has been studied for various medically important effects including hypocholesterolaemic, anti-atherosclerotic, antioxidant and cardioprotective (Bayan et al, 2013). Garlic comprises specific allyl sulphides and other organosulpfur compounds that express the characteristic protective properties of garlic in wide variety of patho-physiological conditions. These sulphide compounds restrict the oxidized

Figure 2. Cardio protective mechanisms of different natural food products

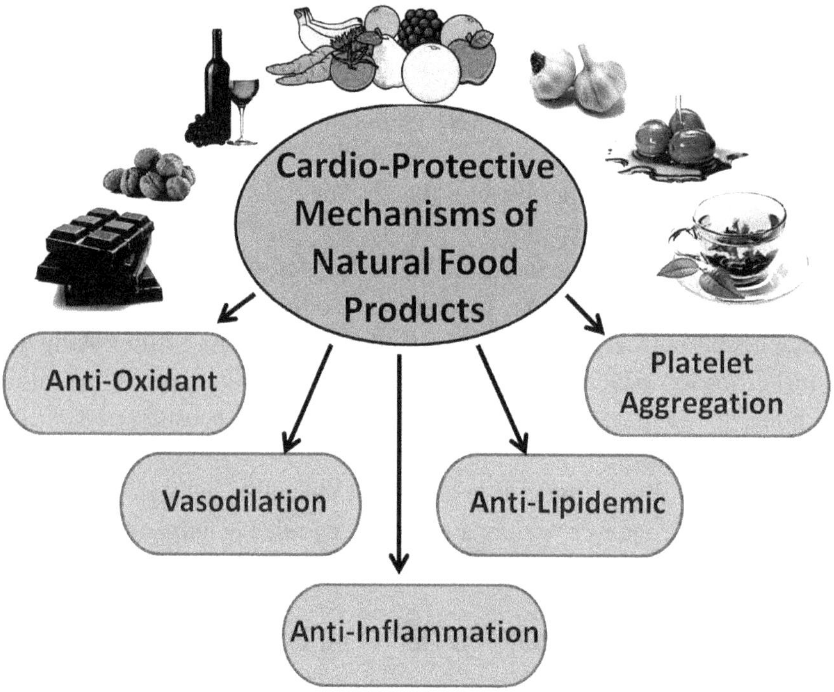

LDL mediated cellular eNOS degradation as well as prevents the vasculae endothelium from oxidative stress mediated effects (Seki & Hosono, 2015). Garlic is well known for reducing total cholesterol and TAG thereby preventing cardiac complications (Tapsell et al, 2006). Garlic consumption decreases mortality and morbidity rates of CVDs through its antithrombotic, hypoglycemic and lipid-lowering properties. Garlic oil is shown to decrease hypercholesterol mediated cardiac hypertrophy *in vivo* by modulating different signaling pathways and molecules including IL-6, p-extracellular signal-regulated kinase-5, p-MAPK-5, calcineurin, p-GATA binding protein 4 thereby improving hypertrophy-associated cardiovascular complications (Hseieh et al., 2014). It is also known for maintaining the homeostasis of the immune system by stimulating specific cell types and other mechanisms important for the development and advancement of various diseases including CVDs. Garlic modulates cytokine secretion thereby contributing to its action for many of the therapeutic effects (Arreola et al., 2015). Garlic supplements have also shown to reduce the high blood pressure. In a meta-analysis conducted by Wang et al., it was observed that garlic consumption directly modulates blood pressure and it is significantly effective in the hypertensive patients (Wang et al., 2015). Preventive effects of garlic powder on CVDs and risk factors were studied in another meta-analysis where it was found that garlic significantly reduces blood total cholesterol and LDL-C levels. Garlic was also found to decrease systolic and diastolic blood pressure (Kwak et al, 2014).

Green Tea, derived from *Camellia sinensis*, is well studied for its role in cardiac protection and CVD prevention (Cooper & Morre, 2005; Kuriyama et al., 2006; Sumpio et al., 2006). Green tea consumption has shown to inhibits cardiomyocyte apoptosis, a critical factor in the transition from hypertrophy to heart failure, prevents cellular damage caused by oxidative stress, p53 modulation and decrease in

Bcl-2 expression (Sheng at al., 2007). It also reduces LDL-C levels thereby directly reducing different cardiac complications.

Syzygium cumini, also known as black plum or jamun, is a well-known for its medicinal properties including anti-inflammatory, hypoglycemic, anti-oxidant, antibacterial and cardioprotective (Chagas et al., 2015). Various *in vitro* and *in vivo* studies have demonstrated the cardioprotective potential of *S. cumini*. It has been shown to reduce isoproterenol-induced myocardial infarction in rats by inducing biochemical alterations (Mastan et al., 2009). It also exerts cardioprotective effects against glucose induced oxidative stress on cardiac myocytes by exerting free radical scavenging activity (Atale et al., 2013).

In studies, nuts consumption as a part of diet has shown different potential health benefits despite of their high fat content (Coates & Howe, 2007). Nuts intake markedly decrease the risk of sudden cardiac arrest and other associated heart problems like high cholesterol levels. Walnuts, almonds and hazelnuts have drawn ample attention in the recent years for their cardio protective and other health benefits.

Oil derived from olives has been shown to decrease CVD risk by reducing LDL oxidizability and downregulate CD40-ligand expression and their downstream products (Castaner et al., 2012). Canola oil can reduce plasma cholesterol levels and influences various biological functions and biomarkers of cardiac disease risks. Canola oil consumption also increases tocopherol levels and effects insulin sensitivity, lipid peroxidation, inflammation, energy metabolism, and cancer cell growth (Lin et al., 2013).

In a recent study, it has been shown that the consumption of beans have hypercholesterolaemic with resulting in reducing the LDL-C levels without disturbing the HDL-c levels (Winham & Hutchins, 2007).

Xuezhikang, Chinese red-yeast rice, comprises statins that are used to supplement the diet for the prevention of cardio vascular diseases. Studies have shown that this rice can prevent the occurrence of cardiac complications in diabetic patients by 50% (Zhao et al., 2004). It has no adverse effects associated with the regular consumption and its commercial production should be encouraged in the other parts of the world as well. Buttermilk consumption has shown to be associated with reduced cholesterol and triglycerides concentrations in men and women by inhibiting intestinal absorption of cholesterol. Therefore, it should be recommended as a natural and low cost dietary product for improving lipid profiles in low risk patients (Conway et al., 2013).

These remarkable effects of natural food products thus reinforce the recommendation to raise the intake for the cardiovascular protection.

FUNCTIONAL FOOD AND CARDIAC HEALTH

Functional food displays advantageous effect on different body functions by improving the state of health and reducing the disease risk apart from its nutritional importance. Functional food comprises the food that we consume as a part of our diet with beneficial effects. It has been observed in various clinical and epidemiological studies that protective nutritional practices can reduce the risk of chronic heart disease upto 60% (Everitt et al., 2006; Kris-Etherton et al., 2002; Habauzit & Morand, 2012). These protective ingredients in our food reduce the major risk factors of cardiac abnormalities like reduction in blood cholesterol levels, hypertension and diabetes. Functional foods majorly comprise soluble fibres, phytostenols, sterols, long-chain *n*-3 fatty acids, soya proteins etc. These components majorly act upon the serum lipids and reduce the risk of heart diseases. The major classes of functional foods along with their main sources are illustrated in the Figure 3.

Figure 3. Major categories of different functional foods and their sources

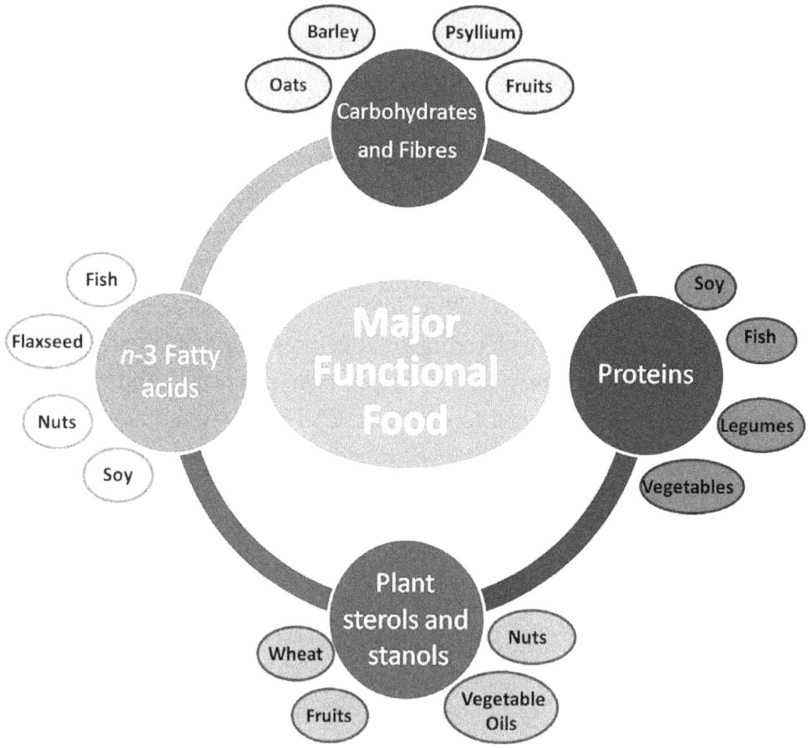

Dietary fibres help in reducing the cholesterol levels and considered as a safe approach for the prevention as well as cure of high cholesterol levels (Erkkila & Lichtenstein, 2006). Soluble fibres decrease the LDL-C levels thereby exerting hypocholestrolaemic effects and hence, recommended harmless. They are majorly present in fruits, oat bran, barley, flaxseed and psyllium.

β-glucan from soluble oats and barley is also well known for the reduction of LDL-C levels. It is primarily associated with the reduction in the bile acid absorption and cholesterol levels. Its consumption in the form of a fruit drink has shown significant reduction in cholesterol levels (Naumann et al, 2006; Nwachukwu et al., 2015).

Long-chain fatty acids of the *n*-3 series are essential dietary compounds as they cannot be synthesized in mammals. They play an important role in modulation of membrane properties and lipid mediated signaling pathways by incorporating into the structural lipids (Sirtori et al, 2009). Intake of *n*-3 fatty acids, like eicosapentaenoic and docosahexaenoic acids result in decreased incidence of coronary heart disease and unexpected cardiac death (von Schacky C, 2004). They are generally present in animal diets, especially fish, with few exceptions of certain seeds like nuts, flaxseeds, linseed, rapeseed and soy. The role of fish consumption in reducing the risk of cardiovascular diseases was established several years back and has become the basis of using fish oils and other fish derived products in purified forms for supplementing the diet for the disease prevention (Elvevoll et al, 2006). It has been observed that *n*-3 fatty acids from fish oil are involved in a number of nuclear receptor-regulated mechanisms thereby regulating tissue lipid metabolism and other associated metabolic and lipoprotein disorders (Dubey & Cheema, 2006). The *n*-3 fatty acids also help in improving atherosclerosis risk factors like hypertension apart from triacylglycerolaemia and HDL-cholesterolaemia (Borghi & Cicero, 2006). Because of these beneficial effects, different forms of n-3 fatty acids have been incorporated into variety of easily available food items, for example, cow's milk and bread spreads.

Sterol compounds produced by plants can decrease the intestinal absorption of dietary and biliary cholesterol by interfering with their transporters thereby altering the cholesterol metabolism. Stanols are formed by saturating β-sitosterol and campesterol and incorporated in the different varieties of functional foods (Winter, 2005). Phytosterols and phytostanols have hypocholesterolaemic efficacy as the esterification of the fatty acids with plant sterols, improve the LDL-C:HDL-C ratio (Chan et al., 2007).

Soya proteins have shown various cardio protective effects in various animal and human studies mainly by reducing the total cholesterol, LDL-C and ischaemic events. Consumption of low carbohydrate diet including either soya or vegetable proteins have shown to reduce the cardiovascular risk (Halton et al, 2006). In 1999, US Food and Drug Administration approved the health claim for the role of soya protein intake in cardiovascular disease risk reduction based on the cholesterol lowering effect of soya proteins. Similarly to soya protein, fish protein also reduces cholestrolaemia and blood pressure thereby preventing cardiovascular risk. Protein derived from lupin seeds has also shown remarkable cholesterol-lowering effects in various studies (Martins et al, 2005). Lupin has an advantage of having the whole protective ingredients for the cardiac protection including fibres, phtosterols and protein. Lupin protein isolates have also shown to decrease the development of hypertension (Pilvi et al, 2006). Red wine and purple-grape juice has shown to exert platelet-inhibitory properties. The antioxidant potential of red wine provides cardioprotection by reducing oxidative stress in different pathological conditions of cardiac system (Das et al., 2007).

BIOACTIVE COMPOUNDS FROM FOOD AS CARDIOPROTECTANTS

Bioactive compounds are defined as the extranutritional components that are present in food in small quantities. Phytochemicals are the bioactive nonnutrient plant compounds present in fruits, vegetables and other plant based foods. They are known to reduce the risk of various chronic diseases directly or indirectly. Phenolic compounds and flavonoids are the extensively studied bioactive compounds as they are present in all the plants. They have been studied widely in cereals, nuts, olive oil, legumes, vegetables, fruits, tea etc. Studies have reported protective relationship among flavonoids and CVD. Their antioxidant potential reflects favorable effects on CVD risk factors. Different classes of bioactive compounds along with their natural sources and protective roles have been summarized in Table 1.

Various plant-derived foods and drinks, comprising chocolate, wine, berry juices, tea, coffee etc., have been extensively studied *in vitro* and *in vivo* for their potential benefits on cardiovascular health. They hold a wide range of phenolic compounds, including flavonols, flavanols, procyanidins and anthocyanins (Pascual-Teresa et al, 2010).

Flavonoids are the most common polyphenolic compounds present in plant derived food products. The reduction in CVD risk as observed after flavonoid intake is clinically significant (Hooper et al, 2008; Mursu et al, 2008). Based on an hypothesis for understanding the polyphenols portective effect, acidic nature of flavonoids may act as chemical uncouplers in the mitochondria leading to an increased resting energy expenses and results in the increased cell longevity (Modriansky & Gabrielova, 2009). Cocoa is rich in flavonoid content that has been well studied for its protective role in cardio vascular disorders (Ding et al., 2006). Other than flavonoids, Cocoa also contains catechins and procyanidins, which can

Table 1. Bioactive compounds, their natural sources, and protective roles in human health

Bioactive Molecules	Major Natural Sources	Protective Roles
Anthocyanins	Red, blue and purple berries	Anti-oxidant, cardio protective, DNA damage protection
Proanthocyanins and Procyanidins	Cocoa, grapes, apple, cinnamon	Anti-oxidant, anti-carcinogenic
Phytoestrogen	Soy, flaxeed oil, whole grains, fruits and vegetables	Anti-oxidant, cardio protective
Hydroxytyrosol	Olive oil	Anti-oxidant, cardio protective
Reserveratol	Nuts, red wine	Anti-oxidant, anti-thrombonic, anti-inflamatory, anti-carcinogenic
Lycopene	Carotenoid fruits including tomatoes	Anti-cancerous
Organosulphur	Onion, garlic	Anti-carcinogenic, cardio protective, anti-oxidant
Isothiocyanates	Cruciferous vegetable	Anti-carcinogenic, cardio protective
Monoterpenes	Citrus fruits, cherries, herbs	Anti-carcinogenic, cardio protective
Quercetin	Onions, fruits, broccoli	Anti- inflammatory, cardio protective, anti-hypertensive, anti diabetic, anti cancerous
Myricetin	Berries, fruits, vegetables, herbs, tea and wine	Anti-oxidant, anti diabetic, anti cancerous
Kaempferol	Aloe vera, fruits	Anti-inflammatory, anti-apoptotic, anti oxidant, anti cancerous, anti bacterial
Luteolin	Fruits, vegetables, medicinal herbs	Anti cancerous, anti oxidant, anti- inflammatory, anti-hypertensive
Fisetin	Strawberry, onion, grapes, wine	Bone protective, neuro protective
Catechin and Epicatechin	Tea, chocolate, apples, pears, grapes and red wine	Anti oxidant, anti-obese, cardio protective
Tannins or Proanthocyanidins	Fruits and vegetables	Anti oxidant, cardio protective, anti-inflammatory, anti-carcinogenic and anti-mutagenic

reduce the oxidant-induced peroxynitrite production in vitro, enhance the NO synthase expression and NO-dependent vasodilation in the aorta and prevent hypertension (Grassi et al, 2005; Kurosawa et al, 2005). Cocoa polyphenols exhibit antioxidant, anti-inflammatory and anti-atherogenic activity and targets NF-κB and iNOS (Rimbach et al, 2009). These benefits make dark chocolate consumption, either in powder, as chocolate or from different cocoa flavanol-rich drinks, a very important measure for reducing cardiovascular risks (Corti et al., 2009).

Phenolic compounds and polyphenols have shown to regulate various signaling pathways involved in cell survival, growth and differentiation. Polyphenols represents the major contender to explain the protective effects of plant-derived food products. The anti-inflammatory action of phytochemicals present in wide variety of plants may play an important role in the prevention of CVDs. Phytochemicals have also been shown to have roles in the reducing platelet aggregation, cholesterol synthesis modulation and blood pressure maintenance.

Catechin and epicatechin are the most common flavonoids. Catechins are also called monomeric flavonols and they are the biosynthetic precursor of proanthocyanidins and well known for their antioxidant potential, but their protective effect on cardiovascular health is also accounted by other effects including mediating important mechanisms like hypertension, inflammation, cellular proliferation, hyperglycaemia and hypercholesterolemia. Epigallocatechin gallate is a major catechin of green tea and it has been shown to decrease vascular inflammation by synthesizing more of nitric oxide thereby blocking endothelial vascular inflammation (Yamakuchi et al, 2008). Nitric oxide production is also restricted by PPAR receptors in response to catechins (Danesi et al, 2009). Catechin consumption has also shown to decrease decreased atherosclerotic factors including TNF-α, sICAM-1, MCP-1 and CRP suggesting the effective role in reducing atherosclerosis and proinflammation (Hsu et al, 2007).

Quercetin is another flavonoid present in fruits, vegetables, nuts, seeds and flowers and has epidemiologic evidence for a protective effect against CVDs. It inhibits platelet aggregation and reduces thromboxane synthesis and may be helpful in reducing CVD risks (Egert et al., 2009).

Oligomeric procyanidins or flavan-3-ols have shown to activate of eNOS and mediating an endothelium dependent relaxant effect that modulates the NO/cGMP pathway (DalBo et al., 2008). Proanthocyanidins present in grape seeds have demonstrated to reduce the levels of proinflammatory markers such as CRP, IL-6, TNF-α and an increase in the production of antiinflammatory cytokines thereby suggesting the obesity-related adipokine dysregulation to manage cardiovascular and metabolic risk factors (Terra et al., 2009). In an *in vitro* study, catechin and proanthocyanidins have shown the cardioprotective effects on myocardial cells against the toxicity originated by the administration of anticancer drugs like doxorubicin (Du et al., 2008).

Anthocyanins are the bioactive compounds with dual benefits, firstly for their impact on the sensorial characteristics of food products and secondly for their health related properties with proposition on cardiovascular disease risk protection. Anthocyanins are the pigments responsible for the bright colors of many fruits and vegetables. (de Pascual-Teresa & Sanchez-Ballesta, 2008). They can act upon different cells involved in the pathogenesis of atherosclerosis, in addition to the effects on cholesterol distribution thereby protecting endothelial cells from CD40- induced proinflammatory signaling (Wallace, 2011; Xia et al., 2007). Anthocyanins have also shown decrease in NF-kB–related proinflammatory chemokines, cytokines, and inflammatory mediator responses in the plasma suggesting inhibition of NFkB activation by anthocyanins (Karlsen et al, 2007).

Curcumin or diferuoylmethane is an active ingredient of and well known for its different protective properties including anti-inflammatory, antioxidative and cardiovascular effects (Miriyala et al., 2007; Ahuja et al., 2011). Curcumin treatment reduces free radical generation, monocyte adhesion to activated endothelial cells and phosphorylation of c-Jun N-terminal kinase, p38 mitogen activated protein kinases. These effects results in the prevention of myocardial function following ischemic or biochemical stress to the heart. Curcumin can also reduce cardiac remodeling and suppresses cardiac hypertrophy (Kohli et al., 2013; Srivastava & Mehta, 2009).

Various phytoestrogens are present in soy, but also in flaxseed oil, whole grains, fruits, and vegetables. Many phenolic compounds have antioxidant properties Hydroxytyrosol is a phenolic compound present in olives and olive oil and well known as a potent antioxidant. Resveratrol is found in nuts and red wine and exhibits antioxidant, antithrombotic and anti-inflammatory properties. Lycopene is also an effective antioxidant present in tomatoes and other fruits. Organosulfur compounds present in garlic, isothiocyanates in cruciferous vegetables and monoterpenes in citrus fruits, cherries, and herbs are few other examples of cardioprotective effects mediating bioactive compounds.

CONCLUSION

Prevention is better than treatment and the same applies to the onset of CVDs. Novel dietary advances for cardiovascular prevention are of major significance at present as there is an increasing despise in primary prevention of CVDs by chronic drug usage. A correlation between CVD prevention and healthy diet has been demonstrated from the various studies. There are sufficient evidences recommending the consumption of food sources rich in bioactive compounds including flavonoids, fibres, plant proteins and phytosterols, polyphenols etc. Integrating plant foods with high levels of flavanols in the diet of healthy individuals can decrease the risk of CVD significantly. The active compounds present in the plants have huge potential to reduce serum total cholesterol and LDL-C levels, thus directly improving cardiac health. Phenolic compunds are potent effectors of biological processes and influence CVD risk via modulating cellular pathways like MAPK signaling pathway and important mediators like NF-κB, AP-1 and Nrf.

There are sufficient evidences for recommending the consumption of food sources rich in bioactive compounds, that is, recommending a diet including variety of fruits, vegetables, whole grains, legumes, oils, and nuts. Various mechanisms of action of most the bioactive compounds have been conducted but more scientific research is need to be done to embark on science based dietary recommendations. Well-designed future investigations with the isolated bioactive compounds are needed to be done to derive the valuable information regarding the mechanism of action and doses to be taken. This will lead to commence recommendations for both the nature of the compounds and the optimal dose and better targets can be achieved in the area of cardiovascular health protection.

ACKNOWLEDGMENT

We acknowledge Department of Biotechnology (DBT), Government of India (BT/PR3978/17/766/2011) for the research grant awarded to Dr. Vibha Rani. We also acknowledge the Department of Biotechnology, Jaypee Institute of Information Technology, Deemed to be University for providing the literature and infrastructural support.

REFERENCES

Ahuja, S., Kohli, S., Krishnan, S., Dogra, D., Sharma, D., & Rani, V. (2011). Curcumin: A potential therapeutic polyphenol, prevents noradrenaline-induced hypertrophy in rat cardiac myocytes. *The Journal of Pharmacy and Pharmacology*, *63*(12), 1604–1612. doi:10.1111/j.2042-7158.2011.01363.x PMID:22060292

Arreola, R., Quintero-Fabian, S., Lopez-Roa, R.I., Flores-Gutierrez, E.O., Reyes-Grajeda, J.P., Carrera-Quintanar, L.C., & Ortuno-Sahagun, D. (2015). Immunomodulation and Anti-Inflammatory Effects of Garlic Compounds. *Journal of Immunology Research*, 1-13.

Atale, N., Chakraborty, M., Mohanty, S., Bhattacharya, S., Nigam, D., Sharma, M., & Rani, V. (2013). Cardioprotective Role of Syzygium cumini Against Glucose- Induced Oxidative Stress in H9C2 Cardiac Myocytes. *Cardiovascular Toxicology*, *13*(3), 278–289. doi:10.1007/s12012-013-9207-1 PMID:23512199

Bayan, L., Koulivand, P. H., & Gorji, A. (2013). Garlic: A review of potential therapeutic effects. *The American Journal of Physiology*, *4*, 1–14. PMID:25050296

Borghi, C., & Cicero, A. (2006). Recent evidence of the role of omega-3 polyunsaturated fatty acids on blood pressure control and hypertension-related complications. *Future Lipidology*, *1*(5), 569–577. doi:10.2217/17460875.1.5.569

Castaner, O., Covas, M. I., Khymenets, O., Nyyssonen, K., Konstantinidou, V., Zunft, H. F., & Fito, M. et al. (2012). Protection of LDL from oxidation by olive oil polyphenols is associated with a downregulation of CD40-ligand expression and its downstream products in vivo in humans. *The American Journal of Clinical Nutrition*, *95*(5), 1238–1244. doi:10.3945/ajcn.111.029207 PMID:22440854

Chagas, V.T., Franca, L.M., Malik, S., & Paes, A.M.D. (2015). Syzygium cumini (L.) skeels: a prominent source of bioactive molecule against cardiometabolic disease. *Frontiers in Pharmacology, 6*(259), 1-8.

Chan, Y., Demonty, I., Pelled, D., & Jones, P. J. (2007). Olive oil containing olive oil fatty acid esters of plant sterols and dietary diacylglycerol reduces low-density lipoprotein cholesterol and decreases the tendency for peroxidation in hypercholesterolaemic subjects. *The British Journal of Nutrition*, *98*(03), 563–570. doi:10.1017/S0007114507730775 PMID:17559697

Coates, A. M., & Howe, P. R. (2007). Edible nuts and metabolic health. *Current Opinion in Lipidology*, *18*(1), 25–30. doi:10.1097/MOL.0b013e3280123a47 PMID:17218828

Conway, V., Couture, P., Richard, C., Gauthier, S. F., Pouliot, Y., & Lamarche, B. (2013). Impact of buttermilk consumption on plasma lipids and surrogate markers of cholesterol homeostasis in men and women. *Nutrition, Metabolism, and Cardiovascular Diseases*, *23*(12), 1255–1262. doi:10.1016/j.numecd.2013.03.003 PMID:23786821

Cooper, R., Morre, D. J., & Morre, D. M. (2005). Medicinal benefits of green tea: Part I. Review of noncancer health benefits. *Journal of Alternative and Complementary Medicine (New York, N.Y.)*, *11*(3), 521–528. doi:10.1089/acm.2005.11.521 PMID:15992239

Corti, R., Flammer, A. J., Hollenberg, N. K., & Luscher, T. F. (2009). Cocoa and Cardiovascular Health. *Circulation*, *119*(10), 1433–1441. doi:10.1161/CIRCULATIONAHA.108.827022 PMID:19289648

Danesi, F., Di Nunzio, M., Boschetti, E., & Bordoni, A. (2009). Green tea extract selectively activates peroxisome proliferator-activated receptor beta/delta in cultured cardiomyocytes. *The British Journal of Nutrition*, *101*(12), 1736–1739. doi:10.1017/S0007114508145871 PMID:19055854

Das, S., Santani, D. D., & Dhalla, N. S. (2007). Experimental evidence for the cardioprotective effects of red wine. *Experiments in Clinical Cardiology*, *12*(1), 5–10. PMID:18650973

de Pascual-Teresa, S., Moreno, D. A., & Garcia-Viguera, C. (2010). Flavanols and Anthocyanins in Cardiovascular Health: A Review of Current Evidence. *International Journal of Molecular Sciences*, *11*(4), 1679–1703. doi:10.3390/ijms11041679 PMID:20480037

de Pascual-Teresa, S., & Sanchez-Ballesta, M. T. (2008). Anthocyanins: From plant to health. *Phytochemistry Reviews*, *7*(2), 281–299. doi:10.1007/s11101-007-9074-0

Ding, E. L., Hutfless, S. M., Ding, X., & Girotra, S. (2006). Chocolate and prevention of cardiovascular disease: A systematic review. *Nutrition & Metabolism*, *3*(1), 2. doi:10.1186/1743-7075-3-2 PMID:16390538

Du, Y., & Lou, H. (2008). Catechin and proanthocyanidin B4 from grape seeds prevent doxorubicin induced toxicity in cardiomyocytes. *European Journal of Pharmacology*, *591*(1-3), 96–101. doi:10.1016/j.ejphar.2008.06.068 PMID:18611398

Dubey, P., & Cheema, S. K. (2006). Molecular mechanisms involved in the regulation of lipid and lipoprotein metabolism by fish oil. *Future Lipidology*, *1*(5), 559–568. doi:10.2217/17460875.1.5.559

Egert, S., Bosy-Westphal, A., Seiberl, J., Kurbitz, C., Settler, U., Plachta-Danielzik, S., & Muller, M. J. et al. (2009). Quercetin reduces systolic blood pressure and plasma oxidised low-density lipoprotein concentrations in overweight subjects with a high-cardiovascular disease risk phenotype: A double-blinded, placebo-controlled cross-over study. *The British Journal of Nutrition*, *102*(7), 1065–1074. PMID:19402938

Elvevoll, E. O., Barstad, H., Breimo, E. S., Brox, J., Eilertsen, K. E., Lund, T., & Osterud, B. et al. (2006). Enhanced incorporation of n-3 fatty acids from fish compared with fish oils. *Lipids*, *41*(12), 1109–1114. doi:10.1007/s11745-006-5060-3 PMID:17269556

Erkkila, A., & Lichtenstein, A. (2006). Fiber and cardiovascular disease risk: How strong is the evidence? *The Journal of Cardiovascular Nursing*, *21*(1), 3–8. doi:10.1097/00005082-200601000-00003 PMID:16407729

Everitt, A. V., Hilmer, S. N., Brand-Miller, J. C., Jamieson, H. A., Truswell, A. S., Sharma, A. P., & Le Couteur, D. G. et al. (2006). Dietary Approaches that Delay Age-Related Diseases. *Journal of Clinical Interventions in Aging*, *1*(1), 11–31. doi:10.2147/ciia.2006.1.1.11 PMID:18047254

Grassi, D., Necozione, S., Lippi, C., Croce, G., Valeri, L., Pasqualetti, P., & Ferri, C. et al. (2005). Cocoa reduces blood pressure and insulin resistance and improves endothelium-dependent vasodilation in hypertensives. *Hypertension*, *46*(2), 398–405. doi:10.1161/01.HYP.0000174990.46027.70 PMID:16027246

Habauzit, V., & Morand, C. (2012). Evidence for a protective effect of polyphenols-containing foods on cardiovascular health: An update for clinicians. *Therapeutic Advances in Chronic Diseases*, *3*(2), 87–106. doi:10.1177/2040622311430006 PMID:23251771

Halton, T. L., Willett, W. C., Liu, S., Manson, J. E., Albert, C. M., Rexrode, K., & Hu, F. B. (2006). Low carbohydrate-diet score and the risk of coronary heart disease in women. *The New England Journal of Medicine*, *355*(19), 1991–2002. doi:10.1056/NEJMoa055317 PMID:17093250

Hooper, L., Kroon, P. A., Rimm, E. B., Cohn, J. S., Harvey, I., Le Cornu, K. A., & Cassidy, A. et al. (2008). Flavonoids, flavonoid-rich foods, and cardiovascular risk: A meta-analysis of randomized controlled trials. *The American Journal of Clinical Nutrition*, *88*, 38–50. PMID:18614722

Hsieh, Y. L., Pai, P., Ho, T. J., Chung, L. C., Cheng, Y. C., Wu, C. H., & Huang, C. Y. et al. (2014). Effects of Garlic Oil on Interleukin-6 Mediated Cardiac Hypertrophy in Hypercholesterol-Fed Hamsters. *The Chinese Journal of Physiology*, *57*(6), 320–328. doi:10.4077/CJP.2014.BAC261 PMID:25575520

Hsu, S. P., Wu, M. S., Yang, C. C., Huang, K. C., Liou, S. Y., Hsu, S. M., & Chien, C. T. (2007). Chronic green tea extract supplementation reduces hemodialysis-enhanced production of hydrogen peroxide and hypochlorous acid, atherosclerotic factors, and proinflammatory cytokines. *The American Journal of Clinical Nutrition*, *86*, 539–547. PMID:17991670

Karlsen, A., Retterstol, L., Laake, P., Paur, I., Kjolsrud-Bohn, S., Sandvik, L., & Blomhoff, R. (2007). Anthocyanins inhibit nuclear factor-kB activation in monocytes and reduce plasma concentrations of pro-inflammatory mediators in healthy adults. *The Journal of Nutrition*, *137*, 1951–1954. PMID:17634269

Kohli, S., Chhabra, A., Jaiswal, A., Rustagi, Y., Sharma, M., & Rani, V. (2013). Curcumin Suppresses Gelatinase B Mediated Norepinephrine Induced Stress in H9c2 Cardiomyocytes. *PLoS ONE*, *8*(10), e76519. doi:10.1371/journal.pone.0076519 PMID:24116115

Kris-Etherton, P. M., Etherton, T. D., Carlson, J., & Gardner, C. (2002). Recent discoveries in inclusive food-based approaches and dietary patterns for reduction in risk for cardiovascular disease. *Current Opinion in Lipidology*, *13*(4), 397–407. doi:10.1097/00041433-200208000-00007 PMID:12151855

Kuriyama, S., Shimazu, T., Ohmori, K., Kikuchi, N., Nakaya, N., Nishino, Y., & Tsuji, I. et al. (2006). Green tea consumption and mortality due to cardiovascular disease, cancer, and all causes in Japan: The Ohsaki study. *Journal of the American Medical Association*, *296*(10), 1255–1265. doi:10.1001/jama.296.10.1255 PMID:16968850

Kurosawa, T., Itoh, F., Nozaki, A., Nakano, Y., Katsuda, S., Osakabe, N., & Itakura, H. et al. (2005). Suppressive effect of cocoa powder on atherosclerosis in Kurosawa and Kusanagi-hypercholesterolemic rabbits. *Journal of Atherosclerosis and Thrombosis*, *12*(1), 20–28. doi:10.5551/jat.12.20 PMID:15725692

Kwak, J. S., Kim, J. Y., Paek, J. E., Lee, Y. J., Kim, H. R., Park, D. S., & Kwon, O. (2014). Garlic powder intake and cardiovascular risk factors: A meta-analysis of randomized controlled clinical trials. *Nutrition Research and Practice*, *8*(6), 644–654. doi:10.4162/nrp.2014.8.6.644 PMID:25489404

Lai, H. T. M., Threapleton, D. E., Day, A. J., Williamson, G., Cade, J. E., & Burley, V. J. (2015). Fruit intake and cardiovascular disease mortality in the UK Women's Cohort Study. *European Journal of Epidemiology*, *30*(9), 1035–1048. doi:10.1007/s10654-015-0050-5 PMID:26076918

Lin, L., Allemekinders, H., Dansby, A., Campbell, L., Durance-Tod, S., Berger, A., & Jones, P. J. (2013). Evidence of health benefits of canola oil. *Nutrition Reviews*, *71*(6), 370–385. doi:10.1111/nure.12033 PMID:23731447

Martins, J. M., Riottot, M., de Abreu, M. C., Viegas-Crespo, A. M., Lança, M. J., Almeida, J. A., & Bento, O. P. et al. (2005). Cholesterol-lowering effects of dietary blue lupin (Lupinus angustifolius L.) in intact and ileorectal anastomosed pigs. *Journal of Lipid Research*, *46*(7), 1539–1547. doi:10.1194/jlr.M500129-JLR200 PMID:15834122

Mastan, S. K., Chaitanya, G., Latha, T. B., Srikanth, A., Sumalatha, G., & Kumar, K. E. (2009). Cardio-protective effect of methanolic extract of Syzygium cumini seeds on isoproterenol-induced myocardial infarction in rats. *Der Pharmacia Lettre*, *1*(1), 143–149.

Miriyala, S., Panchatcharam, M., & Rengarajulu, P. (2007). Cardioprotective effects of curcumin. *Advances in Experimental Medicine and Biology*, *595*, 359–377. doi:10.1007/978-0-387-46401-5_16 PMID:17569220

Modriansky, M., & Gabrielova, E. (2009). Uncouple my heart: The benefits of inefficiency. *Journal of Bioenergetics and Biomembranes*, *41*(2), 133–136. doi:10.1007/s10863-009-9212-z PMID:19365715

Mursu, J., Voutilainen, S., Nurmi, T., Tuomainen, T. P., Kurl, S., & Salonen, J. T. (2008). Flavonoid intake and the risk of ischaemic stroke and CVD mortality in middle-aged Finish men: The Kuopio Ischaemic Heat Disease Risk Factor Study. *The British Journal of Nutrition*, *100*(04), 890–895. doi:10.1017/S0007114508945694 PMID:18377681

Naumann, E., van Rees, A. B., Onning, G., Oste, R., Wydra, M., & Mensink, R. P. (2006). Beta-Glucan incorporated into a fruit drink effectively lowers serum LDL-cholesterol concentrations. *The American Journal of Clinical Nutrition*, *83*, 601–605. PMID:16522906

Nwachukwu, I. D., Devassy, J. G., Aluko, R. E., & Jonesab, P. J. (2015). Cholesterol-lowering properties of oat β-glucan and the promotion of cardiovascular health: Did Health Canada make the right call? *Applied Physiology, Nutrition, and Metabolism*, *40*(6), 535–542. doi:10.1139/apnm-2014-0410 PMID:25933163

O'Toole, T. E., Conklin, D. J., & Bhatnagar, A. (2008). Environmental risk factors for heart disease. *Reviews on Environmental Health*, *23*, 167–202. PMID:19119685

Pandey, K. B., & Rizvi, S. I. (2009). Plant polyphenols as dietary antioxidants in human health and disease. *Oxidative Medicine and Cellular Longevity*, *2*(5), 270–278. doi:10.4161/oxim.2.5.9498 PMID:20716914

Pilvi, T. K., Jauhiainen, T., Cheng, Z. J., Mervaala, E. M., Vapaatalo, H., & Korpela, R. (2006). Lupin protein attenuates the development of hypertension and normalises the vascular function of NaCl-loaded Goto- Kakizaki rats. *Journal of Physiology and Pharmacology*, *57*, 167–176. PMID:16845223

Rimbach, G., Melchin, M., Moehring, J., & Wagner, A. E. (2009). Polyphenols from cocoa and vascular health-a critical review. *International Journal of Molecular Sciences*, *10*(10), 4290–4309. doi:10.3390/ijms10104290 PMID:20057946

Seki, T., & Hosono, T. (2015). Prevention of cardiovascular diseases by garlic-derived sulphur compounds. *Journal of Nutritional Science and Vitaminology*, *61*(Supplement), S83–S85. doi:10.3177/jnsv.61.S83 PMID:26598900

Sheng, R., Gu, Z. L., Xie, M. L., Zhou, W. X., & Guo, C. Y. (2007). EGCG inhibits cardiomyocyte apoptosis in pressure overload-induced cardiac hypertrophy and protects cardiomyocytes from oxidative stress in rats. *Acta Pharmacologica Sinica*, *28*(2), 191–201. doi:10.1111/j.1745-7254.2007.00495.x PMID:17241521

Shrivastava, A. K., Singh, H. V., Raizada, A., & Singh, S. K. (2015). C-reactive protein, inflammation and coronary heart disease. *The Egyptian Heart Journal*, *67*(2), 89–97. doi:10.1016/j.ehj.2014.11.005

Sirtori, C. R., Galli, C., Anderson, J. W., Sirtori, E., & Arnoldi, A. (2009). Functional foods for dyslipidaemia and cardiovascular risk prevention. *Nutrition Research Reviews*, *22*(02), 244–261. doi:10.1017/S0954422409990187 PMID:20003590

Srivastava, G., & Mehta, J. L. (2009). Currying the heart: Curcumin and cardioprotection. *Journal of Cardiovascular Pharmacology and Therapeutics*, *14*(1), 22–27. doi:10.1177/1074248408329608 PMID:19153099

Sumpio, B. E., Cordova, A. C., Berke-Schlessel, D. W., Qin, F., & Chen, Q. H. (2006). Green tea, the 'Asian paradox,' and cardiovascular disease. *Journal of the American College of Surgeons*, *202*(5), 813–825. doi:10.1016/j.jamcollsurg.2006.01.018 PMID:16648021

Tapsell, L. C., Hemphill, I., Cobiac, L., Patch, C. S., Sullivan, D. R., Fenech, M., & Inge, K. E. et al. (2006). Health benefits of herbs and spices: The past, the present, the future. *The Medical Journal of Australia*, *185*, 4–24. PMID:17022438

Terra, X., Montagut, G., Bustos, M., Llopiz, N., Ardevol, A., Blade, C., & Blay, M. et al. (2009). Grapeseed procyanidins prevent low-grade inflammation by modulating cytokine expression in rats fed a high-fat diet. *The Journal of Nutritional Biochemistry*, *20*(3), 210–218. doi:10.1016/j.jnutbio.2008.02.005 PMID:18602813

Visioli, F., & Hagen, T. M. (2007). Nutritional strategies for healthy cardiovascular aging: Focus on micronutrients. *Pharmacological Research*, *55*(3), 199–206. doi:10.1016/j.phrs.2007.01.008 PMID:17317208

von Schacky, C. (2004). Omega-3 fatty acids and cardiovascular disease. *Current Opinion in Clinical Nutrition and Metabolic Care*, *7*(2), 131–136. doi:10.1097/00075197-200403000-00005 PMID:15075702

Wallace, T. C. (2011). Anthocyanins in Cardiovascular Disease. *Advances in Nutrition*, *2*(1), 1–7. doi:10.3945/an.110.000042 PMID:22211184

Wang, H. P., Yang, J., Qin, L. Q., & Yang, X. J. (2015). Effect of Garlic on Blood Pressure: A Meta-Analysis. *Journal of Clinical Hypertension*, *17*(3), 223–231. doi:10.1111/jch.12473 PMID:25557383

Winham, D. M., & Hutchins, A. M. (2007). Baked bean consumption reduces serum cholesterol in hypercholesterolemic adults. *Nutrition Research (New York, N.Y.)*, *27*(7), 380–386. doi:10.1016/j.nutres.2007.04.017

Winter, J. (2005). The phytosterol phenomenon. *Func Food Nutraceutic*., 24–30.

World Health Organization (W.H.O.). (2009). *Cardiovascular diseases (CVDs). Fact sheet Nº 317.* Available at: http://www.who.int/mediacentre/factsheets/fs317/en/ index.html

Xia, M., Ling, W., Zhu, H., Wang, Q., Ma, J., Hou, M., & Ye, Q. et al. (2007). Anthocyanin prevents CD40-activated proinflammatory signaling in endothelial cells by regulating cholesterol distribution. *Arteriosclerosis, Thrombosis, and Vascular Biology*, *27*(3), 519–524. doi:10.1161/01.ATV.0000254672.04573.2d PMID:17158355

Yamakuchi, M., Bao, C., Ferlito, M., & Lowenstein, C. J. (2008). Epigallocatechin gallate inhibits endothelial exocytosis. *Biological Chemistry*, *389*(7), 935–941. doi:10.1515/BC.2008.095 PMID:18627310

Zhao, S. P., Liu, L., Cheng, Y. C., Shishehbor, M. H., Liu, M. H., Peng, D. Q., & Li, Y. L. (2004). Xuezhikang, an extract of cholestin, protects endothelial function through antiinflammatory and lipid-lowering mechanisms in patients with coronary heart disease. *Circulation*, *110*(8), 915–920. doi:10.1161/01.CIR.0000139985.81163.CE PMID:15313947

Chapter 2
Functional Foods and Cardiac Health

Santosh Jain Passi
University of Delhi, India

ABSTRACT

Functional foods containing physiologically-active components, have been reported to confer several health benefits. Longitudinal cohort studies indicate that certain foods and dietary patterns play an important role in primary prevention of numerous disease conditions and this has led to the identification of putative functional foods. Research is necessary to substantiate the potential health benefits of various functional foods for which the diet–health relationships have yet not been scientifically validated. The term 'functional foods' may include health/functional health foods, foods fortified with minerals/vitamins, dietary supplements or even the traditional medicines (Zawistowski, 2014).

INTRODUCTION

Functional foods containing physiologically-active components, have been reported to confer several health benefits. Longitudinal cohort studies indicate that certain foods and dietary patterns play an important role in primary prevention of numerous disease conditions and this has led to the identification of putative functional foods. Research is necessary to substantiate the potential health benefits of various functional foods for which the diet–health relationships have yet not been scientifically validated. The term 'functional foods' may include health/functional health foods, foods fortified with minerals/vitamins, dietary supplements or even the traditional medicines (Zawistowski, 2014).

A food can be regarded as 'functional', if beyond nutritional benefits, it demonstrates suitably the beneficial effects on one or more target functions in the body through improvements in health status and overall well-being and/or by reducing the disease risk. Hence, functional foods can be defined as the foods that provide health benefits beyond the basic nutrition. All foods containing one or more substances possessing physiological/biochemical functions for benefitting the human health, are known as functional foods. Functional foods that are marketed with claims to reduce heart disease focus primarily on the risk factors linked to blood cholesterol and homocysteine levels as well as hypertension. The most

DOI: 10.4018/978-1-5225-0591-4.ch002

common protective ingredients include dietary fibre, soya, omega-3 fatty acids, phytosterols, phytostanols and antioxidants. A critical issue in the regulation of functional foods is the identification of the active components responsible for proposed health benefits (Arnoldi, 2005).

Bioactive compounds' present in foods are the extra/non-nutritional constituents occurring in small quantities and appear to accord beneficial health effects.

The American Dietetic Association has prepared a glossary of major basic definitions of functional foods which include chemopreventive agents, designer foods, pharma-foods, phytochemicals, nutraceutics/nutraceuticals etc.

- *Functional food refers to any food or modified ingredient that can make a beneficial effect beyond that provided by the common nutrients;*
- *Designer foods are the processed foods supplemented with food ingredients, naturally rich in substances that prevent diseases; and this includes genetic engineering of the foods;*
- *Pharma-food is the food or nutrient with potential health or medical use, including prevention and treatment of diseases;*
- *Chemopreventive agents are the nutrient or non-nutrient food components that have been scientifically investigated as potential inhibitors of carcinogenesis;*
- *Phytochemicals are the substances present in fruits and vegetables that can be ingested on daily-basis in appreciable amounts and exhibit a potential to modulate human metabolism by favouring prevention of CVDs, cancer and other diseases;*
- *Nutraceuticals are the substances considered as food or a part of food which offer health or medical benefits, including prevention and treatment of diseases. (Ferrari & Torres, 2003)*

Functional foods, in the form of palatable and ready to use food items, have a huge market due to their health potentials (Arnoldi, 2005).

FUNCTIONAL FOODS AND CVDs

Noncommunicable diseases (NCDs) account for nearly 38 million deaths each year (WHO, n.d.). Cardiovascular disease (CVD) is still a major cause of mortality in western population and is becoming an important cause of morbidity and mortality the world over including the developing countries and the South-east Asian nations where populations are undergoing significant life-style changes. CVD accounting for nearly 20% of global deaths each year comprises disease conditions such as atherosclerosis, hypertension, congestive heart failure, cardiomyopathy, coronary heart disease, hypertrophy, arrhythmias, ventricular fibrillation, ventricular tachycardia, myocardial infarction, and stroke (Kaliora & Dedoussis, 2007).

The major CVD risk factors include smoking, diabetes, insulin resistance, dyslipidemia, obesity and hypertension. Epidemiological studies indicate that after adjustment for various confounding factors, hypertension remains an important risk factor for CVD. On the other hand, clinical intervention trials demonstrate that treatment of hypertension reduces the CVD risk; and the lifestyle intervention studies among mild hypertensives have been found to be effective in reducing the CVD risk (McInnes, 2004).

The underlying mechanism associated with the health effects of hypertension leading to CVD is perhaps linked to acceleration of the atherosclerotic process due to high blood BP; and the elevated BP leading to progressive dilation followed by rupture of small/large vessels. Increased glucose intolerance also plays a crucial role in the progression of CVD; and it is directly associated with overweight/obesity as well as hypertension, hypertriglyceridemia, increased LDL-c and lowered HDL-c. It is an established fact that diabetes mellitus leads to instantaneous peripheral vascular disease; the most common manifestations, however, remain CHD and stroke. Barrett-Connor and Orchard (1985) had reported that the risk of CVD is three times higher among diabetic women as compared to the non-diabetic ones; and the CVD risk is two-fold among diabetic men as against their non-diabetic counterparts. The pathophysiology of atherosclerosis and CVD comprises a combination of chronic processes and acute events such as dyslipidemia, hypertension, endothelial dysfunction, diabetes and cardiac/vascular hypertrophy. A majority of these are determined partly by the genetic factors and partly by the environmental conditions (Kaliora & Dedoussis, 2007).

Appropriate dietary intake is a key strategy in the prevention and regression of CVDs (Sarrafzadegan & Najafian, 1998; Stradling et al., 2013). Meta-analysis by Sofi et al (2008) indicates that adherence to Mediterranean diet (high in legumes, cereals, fruits and vegetables; low in meat and dairy products; having high MUFA:SFA and alcohol in moderation) significantly reduces the CVD mortality risk. The diet and lifestyle-related goals for CVD prevention have ominously been supported by the dietary recommendations of various nations. In many countries, emphasis is laid on reducing serum total cholesterol and LDL-C by incorporating adequate amounts of foods rich in dietary fibre, plant proteins, nuts and phytosterols in daily diets (Jenkins et al., 2005) [264].

Mediterranean diet is a traditional diet based nutritional model adopted in the countries surrounding Mediterranean Sea (central/southern Italy, Greece and Spain). It has been associated with a lower incidence of cardiovascular diseases as compared to the North American diets high in animal fats. (Assmann et al., 2014)

During the last decades, the concept of CVD has changed and the nature of this multifactorial disease has become clearer. For all practical purposes, the CVD risk factors can be divided into three categories - personal traits, lifestyle related factors and biochemical factors. Of these, lifestyle related factors play an important role in modifying the CVD risk both at the individual and the population level (Kaliora & Dedoussis, 2007).

The personal traits such as age, gender, heredity and to some extent the personality type (type A) play a significant role in the development of CVD; however, these factors cannot be addressed through the available treatment choices and are commonly known as the non-modifiable risk factors.

The lifestyle related factors include inappropriate dietary patterns, physical inactivity, overweight/obesity, tobacco smoking, excess alcohol consumption and psychological stress. If addressed effectively, these factors can significantly lower the CVD risk; however, it is often difficult to modify and sustain the changes.

Numerous cohort studies and clinical trials have indicated that certain dietary patterns when followed over long periods can predict the occurrence/non-occurrence of cardiovascular and other inflammatory diseases in due course. Dietary patterns characterised by high intake of vegetables, fruit, legumes, whole grains, nuts/oilseeds, berries and fish; and moderate amounts of dairy products, tea, coffee, cocoa, chocolate and alcohol; and low intake of meat (particularly red meat) and processed foods are associated with reduced incidence of CVD as well as lowered non-cardiovascular and non-cancer mortality. The Mediterranean diets as well as the prudent diets are mainly plant based and include a variety of these foods; therefore, these dietary patterns are associated with lowered incidence of CVD and related mortality (Jacobs & Tapsell, 2015).

In the current dietary recommendations laid down by various nations, diet and lifestyle goals for the prevention of CVD have been given specific attention. These emphasise on including adequate amounts of dietary fibre rich foods, plant proteins, nuts and phytosterols for reducing the serum total cholesterol and LDL-C (Jenkins et al., 2005). It is envisaged that certain functional foods will be able to impact gene polymorphisms which plays an important role in the development of chronic diseases. Although fortification of some commonly consumed foods with vitamins and minerals has been going on for the last many years, introduction of unconventional/innovative functional foods particularly targeting cardiovascular health is on a rise, both in the developed and the developing countries (Weststrate et al., 2002).

Functional foods designed with health claims to curb CVDs primarily focus on reducing various risk factors like total cholesterol and homocysteine levels as well as hypertension. In such functional foods, the major protective ingredients commonly found are soy/soy components, dietary fibre, antioxidants, omega-3 fatty acids, phytosterols and phytostanols. However, as per the regulations relating to functional foods, it is imperative to identify the active components responsible for the proposed health benefits (Arnoldi, 2005).

For preventing CVDs, majority of the dietary recommendations advocate replacing trans fats and saturated fats with non-hydrogenated unsaturated oils; increasing omega-3 fatty acid intake (fish/plant sources), attaining balanced omega-6:omega-3 ratio; consuming plenty of fresh fruits/vegetables, nuts and whole grains; and alongside restricting the intake of refined cereals and de-husked pulses (Mohamed, 2014).

The chapter will highlight the functional role of various food constituents like carbohydrates, proteins (esp. soy proteins), fats/oils, dietary fibre, probiotics, prebiotics, synbiotics, phenolic compounds, phytosterols/plant stanols, antioxidants particularly vitamin E and selenium, flavanols, flavones, isoflavones and curcumin in maintaining cardiac health.

Further, the significance of various functional foods in disease prevention particularly the cardiovascular diseases has been discussed at length. Some of such functional foods include garlic, nuts, vegetables, caffeine, cocoa powder and chocolate, grapes, wines and beer, green tea etc.

FUNCTIONAL ROLE OF VARIOUS FOOD CONSTITUENTS

Dietary Fibre

Large and medium prospective cohort follow-up studies provide enough evidence to support the hypothesis that dietary fibre intake is inversely related to the CVD risk and myocardial infarction (Sánchez-Muniz, 2012). Based on the data from various other cohort studies, Pereira et al (2004) have reported that for every 10 g increase in total dietary fibre intake per day, the coronary risk is lowered by nearly 10–30%. Further, they have documented that the dietary fibre present in whole-grains and fruits is more effective. Data from large prospective studies also endorses that the consumption of whole grain food products decreases the risk of CVDs as well as diabetes (Jacobs & Gallaher, 2004). Improving lipid profile, particularly lowering the LDL-c, positively impacting the glucose and insulin metabolism, controlling blood pressure and bringing about weight reduction contribute to the cardio-protective effects of dietary fibre (Erkkila & Lichtenstein, 2006). Epidemiological and cohort studies have documented that intake of dietary fibre as high as 25-50 g/day was associated with a modest but significant reduction in the CVD risk; and that the effect is brought about by lowering of the TC and LDL-c levels (Kushi, Meyer & Jacobs, 1999).

As per the findings of Third National Health and Nutrition Examination Survey (NHNES-3: 1988-94) the mean dietary fibre intake among men in the US was merely 17g/day (Alaimo, McDowell & Briefel, 1994). On the other hand, dietary fibre intake among the Finnish male cohorts was much higher and it was found to be associated with reduced risk of mortality from coronary artery disease. Pietinen et al. (1996) have reported that men consuming 27 g dietary fibre/day had a lower relative risk of dying from coronary artery disease (RR 0.83, 95% CI; 0.80–0.86) compared to those from the same cohort but having lower consumption of dietary fibre by nearly 10 g/day on an average.

Studies have concluded that wholegrain consumption provides protection against CHD and CVD. Further, it has been reported that a habitual intake of wholegrain foods results in 20% to 40% reduction in CHD risk as compared to rare consumption of these food-items which highlights that fibre from wholegrain sources is best suited for CHD prevention. Although wholegrain products possess strong antioxidant activity and contain phytoestrogens, the evidence is yet not sufficient to prove its beneficial effects in CHD prevention. However, it is well documented that soluble fibre has a small but significant cholesterol lowering effect and perhaps this is responsible for the reduction in CHD events (Flight & Clifto, 2006).

Omega-3 Fatty Acids

Polyunsaturated fatty acids present in fish/fish oils have gained interest in view of their favourable role in the prevention and management of cardiovascular disease. The omega-3 fatty acids play a potent role in the management of CVD; their major mechanism of action includes:

- Prevent arrhythmias (ventricular tachycardia and fibrillation);
- Are the precursors of prostaglandins and leukotrienes;
- Possess anti-inflammatory properties;
- Inhibit the synthesis of cytokines and mitogens;
- Stimulate the release of endothelium-derived nitric oxide;
- Possess antithrombotic properties;
- Confer hypo-lipidemic effects - particularly on TG and VLDL-c and thus, inhibit the formation of plaques (Connor, 2000; 1994).

Studies indicate that the long chain PUFA such as ecosapentanoic acids (EPA) and docosahexanoic acids (DHA) accord protection against cardiac arrhythmias (Serra et al., 2004; Psaltopoulou et al., 2004). In functional foods, incorporation of fatty acids derived from fish oil is an effective strategy in the prevention of various commonly occurring diseases (Jones, 2002). Khandelwal et al (2009) carried out a double-blind randomized control trial among industrial workers (n=178) and found that supplementation with 2g of omega-3 fatty acids per day in the form of fish oil capsules (each capsule containing 1g omega-3) over a period of 28 days brought about a significant increase in HDL-C concentrations (+5.4%) in addition to a 15% reduction in TG levels.

Several clinical trials have demonstrated that the intake of fish oil reduces serum TG concentrations as well as the blood pressure - both in normal individuals and the hypertriglyceridemics. It also reduces the frequency of arrhythmia and the progression of atherosclerosis. Miles et al (2004) have reported that a daily intake of 0.5 to 1.8 g of EPA/DHA decreases the CVD mortality; and that a sufficient intake of omega-3 fatty acids can be reached by consuming fatty fish at least twice a week. Long back the American Heart Association had recommended that adults should eat fish, particularly the fatty fish, at least twice a week; and along with this, they should also consume ALA rich foods such as tofu, soybeans, walnuts, flaxseeds/flaxseed oil and canola oil. Further, the Association had recommended the intake of 1g EPA and DHA per day by the individual suffering from CAD, and a daily intake of 2-4 g of EPA and DHA was advocated to decrease the TG levels by 20-40% (Stone, 1996).

Olive oil is an integral component of Mediterranean diet. Strong evidence indicates that olive oil can confer many health benefits such as reduction in the risk factors of CHD, prevention of various types of cancers and modification in the immune/inflammatory responses. Thus, olive oil is a functional food with varied components that contribute to its overall therapeutic characteristics. It is well known for its high MUFA content and is also a good source of phytochemicals - polyphenolic compounds, squalene and alphatocopherol (Stark & Madar, 2002). Fielding et al (2005) have reported that addition of olive oil to tomatoes during cooking greatly enhances the absorption of lycopene (a carotenoid) which is already known to reduce the risk of CVDs.

Hornych et al (2001) have reported that among older individuals, a daily supplementation of 320mg of gamma linolenic acid (GLA) was found to decrease the arterial blood pressure as well as TC concentrations while it increased the HDL-c and apoA-1 cholesterol fractions.

Antioxidants

Numerous epidemiological, case-control and prospective/retrospective cohort studies have linked dietary antioxidants with the prevention of cardiovascular diseases. The most established studies include:

- The CHAOS study, which documented an inverse correlation between vitamin E intake and mortality due to myocardial infarction (Stephens, 1996).
- The WHO-MONICA project, one of the largest studies, analysed the impact of vitamin E intake by the populations with differences in the incidence of CHD mortality (Gotto, 2003). The study found that in populations with similar serum cholesterol concentrations and blood pressure levels, there was an inverse correlation between CHD mortality and plasma vitamin E values; however, no such relationship existed between CHD mortality and the intake of other vitamins.
- The ARIC study reported an inverse association between vitamin C intake and the carotid wall thickness (Kritchevsky et al., 1995).
- The Kuopio Atherosclerosis study indicated that vitamin C deficiency may be associated with an increased risk of myocardial infarction (Nyyssonen et al., 1997).
- The Zutphen Elderly study found that a daily intake of 30 mg flavonoids had resulted in 50% reduction in CVD mortality as compared to a daily intake of 19 mg flavonoids (Hertog et al., 1993).
- The John Hopkins University study had reported an inverse relation between carotenoid intake and myocardial infarction (Street, Comstock & Salkeld, 1994).
- The EURAMIC study documented a negative relationship between adipose tissue lycopene and the risk for myocardial infarction (Kohlmeier et al., 1997).

- The large prospective Physicians' Health Study, however, did not find sufficient evidence indicating that a higher baseline plasma carotenoid concentrations accord a protective effect against myocardial infarction (Hak et al., 2003).

Measurement of arterial wall intima-media thickness (IMT) is employed to assess the early onset of CVD/atherosclerosis during subclinical stages.

- In the EVA study (N=1384), after adjusting for the normal CVD risk factors, it was found that optimum plasma vitamin E levels, but not that of the carotenoids, were associated with lowered thickening of the arterial walls (Bonithon-Kopp et al., 1997).

Many researches have indicated that the antioxidant vitamins protect the blood vessels against changes induced during atherosclerosis (Ferrari, 1998; Gutteridge, 1995; Halliwell & Chirico, 1993).

Gianetti (2002) has reported an inverse relationship between plasma lycopene concentrations and IMTmax hypothesizing its protective role in atherosclerosis. The study by Aviram et al. (2004) has indicated that the consumption of pomegranate juice (rich in potent tannins and anthocyanins) by atherosclerotic patients with carotid artery stenosis over a period of one year decreased the carotid IMT.

The physiological and medicinal properties of many of the food components gained due recognition only during the twentieth century and a lot of investigations discovered their possible functional role (such as antioxidant properties) which could be effective in preventing various diseases like CVDs, hyperglycemia, brain dysfunctions and cancer. Such functional food components include numerous limonoids and ascorbic acid in citrus fruits; isoflavonoids in soy; tocotrienols in cereals, grains and vegetables; phenolic compounds in ginger and green/black tea; lycopenes in tomatoes, watermelon and guava; anthocyanins in beans, cherries, blackberry, black grapes and strawberry; quercetin in onion, broccoli, red grape (wine), cherries, apple and certain cereals; resveratrol in grape peels and antioxidants in various herbs like rosemary, sage, thyme and oregano (Craig and Beck, 1999; Weisburger, 1999). Hydroxytyrosol - a phenolic compound found in olives/olive oil and lycopene - a carotenoid present in tomatoes/other fruits are potent antioxidants. Resveratrol, existing in nuts and red wine has antioxidant, antithrombotic, and anti-inflammatory properties. Similarly, organosulfur compounds found in garlic and onions, isothiocyanates in cruciferous vegetables, and monoterpenes in citrus fruits, cherries and herbs have demonstrated cardio-protective effects in experimental models (Kris-Etherton et al., 2002).

Epidemiologic studies reveal that the intake of antioxidants, both as dietary components or as supplements, curbs the development of atherosclerotic changes; and therefore, lowers the risk of CVDs (Miller et al., 1997). Clinical trials also validate the findings that antioxidants prevent the formation of atherosclerotic lesions (Ness, Powles & Khaw, 1996)[99]. A meta-analysis has indicated the pooled relative risk reduction for CVD deaths among high vs. low consumers of β-carotene to be 31% (95% CI: 41-20%). On the contrary, another meta-analysis of four randomised trials has reported a moderate adverse effect of β-carotene supplementation based on 12% increase in the relative risk of CVD deaths (Reddy & Katan, 2004; Ness, 2001)[41, 135].

Tocopherol has been reported to be beneficial in inhibiting Cu^{2+} induced LDL oxidation and that for each LDL molecule, six molecules of vitamin E are required to accord an efficient anti-atherogenic antioxidant activity (Ziouzenkova et al., 1996; Halliwell & Chirico, 1993; Duriez & Fruchart, 1993). Long-term supplementation study among animal models indicate that vitamin E intake decreases the risk of atherosclerosis; and that, the diets high in vitamin E and strawberry decreased the lipid peroxidation markers in the animal liver as compared to the control group (Meydani et al., 1998).

Numerous large cohort studies indicate a significant reduction in the incidence of cardiac events both in men and women consuming high amounts of vitamin E as supplements (Rimm & Stampfer, 2000)[136]. However, the HOPE trial indicated that vitamin E supplementation to the tune of 400 IU/d with a mean follow-up period of 4.5 years had no effect on MI, stroke or CVD related mortality among men/women (Yusuf et al., 2000)[137]. Similarly, Collaborative group of the primary prevention project (2001)[138] commented that many other trials had also failed to demonstrate the cardio-protective effect of vitamin E supplementation.

Epidemiological studies have revealed a markedly elevated risk of CVDs at suboptimal levels of essential antioxidants in the plasma as compared with the optimal concentrations of vitamin C (>50 μmol/l), vitamin E (> 30 μmol/l or tocopherol/cholesterol ratio > 5.2 μmol/mmol) and beta carotene (> 0.4 μmol/l). Low levels of any single essential antioxidant can increase the risk; and the combined sub-optimal levels lead to additive or sometimes evn a multiplier effect on the CVD risk. Thus, it has been concluded that antioxidants are crucial components of fruit/vegetable rich diets which have unanimously been linked with a lowered risk of CVD related premature mortality (Gey, Stähelin & Ballmer, 1994).

Multivitamins

A French study (SU.VI. MAX) carried out among healthy individuals has reported that the antioxidant vitamins and mineral intake did not lower the incidence of ischemic heart disease (Hercberg et al., 2004; Hercberg et al., 2010). Similarly, the data pertaining to the American healthy male physicians who were a part of Physicians' Health Study indicate that the multivitamin intake did not lower the cardiovascular or the CHD mortality (Sesso et al., 2008). Several cohort studies, including the Nurses' Health Study have highlighted that there was no positive impact of the usage of multivitamins on the CVD risk (Prentice, 2007; Stampfer et al., 1993; Rimm et al., 1998). A Cochrane review reported that there is no evidence to support antioxidant supplements for primary/secondary prevention of chronic degenerative diseases; and rather implicated β-carotene, vitamin E and vitamin A supplements seem to increase the mortality rate. In view of these findings, it has been suggested that the antioxidant supplements be considered as medicinal products rather than the nutrient supplements (Bjelakovic et al., 2008).

Polyphenols and Phytosterols

This vast heterogeneous group comprises around 8000 species of phenolic compounds (flavonoids, anthraquinones, and phenylpropanoids), about 25,000 terpenoids (terpenes, carotenoids, xanthophylls, and iridoids), 12,000 alkaloids, and several sulfate-containing chemicals such as isothiocyanates (Pang et al., 2012). These phytochemicals confer a variety of metabolic and cardioprotective effects; and exert numerous bioactive functions including antioxidant actions in scavenging the ROS. They play a dynamic role in regulating the metabolic functions of proteins, enzymes, transporters, receptors as well as in signaling the transduction proteins related to various lifestyle-related diseases (Thomas & Pfeiffer, 2012; Lamy et al., 2012; Vittorio et al., 2012). Researches indicate that the phenolic compounds inhibit LDL oxidation both in vitro as well as ex-vivo (Lamuela-Raventos et al., 2004).

Plant sterols/stanols and their esters epitomise another class of functional foods. Chemically, these are quite similar to cholesterol but do not exist in eukaryotic cells in significant amounts. Plant sterols and their derivatives competitively inhibit the absorption of cholesterol in the small intestines (Miettinen et al., 2000; Jones et al., 2000; Ostlund, Spilburg & Stenson, 1999). Studies indicate that the plant sterols and stanols were equally effective in their ability to lower the LDL-C levels highlights their efficacy with/without the presence of fatty acid esters in the sterol ring (Jone & Raeini-Sarjaz, 2001; Law, 2000). A meta-analysis of 18 clinical trials documents that, compared to margarine alone, a regular daily consumption of plant sterols and stanols (equivalent to 2 g of their unesterified components) in the form of spreads lowered LDL-C concentrations by 0.4-0.5 mmol/L among the subjects aged 40–59 years. The researcher has concluded that with the lowering of LDL-C at such levels, a 25% reduction in the heart disease risk can be expected at the population level (Law, 2000). In view of beneficial effects of sterols/stanols, these are commonly being added to the functional foods (Jones, 2002).

Expert groups like National Cholesterol Education Program (NCEP), American Heart Association (AHA) and International Atherosclerosis Society have recommended a daily intake of 2 g phytosterols (plant sterols/stanols) as a part of heart-healthy diet so as to bring about a reduction in the LDL-C concentrations. At this level, phytosterols were found to lower the plasma LDL-C levels by nearly 10% while there was a negligible effect on TG concentrations both among the normocholesterolaemics as well as the hypercholesterolaemics (Katan et al., 2003). In the case of hypertriglyceridemics, however, the evidence supports that phytosterols can lower triglyceride concentrations too (Naumann et al., 2008).

In a study, Micallef and Garg (2008) have reported that phytosterol and omega-3 supplementation resulted in a greater reduction in the LDL-C concentrations than that by phytosterols alone (in spite of an increase in the LDL-C levels by omega-3 supplements); highlighting a positive interaction between phytosterols and omega-3 fatty acids. In a double-blind RCT conducted among industrial workers (N=178), supplementation with 2g plant sterols/day (given as a yoghurt drink) for a duration of 28 days was found to lower the plasma LDL-C by 4.5% and the TG concentrations by 15%. The findings indicate that plant sterol supplementation can help in attenuating the risk of heart disease. A combination of plant sterols (2g/d) and omega-3 (2g/d; this itself had raised the HDL-C by 5·4% and lowered TG by ~15%) indicated no additive effect in reducing the TG (-15%) levels; however, the combination can significantly contribute in reducing the risk of coronary artery disease by way of reduced LDL-C and TG coupled with an increase in the HDL-C concentrations (Khandelwal et al., 2009).

Intake of flavonols and flavones (present in wine, tea, apple and onion) is inversely associated with CHD mortality (Kinsella et al., 1993; Hollman & Katan, 1999). The Zutphen Elderly Study has reported that, of the 805 elderly men, subjects in the highest tertile of flavonoid intake were 68% less likely to have CHD deaths compared to those in the lowest tertile (Hertog et al., 1993)[118]. In the Iowa Women's Health Study (covering 34 489 women) with a follow-up of 16 years, it was reported that the intake of flavanones and anthocyanidins but not the total flavonoids were found to be associated with a decreased risk of CHD, CVD and all-cause mortality (Mink et al., 2007)[119]. Mursu et al (2008)[117] have also reported an inverse association between flavanone/flavone intakes (but not total flavonoid intake) and the CVD mortality. A meta-analysis of prospective cohort studies has shown that a high flavonol intake can perhaps be linked with a modestly lowered risk of CHD mortality (Huxley and Neil, 2003)[120]. However, the US Health Professionals Follow-up Study did not find flavonoid intake to be associated with the CHD mortality risk (Rimm et al.,1996)[121]. However, the Seven Countries Study (25-year follow-up data from 16 cohorts) revealed an inverse association between average flavonoid intake and the age-adjusted CHD mortality (Hertog et al., 1995)[122].

Several clinical studies have examined the effect of dietary phytoestrogens on CVD. Cornwell, Cohick and Raskin (2004) in a systematic review examined 105 clinical studies highlighting the effect of phytoestrogens on cardiovascular health, cancer prevention, cognition, bone mineralization and symptoms relating to menopause. Numerous phytoestrogens present in soy, flaxseeds, whole grains, fruits and vegetables possess antioxidant properties and demonstrate favourable effects on various CVD risk factors. However, since phytoestrogens act as partial estrogen agonists and antagonists, their effects on cancer are rather complex (Kris-Etherton et al., 2002)

Probiotics, Prebiotics, Synbiotics

For reducing CHD risk, the focus of public health strategies has been on lowering the plasma lipids, particularly the TC and LDL-c levels. This includes supplementation of the diet with probiotics, prebiotics and/or synbiotics which presumably improve the lipid profile and glycaemic control by selectively promoting the growth of beneficial bacteria in the gut and consequently their metabolic by-products (Lovegrove & Jackson, 2011).

Animal models have demonstrated that the probiotics (live microbes) exert cholesterol lowering effects while the prebiotics (non-digestible fermentable carbohydrates) reduce the triacylglycerol levels. However, human studies using prebiotics and probiotics have registered favourable outcomes but with regard to the changes in lipid profile, there are conflicting findings (Jackson & Lovegrove, 2002).

Synbiotics are a combination of both the probiotic organisms and the probiotic compounds. In a randomised placebo controlled crossover study, the effect of fermented milk product with/without the addition of *Lactobacillus acidophilus* and fructooligosaccharides was examined among healthy men. The duration of treatment period was 3 weeks and that of the washout period one week. The findings indicated a significant reduction in total and LDL-c after feeding fermented milk containing both the probiotic and prebiotic, as compared to the placebo - fermented milk only (Schaafsma et al. 1998). Many studies have highlighted the role of probiotics and prebiotics in reducing the CVD risk (Al-Sheraji et al., 2012; Pereira & Gibson, 2002).

Inulin has been reported to reduce the cholesterol and triglyceride levels, and thus, exerts beneficial effect on lipid profile and the cardiovascular system (Roberfroid, 2003). Animal studies have demonstrated that inulin influences blood cholesterol and triglyceride levels by reducing the number of very low-density lipoprotein (VLDL) particles and by curtailing the lipogenic enzyme activity (Roberfroid, 2003). However, the findings of human studies are equivocal.

Soy

Consumption of soy protein is associated with a reduced risk of CHD. FDA has concluded that soy protein incorporated in a low saturated fat and low cholesterol diet may decrease the CHD risk by lowering blood cholesterol levels (FDA, 1999), which to some extent can be attributed to the amino acid profile of soy which being different from that of the animal proteins, results in reducing the plasma LDL-C (Costa & Summa, 2000). A meta-analysis of studies assessing the effect of soy protein on serum lipids has revealed that, soy protein ingestion led to a decrease in TC (9.3%), LDL-C (12.9%) and TG (10.5%) as compared to the control group (in most of these studies, total energy, fat, saturated fat and cholesterol intake of the control and the experimental group was similar; and the mean soy protein intake was 47g/day). However, the hypocholesterolemic effect was directly correlated with the subject's serum cholesterol levels; at $\leq$ 6 mmol cholesterol /L, there was minimal or no effect while subjects serum cholesterol levels $\geq$ 7 mmol/L demonstrated the maximum benefit. It is anticipated that soy protein lowers the cholesterol concentrations through activation of the LDL receptor pathway (Sirtori & Lovati, 2001). Additionally, the health effects are also conferred by soy isoflavonoids, specifically the genistein and daidzein, which possess antioxidant properties and are also involved in the regulation of circulating lipid concentrations (van der Schouw et al., 2000). In a randomized controlled trial, Crouse et al (1999) have reported that isolated soy protein containing as little as 37 mg of isoflavones lowered the LDL cholesterol by 8%; and that there was a dose–response effect of isoflavones on TC and LDL-C concentrations. The plausible mechanisms associated with the soy isoflavones inhibiting atherosclerotic development independent of the lipoprotein factor include antioxidant, antiproliferative and antimigratory effects on smooth muscle cells as well as the effects on thrombus formation and maintenance of normal vascular reactivity (Anthony, Clarkson & Williams, 1998) It has been postulated that soy protein consumption specifically increases the circulating genistein concentrations which inhibit the tyrosine kinase activity - an enzyme associated with the development of plaques (Wilcox and Blumenthal, 1995). To reduce the CVD risk, Gibaldi (2001) has proposed a daily intake of estimated 25-50 mg isoflavones.

Nuts and Oilseeds

Nuts are particularly rich in phenols, flavonoids, isoflavonoids, phytosterols and phytic acid. Studies have documented that nut consumption helps in reducing the plasma lipids and thus, provides protection against CVDs (Serra et al., 2004). Numerous epidemiological studies indicate that frequent consumption of nuts helps in lowering the CHD risk (Kris-Etherton et al., 2001; Fraser et al., 1992; Fraser, Lindsted & Beeson, 1995). Various intervention trials and epidemiological studies have documented that nut consumption results in a favourable plasma lipid response (Coates & Howe, 2007; Kris-Etherton et al., 2001). Hu et al (1998) had also reported that a high consumption of nuts, which contains ample amounts of vitamin E, α-linolenic acid and many other bioactive components resulted in a 62% reduction in the CHD risk among women.

In Physicians' Health Study, it has been reported that nut consumption is associated with an appreciable reduction in the risk of sudden cardiac death (Albert et al., 2002). Kris-Etherton et al (2008) have also reported that high intake of nuts had resulted in approximately 35% decrease in the CHD risk. Based on a systematic review of several clinical studies relating to nut consumption, Mukuddem-Petersen, Oosthuizen and Jerling (2005) have concluded that nearly 50-100 g nuts (~1·5-3·5 servings) consumed at least five times a week, as a constituent of a heart-healthy diet (providing ample amounts of MUFA and/or PUFA), can lower the TC by 2-16% and LDL-C by 2-19% among the normo- and hyperlipidaemics. In a controlled investigation carried out by Mercanligil et al (2007) among hypercholesterolaemic men (n=15) kept on a diet providing 40 g hazelnuts/day contributing to 11·6% of the total energy intake, it was found that while the subjects did not register change in their body weight, they had attained a positive change in the blood lipid levels; there was a significant reduction in the VLDL-C (- 29·5%), TG (- 31·8%) and apo B (-9·2%) levels; a small reduction in total cholesterol (- 5·2%) and LDL-C (- 3·3%) levels coupled with a significant increase in HDL-C (+12·6%) concentrations.

Peanuts - the most widely consumed 'nut' (botanically, a legume) has yet not gained enough recognition regarding its beneficial impact on the CVD risk factors. A regular consumption of peanuts (rich in

MUFA, magnesium and folate) reduces serum TG and elevates the plasma magnesium concentrations alongside it reduces the CVD risk (Alper & Mattes, 2003)[195]. Various clinical trials have demonstrated that the nuts, including peanuts (being good sources of numerous cardio-protective nutrients) when consumed regularly can markedly lower the CHD risk. Epidemiological evidence and clinical trials have consistently demonstrated the beneficial effect of peanut consumption on CHD risk and the associated risk factors (Kris-Etherton et al., 2008). In the year 2003, Food and Drug Administration had approved the health claim highlighting the association between nut consumption and decreased CHD risk (FDA, 2003).

Studies have reported that the consumption of sesame or its lignans is helpful in reducing the CVD risk. Alipoor et al (2012) have commented that the sesame seeds containing diets significantly lower the serum TC, LDL-C and TC/HDL-C ratio along with a decrease in lipid peroxidation (assessed by TBARS - thiobarbituric acid reactive substances); however, the activity of glutathione peroxidase and superoxide dismutase had registered an increase. Thus, sesame supplementation among hyperlipidemics can help to lower the serum TC, LDL-C and lipid peroxidation along with improved antioxidant status.

Likewise, flaxseeds and its components can greatly improve the cardiovascular health. Of the 35% oil present in flaxseeds, more than half is in the form of omega-3 or α-linolenic acid (Prasad, 2009). Flaxseed consumption suppresses atherosclerosis; and this is mainly attributed to the presence of lignans which bring about a reduction in serum TC and LDL-C along with an increase in the serum HDL-C. In addition, lignan SDG (secoisolariciresinol diglucoside) and its metabolites also possess antioxidant activity. The lipid lowering property and antioxidant characteristic of lignans are mainly responsible for suppressing the atherosclerotic changes. The cardio-protective effect of flaxseed is primarily attributed to its high omega-3, phytoestrogens, lignans and soluble dietary fibre content. Further, flaxseed consumption not only brings about a reduction in serum TC and LDL-C concentrations, but it also restricts the postprandial glucose absorption as well as decreases certain biomarkers of inflammation; in addition, it increases the serum omega-3 fatty acid (ALA and EPA) levels too (Bloedon & Szapary, 2004).

Fruits and Vegetables

Over the years, copious literature has endorsed the potential public health significance of increasing the consumption of fruits and vegetables; and this has gained wide acceptance in the prevention of CVD (Ness & Powles, 1997). The cardio-protective effects are mainly attributed to numerous bioactive compounds present in fruits and vegetables such as dietary fibre, vitamin C, carotenoids and other components like glucosinolates, folic acid and (iso)flavonoids (Steinmetz & Potter, 1991). Ortega et al (2006) have commented that fruits and vegetables being a significant source of phytosterols bring about reductions in serum cholesterol concentrations as well as the CVD risk. Veer et al (1999) had commented that if the populations adhere to consuming appropriate amounts of a variety of fruits and vegetables, nearly 6-22% of CVD mortality can be averted.

The Health Professionals Follow-up Study covering 39,876 females over a period of 5-years reported that there was a significant inverse association between fruit/vegetable intake and the CVD risk (Liu et al., 2000). Based on a systematic review of a number of ecological, case-control and cohort studies, Ness and Powles (1997) had revealed that there is a significant protective association between fruit/vegetable consumption and the occurrence of CHD Dauchet et al (2006) conducted a meta-analysis of various studies and reported that, an overall relative risk of 0.96 for ischaemic heart disease was associated with each portion of fruit/vegetable consumption in a day.

Beverages

A cross-sectional survey covering 8,821 male/female Polish subjects concluded that tea and coffee consumption was negatively associated with metabolic syndrome/some of its components (Grosso et al., 2014). Green tea, in particular, is rich in antioxidants; therefore tea consumption can accord a number of health benefits (Dasgupta & Klein, 2014). An important constituent of tea - epigalocatechin gallate possesses strong antioxidant, immunostimulatory, anti-inflammatory and antimicrobial properties. Moderately high intake of tea, more than 4 cups per day, is reported to reduce the CVD risk; however, its effect on serum lipoproteins is yet not clear (Yang & Landau, 2000; McKay & Blumberg, 2002). Oriental tea, especially the green tea, is rich in polyphenols that confer a number of positive health effects; its consumption decreases TC concentrations and reduces the oxidation of lipoprotein fractions; while it increases the HDL-C concentrations (Weisburger, 1999; Dreosti, 2000; Weisburger, 1999; Mathé, 1999; Sato & Miyata, 2000).

It has been reported that caffeic and ferulic acids – the two phenolic compounds are able to block the increase in intracellular calcium as well as apoptosis of human endothelial cells induced by oxidized LDLs (Vieira et al., 1999). The well-established effects of caffeine on blood pressure seems to increase the plasma homocysteine levels, which is an independent CVD risk factor (Urgert et al., 2000).

Regarding coffee consumption and CHD risk, meta-analysis of large prospective cohort studies had yielded inconsistent results. In a longitudinal study with a follow-up period of nearly 10 years, Wu et al (2009) have reported that moderate amounts of habitual coffee consumption is associated with a significantly lowered risk of CHD among women (RR 0.82, 95% CI, 0.73-0.92) and men (RR 0.87, 95% CI, 0.80-0.86). In a meta-analysis covering case-control and cohort studies with varying follow-up period of nearly 3-44 years, the case–control studies indicated a significant association between high coffee intake and CHD; however, the long-term prospective cohort studies failed to demonstrate any such association (Sofi et al., 2007). Dasgupta and Klein (2014) have commented that although coffee contains various antioxidants (but lesser than tea), its excessive intake (due to high caffeine content) may produce a number of adverse effects including increase in blood pressure.

Cocoa and chocolate can inhibit in vitro LDL oxidation (Dreosti, 2000). Dark chocolate consumption is reported to be inversely associated with CAD; its blood pressure lowering and anti-inflammatory activities indicate its potential use as a prophylactic/therapeutic agent. While coffee and chocolate consumption in moderation is reported to confer beneficial effects in CAD, these health benefits are lost with heavy consumption (Castelnuovo et al., 2012).

Grapes, wines and beer polyphenolics possess potent antioxidant activity that can protect cellular membranes as well as inhibit LDL oxidation; and thus, averting atherosclerosis (Lampe, 1999; Kinsella et al., 1993). It has been reported that wine consumption in moderation decreases CHD by inhibiting platelet aggregation; this endorses the French paradox explaining a smaller CHD mortality in France than the United States (Renaud & de Lorgeril,1992).

On the contrary, alcohol intake is deleterious in majority of the CVDs such as hypertension, haemorrhagic stroke and atrial fibrillation (Taylor et al., 2009; Patra et al., 2010; Samokhvalov, Irving & Rehm, 2010). Habitual alcohol consumption in large amounts is strongly linked to adverse CVD events; however, moderate consumption may reduce the risk of CVD (Rehm et al., 2010; Maclure, 1993). It has been reported that although restricted consumption may marginally reduce the risk of ischaemic stroke, excessive alcohol intake usually elevates the risk of haemorrhagic stroke (Corrao et al., 2000). Roerecke and Rehm (2010) have also endorsed that light to moderate alcohol consumption usually provides protection against ischaemic diseases; however, this protective effect is lost among heavy drinkers even when alcohol in excess is consumed irregularly. In the patients of ischemic disease, heavy drinking is associated with increased incidence of blood clotting coupled with reduced threshold for ventricular fibrillation which occur immediately after heavy drinking (Rehm et al., 2010).

Spices, condiments and herbs are another class of functional foods that confer a variety of cardio-protective effects. Studies indicate that habitual intake of garlic can help to curb the risk of heart attack and stroke due to its lipid-lowering effects on TC, LDL-C and TG without affecting the HDL-C concentrations (Warshafsky, Kramer & Sivak, 1993; Kleijnen, Knipschild & ter Riet, 1989). Anti-inflammatory and antioxidant attributes of turmeric/curcumin are supposedly responsible for its beneficial effects in several disorders and diseases including myocardial infarction (Krishnaswamy, 2006).

It is expected that over the years, some functional foods will be designed and marketed taking into account the gene polymorphisms that may be relevant for the causation of chronic diseases, particularly the CVDs. In developing economies of South East Asia, Africa and Latin America, the health driven food sector will develop and propagate. This is already existing in many of the nations in the form of vitamin-mineral fortification of commonly consumed foods for the masses in general; however, the emergence of advanced functional foods targeting many of the health related disorders and diseases, particularly the chronic degenerative lifestyle related diseases including the CVDs, overweight/obesity, type 2 diabetes and cancers is on the anvil to tackle the exorbitantly escalating prevalence of these disorders in the developing world (Weststrate et al., 2002).

CONCLUSION

Cardiovascular diseases are a leading cause of morbidity and mortality across the world. These are not only affecting the industrialized and developed nations but even the developing countries where populations are undergoing significant life-style changes. In the prevention and management of CVDs, lifestyle modifications play a significant role that include dietary modifications, regular physical activity, weight management, restricting alcohol intake, abstaining substance abuse and stress management. Dietary modifications are a key component in averting the cardiovascular events and reducing the risk factors. In this regard, the functional foods, in view of their health potentials have a huge market provided they are made available in the form of palatable and ready to use food items. The advent of specifically designed functional foods targeting the lifestyle related diseases (CVDs in particular) is urgently needed to tackle the mounting epidemic of cardiovascular related health issues/diseases.

REFERENCES

Al-Sheraji, S. H., Ismail, A., Manap, M. Y., Mustafa, S., Yusof, R. M., & Hassan, F. A. (2012). Hypocholesterolemic effect of yoghurt containing Bi fidobacterium pseudocatenulatum G4 or Bi fido bacterium longum BB536. *Food Chemistry*, *135*(2), 356–361. doi:10.1016/j.foodchem.2012.04.120 PMID:22868099

Alaimo, K., McDowell, M. A., & Briefel, R. R. (1994). Dietary intake of vitamins, minerals, and fiber of persons ages 2 months and over in the United States: The Third National Health and Nutrition Examination Survey, Phase 1, 1988–1991. *Advance Data*, *258*, 1–26. PMID:10138938

Albert, C. M., Gaziano, J. M., Willett, W. C., & Manson, J. E. (2002). Nut consumption and decreased risk of sudden cardiac death in the Physicians' Health Study. *Archives of Internal Medicine*, *162*(12), 1382–1387. doi:10.1001/archinte.162.12.1382 PMID:12076237

Alipoor, B., Haghighian, M. K., Sadat, B. E., & Asghari, M. (2012). Effect of sesame seed on lipid profile and redox status in hyperlipidemic patients. *International Journal of Food Sciences and Nutrition*, *63*(6), 674–678. doi:10.3109/09637486.2011.652077 PMID:22263599

Alper, C. M., & Mattes, R. D. (2003). Peanut consumption improves indices of cardiovascular disease risk in healthy adults. *Journal of the American College of Nutrition*, *22*(2), 133–141. doi:10.1080/07315724.2003.10719286 PMID:12672709

Anderson, J. W. (1995). Dietary fibre, complex carbohydrate and coronary artery disease. *Canadian Journal Cardiology*, *11*(SG):55G – 62G.

Anderson, J. W. (2002). Dietary fiber prevents carbohydrate-induced hypertriglyceridemia. *Current Atherosclerosis Report*, 536 – 541.

Anonymous, . (2000). Counting the benefits of soy. *Agri-Food Res Ontario.*, *24*, 28–29.

Anthony, M. S., Clarkson, T. B., & Williams, J. K. (1998). Effects of soy isoflavones on ather-osclerosis: Potential mechanisms. *The American Journal of Clinical Nutrition*, *68*, 1390S–1393S. PMID:9848505

Arnoldi, A. (2005). Functional Foods, Cardiovascular Disease and Diabetes, Woodhead Publishing Ltd, Cambridge, UK. *Carbohydrate Polymers*, *61*(4), 480–485. doi:10.1016/j.carbpol.2005.05.012

Assmann, G., Buonob, P., Daniele, A., Valle, E. D., Farinaro, E., Ferns, G., & Vetrani, C. et al. (2014). Functional foods and cardiometabolic diseases: International Task Force for Prevention of Cardiometabolic Diseases. *Nutrition, Metabolism, and Cardiovascular Diseases*, *24*(12), 1272–1300. doi:10.1016/j.numecd.2014.10.010 PMID:25467217

Assmann, G., & Schulte, H. (1992). Relation of high-density lipoprotein cholesterol and triglycerides to incidence of atherosclerotic coronary artery disease (the PROCAM experience). *The American Journal of Cardiology*, *70*(7), 733–737. doi:10.1016/0002-9149(92)90550-I PMID:1519522

Aviram, M., Rosenblat, M., Gaitini, D., Nitecki, S., Hoffman, A., Dornfeld, L., & Hayek, T. et al. (2004). Pomegranate juice consumption for 3 years by patients with carotid artery stenosis reduces common carotid intima-media thickness, blood pressure and LDL oxidation. *Clinical Nutrition (Edinburgh, Lothian)*, *23*(3), 423–433. doi:10.1016/j.clnu.2003.10.002 PMID:15158307

Barrett-Connor, E., & Orchard, T. J. (1985). Insulin-dependent diabetes mellitus and ischemic heart disease. *Diabetes Care*, *8*(Supplement_1), S65–S70. doi:10.2337/diacare.8.1.S65 PMID:4053956

Block, G., Patterson, B., & Subar, A. (1992). Fruit, vegetables, and cancer prevention: A review of the epidemiological evidence. *Nutrition and Cancer*, *18*(1), 1–29. doi:10.1080/01635589209514201 PMID:1408943

Bloedon, L. T., & Szapary, P. O. (2004). Flaxseed and Cardiovascular Risk. *Nutrition Reviews*, *62*(1), 18–27. doi:10.1111/j.1753-4887.2004.tb00002.x PMID:14995053

Bonithon-Kopp, C., Coudray, C., Berr, C., Touboul, P. J., Feve, J. M., Favier, A., & Ducimetiere, P. (1997). Combined effects of lipid peroxidation and antioxidant status on carotid atherosclerosis in a population aged 59–71 year. The EVA study. Etude sur le Vieillisement Arteriel. *The American Journal of Clinical Nutrition*, *65*, 121–127. PMID:8988923

Calabrese, V., Cornelius, C., Dinkova-Kostova, A. T., Iavicoli, I., Di Paola, R., Koverech, A., & Calabrese, E. J. (1822). (2012) Cellular stress responses, hormetic phytochemicals and vitagenes in aging and longevity. *Biochimica et Biophysica Acta*, 753–783.

Castelnuovo, A. D. (2012). Consumption of cocoa, tea and coffee and risk of cardiovascular disease. *European Journal of Internal Medicine*, *23*(1), 15–25. doi:10.1016/j.ejim.2011.07.014 PMID:22153525

Coates, A. M., & Howe, P. R. (2007). Edible nuts and metabolic health. *Current Opinion in Lipidology*, *18*(1), 25–30. doi:10.1097/MOL.0b013e3280123a47 PMID:17218828

Collaborative group of the primary prevention project (PPP). (2001). Low-dose aspirin and vitamin E in people at cardiovascular risk: a randomized trial in general practice. *Lancet*, *357*, 89-95.

Connor, W. E. (1994). n-3 Fatty acids and heart disease. In: Kritchevsky D, Carroll KK, editors. Nutrition and disease update: heart disease. Champaign, IL: American Oil Chemists' Society.

Connor, W. E. (2000). Importance of n-3 fatty acids in health and disease. *The American Journal of Clinical Nutrition*, *71*, 171S–175S. PMID:10617967

Cornwell, T., Cohick, W., & Raskin, I. (2004). Dietary phytoestrogens and health. *Phytochemistry*, *65*(8), 995–1016. doi:10.1016/j.phytochem.2004.03.005 PMID:15110680

Corrao, G., Rubbiati, L., Bagnardi, V., Zambon, A., & Poikolainen, K. (2000). Alcohol and coronary heart disease: A meta-analysis. *Addiction (Abingdon, England)*, *95*(10), 1505–1523. doi:10.1046/j.1360-0443.2000.951015056.x PMID:11070527

Costa, R. L., & Summa, M. A. (2000). Soy protein in the management of hyperlipidemia. *Annales Pharmaceutiques*, *34*, 931–935. doi:10.1345/aph.19371 PMID:10928406

Craig, W., & Beck, L. (1999). Phytochemicals: Health protective effects. *Canadian Journal of Dietetic Practice and Researc*, *60*, 78–84. PMID:11551345

Crouse, J. R. III, Morgan, T., Terry, J. G., Ellis, J., Vitolins, M., & Burke, G. L. (1999). A ran-domized trial comparing the effect of casein with that of soy protein contain-ing varying amounts of isoflavones on plasma concentrations of lipids and lipoproteins. *Archives of Internal Medicine*, *159*(17), 2070–2076. doi:10.1001/archinte.159.17.2070 PMID:10510993

Dasgupta, A., & Klein, K. (2014). *Tea, Coffee, and Chocolate: Rich Sources of Antioxidants*. Antioxidants in Food, Vitamins and Supplements Prevention and Treatment of Disease. doi:10.1016/B978-0-12-405872-9.00013-6

Dauchet, L., Amouyel, P., Hercberg, S., & Dallongeville, J. (2006). Fruit and vegetable consump-tion and risk of coronary heart disease: A meta-analysis of cohort studies. *The Journal of Nutrition*, *136*(10), 2588–2593. PMID:16988131

Delzenne, N. M., Daubioul, C., Neyrinck, A., Lasa, M., & Taper, H. S. (2002). Inulin and oligofructose modulate lipid metabolism in animals: Review of biochemical events and future prospects. *The British Journal of Nutrition*, *87*(S2), S255–S259. doi:10.1079/BJN/2002545 PMID:12088526

Dreosti, I. E. (2000). Antioxidant polyphenols in tea, cocoa, and wine. *Nutrition (Burbank, Los Angeles County, Calif.)*, *16*(7/8), 692–694. doi:10.1016/S0899-9007(00)00304-X PMID:10906600

Duriez, P., & Fruchart, J.-C. (1993). Vitamine E et athérosclerose. *Méd Nutr.*, *29*, 17–19.

Erkkila, A., & Lichtenstein, A. (2006). Fiber and cardiovascular disease risk: How strong is the evidence? *The Journal of Cardiovascular Nursing*, *21*(1), 3–8. doi:10.1097/00005082-200601000-00003 PMID:16407729

Erkkila, A., & Lichtenstein, A. (2006). Fiber and cardiovascular disease risk: How strong is the evidence? *The Journal of Cardiovascular Nursing*, *21*(1), 3–8. doi:10.1097/00005082-200601000-00003 PMID:16407729

Ferrari, C. K. B. (1998). Oxidação lipídica em alimentos e sistemas biológicos: Mecanismos gerais e conseqüências nutricionais e patológicas. *Rev Nutr*, *11*(1), 3–14. doi:10.1590/S1415-52731998000100001

Ferrari, C. K. B., & Torres, E. A. F. S. (2003). Biochemical pharmacology of functional foods and prevention of chronic diseases of aging. *Biomedicine and Pharmacotherapy*, *57*(5-6), 251–260. doi:10.1016/S0753-3322(03)00032-5 PMID:12888262

Fielding, J. M., Rowley, K. G., Cooper, P., & O'Dea, K. (2005). Increases in plasma lycopene concentration after consumption of tomatoes cooked with olive oil. *Asia Pacific Journal of Clinical Nutrition*, *14*, 131–136. PMID:15927929

Fiordaliso, M., Kok, N., Desager, J. P., Goethals, F., Deboyser, D., Roberfroid, M., & Delzenne, N. (1995). Dietary oligofructose lowers triglycerides, phospholipids and cholesterol in serum and very low density lipoproteins of rats. *Lipids*, *30*(2), 163–167. doi:10.1007/BF02538270 PMID:7769973

Food and Drug Administration. (1999). Food labeling: Health claims; soy protein and coronary heart disease. Food and Drug Administration, HHS. Final rule. *Federal Register*, *64*, 57700–57733. PMID:11010706

Food and Drug Administration. (2003). *Qualified Health Claims: Letter of Enforcement Discretion – Nuts and Coronary Heart Disease. docket no. 02P-0505*. Washington, DC: FDA.

Fraser, G. E., Lindsted, K. D., & Beeson, W. L. (1995). Effect of risk factor values on lifetime risk of and age at that first coronary event. The Adventist Health Study. *American Journal of Epidemiology*, *142*, 746–758. PMID:7572946

Fraser, G. E., Sabate, J., Beeson, W. L., & Strahan, T. M. (1992). A possible protective effect of nut consumption on risk of coronary heart disease. The Adventist Health Study. *Archives of Internal Medicine*, *152*(7), 1416–1424. doi:10.1001/archinte.1992.00400190054010 PMID:1627021

Gale, C. R., Ashurst, H. E., Powers, H. J., & Martyn, C. N. (2001). Antioxidant vitamin status and carotid atherosclerosis in the elderly. *The American Journal of Clinical Nutrition*, *74*, 402–408. PMID:11522566

Gianetti, J., Pedrinelli, R., Petrucci, R., Lazzerini, G., De Caterina, M., Bel-lomo, G., & De Catarina, R. (2002). Inverse association between carotid intima-media thickness and the antioxidant lycopene in atherosclerosis. *American Heart Journal, 143*(3), 467–474. doi:10.1067/mhj.2002.120776 PMID:11868053

Gibaldi, M. (2001). Are phytoestrogens a "natural alternative" to estrogen replacement therapy? *The Western Journal of Medicine, 173*(4), 273. doi:10.1136/ewjm.173.4.273 PMID:11017999

Gotto, A. M. Jr. (2003). Antioxidants, statins, and atherosclerosis. *Journal of the American College of Cardiology, 41*(7), 1205–1210. doi:10.1016/S0735-1097(03)00082-2 PMID:12679223

Grassi, D., Necozione, S., Lippi, C., Croce, G., Verli, L., Pasqualetti, P., & Ferri, C. et al. (2005). Cocoa reduces blood pressure and insulin resistance and improves endothelium-dependent vasodilation in hypertensives. *Hypertension, 46*(2), 398–405. doi:10.1161/01.HYP.0000174990.46027.70 PMID:16027246

Gutteridge, J. M. (1995). Lipid peroxidation and antioxidants as biomarkers of tissue damage. *Clinical Chemistry, 41*, 1819–1828. PMID:7497639

Hak, A. E., Stampfer, M. J., Campos, H., Sesso, H. D., Gaziano, J. M., Willett, W., & Ma, J. (2003). Plasma carotenoids and tocopherols and risk of myocardial infarction in a low-risk population of US male physicians. *Circulation, 108*(7), 802–807. doi:10.1161/01.CIR.0000084546.82738.89 PMID:12900344

Halliwell, B., & Chirico, S. (1993). Lipid peroxidation: Its mechanism, measure-ment, and significance. *The American Journal of Clinical Nutrition, 57*(Suppl), 715–725. PMID:8475889

Harland, J., & Haffner, T. (2008). Systematic review, meta-analysis and regression of randomised controlled trials reporting an association between an intake of circa 25 g soya protein per day and blood cholesterol. *Atherosclerosis, 200*(1), 13–27. doi:10.1016/j.atherosclerosis.2008.04.006 PMID:18534601

Hertog, M. G., Feskens, E. J., Hollman, P. C., Katan, M. B., & Kromhout, D. (1993). Dietary antioxidant flavonoids and risk of coronary heart disease: The Zutphen Elderly study. *Lancet, 342*(8878), 1007–1011. doi:10.1016/0140-6736(93)92876-U PMID:8105262

Hertog, M. G. L., Feskens, E. J. M., Hollman, P. C. H., Katan, M. B., & Kromhout, D. (1993). Dietary antioxidant flavonoids and risk of coronary heart disease: The Zutphen Elderly Study. *Lancet, 342*(8878), 1007–1011. doi:10.1016/0140-6736(93)92876-U PMID:8105262

Hertog, M. G. L., Feskens, E. J. M., Hollman, P. C. H., Katan, M. B., & Kromhout, D. (1993). Dietary antioxidant flavonoids and risk of coronary heart disease: The Zutphen Elderly Study. *Lancet, 342*(8878), 1007–1011. doi:10.1016/0140-6736(93)92876-U PMID:8105262

Hertog, M. G. L., Kromhout, D., Aravanis, C., Blackburn, H., Buzina, R., Fidanza, F., & Nedeljkovic, S. et al. (1995). Flavonoid intake and long-term risk of coronary heart disease and cancer in the Seven Countries Country. *Archives of Internal Medicine, 155*(4), 381–386. doi:10.1001/archinte.1995.00430040053006 PMID:7848021

Hertog, M. G. L., Kromhout, D., Aravanis, C., Blackburn, H., Buzina, R., Fidanza, F., & Nedeljkovic, S. et al. (1995). Flavonoid intake and long-term risk of coronary heart disease and cancer in the Seven Countries Country. *Archives of Internal Medicine, 155*(4), 381–386. doi:10.1001/archinte.1995.00430040053006 PMID:7848021

Hollman, P. C. H., & Katan, M. B. (1999, September). (199) Dietary flavonoids: Intake, health effects and bioavailability. *Food and Chemical Toxicology*, *37*(9-10), 937–942. doi:10.1016/S0278-6915(99)00079-4 PMID:10541448

Hornych, A., Girault, F., Oravec, S., Forette, B., & Horrobin, D. (2001). Effect of gamma-linolenic acid on plasma and membrane lipids and renal prostaglandins in old subjects. *Klin Biochem Metab*, *9*, 28–34.

Hu, F. B., Stampfer, M. J., Manson, J. E., Rimm, E. B., Colditz, G. A., Ros-ner, B. A., & Willet, W. et al. (1998). Frequent nut consumption and risk of coronary heart disease in women: Prospective cohort study. *British Medical Journal*, *317*(7169), 1341–1345. doi:10.1136/bmj.317.7169.1341 PMID:9812929

Huxley, R. R., & Neil, H. A. (2003). The relation between dietary flavonol intake and coronary heart disease mortality: A meta-analysis of prospective cohort studies. *European Journal of Clinical Nutrition*, *57*(8), 904–908. doi:10.1038/sj.ejcn.1601624 PMID:12879084

Huxley, R. R., & Neil, H. A. (2003). The relation between dietary flavonol intake and coronary heart disease mortality: A meta-analysis of prospective cohort studies. *European Journal of Clinical Nutrition*, *57*(8), 904–908. doi:10.1038/sj.ejcn.1601624 PMID:12879084

Jackson, K. G., & Lovegrove, J. A. (2002). Functional foods, blood lipids and coronary heart disease. *Fd Sci Tech Bull.*, 1-11.

Jacobs, D. R. Jr, & Gallaher, D. D. (2004). Whole grain intake and cardiovascular disease, a review. *Current Atherosclerosis Reports*, *6*(6), 414–423. doi:10.1007/s11883-004-0081-y PMID:15485586

Jain, S. K., McVie, R., Jaramillo, J. J., Palmer, M., Smith, T., Mea-chum, Z. D., & Little, R. L. (1996). The effect of modest vitamin E supplementation on lipid peroxidation products and other cardiovascular risk factors in diabetic patients. *Lipids*, *31*(1Suppl), 87–90. doi:10.1007/BF02637057 PMID:8729100

Jenkins, D. J., Kendall, C. W., Marchie, A., Faulkner, D. A., Wong, J. M., de Souza, R., & Connelly, P. W. et al. (2005). Direct comparison of a dietary portfolio of cholesterol-lowering foods with a statin in hyper-cholesterolemic participants. *The American Journal of Clinical Nutrition*, *81*, 380–387. PMID:15699225

Jones, P. J. (2002). Clinical nutrition: 7. Functional foods — more than just nutrition. *Canadian Medical Association Journal*, *166*(12), 1555–1563. PMID:12074125

Jones, P. J., Raeini-Sarjaz, M., Ntanios, F. V., Vanstone, C. A., Feng, J. Y., & Parsons, W. E. (2000). Modulation of plasma lipid levels and cholesterol kinetics by phytosterol versus phytostanol esters. *Journal of Lipid Research*, *41*(5), 697–705. PMID:10787430

Jones, P. J. H., & Raeini-Sarjaz, M. (2001). Plant sterols and their derivatives; the current spread of results. *Nutrition Reviews*, *59*(1), 21–24. doi:10.1111/j.1753-4887.2001.tb01901.x PMID:11281249

Kaliora, A. C., & Dedoussis, G. V. Z. (2007). Natural antioxidant compounds in risk factors for CVD. *Pharmacological Research*, *56*(2), 99–109. doi:10.1016/j.phrs.2007.04.018 PMID:17572098

Katan, M. B., Grundy, S. M., Jones, P., Law, M., Miettinen, T., & Paoletti, R. (2003). Efficacy and safety of plant stanols and sterols in the management of blood cholesterol levels. *Mayo Clinic Proceedings*, *78*(8), 965–978. doi:10.1016/S0025-6196(11)63144-3 PMID:12911045

Khandelwal, S., Demonty, I., Jeemon, P., Lakshmy, R., Mukherjee, R., Gupta, R., & Reddy, K. S. et al. (2009). Independent and interactive effects of plant sterols & fish oil n-3 long chain polyunsaturated fatty acids on the plasma lipid profile of mildly hyperlipidemic Indian adults. *The British Journal of Nutrition*, *102*(5), 722–732. doi:10.1017/S0007114509297170 PMID:19296875

Kinsella, J. E., Frankel, E., German, B., & Kanner, J. (1993). Possible mechanisms for the protective role of antioxidants in wine and plant foods. *Food Technology*, *47*(4), 85–89.

Kleijnen, J., Knipschild, P., & ter Riet, G. T. (1989). Garlic, onions and cardiovascular risk factors. A review of the evidence from human experiments with emphasis on commercially available preparations. *British Journal of Clinical Pharmacology*, *28*(5), 535–544. doi:10.1111/j.1365-2125.1989.tb03539.x PMID:2686739

Kohlmeier, L., Kark, J. D., Gomez-Gracia, E., Martin, B. C., Steck, S. E., Kardinaal, A. F., & Kok, F. J. et al. (1997). Lycopene and myocardial infarction risk in the EURAMIC study. *American Journal of Epidemiology*, *146*(8), 618–626. doi:10.1093/oxfordjournals.aje.a009327 PMID:9345115

Kris-Etherton, P. M., Hu, F. B., Ros, E., & Sabaté, J. (2008). The role of tree nuts and peanuts in the prevention of coronary heart disease: Multiple potential mechanisms. *The Journal of Nutrition*, *138*(9), 1746S–1751S. PMID:18716180

Kris-Etherton, P. M., Zhao, G., Binkoski, A. E., Coval, S. M., & Etherton, T. D. (2001). The effects of nuts on coronary heart disease risk. *Nutrition Reviews*, *59*(4), 103–111. doi:10.1111/j.1753-4887.2001.tb06996.x PMID:11368503

Krishnaswamy, K. (2006). *Turmeric-The salt of the orient is the spice of life*. New Delhi, India: Allied Publishers Pvt. Ltd.

Kritchevsky, S. B., Shimakawa, T., Tell, G. S., Dennis, B., Carpenter, M., Eck-feldt, J. H., & Heiss, G. et al. (1995). Dietary antioxidants and carotid artery wall thickness. The ARIC study. Atherosclerosis Risk in Communities study. *Circulation*, *92*(8), 2142–2150. doi:10.1161/01.CIR.92.8.2142 PMID:7554194

Kushi, L. H., Meyer, K. A., & Jacobs, D. R. Jr. (1999). Cereals, legumes, and chronic disease risk reduction: Evidence from epidemiologic studies. *The American Journal of Clinical Nutrition*, *70*, 451S–458S. PMID:10479217

Lampe, J. W. (1999). Health effects of vegetables and fruit: Assessing mecha-nisms of action in human experimental studies. *The American Journal of Clinical Nutrition*, *70*(Suppl), 475–490. PMID:10479220

Lamuela-Raventos, R. M., Gimeno, E., Fito, M., Castellote, A. I., Covas, M., de la Torre-Boronat, M. C., & Lopez-Sabater, M. C. (2004). Interaction of olive oil phenol antioxidant components with low-density lipo protein. *Biological Research*, *37*(2), 247–252. doi:10.4067/S0716-97602004000200011 PMID:15455654

Lamy, S., Akla, N., Ouanouki, A., Lord-Dufour, S., & Beliveau, R. (2012). Diet-derived polyphenols inhibit angiogenesis by modu-lating the interleukin-6/STAT3 pathway. *Experimental Cell Research*, *318*(13), 1568–1596. doi:10.1016/j.yexcr.2012.04.004 PMID:22522122

Law, M. (2000). Plant sterol and stanol margarines and health. *British Medical Journal, 320*(7238), 861–864. doi:10.1136/bmj.320.7238.861 PMID:10731187

Liu, S., Manson, J. E., Lee, I.-M., Cole, S. R., Hennekens, C. H., Willet, W. C., & Buring, J. E. (2000). Fruit and vegetable intake and risk of cardiovascular disease: The Women's Health Study. *The American Journal of Clinical Nutrition, 72*, 922–928. PMID:11010932

Lovegrove, J. A., & Jackson, K. G. (2011). Functional foods and coronary heart disease (CHD). In Functional Foods - Concept to Product (2nd ed.). Woodhead Publishing Series in Food Science, Technology and Nutrition.

Maclure, M. (1993). Demonstration of deductive meta-analysis: Ethanol intake and risk of myocardial infarction. *Epidemiologic Reviews, 15*(2), 328–351. PMID:8174661

Margetts, B.M., Thompson, R., & Duffy, S. (1994). *A Review of the Epidemiological Literature Linking Fruit and Vegetable Consumption to Risk of Cancer*. Nutritional Epidemiology Working Group on Diet and Cancer.

Mathé, G. (1999). Red wine, green tea and vitamins: Do their antioxidants play a role in immunologic protection against cancer or even AIDS? *Biomedicine and Pharmacotherapy, 53*(4), 165–167. doi:10.1016/S0753-3322(99)80084-5 PMID:10392288

McInnes, G. T. (2004). How important is optimal blood pressure control? *Clinical Therapeutics, 26*, 3–11. doi:10.1016/S0149-2918(04)90140-3 PMID:15291374

McKay, D. L., & Blumberg, J. B. (2002). The role of tea in human health: An update. *Journal of the American College of Nutrition, 21*(1), 1–13. doi:10.1080/07315724.2002.10719187 PMID:11838881

Mercanligil, S. M., Arslan, P., Alasalvar, C., Okut, E., Akgul, E., Pinar, A., & Shahidi, F. et al. (2007). Effects of hazelnut-enriched diet on plasma cholesterol and lipoprotein profiles in hypercholesterolemic adult men. *European Journal of Clinical Nutrition, 61*(2), 212–220. doi:10.1038/sj.ejcn.1602518 PMID:16969381

Meydani, M., Lipman, R. D., Han, S. N., Wu, D., Beharka, A., Mar-tin, K., & Meydani, S. N. et al. (1998). The effect of long-term dietary supplementation with antioxidants. *Annals of the New York Academy of Sciences, 854*(1), 352–360. doi:10.1111/j.1749-6632.1998.tb09915.x PMID:9928443

Micallef, M. A., & Garg, M. L. (2008). The lipid-lowering effects of phytosterols and (n-3) polyunsaturated fatty acids are synergistic and complementary in hyperlipidemic men and women. *The Journal of Nutrition, 138*, 1086–1090. PMID:18492838

Miettinen, T. A., Vuoristo, M., Nissinen, M., Jarvinen, H. J., & Gylling, H. (2000). Serum, biliary, and fecal cholesterol and plant sterols in cholectomized patients before and during consumption of stanol ester margarine. *The American Journal of Clinical Nutrition, 71*(5), 1095–1102. PMID:10799370

Miller, E. R., Appel, L. J., Levander, O. A., & Levine, D. M. (1997). The effect of antioxidant vitamin supplementation on traditional cardiovascular risk factors. *Journal of Cardiovascular Risk, 4*(1), 19–24. doi:10.1177/174182679700400104 PMID:9215516

Mink, P. J., Scrafford, C. G., Barraj, L. M., Harnack, L., Hong, C. P., Nettleton, J. A., & Jacobs, D. R. Jr. (2007). Flavonoid intake and cardio vascular disease mortality: A prospective study in post-menopausal women. *The American Journal of Clinical Nutrition, 85*, 895–909. PMID:17344514

Mohamed, S. (2014). Functional foods against metabolic syndrome (obesity, diabetes, hypertension and dyslipidemia) and cardiovascular disease. *Trends Fd Sci Tech., 35*(2), 114–128. doi:10.1016/j.tifs.2013.11.001

Mukuddem-Petersen, J., Oosthuizen, W., & Jerling, J. C. (2005). A systematic review of the effects of nuts on blood lipid profiles in humans. *The Journal of Nutrition, 135*, 2082–2089. PMID:16140880

Mursu, J., Voutilainen, S., Nurmi, T., Tuomainen, T.-P., Kurl, S., & Salonen, J. T. (2008). Flavonoid intake and the risk of ischaemic stroke and CVD mortality in middle-aged Finnish men: The Kuopio Ischaemic Heart Disease Risk Factor Study. *The British Journal of Nutrition, 100*(04), 890–895. doi:10.1017/S0007114508945694 PMID:18377681

Naumann, E., Plat, J., Kester, A. M., & Mensink, R. P. (2008). The baseline serum lipoprotein profile is related to plant stanol induced changes in serum lipoprotein cholesterol and triacylglycerol concentrations. *Journal of the American College of Nutrition, 27*(1), 117–126. doi:10.1080/07315724.2008.10719683 PMID:18460490

Ness, A. R. (2001). Commentary: Beyond beta-carotene—antioxidants and cardiovascular disease. *International Journal of Epidemiology, 30*(1), 143–144. doi:10.1093/ije/30.1.143 PMID:11171875

Ness, A. R., & Powles, J. W. (1997). Fruit and vegetables, and cardiovascular disease: A review. *International Journal of Epidemiology, 26*(1), 1–13. doi:10.1093/ije/26.1.1 PMID:9126498

Ness, A. R., Powles, J. W., & Khaw, K. T. (1996). Vitamin C and cardiovascular disease: A systematic review. *Journal of Cardiovascular Risk, 3*(6), 513–521. doi:10.1097/00043798-199612000-00006 PMID:9100087

Noncommunicable Diseases. (2015). *Fact sheet*. Retrieved from: www.who.int/mediacentre/factsheets/fs355/en/

Nyyssonen, K., Parviainen, M. T., Salonen, R., Tuomilehto, J., & Salonen, J. T. (1997). Vitamin C deficiency and risk of myocardial infarction: Prospective population study of men from eastern Finland. *BMJ (Clinical Research Ed.), 314*(7081), 634–638. doi:10.1136/bmj.314.7081.634 PMID:9066474

Ortega, R. M., Palencia, A., & Lopez-Sobaler, A. M. (2006). Improvement of cholesterol levels and reduction of cardiovascular risk via the consumption of phytosterols. *The British Journal of Nutrition, 96*(S1Suppl), 89S–93S. doi:10.1079/BJN20061708 PMID:16923260

Ostlund, R. E., Spilburg, C. A., & Stenson, W. F. (1999). Sitostanol administered in lecithin micelles potently reduces cholesterol absorption in humans. *The American Journal of Clinical Nutrition, 70*, 826–831. PMID:10539742

Pang, G., Xie, J., Chen, Q., & Hu, Z. (2012). How functional foods play critical roles in human health. *Food Science and Human Wellness, 1*(1), 26–60. doi:10.1016/j.fshw.2012.10.001

Park, S. H., Kyeong, M. S., Hqang, Y., Ryu, S. Y., Han, S. B., & Kim, Y. (2012). Inhibition of LPS binding to MD-2 co-receptor for suppressing TLR4-mediated expression of inflammatory cytokine by 1-dehydro-10-gingerdione from dietary ginger. *Biochemical and Biophysical Research Communications, 419*(4), 735–740. doi:10.1016/j.bbrc.2012.02.091 PMID:22387540

Patra, J., Taylor, B., Irving, H., Roerecke, M., Baliunas, D., Mohapatra, S., & Rehm, J. (2010). Alcohol consumption and the risk of morbidity and mortality from different stroke types -a systematic review and meta-analysis. *BMC Public Health, 10*(1), 258. doi:10.1186/1471-2458-10-258 PMID:20482788

Pedersen, A., Sandström, B., & Amelsvoort, J. M. M. V. (1997). The effect of ingestion of inulin on blood lipids and gastrointestinal symptoms in healthy females. *The British Journal of Nutrition, 78*(02), 215–222. doi:10.1079/BJN19970141 PMID:9301412

Pereira, D. I. A., & Gibson, G. R. (2002). Effects of consumption of probiotics and prebiotics on serum lipid levels in humans. *Critical Reviews in Biochemistry and Molecular Biology, 37*(4), 259–281. doi:10.1080/10409230290771519 PMID:12236466

Pereira, M. A., O'Reilly, E., Augustsson, K., Fraser, G. E., Goldbourt, U., Heitmann, B. L., & Ascherio, A. et al. (2004). Dietary fiber and risk of coronary heart disease: A pooled analysis of cohort studies. *Archives of Internal Medicine, 164*(4), 370–376. doi:10.1001/archinte.164.4.370 PMID:14980987

Pietinen, P., Rimm, E. B., Korhonen, P., Hartman, A. M., Willett, W. C., Albanes, D., & Virtamo, J. et al. (1996). Intake of dietary fiber and risk of coronary heart disease in a cohort of Finnish men. The Alpha-Tocopherol, Beta-Carotene Cancer Prevention Study. *Circulation, 94*(11), 2720–2727. doi:10.1161/01.CIR.94.11.2720 PMID:8941095

Prasad, K. (2009). Flax seed and Cardiovascular Health. *Journal of Cardiovascular Pharmacology, 54*(5), 369–377. doi:10.1097/FJC.0b013e3181af04e5 PMID:19568181

Psaltopoulou, T., Naska, A., Orfanos, P., Trichopoulos, D., Mountokalakis, T., & Trichopoulou, A. (2004). Olive oil, the Mediterranean diet, and arterial blood pressure: The Greek European prospective investigation into cancer and nutrition (EPIC) study. *The American Journal of Clinical Nutrition, 80*, 1012–1018. PMID:15447913

Rehm, J., Baliunas, D., Borges, G. L. G., Graham, K., Irving, H. M., & Kehoe, T. (2010). The relation between different dimensions of alcohol consumption and burden of disease -An overview. *Addiction (Abingdon, England), 105*, 817–843. PMID:20331573

Reinhart, K., Talati, R., White, C., & Coleman, C. I. (2009). The impact of garlic on lipid parameters: A systematic review and meta-analysis. *Nutrition Research Reviews, 22*(01), 39–48. doi:10.1017/S0954422409350003 PMID:19555517

Renaud, S., & de Lorgeril, M. (1992). Wine, alcohol, platelets, and the French paradox for coronary hearth disease. *Lancet, 339*(8808), 1523–1526. doi:10.1016/0140-6736(92)91277-F PMID:1351198

Rimm, E. B., Katan, M. B., Ascherio, A., Stampfer, M. J., & Willett, W. C. (1996). Relation between intake of flavonoids and risk for coro-nary heart disease in male health professionals. *Annals of Internal Medicine, 125*(5), 384–389. doi:10.7326/0003-4819-125-5-199609010-00005 PMID:8702089

Rimm, E. B., & Stampfer, M. J. (2000). Antioxidants for vascular disease. *The Medical Clinics of North America, 84*(1), 239–249. doi:10.1016/S0025-7125(05)70216-9 PMID:10685137

Roberfroid, M. B. (2003). Introducing inulin-type fructans. *The British Journal of Nutrition, 93*(S1), 13–26. doi:10.1079/BJN20041350 PMID:15877886

Roerecke, M., & Rehm, J. (2010). Irregular heavy drinking occasions and risk of ischemic heart disease: A systematic review and meta-analysis. *American Journal of Epidemiology, 171*(6), 633–644. doi:10.1093/aje/kwp451 PMID:20142394

Samokhvalov, A. V., Irving, H. M., & Rehm, J. (2010). Alcohol as a risk factor for atrial fibrillation: A systematic review and meta-analysis. *European Journal of Cardiovascular Prevention and Rehabilitation, 17*, 706–712. doi:10.1097/HJR.0b013e32833a1947 PMID:21461366

Sánchez-Muniz, F. J. (2012). Dietary fibre and cardiovascular health. *Nutricion Hospitalaria, 27*(1), 31–45. PMID:22566302

Sarrafzadegan, N., & Najafian, J. (1998). Prionties in cardiovascular prevention in Iran. *Iran Health Journal., 1*(Supp 1), 131.

Sato, T., & Miyata, G. (2000). The nutraceutical benefit, Part I: Green tea. *Nutrition (Burbank, Los Angeles County, Calif.), 16*(4), 315–317. doi:10.1016/S0899-9007(99)00301-9 PMID:10758375

Schaafsma, G., Meuling, W. J. A., van Dokkum, W., & Bouley, C. (1998). Effects of a milk product, fermented with Lactobacillus acidophilus and with fructo-oligosaccharides added, on blood lipids in male volunteers. *European Journal of Clinical Nutrition, 52*(6), 436–440. doi:10.1038/sj.ejcn.1600583 PMID:9683397

Sirtori, C. R., & Lovati, M. R. (2001). Soy proteins and cardiovascular disease. *Current Atherosclerosis Reports, 3*(1), 47–53. doi:10.1007/s11883-001-0010-2 PMID:11123848

Sofi, F., Cesari, F., Abbate, R., Gensini, G. F., & Casini, A. (2008). Adherence to Mediterranean diet and health status: Meta-analysis. *BMJ (Clinical Research Ed.), 337*(sep11 2), a1344. doi:10.1136/bmj.a1344 PMID:18786971

Sofi, F., Conti, A. A., Gori, A. M., Luisi, M. L. E., Casini, A., Abbate, R., & Gensini, G. F. (2007). Coffee consumption and risk of coronary heart disease: A meta-analysis. *Nutrition, Metabolism, and Cardiovascular Diseases, 17*(3), 209–223. doi:10.1016/j.numecd.2006.07.013 PMID:17156982

Stark, A. H., & Madar, Z. (2002). Olive oil as a functional food: Epidemiology and nutritional approaches. *Nutrition Reviews, 60*(6), 170–176. doi:10.1301/002966402320243250 PMID:12078915

Steinmetz, K. A., & Potter, J. D. (1991). Vegetables, fruit, and cancer. I. Epidemiology. *Cancer Causes & Control, 2*(5), 325–357. doi:10.1007/BF00051672 PMID:1834240

Steinmetz, K. A., & Potter, J. D. (1991). Vegetables, fruit, and cancer. II. Mechanisms. *Cancer Causes & Control, 2*(6), 427–442. doi:10.1007/BF00054304 PMID:1764568

Stephens, N. G., Parsons, A., Schofield, P. M., Kelly, F., Cheeseman, K., & Mitchinson, M. J. (1996). Randomised controlled trial of Vitamin E in patients with coronary disease: Cambridge Heart Antioxidant Study (CHAOS). *Lancet*, *347*(9004), 781–786. doi:10.1016/S0140-6736(96)90866-1 PMID:8622332

Street, D. A., Comstock, G. W., Salkeld, R. M., Schuep, W., & Klag, M. J. (1994). Serum antioxidants and myocar-dial infarction. Are low levels of carotenoids and α-tocopherol risk factors for myocardial infarction? *Circulation*, *90*(3), 1154–1161. doi:10.1161/01.CIR.90.3.1154 PMID:8087925

Taylor, B., Irving, H. M., Baliunas, D., Roerecke, M., Patra, J., Mohapatra, S., & Rehm, J. (2009). Alcohol and hypertension: Gender differences in dose-response relationships determined through systematic review and meta-analysis. *Addiction (Abingdon, England)*, *104*(12), 1981–1990. doi:10.1111/j.1360-0443.2009.02694.x PMID:19804464

Urgert, R., van Vliet, T., Zock, P. L., & Katan, M. B. (2000). Heavy coffee consumption and plasma homocysteine: A randomized controlled trial in healthy volunteers. *The American Journal of Clinical Nutrition*, *72*, 1107–1110. PMID:11063436

van der Schouw, Y. T., de Kleijn, M. J., Peeters, P. H., & Grobbee, D. E. (2000). Phyto-oestro-gens and cardiovascular disease risk. *Nutrition, Metabolism, and Cardiovascular Diseases*, *10*, 154–167. PMID:11006924

Veer, P.V., Jansen, M.C.J.F., Klerk, M., & Kok, F.J. (1999). Fruits and vegetables in the prevention of cancer and cardiovascular disease. *Public Health Nutrition*, *3*(1), 103–107. PMID:10786730

Vieira, A. J. S. C., Telo, J. P., Pereira, H. F., Patrocínio, P. F., & Dias, R. M. B. (1999). Antioxi-dant effect of naturally occurring xanthines on the oxidative damage of DNA bases. *The Journal of Chemical Physics*, *96*, 116–123.

Wang, C., Harris, W., Chung, M., Lichtenstein, A. H., Balk, E. M., Kupelnick, B., & Lau, J. et al. (2006). n-3 Fatty acids from fish or fish-oil supplements, but not a-linolenic acid, benefit cardiovascular disease outcomes in primary- and secondary-prevention studies: A systematic review. *The American Journal of Clinical Nutrition*, *84*, 5–17. PMID:16825676

Warshafsky, S., Kramer, R. S., & Sivak, S. L. (1993). Effect of garlic on total serum cholesterol: A meta-analysis. *Annals of Internal Medicine*, *119*(7_Part_1), 599–605. doi:10.7326/0003-4819-119-7_Part_1-199310010-00009 PMID:8363171

Weisburger, J. H. (1999). Mechanisms of action of antioxidants as exemplified in vegetables, tomatoes and tea. *Food and Chemical Toxicology*, *37*(9-10), 943–948. doi:10.1016/S0278-6915(99)00086-1 PMID:10541449

Weststrate, J. A., Poppel, G. V., & Verschuren, P. M. (2002). Functional foods, trends and future. *The British Journal of Nutrition*, *88*(S2), S233–S235. doi:10.1079/BJN2002688 PMID:12495465

Wilcox, J. N., & Blumenthal, B. F. (1995). Thrombotic mechanisms in atherosclerosis: Po-tential impact of soy proteins. *The Journal of Nutrition*, *125*, 631S–638S. PMID:7884545

World Health Organization (WHO). (n.d.) Fact Sheet. Retrieved from: www.who.int/mediacentre/factsheets/fs355/en/)

Wu, J., Ho, S. C., Zhou, C., Ling, W. H., Chen, W. Q., Wang, C. L., & Chen, Y. M. (2009). Coffee consumption and risk of coronary heart diseases: A meta-analysis of 21 prospective cohort studies. *International Journal of Cardiology*, *137*(3), 216–225. doi:10.1016/j.ijcard.2008.06.051 PMID:18707777

Yang, C. S., & Landau, J. M. (2000). Effects of tea consumption on nutrition and health. *The Journal of Nutrition*, *130*, 2409–2412. PMID:11015465

Yusuf, S., Dagenais, G., Pogue, J., & Sleight, P. (2000). Vitamin E supplementation and cardiovascular events in high-risk patients. The Heart Outcomes Prevention Evaluation Study Investigators. *The New England Journal of Medicine*, *345*, 154–160. PMID:10639540

Zawistowski, J. (2014). Regulation of Functional Foods in Selected Asian Countries in the Pacific Rim. In Nutraceutical and Functional Food Regulations in the United States and Around the World (2nd ed.). Food Science and Technology. doi:doi:10.1016/B978-0-12-405870-5.00024-4 doi:10.1016/B978-0-12-405870-5.00024-4

Ziouzenkova, O., Gieseg, S. P., Ramos, P., & Esterbauer, H. (1996). Factors affecting resistance of low density lipoproteins to oxidation. *Lipids*, *31*(1Suppl), 71–76. doi:10.1007/BF02637054 PMID:8729097

Chapter 3
Lentils (*Lens culinaris*, L.): A Novel Functional Food

Mo'ez Al-Islam Ezzat Faris
University of Sharjah, UAE

Amita Attlee
University of Sharjah, UAE

ABSTRACT

Lentils have been part of human diet from ancient times. This chapter focuses on the nutritional composition, presence of bioactive substances, antioxidants and health rendering properties of lentils. Recent definitions have considered lentils as a prophylactic and therapeutic functional food due to its considerable content of essential macronutrients, namely functional proteins and carbohydrates, and essential micronutrients, as well as bioactive phytochemicals such as phytates and polyphenols. Indeed, the presence of an impressive arsenal of secondary metabolites, minerals and bioactive constituents in lentils have shown to be promising contributors in the management and prevention of several human chronic diseases, attributed to their anticarcinogenic, hypoglycemic, hypocholesterolemic and blood-pressure lowering properties.

INTRODUCTION

Lentils are a part of legume family and form an important constituent of traditional diets. There has been an emerging interest in lentils as functional food due to their high nutritional value, presence of bioactive components, antioxidants and other phytochemicals that render health properties to lentils. Evidence supports that consumption of lentils is related to reduced incidence of chronic diseases such as cardio-vascular disease, overweight and obesity, diabetes and cancers. This chapter aims to highlight the importance of human consumption of lentils and emphasize their contribution as a functional food in the diets. Specifically, the chapter is logically organized to provide an in-depth review and update about nutritional composition, presence of bioactive substances, antioxidants and other phytochemicals in lentils, followed by evidence on their vital role in promoting health of body systems, and reduction in incidence of chronic diseases and in alleviating their symptoms.

DOI: 10.4018/978-1-5225-0591-4.ch003

BACKGROUND

Food and Agricultural Organization (FAO) has defined the terms legumes, pulses and lentils. A legume is a simple dry fruit which develops from a simple carpel and usually dehisces (opens along a seam) on two sides. Pulses are important food crops due to their high protein and essential amino acid content. Like many leguminous crops, pulses play a key role in crop rotation through their ability to fix atmospheric nitrogen. Lentils (*Lens culinaris* L.) are a member of the Leguminoceae family. Lentil plant is an annual plant with flattened edible seeds that constitutes one of the most important traditional dietary components (FAO, 1988). Its lens-shaped seeds exist with a spectrum of colors including yellow, red, orange, green, brown or black depending on the cultivar, and subsequently the composition of the seed coats and cotyledons (Xu & Chang, 2010).

Lentils are relatively tolerant to drought and are grown in all five continents of the world. FAO (2008) reported that world's production of lentils was about 2.83 million metric tons, primarily coming from Canada (36.9%) and India (28.7%), followed by Nepal, China and Turkey.

Lentils have been incorporated into different world cuisines throughout the globe. For example, lentils are commonly mixed with cereals such as rice, as in the South Asian dish "Khitchri", the Egyptian dish "Koshari", and the Syriandish "Mjaddara". It is also consumed as dehulled split lentil soup, the most customarily consumed form of lentils in many Middle Eastern countries (Dagher, 1991).

Legumes (pulses) are gaining enough interest as emerging functional foods. Several authors explicitly revised the chemical and nutritional values of lentils, as well as bioactive phytochemicals in pulses and their health benefits (Campos-Vega et al., 2010; Champ, 2002; Duranti, 2006; Rochfort & Panozzo, 2007; Roy et al., 2010; Scarafoni et al., 2007; Tharanathan & Mahadevamma, 2003). The health-improving and disease-preventing aspects of lentils have been supported by a large body of evidence, and have been critically reviewed elsewhere (Faris et al., 2013).

Interestingly, lentils had been mentioned in ancient treatment remedies and were documented by Dioscorides as one of the therapeutic plants (Lardos, 2006). Lentil seeds are used in the folk medicine of many ethnicities to treat different illnesses. They are used orally to treat diabetes (Giday et al., 2007), topically as a water paste to treat skin infections (Teklehaymanot et al., 2007) and for the treatment of burns, after being roasted, milled and applied directly to affected areas (Sezik et al., 2001). In addition, lentils are used as a source of lectins for the treatment and prophylaxis of retroviral infections including human immunodeficiency virus (HIV) infections (Alexandre et al., 2010). Ethnopharmacologically, lentil soup was a staple meal in the ancient world, and it was especially prepared for the ailing individual(s) and not for all members of the household unit (Totelin, 2015).

MAIN FOCUS OF THE CHAPTER

Macro and Micro Nutrients

The chemical composition and individual constituents of whole and split lentils are summarized in Table 1 (USDA, 2010).

- **Carbohydrates:** Total carbohydrates represent the major component of lentil seeds (Padovani et al., 2007) with starches occupying most of the carbohydrate mass (Table 1). Among twenty-three

Table 1. Nutrient content of whole and split lentils, g/100 g FM[a]

Nutrient	Unit	Whole Lentils	Split lentils
Water	g	10.4	11.8
Energy	Kcal	353	327
Protein	g	25.8	25
Total lipids (Fat)	g	1.1	2.2
Ash	g	2.7	1.9
Carbohydrates, by difference	g	60.1	59.2
Fibres, total dietary	g	30.5	10.8
Sugars, total	g	2.0	-
Sucrose	g	1.5	-
Glucose (Dextrose)	g	0.0	-
Fructose	g	0.3	-
Lactose	g	0.0	-
Maltose	g	0.3	-
Galactose	g	0.0	-
Calcium, Ca	mg	56	41
Iron, Fe	mg	7.5	7.6
Magnesium, Mg	mg	122	72
Phosphorus, P	mg	451	294
Potassium, K	mg	955	578
Sodium, Na	mg	6	7
Zinc, Zn	mg	4.8	3.9
Copper, Cu	mg	0.5	1.3

continued in following column

Table 1. Continued

Nutrient	Unit	Whole Lentils	Split lentils
Manganese, Mn	mg	1.3	1.4
Selenium, Se	mg	8.3	8.2
Vitamin C, total ascorbic acid	mg	4.4	1.7
Thiamin	mg	0.9	0.5
Riboflavin	mg	0.2	0.1
Niacin	mg	2.6	1.5
Pantothenic acid	mg	2.1	0.3
Pyridoxine (B_6)	mg	0.5	0.4
Folate, total DFE	mg	479	204
Vitamin A, IU	IU	39	58
Vitamin A, RAE	µg	2	3
Carotene, beta	mg	23	35
Vitamin E (α-tocopherol)	mg	0.5	-
Tocopherol, (γ-tocopherol)	mg	4.2	-
Vitamin K (phylloquinone)	mg	5.0	-
Choline, total	mg	96.4	-
Fatty acids, total SFA	g	0.2	0.4
Fatty acids, total MUFA	g	0.2	0.5
Fatty acids, total PUFA	g	0.5	1.1
Cholesterol	mg	0.0	0.0

[a]Source: United States Department of Agriculture (USDA) National Nutrient Database for Standard Reference, Release 23 (2010). (Accessed Dec 2010).

pulse grains, starch yield percent from lentils is the second highest, up to 47.1% (Hoover et al., 2010). In lentils, amylose represents only about 23.5-24.7% of total starch (Hoover & Ratnayake, 2002). This content is lower than in most other pulses but is similar to most grains. Furthermore, lentils are a valuable source of total dietary fibers, with insoluble dietary fiber of approximately 93-99.7% of total dietary fiber (USDA, 2010; Bednar et al., 2001) (Table 1).

Lentils are considered among the best sources of prebiotics (Dwivedi et al., 2014), and contain nutritionally significant amounts of prebiotic carbohydrates, including raffinose-family oligosaccharides (RFO), sugar alcohols, fructooligosaccharides (FOS), and resistant starch (RS) carbohydrates (Johnson et al., 2013). The functional significance of these carbohydrates arises from the fact that oligosaccharides work as selective promoters for the growth of beneficial gut microbes (prebiotics) that aid in improving gut health, restoring microbial balance, and preventing intestinal diseases (Fooks et al., 1999). Johnson et al. (2013) found that total prebiotic carbohydrate concentrations of lentils suggest that a 100 g serving of lentils may provide over 13 g (12.3 g-14.1 g) of prebiotics, thus emphasizing on the role of lentils as a leading source for these prebiotic carbohydrates.

Quantitatively, α-galactosides or raffinose family oligosaccharides account for 53.0% of the total sugars and oligosaccharides content in lentils (Vidal-Valverde et al., 2002). In these oligosaccharides, stachyose represents the major oligosaccharide, followed by ciceritol and raffinose (El-Adawy et al., 2003; Vidal-Valverde et al., 2002). The functional significance of these carbohydrates arises from the fact that oligosaccharides work as selective promoters for the growth of beneficial gut microbes that aid in improving gut health and preventing intestinal diseases (Fooks et al., 1999). Han (2005) found that among different legume pulses, ciceritol was uniquely identified in lentils and chickpeas, whereas verbascose was uniquely identified in lentils and peas.

- **Proteins:** Lentils and pulses are considered to be a good source of proteins that makes them a significant food source for developing countries and low-income people (Hoover et al., 2010; Lombardi-Boccia et al., 2003).

In addition to providing essential and nonessential amino acids and carbon skeletons for the metabolic needs of the human body, lentils are sources of some storage proteins that are usually consumed by the germ during seed germination. The most abundant class of storage proteins in pulses is the water-insoluble fraction, globulins, which forms an average of 47% of the total seed proteins, while the water-soluble protein fraction, predominantly albumins, contributes only 3.8% (Lombardi-Boccia et al., 2003). These storage proteins are described as biologically active proteins. These proteins have been historically referred to as ''anti-nutritional'' compounds such as lectins and protease inhibitors. These anti-nutrients result in reducing the digestibility of lentil proteins to about 79-92% (Grant et al., 2003).

The major amino acids in lentils are Glu, Asp, Arg, Leu, and Lys (Bamdad et al., 2006), with Glu and Asp making about 48% of the total amino acids in three cultivars of *L. culinaris*. Since lentil proteins are rich in lysine and limited in sulfur-containing amino acids, Met and Cys, and Trp, lentil proteins need to be nutritionally complemented with other sulfur amino acid-rich proteins such as those found in grains. Interestingly, such mutual complementation is quite common in Mediterranean and South-Asian cuisines (Faris & Takruri, 2003). On the other hand, the protein fraction of total lentil nitrogen, protein nitrogen (PN), is considerably high (4.49 g N/100g dry matter (DM)) representing about 89% of total nitrogen (5.03 g), while the non-protein nitrogen (NPN) part accounts for the remaining part (0.54 g N/100g DM) (El-Adawy et al., 2003), indicating better nitrogen usability than in high NPN foods.

- **Fats:** Lentils have relatively low fat and therefore low energy content (Table 1) (USDA, 2010). Ryan and colleagues found that lentil seeds contained a total fat of about 1.4 g/100 g, distributed unevenly over the fatty fractions as follows: saturated fatty acids (SFA), 16.7%; monounsaturated fatty acids (MUFA), 23.7% and polyunsaturated fatty acids (PUFA), 58.8% (Ryan et al., 2007).
- **Minerals:** Ash content of lentils is relatively high, with a range value of 3-5 g/100 g on dry matter (DM) basis. Indeed, the mineral content of lentils is comprised of relatively high levels of Mg, P, Ca and S (Demirbas, 2005; Padovani et al., 2007). In addition, lentils have a low Na and relatively high K contents, with a K: Na ratio of about 30:1 to 90:1. This differential Na: K ratio makes lentils quite appealing as a constituent of a healthy diet for patients with hypertension.

Iron (Fe) is also present in significant quantity in lentils (Demirbas, 2005; El-Adawy et al., 2003). However, the bioavailability of the iron in lentils is known to be reduced by iron-chelating phytochemicals, such as tannins, oxalates and phytates (Sandberg, 2002). These natural chelating agents could be minimized by cooking, germination and fermentation of lentils prior to ingestion (Rodríguez et al., 2008; Umeta et al., 2005). Lentils also contain Zn ranging between 3.2 to 6.3 mg/100 g (Demirbas, 2005; Umeta et al., 2005). Several other trace minerals have been reported in lentils including Cu, Mn, Mo, and B (Demirbas, 2005; Rodríguez et al., 2008; Umeta et al., 2005). Overall, lentils are considered a good dietary source of the aforementioned minerals. It is well noticed that lentil content of major and trace minerals is subject to a wide variation due to differences in soil conditions and agricultural practices.

Selenium content of lentils is directly related to the soil content in the land of origin. For example, it has been found that lentils grown in Saskatchewan province/Canada contain 425–673 µg Se/kg depending on location, soil characteristics, and growing conditions (Thavarajah et al., 2008). The latter quantities provide 80–120% of the Se recommended dietary allowance (RDA) in just a 100 g of dry lentils. In fact, the uniqueness of lentils as a rich natural source of Se has drawn significant interest as a target crop for Se biofortification to be used as a food-based solution for populations with Se deficiencies (Thavarajah et al., 2011).

- **Vitamins:** Lentils are a significant dietary source of a plethora of vitamins including folate, thiamin (B_1) and riboflavin (B_2) (USDA, 2010). Other water-soluble vitamins have also been reported in lentils as follows: niacin; pantothenic acid and pyridoxine. In addition, vitamin E (α, β and γ tocopherols) was measured in lentils by Ryan et al. (2007). The α-tocopherol, and β and γ-tocopherols contents were 1.6 and 4.5 mg/100 g, respectively. This, however, is far from the RDA value of α-tocopherol (15 mg/d). Further, phylloquinone, vitamin K, as reported by USDA (2010) averages about 5 µg/100 g. The daily value of vitamin K is about 80 µg (Table 1). The low vitamin K content renders lentils safe in cardiovascular patients on anticoagulant treatment.

Bioactive Functional Components

Considering the vast number of the ethnopharmacological uses of lentils, it is not surprising that bioactive phytochemicals or plant secondary metabolites have been identified and quantified in leguminous seeds. Based on their chemical structures, bioactive components in lentil seeds could be categorized into different functional bioactive compounds (Issa et al., 2006) as represented in Table 2.

1. **Phytosterols:** Phytosterols are nonnutritive compounds or phytochemicals with the same basic functions in plants as cholesterol in animals; that is, they regulate the membrane fluidity of plant cells and other physiologic functions associated with plant biology (Rao et al., 1998). Legumes are one of the major natural sources of phytosterols. Indeed, phytosterols have shown to be abundant in lentil seeds. Researchers (Kalogeropoulos et al., 2010) reported that β-sitosterol represents the predominate phytosterol (about 15.0-24.0 mg/100 g FM) in cooked dry legumes.
2. **Squalene:** Squalene is a non-phenolic hydrocarbon phytochemical compound with chemopreventive potential against colorectal cancer (CRC) (Rao et al., 1998). It is a triterpene that contains six isoprene units and works as a key intermediate in the biosynthetic pathway to steroids in plants and animals. Lentils contain about 0.7 mg/100 g squalene, 0.0007% (Ryan et al., 2007). In other

Table 2. Bioactive functional components in lentils[a]

Category	Individual Compounds
Proteins Trypsin inhibitors Lectins	Bowman-Birk Trypsin Inhibitors (BBI)
Polyphenolics Non-flavonoid Flavonoids	Hydroxybenzoic acid, Hydroxycinnamic acid Flavonols, Flavones, Trans-resveratrol-3- *O*-glucoside, Proanthocyanidins, Flavan-3-ols
Anthocyanins	Catechins, Gallocatechin
Tannins and tannin-related monomers	*p*-Coumaric acid, Ferulic acid, Sinapic acid, Quercetin, Kaempferol, Delphinidin, Cyanidins
Phytate	Phytic acid
Hydrocarbons	Squalene
Carotenoids Saponins	β-carotene

[a]Faris et al., 2013.

reports, squalene was found to be 0.14-0.16 mg/100 g FM, and 0.00015%, in cooked dry legumes. Thus, lentils could be described as a poor source for squalene.

3. **Phytic Acid:** Phytic acid (myo-inositol-1,2,3,4,5,6, hexabisphosphates, IP_6) is aubiquitous plant component that constitutes 1-5% by weight of most cereals, nuts, legumes, oil seeds, spores, needles and pollen (Graf & Eaton, 1990), and is considered as the major source of phosphorous in pulses (Morris & Hill, 1996). It usually occurs as a mixed Ca-Mg-K salt in discrete regions of the seeds. In the past, its primary functions during dormancy were believed to be the storage of cations and phosphorus, a cell wall precursor and as storehouse for potential energy (Graf & Eaton, 1990). However, nowadays phytic acid has been proposed to serve a vital role in protecting the seeds against the deleterious effects of oxygen and iron. Lentils are considered good sources for phytic acid and its related phytates (Ayet et al., 1997).
4. **Saponins:** Saponins are naturally occurring surface-active glycosides. They include a diverse group of compounds characterized by their structure containing a steroid or triterpenoid aglycone and one or more *ose* chains. Several reports have revealed that the hypoglycemic activity of most antidiabetic medicinal plants has been attributed to the presence of saponins (Elekofehinti, 2015). Lentils, like other legumes, are considered among the best sources of saponins. The lentil content of saponins could be as low as 25 mg depending on germination conditions (Güçlü-Üstündağ & Mazza, 2007).
5. **Lectins:** Hemagglutinins, or lectins, are a very important group of biologically active proteins or glycoproteins found in almost all organisms (De Mejía & Prisecaru, 2005). Their ability to agglutinate erythrocytes is a recognized physiological effect that depends on their specificity and high binding affinity for a particular carbohydrate moiety on the cell surface (De Mejía & Prisecaru, 2005). Lectins are found naturally in lentils. From lentil seed storage proteins, two lectin-binding fractions were isolated (Freier & Rüdiger, 1990). These lectin-binding proteins were found to be strong stimulators of murine B lymphocyte proliferation.
6. **Defensins:** Defensins form a class of host defense peptides in plants and animals, and participate in development of the innate immune response. Plant defensins are small basic, cysteine-rich peptides.

Recently, defensin has been characterized in germinated lentil seeds (Finkina et al., 2008), and was termed Lc-def. The Lc-def consists of 47 amino acid residues and has eight cysteines forming four disulfide bonds.

7. **Protease Inhibitors:** Protease inhibitors have been widely investigated in legumes. Trypsin inhibitors have been identified in lentil seeds with a range of 3–8 trypsin inhibitor unit (TIU)/mg in four different cultivars (Guillamon et al., 2008). From a historic point of view, the proteinase or protease inhibitors are considered as anti-nutritional components of legume seeds, due to their property of decreasing the digestibility of dietary proteins.

In legume seeds, Bowman-Birk type trypsin-chymotrypsin inhibitor (BBI) is present at higher concentrations compared to other plant families and tissues (Cheung & Ng, 2007). Unlike other legumes, however, kinetic studies have shown that the isolated BBI from *L. culinaris* seeds, *L. culinaris* trypsin inhibitor (LCTI) is characterized by unusual strong binding affinity to its target (Scarafoniet al., 2007). In addition; LCTI has been shown to be resistant to thermal denaturation over a wide range of temperature and pH values. The latter could be due to a generally conserved tertiary structure and hydrogen bond network. Such a unique stability explains the potential beneficial effects of BBIs even after the lentils are cooked (Lajolo & Genovese, 2002). Due to their proteolytic effect against reverse transcriptase enzyme involved in viral replication, trypsin inhibitors have been suggested in different medical applications, including inhibition of cancer and utilization in acquired immunodeficiency syndrome (AIDS) (de Almeida Costa et al., 2006).

8. **Dietary Fibers:** Lentils could be considered as a valuable source of dietary fibers (Table 1), most of which (93-99.7%) is insoluble and less than 7% soluble (USDA, 2010; Bednar et al., 2001; de Almeida Costa et al., 2006). The β-glucan component of soluble fibers in lentils is relatively low as compared to its good sources such as oats. However, it is relatively higher than that of peas, winter wheat and flaxseeds (Demirbas, 2005). This functional ingredient had been found to have a hypocholesterolemic effect, an ability to increase HDL-cholesterol and decrease LDL-cholesterol in addition to potential cancer preventive, antitumor, antibacterial and glucose control effects (Demirbas, 2005). Further, by virtue of their fiber content, green lentils supplemented to healthy subjects consuming typical Western diet had been found to increase their fecal weights significantly, thus aiding in protecting their gut from constipation and its harmful complications (Stephen et al., 1995).
9. **Resistant Starches:** Based on starch digestibility, starch had been classified into three groups, namely readily digestible starch (RDS), partially resistant or slowly digestible starch (SDS), and resistant starch (RS). According to this classification, starches that resist the hydrolytic effect of digestive enzymes are collectively called resistant starches. Thus, RS are defined as "the sum of starch and starch-degradation products that, on average, reach the human large intestine" (Perera et al., 2010), and being recognized as a significant contributor to gastrointestinal health.

Lentils contain about 25.4 g RS/100 g total starch on FM, representing about 47.7% of total starch content (García-Alonso et al., 1998), with an average value of 43.7–65.2% (Hoover et al., 2010). Other fractions of starch, RDS and SDS, were found to be 5.2–14.8 and 29.7–41.5% of total starch, respectively (Hoover et al., 2010). It has been reported that although lentils contain good quantities of fermentable soluble dietary fibers and RS, they exhibited the lowest bifidogenic effect when compared with that of other legumes such as peas and chickpeas after being cooked by similar procedures (Queiroz-Monici et al., 2005). Queiroz-Monici et al. (2005) reviewed the bifidogenic effect of dietary fibers and RS, assessed on the intestinal microbiota of rats fed diets based on different pulses including lentils. Later, other researchers (Hernández-Salazar et al., 2010) evaluated the antioxidant capacity and the *in vitro* fermentation by human fecal microflora of the indigestible fraction of cooked lentils and other pulses. They found that the insoluble indigestible fraction (IIF) was higher than the soluble counterpart, soluble indigestible fraction (SIF) in lentils and other pulses. The indigestible fraction (IF) of lentils and other pulses are fermented by colonic bacteria as shown by *in vitro* fermentation studies (Granito et al., 2001). IF from black bean and lentil were the best substrates for the fermentative production of short chain fatty acids (SCFA), especially butyric acid (Hernández-Salazar et al., 2010). Butyrate had been shown to play a regulatory role on the transepithelial fluid transport, reinforces the epithelial defense barrier, modulates visceral sensitivity and intestinal motility and ameliorates mucosal inflammation and oxidative status. Further, several studies have stressed the role of butyrate in the inhibition and prevention of colorectal cancer (CRC). Extraintestinally, butyrate exerts potentially useful effects on hemoglobinopathies, genetic metabolic diseases, hypercholesterolemia, insulin resistance, and ischemic stroke. The mechanisms of action of butyrate vary, mostly related to its potent regulatory effects on gene expression (Canani et al., 2011).

10. **Polyphenolics:** Lentils have the highest total phenolic content (TPC) in comparison to six other common legumes (Han, 2005; Xu & Chang, 2007). Their TPC based on DM was 759 mg gallic acid equivalents (GAE)/100 g, total flavonoid content of 221 mg catechin equivalents/100 g, and the condensed tannin content of 870 mg catechins equivalents/100 g. Tannins and tannin-related compounds play an important role in protecting seeds against oxidative damage induced by multiple environment factors (Salariya, 2005). These compounds are mainly concentrated in the testa, with lentils being among the richest leguminous seeds in their condensed tannin content, up to 915 mg/100 g (Salariya, 2005). Furthermore, lentils contain different tannin-related phenolic compounds (Troszyńska et al., 2006). It was evident that lentils had the greatest level of condensed tannins linked to the indigestible fraction of the seed, with about 23% of condensed tannins found in this fraction (Hernández-Salazar et al., 2010). Total phenolic content and antioxidant activity in lentils exhibit higher or compatible value with those of fruits or vegetables. In addition, total phenolic content of lentils exhibited significant correlation with total antioxidant activity, implying that phenolic compounds are major antioxidant compounds in lentils (Han, 2005). Recently, lentils scored the highest values among fourteen different types and varieties of legumes for simple polyphenols and the total phenolic contents, with total phenolic content of about 26 mg GAE /100 g FM (Kalogeropoulos et al., 2010).

The distribution of phenolic compounds differs in the cotyledon and the lentil seed coat, with non-flavonoid phenolic compounds, such as free and combined hydroxybenzoic and hydroxycinnamic acids, located mainly in the cotyledon of lentils (Dueñas et al., 2003). On the other hand, flavonoids, such as glycosides of flavonols and flavones, are mainly present in the seed coat of lentils. The coat also contains trans-resveratrol-3-*O*-glucoside, and large amounts of proanthocyanidins, with the major groups of phenolic compounds that are present in the seed coat, but absent in the cotyledon (Dueñas et al., 2002; Dueñas et al., 2003).

Interestingly, seed coat represents only a small percentage of the entire lentil seed weight, ranging from 8% to 11% (Bhattacharya et al., 2005; Duenas et al., 2006) but provides significant contribution to the overall benefits of lentils. It has been found that the darkness of the coat of colored legumes such as lentils is accompanied with their phenolic contents. Xu and coworkers (2007) found that dark colored legumes such as lentils possess higher phenolic content and antioxidant activities than the pale colored ones. Dark colored legumes, such as green or red whole lentils, had a significantly higher phenolic content and antioxidant capacity than that of the pale colored, green, yellow or white, legumes (Xu et al., 2007; Xu & Chang, 2010). Unfortunately, several Asian lentil dishes involve dehulled seeds to improve the texture, thereby reducing the beneficial properties of lentils.

Flavonoids and tannins have been widely investigated for their antioxidant potentials and possible clinical applications in the management and prophylaxis of cardiovascular diseases, diabetes, osteoporosis and neurodegenerative diseases (Scalbert et al., 2005). Flavonoids have also been reported to induce xenobiotic-metabolizing and detoxifying enzymes such as glutathione-S-transferases (GST) (Moon et al., 2006), making the flavonoids appealing candidates for combating carcinogenesis. The cost-effectiveness of lentils and the ease at which flavonoids could be extracted give lentils an advantage over other natural sources of flavonoids.

11. **Minor Antioxidants:** In addition to the total polyphenols, other low molecular weight constituents present in lentils may contribute to their total antioxidant capacity (Fernandez-Orozco et al., 2003). They include tocopherols: α-T (0.56), β-T (0.29), γ-T (9.7), δ-T (0.25 mg/100 g DM), reduced glutathione (0.11 g/100 g DM), and soluble proteins (about 13.9 g/100g DM). It is worth mentioning, however, that the contribution of non-polyphenolic low molecular weight constituents to the total antioxidant capacity of lentils is considered low when compared to that of polyphenolics (Fernandez-Orozco et al., 2003).
12. **Phytoestrogens:** On the other hand, lentils are classified among the poor sources of phytoestrogens, with different isoflavones and lignans as follows: formononetin, daidzein, genistein, glycitein, matairesinol, lariciresinol, pinoresinol, secoisolariciresinol, forcoumestrol, with mean values of total isoflavones (9.5), total lignans (26.6), and total phytoestrogens (36.5 µg/100 g fresh matter (FM) (Thompson et al., 2006). Mazur et al. (1998) found that formononetin, biochanin A, daidzein, genistein, coumestrol, and secoisolariciresinol phytoestrogens contents for whole and split lentils were relatively of low levels in comparison with phytoestrogen-rich sources (Mazur et al., 1998).

Antioxidant Potential of Lentils

Lentils have shown the highest total antioxidant capacity (TAC) among tested pulses (peas, beans, chickpeas and soybeans) measured by ferric reducing antioxidant power (FRAP) and total radical-trapping antioxidant parameter (TRAP) measures, second only to broad beans by Trolox equivalent antioxidant capacity (TEAC) measure (Pellegrini et al., 2006). These findings were also confirmed by Duenas et al. (2006) who found that lentils had a greater antioxidant activity than peas (Duenas et al., 2006).

In another study, Xu and Chang (2008) found that lentils had the highest antioxidant capacity when measured as 2,2-diphenyl-1-picrylhydrazyl (DPPH) free radical scavenging capacity in comparison with green pea, yellow pea and chickpea. The same study also revealed that the oxygen radical absorbing capacity (ORAC) of lentils was significantly higher than that of green pea, yellow pea and chickpea. Lentils had a higher ORAC value than most of the common fruits and vegetables including apples, plums, blackberries, cherries, figs, peaches, pears, oranges, garlic, cabbage and almonds (USDA, 2010). Recently, lentils demonstrated the highest antioxidant activity among the most commonly used pulses such as pea, lentils, and chickpea ecotypes in the Southern of Italy (Fratianni et al., 2014).

Health Improving Effects of Lentils

Cardiovascular Health

Table 3 summarizes the health improving effects of lentils on cardiovascular and other body systems and functions. Legume seeds constitute an important group of protein sources not only in non-ruminant but also in ruminant diets, the bulk of this protein (about 80%) being in the form of storage proteins, mainly conglycinins and glycinins (Rubio, 2000). These storage proteins in beans, peas, and lentils were found by Kingman et al. (1993) to exert a hypocholesterolemic effect in pigs. They concluded that the mechanism for the hypocholesterolemic effect of legume feeding did not involve increased cholesterol clearance via the intestinal route, but rather the effects on plasma amino acids.

Legume consumption had been inversely associated with the incidence of CVD (Flight & Clifton, 2006). Lentils possess angiotensin I-converting enzyme (ACE) inhibitor activity, thereby concluding that red lentil protein hydrolysates could contribute to its blood pressure-lowering effects (Boye et al., 2010). Later, the ACE inhibitory effect in different hydrolysates obtained from protein concentrates of two lentil varieties by using *in vitro* gastrointestinal simulation was confirmed (Barbana & Boye, 2011). This blood-pressure lowering effect was revealed *in vivo* by lentils, which, when compared with dried beans, peas, and chickpeas, solely decreased blood pressure in spontaneously hypertensive rats (SHR), thus supporting the evidence on the important role of lentils in attenuating risk of CVD (Hanson et al., 2014). Recently, specific fragments were identified from legumin, vicilin and convicilin with amino acid sequences contributing to the antioxidant and ACE-inhibitory activity of lentil hydrolysates (Garcia-Mora et al., 2014). Among four types of pulses at 30% w/w concentration in the experimental diet given

Table 3. Health improving effects of lentil components[a]

Health Effect	Responsible Component(s)
Antioxidant	Vitamin E, Vitamin C, Polyphenolics
Anticancer	Flavonoids, BBI, Phytic acid, Phytosterols, Squalene, Defensin, Lectins, RS, Saponins
Antibiotic	Defensin
Anti-inflammatory	Phytosterols, BBI
Hypolipidaemic	Phytosterols, Squalene
Reduction of glycemic load	RS when replacing digestible starch
Blood pressure-lowering effect	K, proteins
Anti atherogenic	Squalene
Laxative	Insoluble dietary fibres, RS
Bifidogenic	Raffinose family oligosaccharides, RS

[a]Faris et al., 2013.

for four weeks to SHR, and using pulse wave velocity (PWV) and blood pressure (BP) measurements, only lentils significantly reduced the rise in BP and large-artery remodeling. Further, lentils were able to decrease the media:lumen ratio and media width of the aorta in the SHR, and led to decrease the levels of total cholesterol (TC) and LDL-cholesterol. These promising findings reinforce the significance of lentils as part of the therapeutic lifestyle changes (TLC) and dietary approaches to stop hypertension (DASH) diet prescribed for hypertensive patients (Hanson et al., 2014).

Accumulating evidence supports the cardioprotective, hypolipidemic, and hypohomocysteinemic effects of pulses, including lentils. Hyperhomocysteinemia has been linked to an increased risk of CVD (Ueland et al., 2000). The Framingham Heart study found that lentils contributed 1.7% of total folate intake; regardless the source of folate, whether food or supplement, serum folate concentrations significantly increased whereas serum homocysteine concentrations significantly decreased in a dose-dependent manner (Tucker et al., 1996). In a recent study conducted on 22 adult males with hypercholesterolemia or coronary artery disease, it was found that daily consumption of folate-rich foods, including 50 g beans of lentils, chickpea, kidney beans or peas, at a combined amount of 500 μg daily for five weeks, significantly decreased plasma total homocysteine (tHyc) to 8% reduction when compared to consumption of similar quantity of supplementary folic acid (Pintó et al., 2005). In Egypt, lentils were found among the leading source of dietary intake of folate, with an average value of 75 μg/100 g (Hefni et al., 2010).

In vivo, lentils were examined for their glycemic and lipidemic effects using the streptozotocin-induced diabetes rat model (Al-Tibi et al., 2010). In this study, the administration of lentils significantly increased HDL cholesterol in diabetic rats. However, the changes had no significant influence on other lipid profile including triacylglycerol (TAG), TC and LDL cholesterol. This discrepancy in the lipidemic effect of lentils may be due to the increase in adipose tissue lipolysis in absence of insulin, and to a decrease in lipoprotein lipase activity (Eidi & Eidi, 2009). The underlying mechanism of the hypocholesterolemic effect of lentils has not yet been studied. However, it has shown that the hypocholesterolemic effect of raw pea was probably due to increased fecal bile acid output and an increased bile acid formation (Martins et al., 2004), a topic that needs to be further investigated. Studies conducted by Jenkins et al. (1983) showed that daily consumption of 140 g of dried lentils and other pulses cooked or canned for 4 months by a group of seven-free living hyperlipidemic males significantly reduced serum TAG by 7% and total cholesterol by 25%, but did not significantly affect LDL- or HDL-cholesterol. Other researchers (Dabai et al., 1996) investigated the effects of different legume species on blood lipids and fecal steroids in Sprague-Dawley rats for 8-weeks. They found that lentils were second to bambara groundnuts in their hypocholesterolemic effect. In addition, their study revealed that plasma TAG concentrations were significantly reduced on lentils and other legume diets, as compared to a control Western-type human diet; similarly, plasma LDL-cholesterol concentration was significantly reduced on lentils and other legume diets, except bambara groundnuts, as compared to the control diet (Dabai et al., 1996). However, Shams et al. (Shams et al., 2010) found that the addition of 50 g cooked lentils to the diet of diabetic patients led to a significant decrease in TC but not in LDL, HDL and TAG.

The latter findings were previously confirmed by a controlled interventional study conducted by Duane (1997). In their cross-over study on 9 male subjects housed in a metabolic ward for 6-7 weeks, consumption of 120 g baked mixed pulses, 60% red, navy, and lima beans, 27% peas and 13% lentils, significantly reduced serum LDL-cholesterol by 8%, from 138 mg/dL at baseline to 126 mg/dL at the end of treatment, as compared to the isoenergetic control diet. However, no other significant change was detected in serum TC, HDL-cholesterol, or VLDL-cholesterol.

In a meta-analysis of randomized controlled trials on the blood cholesterol-lowering effect of non-soy legume consumption conducted by Bazzano and coworkers (Bazzano et al., 2011), it was found that the 10 clinical trials that included 268 participants given diets rich in non-soy pulses, beans, peas, lentils or chickpeas for a minimum duration of 3 weeks, resulted in a significant reduction in total and LDL-cholesterol levels. They recommended that dietary modification strategies that target the reduction of risk factors for CVD should include an increase in legume consumption in addition to other strategies, which have been of proven benefit.

Diabetes

It has been strongly suggested that eating pulses is beneficial in the prevention and management of diabetes. Therefore, consumption of a wide range of carbohydrate foods from cereals, vegetables, pulses, and fruits both for the general population and for people with diabetes, especially those with type II diabetes (Venn & Mann, 2004) is generally recommended. Pulses have shown an ability to improve blood glucose, lipid and lipoprotein metabolism in diabetic and healthy people. The acute metabolic advantage for pulses in glucose handling may partly be due to the intact structure of the pulse grain (Venn & Mann, 2004). Table 4 reviews the clinical trials conducted on the effect of lentils on serum glucose and lipid profile.

In addition to bowel movement improvement due to the high fiber content, lentil-derived leguminous fibers have been found to prevent the impairment of the metabolic control in diabetic rats when total carbohydrates intake was increased, suggesting that lentil carbohydrates, including dietary fibers, could have promising implications for diabetic patients (Wolever et al., 1994).

The hypoglycemic effect, or more accurately the ability to alleviate the glycemic load, of lentil has been demonstrated in experimentally induced diabetic rats, healthy volunteers, and insulin-dependent and non-insulin dependent diabetic patients (Al-Tibi et al., 2010; Shams, et al., 2010; Wolever et al., 1994). Shams et al. (2010) found that addition of 50 g cooked lentils to diabetic patient diet led to a significant decrease in fasting blood glucose. Results of this study were partly confirmed, where lentils were examined for their glycemic effects *in vivo* using the streptozotocin-induced diabetes rat model; wherein, the administration of lentils significantly decreased serum blood glucose (Al-Tibi et al., 2010).

Lentils have shown low glycemic index (GI) in healthy volunteers, with an average value of approximately 29 (Jenkins et al., 1981). Indeed, the values vary from 18 to 52, with an average value of 26 for red lentils (mean of 4 studies), 30 for green lentils (mean of 3 studies), 29 for NS type lentils (mean of 2 studies) and 52 (1 study) for green lentils canned in brine (Foster-Powell et al., 2002).

Increasing the proportion of low GI carbohydrates in the diet has been associated with a range of health benefits, including protection against diabetes type 2, CHD and obesity (Flight & Clifton, 2006; Hodge, English et al., 2004; Liu, 2007). There is a noticeable variation in the reported values of GI for lentils between *in vitro* and *in vivo*(Araya et al., 2002; Chung et al., 2008; Foster-Powell et al., 2002; Germaine et al., 2008; Hodge et al., 2004) that may reflect the effects of many factors such as botanical variation and agricultural conditions of growing lentils, the form of lentils and preparation methods, along with the variation in the *in vitro* assays. Despite this variation between *in vivo* and *in vitro* GI, lentils still had the lowest and the slowest rate of hydrolysis of starches, and the lowest estimated glycemic index (eGI) among tested pulse grains, chickpeas and peas (Chung et al., 2008).

Table 4. Summary of clinical trials on the effect of lentils on blood glucose, lipids, and homocysteine levels

Study	No. and Type of Subjects	Type of Design	Treatment	Tested Variable	Results
Pinto,et al. (2005)	20 male patients with hyperhomocysteinemia and coronary artery disease	Randomized, crossover intervention Trial	500 µg folate from dietary sources, including lentils and other pulses and foods	Plasma total hyperhomocysteinemia	Significantly reduced plasma tHcy concentrations (-8.6%)
Jenkins, et al. (1983)	7 male hyperlipidemic patients	Randomized controlled trials	140 g of dried lentils and other pulses cooked or canned for 4-month period.	Lipid profile	Significantly reduced serum TAG (- 7%) and TC (- 25%)
Duane, et al. (1997)	9 subjects on a metabolic ward during two randomly ordered 6-7 week periods	Cross-over	120 g baked mixed pulses, 60% red, navy, and lima beans, 27% peas and 13% lentils,	Lipid profile	Significantly reduced serum LDL-cholesterol (-8%)
Shams, et al. (2010)	30 patients with type II diabetes mellitus	Randomized cross-over clinical trial	Normal diet with 50 gm cooked lentil and 6 gm canola oil substitute of 30gm bread and 20gm cheese	Serum lipids and glucose levels	Significant reduction of FBS and TC (-3.5%), and improvement of glycemic control (-1.6% blood glucose)
Jenkins et al. (2012)	121 (with DM2)	Parallel RCT	Low-GI legume diet. Control: high wheat-fibre diet, Target: 1 cup/day of cooked beans, chickpeas or lentils (adherence assessed by 7-d FR)		Low-GI legume diet 2 HbA1c (−0.5%), body weight (−2.7 kg), waist circumference (−1.4 cm), and total cholesterol (−8 mg/dL) Blood pressure and heart rate reduced on low-GI legume diet in comparison with control
Meta-Analysis of Clinical Studies					
Bazzano, et al. (2011)	268 in 10 trials	Randomized controlled trials	120-130 g lentil/day for 30-56 days, macronutrient and total energy contents of intervention and control diets are the same	Lipid profile	Significantly reduced serum TC (-11.8 mg/dl) and LDL (-8 mg/dl) for non-soy legumes including lentils

Overweight and Obesity

Obesity control is an important intervention in an effort to reduce the incidence of chronic diseases, including diabetes. Epidemiological and interventional studies have shown that the consumption of phenolic-rich foods is inversely associated with the prevalence of obesity and several chronic diseases (Kris-Etherton et al., 2002).Pulses contain components that have been shown to benefit weight control. Among the pulses that had shown "anti-obesity" effect are lentils. In human subjects, consumption of lentils with pasta and sauce were found to lower food intake when compared with consuming pasta and sauce only or consuming chickpeas with pasta and sauce (Mollard et al., 2012). Further, the high fiber content and low glycemic response of lentils have been looked at as a means for increasing satiety, reducing the food intake, and thus controlling body weight (Mollard et al., 2012). Among four different pulses, lentils exhibited the strongest satiating properties, resulting in lower food intake as compared to other dietary meals. Lentils led to 8% lower cumulative energy intake as compared to a reference mea (Mollard et al., 2012). This evidence improves the observational studies that consistently show an inverse relationship between pulse consumption and BMI or risk for obesity (McCrory et al., 2010).

Arginine has been shown to possess thermogenic properties, thus enhances carbohydrate and fat oxidation via increased mitochondrial biogenesis and modulation of genes that regulate energy expenditure (Trock et al., 1990). Analysis of lentils has demonstrated that arginine is a major amino acid constituent of lentil protein at 11.0–11.3 g/16 g N (Bhatty & Christison, 1984). In addition to arginine, lentils contain significant amounts of glutamine at approximately 15.0 g/16 g N (Bhatty & Christison, 1984), which has been shown to increase postprandial energy expenditure by 49% in human subjects (Marinangeli & Jones, 2012). Other integral factors in lentils that make it useful in preventing obesity and related co-morbidities include the inhibitory effect of lentils against α-glucosidase and lipase enzymes. The inhibition of α-glucosidase reduces intestinal glucose digestion and absorption, consequently controlling the post-prandial glycemic response, which is crucial in the management of type 2 diabetes (Balasubramaniam et al., 2013). The inhibition of lipase is considered to be one of the more effective strategies for managing obesity (Xu et al., 2005). Recently, Zhang et al. (2015) found that flavonols, not the flavanols, in lentils showed the inhibitory activities against α-glucosidase and pancreatic lipase, thus suggesting a potential role of lentil consumption in managing weight and control of blood glucose.

Cancers

Pulses, including lentils, are consumed traditionally in populations where cancers of the colon, breast, and prostate are low (Correa, 1981). In a prospective study on 90,630 women, and among a vast number of flavonoid-rich foods, lentils or beans were the only foods that exhibited an inverse association with the risk of breast cancer (Adebamowo et al., 2005). Consumption of foods with high glycemic index (GI) and high glycemic load (GL) is associated with hyperglycemia and hyperinsulinemia. These foods have also been suggested to cause metabolic disturbances correlated with increased incidence of colorectal cancer (CRC) (Bruce et al., 2000). Hence, the lower incidence of CRC in developing as compared to developed countries could be partially attributed to the consumption of larger quantities of low GI foods, such as pulses.

Lentils have shown significantly the highest polyphenolic content expressed in terms of total phenolic content. Possible mechanisms for chemopreventive activity of phenolic acids include inhibition of carcinogen uptake, inhibition of formation or activation of the carcinogen, deactivation or detoxification of the carcinogen, preventing the carcinogen binding to DNA, and enhancing the level or fidelity of DNA repair. In addition, antioxidant properties include scavenging reactive electrophils and oxygen radicals and inhibiting arachidonic acid metabolism into Prostaglandin-E_2 (PGE_2) by cyclooxygenases 1 & 2 (COX-1 & COX-2) (Nichenametla et al., 2006).

Plant lectins are unique group of proteins and glycoproteins with potent biological activity. Lentils are natural sources of lectins. Several lectins have been found to possess anticancer properties *in vitro*, *in vivo*, and in human case studies (De Mejía & Prisecaru, 2005); they are used as therapeutic agents, preferentially binding to cancer cell membranes or their receptors, causing cytotoxicity, apoptosis, and inhibition of tumor growth. They also affect the immune system by altering the production of various interleukins, or by activating certain protein kinases. Lectins can bind to ribosomes and inhibit protein synthesis, modify the cell cycle by inducing non-apoptotic G1-phase accumulation mechanisms, G2/M phase cell cycle arrest and apoptosis, can activate the caspases cascade, and can also down regulate telomerase activity and inhibit angiogenesis (De Mejía & Prisecaru, 2005). Mechanisms by which lectins exert their tumor suppressor effects were also summarized by Scarafoni et al. (2007). Hence, lectins seem to be promising therapeutic agents against tumorigenesis especially since these compounds have the advantage of being internalized into cells, causing cancer cell agglutination and/or aggregation.

In addition, other investigators (Sames et al., 2001; Wang et al., 2000) confirmed the inhibitory effect of *L. culinaris* Agglutinin (LCA) against hepatoma and skin melanoma cell lines. Interestingly, LCA-reactive fraction of serum α-fetoprotein (AFP-L_3) has been widely investigated as a valuable marker for evaluation of curability of surgical treatment and for improving the accuracy of prognosis. In addition, it has been suggested that lectins could be used as a noninvasive screening tool for colorectal neoplasms and for the early diagnosis of the cancer, as they exhibited ability for binding to human colonocytes, and thus predict the presence of malignant and premalignant lesions in the colon (Desilets et al., 1999). On the other hand, lectins derived from lentils have been shown to be non-toxic, which allows for safe utilization in medical diagnostic kits (Mitchell et al., 1998).

A novel peptide called "defensin" has been characterized recently in germinated lentil seeds (Finkina et al., 2008). Plant defensins are characterized by a broad spectrum of biological activities including antimicorbial activities against bacteria and fungi. The purified lentil defensin possesses an antifungal activity inhibiting the *Aspergillus niger* growth. Further, several reports demonstrated the ability of defensins to modify the activities of digestive enzymes, trypsin and α-amylases, and HIV-1 reverse transcriptase enzyme implicated in viral replication. Some defensins have also been shown to block ion channels and inhibit protein translation. Hence, they have been suggested to aid in halting tumorigenesis. Indeed, defensin exhibited an antiproliferative activity against more than one tumor cell line (Finkina et al., 2008).

Among the bioactive peptides that characterize pulses are the "BBI", for which beneficial biochemical and functional properties have been proved, such as the efficacy of BBI against tumor cells *in vitro* (Losso, 2008; Scarafoni et al., 2007). BBI are present at higher concentrations in pulses as compared to other plant families and tissues. Proteases are considered key factors in cancer progression and metastasis; therefore, suppressing their activities by protease inhibitors appears to be contributing to inhibiting carcinogenesis (Losso, 2008). Indeed, BBIs have shown to possess cancer preventive and suppressing agents in various *in vitro* and *in vivo* model systems (Kennedy, 1998). A compelling body of therapeutic evidence suggests potential clinical applications for BBI in radioprotection, skeletal muscle atrophy, obesity, autoimmune diseases, multiple sclerosis, and inflammation (Armstrong et al., 2000; Kennedy,

1998). In some cases, as in the treatment of oral leukoplakia lesions, the use of BBIs has reached phase II of clinical trials (Armstrong et al., 2000). Unlike other pulses, kinetic studies have shown that the isolated BBI from *L. culinaris* seeds, *L. culinaris* trypsin inhibitor (LCTI), is characterized by unusual strong binding affinity to its target as compared to other natural BBI (Scarafoni et al., 2007). In addition, LCTI has shown to be resistant to thermal denaturation over a wide range of pH, probably due to its generally conserved tertiary structure and hydrogen bond network. Such a unique character explains the potential beneficial effects of BBIs even after cooking the lentils (Lajolo & Genovese, 2002). Mature lentil BBI inhibits cell proliferation of colon cancer cells in a dose dependent manner due to their intrinsic abilities to inhibit serine proteases (Armstrong et al., 2000).

Lentils contain considerably high amount of the folic acid, which is expected to be involved in the cancer preventive effect of lentils. Folate is essential for the *de novo* biosynthesis of purines and thymidylate, which affects DNA replication and cell division, and synthesis of S-adenosyl methionine (SAM) (Milner et al., 2001). Folic acid and SAM work as methylating agents that have the potential to prevent hypomethylation of DNA, which is observed in colorectal neoplasia in humans and may contribute to the loss of normal controls on proto-oncogene expression (Greenwald et al., 2001). Hence, folic acid is considered to be among the potent agents that suppress gene expression by DNA methylation (Chen & Kong, 2005). In humans, higher folate intake has been inversely associated with the risk of colon cancer (Chen & Kong, 2005). Folic acid is considered among the most potent and effective colon cancer chemopreventive agents in experimental rodents, with potency number of seven, in comparison with the most potent chemopreventive factor examined in this context, non-steroidal anti-inflammatory drug (NSAID) Celecoxib, with a potency factor of fourteen (Chen & Kong, 2005; Corpet & Taché, 2002).

Phytic acid (IP_6) is the major source of phosphorous in pulses (Morris & Hill, 1996). Dietary phytates have shown to be effective in halting colorectal carcinogenesis (Marks et al., 2006). Several molecular mechanisms have been suggested for the antineoplastic activities of IP_6. The modification of signal transduction pathways resulting in cell cycle arrest, thus reducing cell proliferation has been demonstrated as one mechanism. It has also been implicated in induction of apoptosis, inhibition of angiogenesis and tumor metastasis, induction of differentiation of malignant cells, and enhancement of immunity. Further, several studies have indicated anti-inflammatory and antioxidant properties, reduction of the expression of phase I xenobiotic metabolizing enzymes over expression of phase II detoxifying enzymes and tumor suppressor genes and suppression of protooncogens (Fox & Eberl, 2002; Verghese et al., 2006; Vucenik & Shamsuddin, 2006). Preliminary studies in human cancer patients have shown that IP_6 and inositol, an adjuvant to chemotherapy, appeared to enhance the anticancer effect of the conventional chemotherapy, control cancer metastases, and improve quality of life by reducing the side effects of common chemotherapy (Vucenik & Shamsuddin, 2006). Similar anti-inflammatory and anticarcinogenic effects induced by resistant-starch (RS)-rich pulses such as lentils could work as additional factors in preventing cancer, especially CRC (Perera et al., 2010).

In recent years, food and non-food sources of saponins have come into renewed focus due to increasing evidence of their positive health implications such as hypocholesterolemic and anticancer properties (Güçlü-Üstündağ & Mazza, 2007). Anticancer activity of saponins has been reported for many triterpenes and steroid saponins including, but not limited to, soya saponins present in pulses, including lentils (Güçlü-Üstündağ & Mazza, 2007). Different forms of saponins isolated from different plant sources have been identified as potential anticancer agents by the National Cancer Institute's anticancer drug screen program.

Soya saponins have been suggested to be potent chemopreventive agents against CRC, an effect that had been evidenced through several epidemiological, *in vivo* and *in vitro* laboratory studies that were critically reviewed by Gurfinkel and Rao (Gurfinkel & Rao, 2003).

Natural chemopreventive nutrients and phytochemicals act at multiple levels of prevention, and exert synergistic and additive effects when combined together by modulating one or several cell signaling pathways involved in the process of carcinogenesis (Issa, et al., 2006). In contrast to pharmacological chemopreventive agents, the dietary natural non-toxic constituents can reach the colon directly, where they will be able to exert their antitumor effects on their targets (Gossé, et al., 2005). Examples of promising and studied diet-derived chemopreventive agents include plant antioxidant nutrients and phytochemicals such as polyphenolic phytochemicals (Nichenametla, et al., 2006).

The presence of a wide spectrum of bioactive phytochemicals and peptides in lentils make it a functional food with chemopreventive effect against CRC. The chemopreventive potential of lentils against colorectal carcinogenesis was investigated (Faris et al., 2009; Shomaf et al., 2011) using azoxymethane (AOM) to chemically induce colon cancer in Fischer 344 rats that were fed different lentil diets- raw whole green, cooked whole green, raw split red and cooked split red, before and after the carcinogen injection, in order to mimic the initiation/promotion and progression model of human sporadic CRC. The lentils significantly reduced the number of dysplastic lesions and neoplasms in the colons of rats when compared with control (Shomaf et al., 2011).

In the other part (Faris et al., 2009), the preneoplastic lesions called aberrant crypt foci (ACF) were used as surrogate endpoints for chemoprevention trials; pre-cancerous lesions count, crypt size and multiplicity were significantly reduced in rat groups fed different lentils in comparison with the control group; cooked whole lentils being the most effective. For lentil diets, cooked whole lentils had a striking 77.8% reduction in large ACF, whereas the reduction was only 26.8% in rats fed with raw whole lentils. As large ACF have shown to predict more accurately preneoplastic potential, this suggested that the lentils, particularly cooked whole lentils, may act by retarding progression of the early aberrant crypts. This preferred effect is elucidated by the substantial reduction in the multicrypt foci, >4AC, by different treatments, and the ability of these dietary factors to considerably reduce the number of aberrant crypts derived from these large foci. Cooked whole lentils resulted in the highest reduction of the AC from large or multicrypt foci, with a percent reduction of about 65%. These findings of Faris et al. (Faris et al., 2009) were confirmed later by Busambwa and colleagues (Busambwa et al., 2014), who found that sprouted and non-sprouted lentils reduced AOM-induced ACF in Fischer 344 male rats, with a concomitant significant increase in glutathione, glutathione-S-transferases (GST) and catalase activities. Further, lentils exhibited greater chemopreventive effect in comparison with other grain legumes such as green and yellow peas (Busambwa et al., 2014).

It is noteworthy to indicate that the ability to reduce total ACF number reflects the ability of tested materials to prevent carcinogenesis initiation or working as blocking agents. According to Chen and Kong (2005), the blocking agents that inhibit colon carcinogenesis could exert their preventive effect by several mechanisms, including: enhancement of detoxification of carcinogens, inhibition of cytochrome P450 (CYP450) mediated activation of carcinogens, scavenging free radicals and halting antioxidant activity, and finally trapping the carcinogen and preventing their interaction with DNA.

For the large ACF, the reduced number of multicrypt foci is pivotal biomarker that reflects the ability of tested materials to prevent cancer promotion, or to work as suppressing agents. The reduction in the high multiplicity ACF has been associated with lowered levels of inducible nitric oxide synthase (iNOS) and COX-2 enzymes (Kwon & Magnuson, 2007; Kwon et al., 2004), and associated in other studies with suppression of proliferation, production of PGE_2, and Cyclin D1 protein expression, and upregulation of apoptosis (Sengupta et al., 2004; Tanaka et al., 2000; Tanaka et al., 2000). Other biomarkers such as urinary levels of oxidative DNA damage and expression of COX genes, COX-2 mRNA, in colonic mucosa have also been used in chemoprevention studies (Lala et al., 2006). So, further research is required to elaborate the molecular, genetic, and epigenetic mechanisms underlying the chemopreventive effect of lentils against CRC.

Faris et al. (2009) reported that the chemopreventive ability of lentils in F344 rats was accompanied with increased activity of the xenobiotic detoxifying liver enzymes glutathione-S-transferases (GSTs) in all lentil-fed groups in comparison with the control.

It has been reported that anticarcinogenic enzyme inducers can be either monofunctional which elevates only the Phase II enzymes involved in xenobiotic detoxification, e.g. GST, or bifunctional, which elevates both the Phase I enzymes that catalyze the metabolic activation of carcinogens, e.g. CYP450, and Phase II xenobiotic detoxifying enzymes (Talalay, 1989). Antioxidant polyphenolics present in lentils and other pulses are among the monofunctional inducers that increase the activity of xenobiotic detoxifying enzymes alone (Pool-Zobel et al., 2005). The finding that hepatic levels of antioxidant enzymes such as GST were significantly greater in rats fed chemopreventive lentil diets than in rats fed control diet implies an increased antioxidant capacity to defend against oxidative stress that was triggered by chemopreventive agents (Pool-Zobel et al., 2005).

Further, the induced GST in livers of rats fed on split lentils could be ascribed partly to the presence of appreciated quantities of phytic acid in the cotyledons. It was found that levels of GST were increased concomitantly with increasing phytic acid, inositol, and polyphenolics content in the tested diets, when compared with the control diet. Phytic acid could reduce colon cancer via chelation of iron and suppression of iron related initiation and promotion of carcinogenesis and it may have potential therapeutic use in cancer due to its property of enhancing the activity of natural killer cells associated with suppressed tumor incidence (Khatiwada et al., 2006).

Finally, the inhibitory action of lentils could be explained, in part, by its putative antioxidant activity, and by the presence of other chemopreventive agents in the cotyledons rather than the antioxidant phytochemicals accumulated in the seed coat, as presented in the rat fed the split lentils. Further, the high selenium content in lentils may also be a contributing factor to anticarcinogenic potential of lentils, as this element is involved in the induction of apoptosis and enhancement of immune system (Arthur et al., 2003).

Thus, it might be speculated that the antioxidant phytochemicals were not the only responsible factors for chemoprevention, as the chemopreventive ability was not restricted to polyphenolic-rich whole, non-split, and lentil seeds. The reduction in colon carcinogenesis in rats fed on split lentils could be attributed to the presence of anticancer macro- and micro-constituents in lentil cotyledons. Industrially, and in an attempt to popularize the consumption of the nutrient-dense, health-improving lentils by different sectors of the community, researchers have attempted to develop healthy snack bars that are based on lentils as a basic ingredient in the form of micronized flaked lentils (Ryland et al., 2010).

SOLUTIONS AND RECOMMENDATIONS

It is clear that lentils have been an integral part of traditional diets consumed for their nutritive value, taste, ease of availability and cooking in variety of cuisines. However, the advanced technology and research have uncovered newer aspects of lentils that direct the importance of considering lentils as functional food. It is, therefore, imperative to emphasize on the consumption of lentils in regular diets so as to benefit from their nutritional value, presence of bioactive components and other phytochemicals as well as reduction in the incidence of chronic diseases. Further, well-designed and larger-scaled randomized-controlled trials could be integrated for better understanding of the therapeutic effects of lentils, and to explain discrepancies in the clinical studies on the specific role of lentils consumption in different human ailments and diseases.

FUTURE RESEARCH DIRECTIONS

With the plethora of evidence emerging on the health benefits of lentils, it is recommended that the direction of future research focuses on the relationship of specific nutritional and bioactive components in lentils with the specific health or disease conditions. Further, the specific amounts of each integral component associated with the health effect must be determined. This will assist in estimating the amount of lentil consumption for therapeutic use. The molecular mechanisms underlying the chemopreventive effect of lentils in chemically-induced chronic diseases in animal models (namely cancer and diabetes) are required for better understanding of the effect of lentils on these diseases. *In vitro*, future research should enhance the information on the mechanisms involved in molecular and cytological modifications induced by lentil bioactive components; that will assist in developing drugs and medications from lentils bioactive functional components.

CONCLUSION

A compelling body of evidence investigating lentils, *L. culinaris,* confirms that lentil is one of the most nutritious and health improving foods known to man. According to recent definitions, lentil could be considered a prophylactic and therapeutic functional food due to its considerable content of essential macronutrients, namely functional proteins and carbohydrates, and essential micronutrients, as well as bioactive phytochemicals such as phytates and polyphenols. Indeed, lentils contain an impressive arsenal of secondary metabolites, minerals and bioactive constituents that have shown to be promising in the management and prevention of several human chronic illnesses due to their anticarcinogenic, hypoglycemic, hypocholesterolemic and blood-pressure lowering properties. Further research is required to improve the nutritional quality of lentil proteins and optimize the agricultural and culinary conditions to ensure maximum utilization of the rich supply of bioactive phytochemicals in lentils.

REFERENCES

Adebamowo, C. A., Cho, E., Sampson, L., Katan, M. B., Spiegelman, D., Willett, W. C., & Holmes, M. D. (2005). Dietary flavonols and flavonol rich foods intake and the risk of breast cancer. *International Journal of Cancer*, *114*(4), 628–633. doi:10.1002/ijc.20741 PMID:15609322

Al-Tibi, A. M., Takruri, H. R., & Ahmad, M. N. (2010). Effect of dehulling and cooking of lentils (Lens culinaris L.) on serum glucose and lipoprotein levels in streptozotocin-induced diabetic rats. *Malaysian Journalof Nutrition*, *16*(3), 409–418. PMID:22691994

Alexandre, K. B., Gray, E. S., Lambson, B. E., Moore, P. L., Choge, I. A., Mlisana, K., & Morris, L. et al. (2010). Mannose-rich glycosylation patterns on HIV-1 subtype C gp120 and sensitivity to the lectins, Griffithsin, Cyanovirin-N and Scytovirin. *Virology*, *402*(1), 187–196. doi:10.1016/j.virol.2010.03.021 PMID:20392471

Araya, H., Contreras, P., Alvina, M., Vera, G., & Pak, N. (2002). A comparison between an in vitro method to determine carbohydrate digestion rate and the glycemic response in young men. *European Journal of Clinical Nutrition*, *56*(8), 735–739. doi:10.1038/sj.ejcn.1601386 PMID:12122549

Armstrong, W. B., Kennedy, A. R., Wan, X. S., Atiba, J., McLaren, C. E., & Meyskens, F. L. (2000). Single-dose administration of Bowman-Birk inhibitor concentrate in patients with oral leukoplakia. *Cancer Epidemiology, Biomarkers & Prevention*, *9*(1), 43–47. PMID:10667462

Arthur, J. R., McKenzie, R. C., & Beckett, G. J. (2003). Selenium in the immune system. *The Journal of Nutrition*, *133*(5), 1457S–1459S. PMID:12730442

Ayet, G., Burbano, C., Cuadrado, C., Pedrosa, M. M., Robredo, L. M., Muzquiz, M., & Osagie, A. et al. (1997). Effect. of Germination, under Different Environmental Conditions, on Saponins, Phytic Acid and Tannins in Lentils (Lens culinaris). *Journal of the Science of Food and Agriculture*, *74*(2), 273–279. doi:10.1002/(SICI)1097-0010(199706)74:2<273::AID-JSFA800>3.0.CO;2-L

Balasubramaniam, V., Mustar, S., Khalid, N. M., Rashed, A. A., Noh, M. F. M., Wilcox, M. D., & Pearson, J. et al. (2013). Inhibitory activities of three Malaysian edible seaweeds on lipase and α-amylase. *Journal of Applied Phycology*, *25*(5), 1405–1412. doi:10.1007/s10811-012-9964-4

Bamdad, F., Goli, A. H., & Kadivar, M. (2006). Preparation and characterization of proteinous film from lentil (Lens culinaris): Edible film from lentil (Lens culinaris). *Food Research International*, *39*(1), 106–111. doi:10.1016/j.foodres.2005.06.006

Barbana, C., & Boye, J. I. (2011). Angiotensin I-converting enzyme inhibitory properties of lentil protein hydrolysates: Determination of the kinetics of inhibition. *Food Chemistry*, *127*(1), 94–101. doi:10.1016/j.foodchem.2010.12.093

Bazzano, L. A., Thompson, A. M., Tees, M. T., Nguyen, C. H., & Winham, D. M. (2011). Non-soy legume consumption lowers cholesterol levels: A meta-analysis of randomized controlled trials. *Nutrition, Metabolism, and Cardiovascular Diseases*, *21*(2), 94–103. doi:10.1016/j.numecd.2009.08.012 PMID:19939654

Bednar, G. E., Patil, A. R., Murray, S. M., Grieshop, C. M., Merchen, N. R., & Fahey, G. C. (2001). Starch and fiber fractions in selected food and feed ingredients affect their small intestinal digestibility and fermentability and their large bowel fermentability in vitro in a canine model. *The Journal of Nutrition*, *131*(2), 276–286. PMID:11160546

Bhattacharya, S., Narasimha, H. V., & Bhattacharya, S. (2005). The moisture dependent physical and mechanical properties of whole lentil pulse and split cotyledon. *International Journal of Food Science & Technology*, *40*(2), 213–221. doi:10.1111/j.1365-2621.2004.00933.x

Bhatty, R., & Christison, G. (1984). Composition and nutritional quality of pea (*Pisumsativum* L.), faba bean (*Viciafaba* L. spp. minor) and lentil (*Lens culinaris* Medik.) meals, protein concentrates and isolates. *Plant Foods for Human Nutrition (Dordrecht, Netherlands)*, *34*(1), 41–51. doi:10.1007/BF01095071

Boye, J. I., Roufik, S., Pesta, N., & Barbana, C. (2010). Angiotensin I-converting enzyme inhibitory properties and SDS-PAGE of red lentil protein hydrolysates. *LWT-Food Science and Technology*, *43*(6), 987–991. doi:10.1016/j.lwt.2010.01.014

Bruce, W. R., Giacca, A., & Medline, A. (2000). Possible mechanisms relating diet and risk of colon cancer. *Cancer Epidemiology, Biomarkers & Prevention*, *9*(12), 1271–1279. PMID:11142411

Busambwa, K., Miller-Cebert, R., Aboagye, L., Dalrymple, L., Boateng, J., Shackelford, L., & Verghese, M. et al. (2014). Inhibitory effect of lentils, green split and yellow peas (sprouted and non-sprouted) on azoxymethane-induced aberrant crypt foci in Fisher 344 male rats. *International Journal of Cancer Research*, *10*(1), 27–36. doi:10.3923/ijcr.2014.27.36

Campos-Vega, R., Loarca-Piña, G., & Oomah, B. D. (2010). Minor components of pulses and their potential impact on human health. *Food Research International*, *43*(2), 461–482. doi:10.1016/j.foodres.2009.09.004

Canani, R. B., Costanzo, M., Leone, L., Pedata, M., Meli, R., & Calignano, A. (2011). Potential beneficial effects of butyrate in intestinal and extra intestinal diseases. *World Journal of Gastroenterology*, *17*(12), 1519–1528. doi:10.3748/wjg.v17.i12.1519 PMID:21472114

Champ, M. M.-J. (2002). Non-nutrient bioactive substances of pulses. *The British Journal of Nutrition*, *88*(S3), 307–319. doi:10.1079/BJN2002721 PMID:12498631

Chen, C., & Kong, A.-N. T. (2005). Dietary cancer-chemopreventive compounds: From signaling and gene expression to pharmacological effects. *Trends in Pharmacological Sciences*, *26*(6), 318–326. doi:10.1016/j.tips.2005.04.004 PMID:15925707

Cheung, A. H., & Ng, T. B. (2007). Isolation and characterization of a trypsin-chymotrypsin inhibitor from the seeds of green lentil (*Lens culinaris*). *Protein and Peptide Letters*, *14*(9), 859–864. doi:10.2174/092986607782110310 PMID:18045226

Chung, H.-J., Liu, Q., Pauls, K. P., Fan, M. Z., & Yada, R. (2008). In vitro starch digestibility, expected glycemic index and some physicochemical properties of starch and flour from common bean (*Phaseolus vulgaris* L.) varieties grown in Canada. *Food Research International*, *41*(9), 869–875. doi:10.1016/j.foodres.2008.03.013

Corpet, D. E., & Taché, S. (2002). Most effective colon cancer chemopreventive agents in rats: A systematic review of aberrant crypt foci and tumor data, ranked by potency. *Nutrition and Cancer*, *43*(1), 1–21. doi:10.1207/S15327914NC431_1 PMID:12467130

Correa, P. (1981). Epidemiological correlations between diet and cancer frequency. *Cancer Research*, *41*(9 Part 2), 3685–3689. PMID:6266659

Dabai, F. D., Walker, A. F., Sambrook, I. E., Welch, V. A., Owen, R. W., & Abeyasekera, S. (1996). Comparative effects on blood lipids and faecal steroids of five legume species incorporated into a semi-purified, hypercholesterolaemic rat diet. *The British Journal of Nutrition*, *75*(04), 557–571. doi:10.1079/BJN19960159 PMID:8672408

Dagher, S. M. (1991). *Traditional Foods in the Near East*. FAO.

de Almeida Costa, G. E., da Silva Queiroz-Monici, K., Reis, S. M. P. M., & de Oliveira, A. C. (2006). Chemical composition, dietary fibre and resistant starch contents of raw and cooked pea, common bean, chickpea and lentil legumes. *Food Chemistry*, *94*(3), 327–330. doi:10.1016/j.foodchem.2004.11.020

De Mejía, E. G., & Prisecaru, V. I. (2005). Lectins as bioactive plant proteins: A potential in cancer treatment. *Critical Reviews in Food Science and Nutrition*, *45*(6), 425–445. doi:10.1080/10408390591034445 PMID:16183566

Demirbas, A. (2005). β-Glucan and mineral nutrient contents of cereals grown in Turkey. *Food Chemistry*, *90*(4), 773–777. doi:10.1016/j.foodchem.2004.06.003

Desilets, D. J., Davis, K. E., Nair, P. P., Salata, K. F., Maydonovitch, C. L., Howard, R. S., & Wong, R. K. et al. (1999). Lectin. binding to human colonocytes is predictive of colonic neoplasia. *The American Journal of Gastroenterology*, *94*(3), 744–750. doi:10.1111/j.1572-0241.1999.00946.x PMID:10086661

Duane, W. (1997). Effects of legume consumption on serum cholesterol, biliary lipids, and sterol metabolism in humans. *Journal of Lipid Research*, *38*(6), 1120–1128. PMID:9215540

Dueñas, M., Hernández, T., & Estrella, I. (2002). Phenolic composition of the cotyledon and the seed coat of lentils (*Lens culinaris* L.). *European Food Research and Technology*, *215*(6), 478–483. doi:10.1007/s00217-002-0603-1

Duenas, M., Hernandez, T., & Estrella, I. (2006). Assessment of in vitro antioxidant capacity of the seed coat and the cotyledon of legumes in relation to their phenolic contents. *Food Chemistry*, *98*(1), 95–103. doi:10.1016/j.foodchem.2005.05.052

Dueñas, M., Sun, B., Hernández, T., Estrella, I., & Spranger, M. I. (2003). Proanthocyanidin composition in the seed coat of lentils (*Lens culinaris* L.). *Journal of Agricultural and Food Chemistry*, *51*(27), 7999–8004. doi:10.1021/jf0303215 PMID:14690386

Duranti, M. (2006). Grain legume proteins and nutraceutical properties. *Fitoterapia*, *77*(2), 67–82. doi:10.1016/j.fitote.2005.11.008 PMID:16406359

Dwivedi, S., Sahrawat, K., Puppala, N., & Ortiz, R. (2014). Plant prebiotics and human health: Biotechnology to breed prebiotic-rich nutritious food crops. *Electronic Journal of Biotechnology*, *17*(5), 238–245. doi:10.1016/j.ejbt.2014.07.004

Eidi, A., & Eidi, M. (2009). Antidiabetic effects of sage (*Salvia officinalis* L.) leaves in normal and streptozotocin-induced diabetic rats. *Diabetes & Metabolic Syndrome: Clinical Research & Reviews*, *3*(1), 40–44. doi:10.1016/j.dsx.2008.10.007

El-Adawy, T., Rahma, E., El-Bedawey, A., & El-Beltagy, A. (2003). Nutritional potential and functional properties of germinated mung bean, pea and lentil seeds. *Plant Foods for Human Nutrition (Dordrecht, Netherlands)*, *58*(3), 1–13. doi:10.1023/B:QUAL.0000040339.48521.75 PMID:12859008

Elekofehinti, O. O. (2015). Saponins: Anti-diabetic principles from medicinal plants–A review. *Pathophysiology*, *22*(2), 95–103. doi:10.1016/j.pathophys.2015.02.001 PMID:25753168

Faris, M. A. I. E., & Takruri, H. R. (2003). Study of the effect of using different levels of tahinah (sesame butter) on the protein digestibility-corrected amino acid score (PDCAAS) of chickpea dip. *Journal of the Science of Food and Agriculture*, *83*(1), 7–12. doi:10.1002/jsfa.1273

Faris, M. A. I. E., Takruri, H. R., & Issa, A. Y. (2013). Role of lentils (*Lens culinaris* L.) in human health and nutrition: A review. *Mediterranean Journal of Nutrition and Metabolism*, *6*(1), 3–16. doi:10.1007/s12349-012-0109-8

Faris, M. A. I. E., Takruri, H. R., Shomaf, M. S., & Bustanji, Y. K. (2009). Chemopreventivc effect of raw and cooked lentils (*Lens culinaris* L) and soybeans (Glycine max) against azoxymethane-induced aberrant crypt foci. *Nutrition Research (New York, N.Y.)*, *29*(5), 355–362. doi:10.1016/j.nutres.2009.05.005 PMID:19555818

Fernandez-Orozco, R., Zieliński, H., & Piskuła, M. K. (2003). Contribution of low-molecular weight antioxidants to the antioxidant capacity of raw and processed lentil seeds. *Food/Nahrung, 47*(5), 291-299.

Finkina, E. I., Shramova, E. I., Tagaev, A. A., & Ovchinnikova, T. V. (2008). A novel defensin from the lentil Lens culinaris seeds. *Biochemical and Biophysical Research Communications*, *371*(4), 860–865. doi:10.1016/j.bbrc.2008.04.161 PMID:18468512

Flight, I., & Clifton, P. (2006). Cereal grains and legumes in the prevention of coronary heart disease and stroke: A review of the literature. *European Journal of Clinical Nutrition*, *60*(10), 1145–1159. doi:10.1038/sj.ejcn.1602435 PMID:16670693

Food and Agriculture Organization (FAO). (1988). *Traditional Food Plants*. Rome: FAO.

Food and Agriculture Organization (FAO). (2011). *Economic and Social Department: The Statistical Division*. Retrieved from http://faostat.fao.org/site/567/DesktopDefault.aspx?PageID=567#ancor

Fooks, L. J., Fuller, R., & Gibson, G. R. (1999). Prebiotics, probiotics and human gut microbiology. *International Dairy Journal*, *9*(1), 53–61. doi:10.1016/S0958-6946(99)00044-8

Foster-Powell, K., Holt, S. H., & Brand-Miller, J. C. (2002). International table of glycemic index and glycemic load values: 2002. *The American Journal of Clinical Nutrition*, *76*(1), 5–56. PMID:12081815

Fox, C., & Eberl, M. (2002). Phytic acid (IP6), novel broad spectrum anti-neoplastic agent: A systematic review. *Complementary Therapies in Medicine*, *10*(4), 229–234. doi:10.1016/S0965-2299(02)00092-4 PMID:12594974

Fratianni, F., Cardinale, F., Cozzolino, A., Granese, T., Albanese, D., Di Matteo, M., & Nazzaro, F. et al. (2014). Polyphenol composition and antioxidant activity of different grass pea (*Lathyrussativus*), lentils (*Lens culinaris*), and chickpea (*Cicer arietinum*) ecotypes of the Campania region (Southern Italy). *Journal of Functional Foods*, *7*, 551–557.

Freier, T. C., & Rüdiger, H. E. (1990). Lectin-binding proteins from lentil seeds as mitogens for murine B lymphocytes. *Phytochemistry*, *29*(5), 1459–1461. doi:10.1016/0031-9422(90)80100-U

García-Alonso, A., Goñi, I., & Saura-Calixto, F. (1998). Resistant starch and potential glycaemic index of raw and cooked legumes (lentils, chickpeas and beans). *ZeitschriftfürLebensmitteluntersuchung und-Forschung A, 206*(4), 284-287.

Garcia-Mora, P., Peñas, E., Frias, J., & Martínez-Villaluenga, C. (2014). Savinase, the most suitable enzyme for releasing peptides from lentil (*Lens culinaris* var. Castellana) protein concentrates with multifunctional properties. *Journal of Agricultural and Food Chemistry*, *62*(18), 4166–4174. doi:10.1021/jf500849u PMID:24738747

Germaine, K. A., Samman, S., Fryirs, C. G., Griffiths, P. J., Johnson, S. K., & Quail, K. J. (2008). Comparison of in vitro starch digestibility methods for predicting the glycaemic index of grain foods. *Journal of the Science of Food and Agriculture*, *88*(4), 652–658. doi:10.1002/jsfa.3130

Giday, M., Teklehaymanot, T., Animut, A., & Mekonnen, Y. (2007). Medicinal plants of the Shinasha, Agew-awi and Amhara peoples in northwest Ethiopia. *Journal of Ethnopharmacology*, *110*(3), 516–525. doi:10.1016/j.jep.2006.10.011 PMID:17101251

Gossé, F., Guyot, S., Roussi, S., Lobstein, A., Fischer, B., Seiler, N., & Raul, F. (2005). Chemopreventive properties of apple procyanidins on human colon cancer-derived metastatic SW620 cells and in a rat model of colon carcinogenesis. *Carcinogenesis*, *26*(7), 1291–1295. doi:10.1093/carcin/bgi074 PMID:15790589

Graf, E., & Eaton, J. W. (1990). Antioxidant functions of phytic acid. *Free Radical Biology & Medicine*, *8*(1), 61–69. doi:10.1016/0891-5849(90)90146-A PMID:2182395

Granito, M., Champ, M., David, A., Bonnet, C., & Guerra, M. (2001). Identification of gas-producing components in different varieties of *Phaseolus vulgaris* by in vitro fermentation. *Journal of the Science of Food and Agriculture*, *81*(6), 543–550. doi:10.1002/jsfa.839

Greenwald, P., Clifford, C., & Milner, J. (2001). Diet and cancer prevention. *European Journal of Cancer*, *37*(8), 948–965. doi:10.1016/S0959-8049(01)00070-3 PMID:11334719

Güçlü-Üstündağ, Ö., & Mazza, G. (2007). Saponins: Properties, applications and processing. *Critical Reviews in Food Science and Nutrition*, *47*(3), 231–258. doi:10.1080/10408390600698197 PMID:17453922

Guillamon, E., Pedrosa, M. M., Burbano, C., Cuadrado, C., de Cortes Sánchez, M., & Muzquiz, M. (2008). The trypsin inhibitors present in seed of different grain legume species and cultivar. *Food Chemistry*, *107*(1), 68–74. doi:10.1016/j.foodchem.2007.07.029

Gurfinkel, D., & Rao, A. (2003). Soyasaponins: The relationship between chemical structure and colon anticarcinogenic activity. *Nutrition and Cancer*, *47*(1), 24–33. doi:10.1207/s15327914nc4701_3 PMID:14769534

Han, I. H. (2005). *Oligosaccharide reduction, protein digestibility improvement, antioxidant activity determination and phenolic compounds identification in legumes*. Washington State University.

Hanson, M. G., Zahradka, P., & Taylor, C. G. (2014). Lentil-based diets attenuate hypertension and large-artery remodelling in spontaneously hypertensive rats. *The British Journal of Nutrition*, *111*(04), 690–698. doi:10.1017/S0007114513002997 PMID:24063808

Hefni, M., Öhrvik, V., Tabekha, M., & Witthöft, C. (2010). Folate content in foods commonly consumed in Egypt. *Food Chemistry*, *121*(2), 540–545. doi:10.1016/j.foodchem.2009.12.044

Hernández-Salazar, M., Osorio-Diaz, P., Loarca-Piña, G., Reynoso-Camacho, R., Tovar, J., & Bello-Pérez, L. A. (2010). *In vitro* fermentability and antioxidant capacity of the indigestible fraction of cooked black beans (*Phaseolus vulgaris* L.), lentils (*Lens culinaris* L.) and chickpeas (*Cicer arietinum* L.). *Journal of the Science of Food and Agriculture*, *90*(9), 1417–1422. doi:10.1002/jsfa.3954 PMID:20549791

Hodge, A. M., English, D. R., O'Dea, K., & Giles, G. G. (2004). Glycemic index and dietary fiber and the risk of type 2 diabetes. *Diabetes Care*, *27*(11), 2701–2706. doi:10.2337/diacare.27.11.2701 PMID:15505008

Hoover, R., Hughes, T., Chung, H., & Liu, Q. (2010). Composition, molecular structure, properties, and modification of pulse starches: A review. *Food Research International*, *43*(2), 399–413. doi:10.1016/j.foodres.2009.09.001

Hoover, R., & Ratnayake, W. (2002). Starch characteristics of black bean, chick pea, lentil, navy bean and pinto bean cultivars grown in Canada. *Food Chemistry*, *78*(4), 489–498. doi:10.1016/S0308-8146(02)00163-2

Issa, A. Y., Volate, S. R., & Wargovich, M. J. (2006). The role of phytochemicals in inhibition of cancer and inflammation: New directions and perspectives. *Journal of Food Composition and Analysis*, *19*(5), 405–419. doi:10.1016/j.jfca.2006.02.009

Jenkins, D., Wolever, T., Taylor, R. H., Barker, H., Fielden, H., Baldwin, J. M., & Goff, D. V. et al. (1981). Glycemi.c index of foods: A physiological basis for carbohydrate exchange Am*erica.n. The Journal of Clinical Nutrition*, *34*(3), 362–366.

Jenkins, D., Wong, G. S., Patten, R., Bird, J., Hall, M., Buckley, G. C., & Little, J. A. et al. (1983). Legumin.ous seeds in the dietary management of hyperlipidemia. *The American Journal of Clinical Nutrition*, *38*(4), 567–573. PMID:6624698

Johnson, C. R., Combs, G. F., & Thavarajah, P. (2013). Lentil (*Lens culinaris* L.): A prebiotic-rich whole food legume. *Food Research International*, *51*(1), 107–113. doi:10.1016/j.foodres.2012.11.025

Kalogeropoulos, N., Chiou, A., Ioannou, M., Karathanos, V. T., Hassapidou, M., & Andrikopoulos, N. K. (2010). Nutritional evaluation and bioactive microconstituents (phytosterols, tocopherols, polyphenols, triterpenic acids) in cooked dry legumes usually consumed in the Mediterranean countries. *Food Chemistry*, *121*(3), 682–690. doi:10.1016/j.foodchem.2010.01.005

Kennedy, A. R. (1998). The Bowman-Birk inhibitor from soybeans as an anticarcinogenic agent. *The American Journal of Clinical Nutrition*, *68*(6), 1406S–1412S. PMID:9848508

Khatiwada, J., Verghese, M., Walker, L., Shackelford, L., Chawan, C., & Sunkara, R. (2006). Combination of green tea, phytic acid, and inositol reduced the incidence of azoxymethane-induced colon tumors in Fisher 344 male rats. *LWT-Food Science and Technology*, *39*(10), 1080–1086. doi:10.1016/j.lwt.2005.07.018

Kingman, S. M., Walker, A. F., Low, A., Sambrook, I., Owen, R., & Cole, T. (1993). Comparative effects of four legume species on plasma lipids and faecal steroid excretion in hypercholesterolaemic pigs. *The British Journal of Nutrition*, *69*(02), 409–421. doi:10.1079/BJN19930043 PMID:8489997

Kris-Etherton, P. M., Hecker, K. D., Bonanome, A., Coval, S. M., Binkoski, A. E., Hilpert, K. F., & Etherton, T. D. et al. (2002). Bioactive compounds in foods: Their role in the prevention of cardiovascular disease and cancer. *The American Journal of Medicine*, *113*(9), 71–88. doi:10.1016/S0002-9343(01)00995-0 PMID:12566142

Kwon, Y., & Magnuson, B. A. (2007). Effect of azoxymethane and curcumin on transcriptional levels of cyclooxygenase-1 and-2 during initiation of colon carcinogenesis. *Scandinavian Journal of Gastroenterology*, *42*(1), 72–80. doi:10.1080/00365520600825216 PMID:17190766

Kwon, Y., Malik, M., & Magnuson, B. A. (2004). Inhibition of colonic aberrant crypt foci by curcumin in rats is affected by age. *Nutrition and Cancer*, *48*(1), 37–43. doi:10.1207/s15327914nc4801_6 PMID:15203376

Lajolo, F. M., & Genovese, M. I. (2002). Nutritional significance of lectins and enzyme inhibitors from legumes. *Journal of Agricultural and Food Chemistry*, *50*(22), 6592–6598. doi:10.1021/jf020191k PMID:12381157

Lala, G., Malik, M., Zhao, C., He, J., Kwon, Y., Giusti, M. M., & Magnuson, B. A. (2006). Anthocyanin-rich extracts inhibit multiple biomarkers of colon cancer in rats. *Nutrition and Cancer*, *54*(1), 84–93. doi:10.1207/s15327914nc5401_10 PMID:16800776

Lardos, A. (2006). The botanical materiamedica of the Iatrosophikon-a collection of prescriptions from a monastery in Cyprus. *Journal of Ethnopharmacology*, *104*(3), 387–406. doi:10.1016/j.jep.2005.12.035 PMID:16459038

Lentils. (2003). InGrant, G. D. M., & Alonso, R. (Eds.), *Encyclopedia of Food Science and Nutrition*. London: Elsevier Science Ltd.

Liu, R. H. (2007). Whole grain phytochemicals and health. *Journal of Cereal Science*, *46*(3), 207–219. doi:10.1016/j.jcs.2007.06.010

Lombardi-Boccia, G., Ruggeri, S., Aguzzi, A., & Cappelloni, M. (2003). Globulins enhance in vitro iron but not zinc dialysability: A study on six legume species. *Journal of Trace Elements in Medicine and Biology*, *17*(1), 1–5. doi:10.1016/S0946-672X(03)80037-8 PMID:12755494

Losso, J. N. (2008). The biochemical and functional food properties of the Bowman-Birk inhibitor. *Critical Reviews in Food Science and Nutrition*, *48*(1), 94–118. doi:10.1080/10408390601177589 PMID:18274967

Marinangeli, C. P., & Jones, P. J. (2012). Pulse grain consumption and obesity: Effects on energy expenditure, substrate oxidation, body composition, fat deposition and satiety. *The British Journal of Nutrition*, *108*(S1), S46–S51. doi:10.1017/S0007114512000773 PMID:22916815

Marks, G., Aydos, R. D., Fagundes, D. J., Pontes, E. R. J. C., Takita, L. C., Amaral, E. G. A. S., & Ynouye, C. M. et al. (2006). Modulation of transforming growth factor beta2 (TGF-beta2) by inositol hexaphosphate in colon carcinogenesis in rats. *Acta Cirurgica Brasileira*, *21*, 51–56. doi:10.1590/S0102-86502006001000012 PMID:17293967

Martins, J. M., Riottot, M., de Abreu, M. C., Lança, M. J., Viegas-Crespo, A. M., Almeida, J. A., & Bento, O. P. et al. (2004). Dietary raw peas (*Pisum sativum* L.) reduce plasma total and LDL cholesterol and hepatic esterified cholesterol in intact and ileorectal anastomosed pigs fed cholesterol-rich diets. *The Journal of Nutrition*, *134*(12), 3305–3312. PMID:15570030

Mazur, W. M., Duke, J. A., Wähälä, K., Rasku, S., & Adlercreutz, H. (1998). Isoflavonoids and lignans in legumes: Nutritional and health aspects in humans. *The Journal of Nutritional Biochemistry*, *9*(4), 193–200. doi:10.1016/S0955-2863(97)00184-8

McCrory, M. A., Hamaker, B. R., Lovejoy, J. C., & Eichelsdoerfer, P. E. (2010). Pulse consumption, satiety, and weight management. *Advances in Nutrition: An International Review Journal*, *1*(1), 17–30. doi:10.3945/an.110.1006 PMID:22043448

Milner, J. A., McDonald, S. S., Anderson, D. E., & Greenwald, P. (2001). Molecular targets for nutrients involved with cancer prevention. *Nutrition and Cancer*, *41*(1-2), 1–16. doi:10.1080/01635581.2001.9680606 PMID:12094610

Mitchell, B. S., Brooks, S. A., Leathem, A. J., & Schumacher, U. (1998). Do HPA and PHA-L have the same binding pattern in metastasizing human breast and colon cancers? *Cancer Letters*, *123*(1), 113–119. doi:10.1016/S0304-3835(97)00414-X PMID:9461027

Mollard, R., Zykus, A., Luhovyy, B., Nunez, M., Wong, C., & Anderson, G. (2012). The acute effects of a pulse-containing meal on glycaemic responses and measures of satiety and satiation within and at a later meal. *The British Journal of Nutrition*, *108*(03), 509–517. doi:10.1017/S0007114511005836 PMID:22054112

Moon, Y. J., Wang, X., & Morris, M. E. (2006). Dietary flavonoids: Effects on xenobiotic and carcinogen metabolism. *Toxicology In Vitro*, *20*(2), 187–210. doi:10.1016/j.tiv.2005.06.048 PMID:16289744

Morris, E. R., & Hill, A. D. (1996). Inositol phosphate content of selected dry beans, peas, and lentils, raw and cooked. *Journal of Food Composition and Analysis*, *9*(1), 2–12. doi:10.1006/jfca.1996.0002

Nichenametla, S. N., Taruscio, T. G., Barney, D. L., & Exon, J. H. (2006). A review of the effects and mechanisms of polyphenolics in cancer. *Critical Reviews in Food Science and Nutrition*, *46*(2), 161–183. doi:10.1080/10408390591000541 PMID:16431408

Padovani, R. M., Lima, D. M., Colugnati, F. A., & Rodriguez-Amaya, D. B. (2007). Comparison of proximate, mineral and vitamin composition of common Brazilian and US foods. *Journal of Food Composition and Analysis*, *20*(8), 733–738. doi:10.1016/j.jfca.2007.03.006

Pellegrini, N., Serafini, M., Salvatore, S., Del Rio, D., Bianchi, M., & Brighenti, F. (2006). Total antioxidant capacity of spices, dried fruits, nuts, pulses, cereals and sweets consumed in Italy assessed by three different in vitro assays. *Molecular Nutrition & Food Research, 50*(11), 1030–1038. doi:10.1002/mnfr.200600067 PMID:17039458

Perera, A., Meda, V., & Tyler, R. (2010). Resistant starch: A review of analytical protocols for determining resistant starch and of factors affecting the resistant starch content of foods. *Food Research International, 43*(8), 1959–1974. doi:10.1016/j.foodres.2010.06.003

Pintó, X., Vilaseca, M. A., Balcells, S., Artuch, R., Corbella, E., Meco, J. F., & Grinberg, D. et al. (2005). A folat.e-rich diet is as effective as folic acid from supplements in decreasing plasma homocysteine concentrations In*terna.tional. Journal of Medical Science*, 2(2), 58.

Pool-Zobel, B., Veeriah, S., & Böhmer, F.D. (2005). Modulation of xenobiotic metabolising enzymes by anticarcinogens-focus on glutathione S-transferases and their role as targets of dietary chemoprevention in colorectal carcinogenesis. *Mutation Research/Fundamental and Molecular Mechanisms of Mutagenesis, 591*(1), 74-92.

Queiroz-Monici, K. S., Costa, G. E., da Silva, N., Reis, S. M., & de Oliveira, A. C. (2005). Bifidogenic effect of dietary fiber and resistant starch from leguminous on the intestinal microbiota of rats. *Nutrition (Burbank, Los Angeles County, Calif.), 21*(5), 602–608. doi:10.1016/j.nut.2004.09.019 PMID:15850967

Rao, C. V., Newmark, H. L., & Reddy, B. S. (1998). Chemopreventive effect of squalene on colon cancer. *Carcinogenesis, 19*(2), 287–290. doi:10.1093/carcin/19.2.287 PMID:9498278

Rochfort, S., & Panozzo, J. (2007). Phytochemicals for health, the role of pulses. *Journal of Agricultural and Food Chemistry, 55*(20), 7981–7994. doi:10.1021/jf071704w PMID:17784726

Rodríguez, C., Frias, J., Vidal-Valverde, C., & Hernández, A. (2008). Correlations between some nitrogen fractions, lysine, histidine, tyrosine, and ornithine contents during the germination of peas, beans, and lentils. *Food Chemistry, 108*(1), 245–252. doi:10.1016/j.foodchem.2007.10.073

Roy, F., Boye, J., & Simpson, B. (2010). Bioactive proteins and peptides in pulse crops: Pea, chickpea and lentil. *Food Research International, 43*(2), 432–442. doi:10.1016/j.foodres.2009.09.002

Rubio, L. (2000). Physiological effects of legume storage proteins. *Nutrition Abstracts andReiew Series A. Human and Experimental, 70*, 531–538.

Ryan, E., Galvin, K., O'Connor, T., Maguire, A., & O'Brien, N. (2007). Phytosterol, squalene, tocopherol content and fatty acid profile of selected seeds, grains, and legumes. *Plant Foods for Human Nutrition (Dordrecht, Netherlands), 62*(3), 85–91. doi:10.1007/s11130-007-0046-8 PMID:17594521

Ryland, D., Vaisey-Genser, M., Arntfield, S. D., & Malcolmson, L. J. (2010). Development of a nutritious acceptable snack bar using micronized flaked lentils. *Food Research International, 43*(2), 642–649. doi:10.1016/j.foodres.2009.07.032

Salariya, A. M. (2005). The effects of hydrothermal processing on antinutrients, protein and starch digestibility of food legumes. *International Journal of Food Science & Technology, 40*(7), 695–700. doi:10.1111/j.1365-2621.2005.00978.x

Sames, K., Schumacher, U., Halata, Z., Damme, E. V., Peumans, W., Asmus, B., & Moll, I. et al. (2001). Lectin. and proteoglycan histochemistry of Merkel cell carcinomas. *Experimental Dermatology*, *10*(2), 100–109. doi:10.1034/j.1600-0625.2001.010002100.x PMID:11260248

Sandberg, A.-S. (2002). Bioavailability of minerals in legumes. *The British Journal of Nutrition*, *88*(S3), 281–285. doi:10.1079/BJN/2002718 PMID:12498628

Scalbert, A., Manach, C., Morand, C., Rémésy, C., & Jiménez, L. (2005). Dietary polyphenols and the prevention of diseases. *Critical Reviews in Food Science and Nutrition*, *45*(4), 287–306. doi:10.1080/1040869059096 PMID:16047496

Scarafoni, A., Magni, C., & Duranti, M. (2007). Molecular nutraceutics as a mean to investigate the positive effects of legume seed proteins on human health. *Trends in Food Science & Technology*, *18*(9), 454–463. doi:10.1016/j.tifs.2007.04.002

Sengupta, A., Ghosh, S., & Das, S. (2004). Modulatory influence of garlic and tomato on cyclooxygenase-2 activity, cell proliferation and apoptosis during azoxymethane induced colon carcinogenesis in rat. *Cancer Letters*, *208*(2), 127–136. doi:10.1016/j.canlet.2003.11.024 PMID:15142670

Sezik, E., Yeşilada, E., Honda, G., Takaishi, Y., Takeda, Y., & Tanaka, T. (2001). Traditional medicine in Turkey X. Folk medicine in central Anatolia. *Journal of Ethnopharmacology*, *75*(2), 95–115. doi:10.1016/S0378-8741(00)00399-8 PMID:11297840

Shams, H., Tahbaz, F., & Abadi, A. (2010). Effects of cooked lentils on glycemic control and blood lipids of patients with type 2 diabetes. *ARYA Atherosclerosis, 4*(1).

Shomaf, M., Takruri, H., & Faris, M. A. I. E. (2011). Lentils (Lens culinaris, L.) Attenuate Colonic Lesions and Neoplasms in Fischer 344 Rats. *Jordan Medical Journal*, *45*, 231–239.

Stephen, A. M., Dahl, W. J., Sieber, G. M., van Blaricom, J. A., & Morgan, D. R. (1995). Effect of green lentils on colonic function, nitrogen balance, and serum lipids in healthy human subjects. *The American Journal of Clinical Nutrition*, *62*(6), 1261–1267. PMID:7491890

Talalay, P. (1989). Mechanisms of induction of enzymes that protect against chemical carcinogenesis. *Advances in Enzyme Regulation*, *28*, 237–250. doi:10.1016/0065-2571(89)90074-5 PMID:2696344

Tanaka, T., Kohno, H., Murakami, M., Shimada, R., Kagami, S., Sumida, T., & Ogawa, H. et al. (2000). Suppres.sion of azoxymethane-induced colon carcinogenesis in male F344 rats by mandarin juices rich in β-cryptoxanthin and hesperidin In*terna.tional. Journal of Cancer*, *88*(1), 146–150.

Tanaka, T., Kohno, H., Shimada, R., Kagami, S., Yamaguchi, F., Kataoka, S., & Ohigashi, H. et al. (2000). Prevention of colonic aberrant crypt foci by dietary feeding of garcinol in male F344 rats. *Carcinogenesis*, *21*(6), 1183–1189. doi:10.1093/carcin/21.6.1183 PMID:10837008

Teklehaymanot, T., Giday, M., Medhin, G., & Mekonnen, Y. (2007). Knowledge and use of medicinal plants by people around DebreLibanos monastery in Ethiopia. *Journal of Ethnopharmacology*, *111*(2), 271–283. doi:10.1016/j.jep.2006.11.019 PMID:17187950

Tharanathan, R., & Mahadevamma, S. (2003). Grain legumes—a boon to human nutrition. *Trends in Food Science & Technology*, *14*(12), 507–518. doi:10.1016/j.tifs.2003.07.002

Thavarajah, D., Ruszkowski, J., & Vandenberg, A. (2008). High potential for selenium biofortification of lentils (*Lens culinaris* L.). *Journal of Agricultural and Food Chemistry*, *56*(22), 10747–10753. doi:10.1021/jf802307h PMID:18954072

Thavarajah, P., Sarker, A., Materne, M., Vandemark, G., Shrestha, R., Idrissi, O., & Vandenburg, A. et al. (2011). A globa.l survey of effects of genotype and environment on selenium concentration in lentils (*Lens culinaris* L): Impli.cations for nutritional fortification strategies. *Food Chemistry*, *125*(1), 72–76. doi:10.1016/j.foodchem.2010.08.038

Thompson, L. U., Boucher, B. A., Liu, Z., Cotterchio, M., & Kreiger, N. (2006). Phytoestrogen content of foods consumed in Canada, including isoflavones, lignans, and coumestan. *Nutrition and Cancer*, *54*(2), 184–201. doi:10.1207/s15327914nc5402_5 PMID:16898863

Totelin, L. (2015). When foods become remedies in ancient Greece: The curious case of garlic and other substances. *Journal of Ethnopharmacology*, *167*, 30–37. doi:10.1016/j.jep.2014.08.018 PMID:25173971

Trock, B., Lanza, E., & Greenwald, P. (1990). Dietary fiber, vegetables, and colon cancer: Critical review and meta-analyses of the epidemiologic evidence. *Journal of the National Cancer Institute*, *82*(8), 650–661. doi:10.1093/jnci/82.8.650 PMID:2157027

Troszyńska, A., Amarowicz, R., Lamparski, G., Wołejszo, A., & Baryłko-Pikielna, N. (2006). Investigation of astringency of extracts obtained from selected tannins-rich legume seeds. *Food Quality and Preference*, *17*(1), 31–35. doi:10.1016/j.foodqual.2005.04.006

Tucker, K. L., Selhub, J., Wilson, P. W., & Rosenberg, I. H. (1996). Dietary intake pattern relates to plasma folate and homocysteine concentrations in the Framingham Heart Study. *The Journal of Nutrition*, *126*(12), 3025. PMID:9001370

Ueland, P. M., Refsum, H., Beresford, S. A., & Vollset, S. E. (2000). The controversy over homocysteine and cardiovascular risk. *The American Journal of Clinical Nutrition*, *72*(2), 324–332. PMID:10919921

Umeta, M., West, C. E., & Fufa, H. (2005). Content of zinc, iron, calcium and their absorption inhibitors in foods commonly consumed in Ethiopia. *Journal of Food Composition and Analysis*, *18*(8), 803–817. doi:10.1016/j.jfca.2004.09.008

USDA. (2010). *USDA Database for the Oxygen Radical Absorbance Capacity (ORAC) of Selected Foods, Release2*. Retrieved from www.ars.usda.gov/SP2UserFiles/Place/12354500/Data/ORAC/ORAC_R2.pdf

USDA. (2010). *USDA National Nutrient Database for Standard Reference, Release 23*. Retrieved from http://www.ars.usda.gov/research/publications/publications.htm?seq_no_115=243584

Venn, B., & Mann, J. (2004). Cereal grains, legumes and diabetes. *European Journal of Clinical Nutrition*, *58*(11), 1443–1461. doi:10.1038/sj.ejcn.1601995 PMID:15162131

Verghese, M., Rao, D., Chawan, C., Walker, L., & Shackelford, L. (2006). Anticarcinogenic effect of phytic acid (IP 6): Apoptosis as a possible mechanism of action. *LWT-Food Science and Technology*, *39*(10), 1093–1098. doi:10.1016/j.lwt.2005.07.012

Vidal-Valverde, C., Frias, J., Sierra, I., Blazquez, I., Lambein, F., & Kuo, Y. H. (2002). New functional legume foods by germination: Effect on the nutritive value of beans, lentils and peas. *European Food Research and Technology*, *215*(6), 472–477. doi:10.1007/s00217-002-0602-2

Vucenik, I., & Shamsuddin, A. M. (2006). Protection against cancer by dietary IP6 and inositol. *Nutrition and Cancer*, *55*(2), 109–125. doi:10.1207/s15327914nc5502_1 PMID:17044765

Wang, H., Ng, T., Ooi, V. E., & Liu, W. (2000). Effects of lectins with different carbohydrate-binding specificities on hepatoma, choriocarcinoma, melanoma and osteosarcoma cell lines. *The International Journal of Biochemistry & Cell Biology*, *32*(3), 365–372. doi:10.1016/S1357-2725(99)00130-2 PMID:10716633

Wolever, T. M., Katzman-Relle, L., Jenkins, A. L., Vuksan, V., Josse, R. G., & Jenkins, D. J. (1994). Glycaemic index of 102 complex carbohydrate foods in patients with diabetes. *Nutrition Research (New York, N.Y.)*, *14*(5), 651–669. doi:10.1016/S0271-5317(05)80201-5

Xu, B., & Chang, S. (2007). A comparative study on phenolic profiles and antioxidant activities of legumes as affected by extraction solvents. *Journal of Food Science*, *72*(2), S159–S166. doi:10.1111/j.1750-3841.2006.00260.x PMID:17995858

Xu, B., & Chang, S. K. (2008). Effect of soaking, boiling, and steaming on total phenolic contentand antioxidant activities of cool season food legumes. *Food Chemistry*, *110*(1), 1–13. doi:10.1016/j.foodchem.2008.01.045 PMID:26050159

Xu, B., & Chang, S. K. (2010). Phenolic substance characterization and chemical and cell-based antioxidant activities of 11 lentils grown in the Northern United States. *Journal of Agricultural and Food Chemistry*, *58*(3), 1509–1517. doi:10.1021/jf903532y PMID:20058926

Xu, B., Yuan, S., & Chang, S. (2007). Comparative analyses of phenolic composition, antioxidant capacity, and color of cool season legumes and other selected food legumes. *Journal of Food Science*, *72*(2), S167–S177. doi:10.1111/j.1750-3841.2006.00261.x PMID:17995859

Xu, B. J., Han, L. K., Zheng, Y. N., Lee, J. H., & Sung, C. K. (2005). In vitro inhibitory effect of triterpenoidal saponins from Platycodi Radix on pancreatic lipase. *Archives of Pharmacal Research*, *28*(2), 180–185. doi:10.1007/BF02977712 PMID:15789748

Zhang, B., Deng, Z., Ramdath, D. D., Tang, Y., Chen, P. X., Liu, R., & Tsao, R. et al. (2015). Phenoli.c profiles of 20 Canadian lentil cultivars and their contribution to antioxidant activity and inhibitory effects on α-glucosidase and pancreatic lipase. *Food Chemistry*, *172*, 862–872. doi:10.1016/j.foodchem.2014.09.144 PMID:25442631

Chapter 4
Health Promoting Effects of Kimchi

Kim Hyun Ju
World Institute of Kimchi, Korea

Han Eung-Soo
World Institute of Kimchi, Korea

ABSTRACT

Kimchi is a traditional Korean food manufactured by fermenting vegetables with probiotic Lactic Acid Bacteria (LAB). Many bacteria are involved in the fermentation of kimchi, but LAB become dominant while the putrefactive bacteria are suppressed during salting of baechu cabbage and the fermentation. The addition of other subingredients and formation of fermentation byproducts of LAB promote the fermentation process of LAB to eventually lead to eradication of putrefactive and pathogenic bacteria, and also increase the functionalities of kimchi. Accordingly, kimchi can be considered a vegetable probiotic food that contributes health benefits in a similar manner as yogurt as a dairy probiotic food. Further, the major ingredients of kimchi are cruciferous vegetables; and other healthy functional foods such as garlic, ginger, red pepper powder, and so on are added to kimchi as subingredients. As all of these ingredients undergo fermentation by LAB, kimchi is regarded as a source of LAB; and the fermentative byproducts from the functional ingredients significantly boost its functionality. Because kimchi is both tasty and highly functional, it is typically served with steamed rice at every Korean meal. Health functionality of kimchi, based upon our research and that of other, includes anticancer, antiobesity, anticonstipation, colorectal health promotion, probiotic properties, cholesterol reduction, fibrolytic effect, antioxidative and antiaging properties, brain health promotion, immune promotion, and skin health promotion. In this review we describe the health functionalities of kimchi and the probiotic properties of its LAB.

DOI: 10.4018/978-1-5225-0591-4.ch004

BLOOD CIRCULATION EFFECTS

Lipid Lowering Effects

Cholesterol in the blood is essential to maintain homeostasis of the human body, being involved in several physiological functions such as producing hormones and vitamins, and maintaining cell membranes, and nerve cells. It is derived from both exogenous dietary sources and endogenous biosynthetic pathways. Dietary cholesterol plays a huge role in serum cholesterol levels, since cholesterol is synthesized to a minimal level for balancing. As diet patterns have been changing towards western style, elevated blood cholesterol is becoming more common. Hypercholesterolemia is one of the major risk factors for cardiovascular disease, and the leading cause of death in many countries (Law et al., 1994). The risk of heart attack is three times higher in those with hypercholesterolemia, compared to those who have normal blood lipid profiles, and it was reported that hypercholesterolemia contributed to 45% of heart attacks in Western Europe and 35% of heart attacks in Central and Eastern Europe from 1999 to 2003 (Yusuf et al., 2004).

In a study investigating blood lipid concentration according to kimchi consumption in middle-aged males, individuals with greater kimchi consumption showed higher dietary fiber and calcium intake, and HDL-cholesterol was positively correlated with kimchi consumption. Meanwhile, there was a positive correlation for salty taste preference with blood neutral lipids and total cholesterol levels, and there was a negative correlation for spicy taste preference with systolic blood pressure, blood neutral lipids, and total cholesterol levels, and these results are consistent with animal studies (Kwon et al., 1999). In one study, the kimchi ingredients known to have a particularly good antioxidant effect were added at 30% the amount of mustard leaf to make cabbage kimchi; this was manufactured into a pill, and when subjects ate 3g per day for 6 weeks, although there was no change in body fat or obesity, blood neutral lipid levels and LDL/HDL-cholesterol ratio significantly decreased. When the water-soluble and water-insoluble fractions of kimchi were made into separate pills, both groups showed a blood lipid-reducing effect, but the water-soluble pill had a greater neutral lipid-reducing effect, and the water-insoluble pill had a greater effect of increasing HDL-cholesterol concentration. Therefore, it is thought that there is a difference in the active ingredients or mechanisms of the two solvent extracts (Choi et al., 2001). These lipid-reducing effects of kimchi and kimchi ingredients have been reported in epidemiological studies, animal studies, and clinical trials. Lactic acid bacteria (LAB) have attracted attention with its cholesterol lowering functionality, especially considering the fact that members of the genera Lactobacillus, Lactococcus, are most commonly given safe or generally recognized as safe (GRAS) status, and the safety of probiotics has been well proved over a long period of experiences. Supplementation of *L. plantarum* CIB 001 can have short-term (6 weeks) effects on blood lipids and liver injury, as well as on the atherogenic index and cardiac risk factors (Cha et al., 2012). Leu. Kimchi GJ2 isolated from kimchi exerts an antiatherosclerotic effect by reducing serum and liver cholesterol levels (Lee et al., 2008). In spite of continued interest in cholesterol lowering potential of LAB strains, all related mechanisms are not fully understood yet, and several hypotheses are still being investigated in an attempt to explain the observed hypocholesterolaemic effects. A study group focused on the effect of 3 LAB strains (*Lactobacillus plantarum* A6a2, *Lactobacillus sakei* C10, *Lactobacillus brevis* J23) isolated from kimchi, for controlling cholesterol efflux in enterocytes, by ATP binding cassette (ABC) transporters, which are direct target genes of liver X receptors (LXR α/ß). *Lactobacillus rhamnosus* LGG was used as control. The treatment of Caco-2 cells with the LAB strains resulted in up-regulation of the LXRs and an increased expression of intestinal sterol efflux transporters ABCG5/ABCG8. Furthermore, cholesterol isotope assay confirmed the results, showing an increase in cholesterol efflux, and therefore, suggesting that up-regulation of LXR-ABCG5/8 is one of the mechanisms for the cholesterol lowering ability of LABs (Kim, 2012). LXRs are ligand-activated transcription factors and key regulators of cholesterol homeostasis. When activated by ligands, they undergo a conformational change that recruits coactivator proteins and regulate transport, catabolism, and elimination of lipid, by enhancing transcription of the target genes. With a microarray analysis of mouse intestine and liver genes, which were up-regulated by a LXR agonist and in vivo studies using knockout mice, it has been proposed that ABCG5 and ABCG8 could promote efflux of cholesterol and sitosterol (plant sterol) (Duan et al., 2004; Jiang et al., 2008)

A *kimchi* pill supplementation (3 g/day) study with 12 middle aged healthy Korean adults showed the atherogenic index for the *kimchi* group decreased compared to placebo group (Choi et al. 2001). High *kimchi* intake (210g/day) improved fasting blood glucose and total serum cholesterol compared to low *kimchi* intake (15g/day) in young healthy adults (Choi et al. 2013, Figure 1).

Antiatherosclerosis Effects

Among serum lipids, cholesterol is the number one risk factor for atherosclerosis. The consumption of kimchi has been reported to have a positive effect on lipid metabolism and the efficacy of kimchi in cholesterol regulation has been confirmed. When lipid metabolism was investigated after feeding white rats with 3%, 5%, and 10% cabbage kimchi feed, blood neutral lipids, blood cholesterol, and phospholipid levels decreases significantly in the kimchi intake groups. In all kimchi groups, the lipid concentration in the liver decreased, and the high-density lipoprotein (HDL) cholesterol levels and fecal lipid excretion function increased. Atherosclerotic index and HMG-CoA reductase activity decreased in the

Figure 1. Changes in plasma biochemical parameters of the subjects after 7 days of kimchi consumption
Source: (Choi et al. 2013).

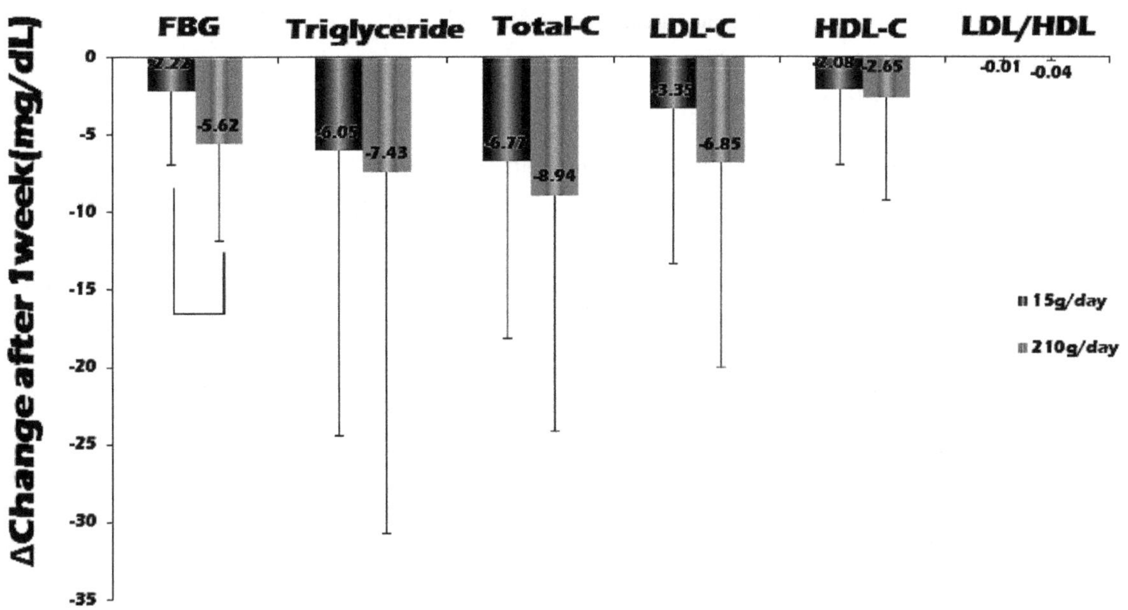

kimchi groups in a concentration-dependent manner. HMG-CoA reductase is an enzyme that controls new cholesterol synthesis, and the fact that its activity decreases with kimchi intake is thought to lead to suppression of new cholesterol synthesis, decreasing blood cholesterol levels (Kwon et al., 1997). In an experiment on rabbits, feeding with kimchi for 12 weeks was reported to have a preventative effect against atherosclerosis, decreasing plasma cholesterol, neutral lipids, very low-density lipoprotein, and LDL concentration, and increasing HDL concentration (Kwon et al., 1998). Oxidative transformation of low-density lipoproteins (LDLs) is highly related to the formation of atherosclerosis. Rabbits that ate cholesterol feed had increase LDL, plasma thiobarbituric acid reactive substance (TBARS), and peroxide value (POV) content by rearing term. However, compared to the control group, these values were decreased in groups that ate cabbage, red pepper powder, and garlic. In particular, lipoperoxide formation was suppressed in chili pepper and garlic groups compared to the control group (Kwon et al., 2003a, 2003b). The active principle, 3-(4'-hydroxyl-3'5'-dimethoxyphenyl) propionic acid (HDMPPA) in *baechu kimchi* responsible for lowering lipid lowering activity also showed anti-atherogenic effects (Lee et al., 2004; Kim et al., 2007; Noh et al., 2013). The β-sitosterol and S-methylcystein sulfoxide in cabbage are reported to have an effect of reducing cholesterol concentration, and the allin and allicin contained in garlic are known to combine with the SH group of coenzyme A to reduce fatty acids, neutral lipids, phospholipids, and cholesterol concentration.

Oxysterols such as 7-ketocholesterol (7-KC) have been reported to be partially responsible for the cytotoxicity of oxLDL and induce endoplasmic reticulum (ER) stress which eventually causes apoptosis. 7-KC causes aberrant ER stress and apoptosis, all of which are inhibited by Kimchi methanol extract (KME) and glutathione. The inhibitory expression of ER stress markers highlights its new protective role against oxLDL-induced ER stress, apoptosis, and subsequent atherosclerosis (Kim et al., 2012). OxLDL strongly induced cell death and lipid peroxidation in THP-1-derived macrophages. However, KME and HDMPPA significantly improved cell viability and inhibited lipid peroxidation induced by oxLDL in THP-1-derived macrophages. Moreover, KME and HDMPPA suppressed CD36 and PPAR-gamma expressions, both of which participate in cholesterol influx. In contrast, KME and HDMPPA augmented LXRα, PPARα, and ABCA1 expression, which are associated with cholesterol efflux. Consequently, KME and HDMPPA suppressed lipid accumulation (Yun et al., 2014, Figure 2).

Antithrombotic Effects

Kimchi consumption has a preventative effect against atherosclerosis because it decreases serum cholesterol levels and has fibrolytic activity, which suppresses blood clotting. Thrombus formation is one of the major causes of atherosclerosis. Accordingly, suppression of thrombosis is known to be an important method for preventing atherosclerosis. In order to investigate the fibrolytic activity of kimchi, white rats were reared for 6 weeks on a diet of 3%, 5%, or 10% added kimchi. When plasma isolated from the blood of these rats was inspected for fibrolytic activity, although there was not a large difference between control group and the 3% and 5% kimchi groups, the 10% kimchi group showed higher fibrolytic activity than the control group. This activity increased with increasing kimchi content. In order to identify the fibrolytic substances in kimchi, based on experimental results such as these, kimchi and kimchi ingredients were first extracted using water and methanol, and the activity of these extract was examined. For water extracts, fibrolytic activity was highest for water dropwort, and was also relatively high in spring onion and radish. Meanwhile, of the methanol extracts, chili pepper showed superior fi-

Figure 2. Inhibitory effect of KME (500 ug/mL) and HDMPPA (50 ug/mL) on lipid accumulation by Oil Red O staining. THP-1-derived macrophages were incubated with or without KME or HDMPPA for 24 h followed by addition of oxLDL (100 mg/mL) for 48 h, following which Oil Red O staining was performed. Stained cells were observed under a microscope (A) and quantified at 510 nm (B). Data are expressed as mean – SD (n = 3, p<0.05). [a~d] *Indicates significant difference*
Source: (Yun et al., 2014).

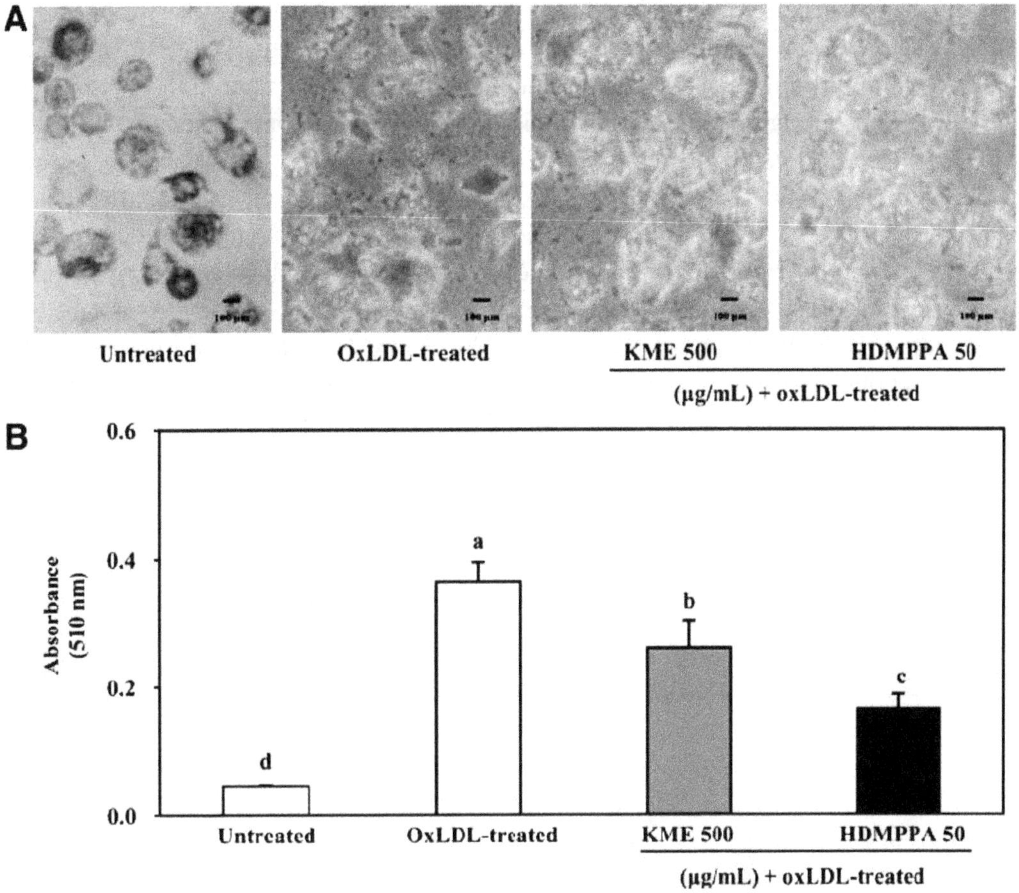

brolytic activity, while radish, kimchi, and spring onion also had high activity. The fibrolytic activity of kimchi methanol extract was higher than water extract, suggesting that the active substances are likely to be non-protein substances. Of the water extracts, fibrolytic activity was highest for water dropwort, followed by spring onion, radish, and cabbage, while for the methanol extracts, activity was highest for red pepper powder, followed by radish, spring onion, and cabbage. The fibrolytic activity of red pepper powder methanol extract was highest of all the ingredients tested (Kim et al., 1998). Meanwhile, when the bacterial strains that produce thrombolytic enzymes were isolated and identified, they were found to be *Bacillus amyloliquefacins*, *Bacillus brevis*, and *Micrococcus luteus* (Noh et al., 1999). Also, of the ingredients in kimchi, garlic in particular has been reported to have thrombolytic properties in clinical studies (Sainani et al., 1979; Ariga et al., 1999), and chilli peppers and salted fish paste are known to have thrombolytic activity (Jang et al., 1998).

Blood Pressure Lowering Effects

Anti-hypertensive effect of Lactobacillus sp. isolated from Kimchi by examining its effects on renal angiotensin-converting enzyme (ACE) inhibitory activity, lipid components and blood pressure using the spontaneously hypertensive rat (SHR) system. Most Lactobacillus sp. extracts (lysozyme, sonication and ethyl acetate extracts) showed higher capacities for the inhibition of ACE activity than those of cultured media. Particularly, LG 7, 8 and 42 of Lactobacillus sp. showed the strongest inhibitory activity among the Lactobacillus sp. extracts. The concentrations of total cholesterol and triglycerides in the serum were lower in the Lactobacillus sp. administration groups than in the control group, but these differences were not significant. The HDL-cholesterol concentrations of the LG 42 administration groups (IX, X) were significantly higher than that of the control group. At 4 weeks, the systolic blood pressure (SBP) in the LG 42 Lactobacillus sp. (1×109 cfu/mL) group (XI) was about 27% lower than that of the control group (V). No adverse effects were observed on the liver and there was no difference in the aspartate aminotransferase (AST) and alanine aminotransferase (ALT) values among groups. The results of this study suggest that long term consumption of LG 42 Lactobacillus sp. may be beneficial to the prevention of high blood pressure (Yu et al., 2009, Figure 3). In leaves of improved Dolsan leaf mustard (DLM) at the 60th day growth, angiotensin converting enzyme (ACE) inhibitory effect was the highest about 94.0%. The cytotoxicity against HepG2 was the highest in roots of DLM. And the anti-oxidative and ACE inhibitory effect in leaves of DLM were higher than those of other parts (Yu, 2004).

*Figure 3. Inhibitory effect of Lactobacillus metabolite (cultured broth) on the ACE; data are expressed as mean ± SD (n=3). *p<0.0005, **p<0.001, ***p<0.005, ****p<0.01, *****p<0.05 (t-test).*
Source: (Yu MH et al., 2009).

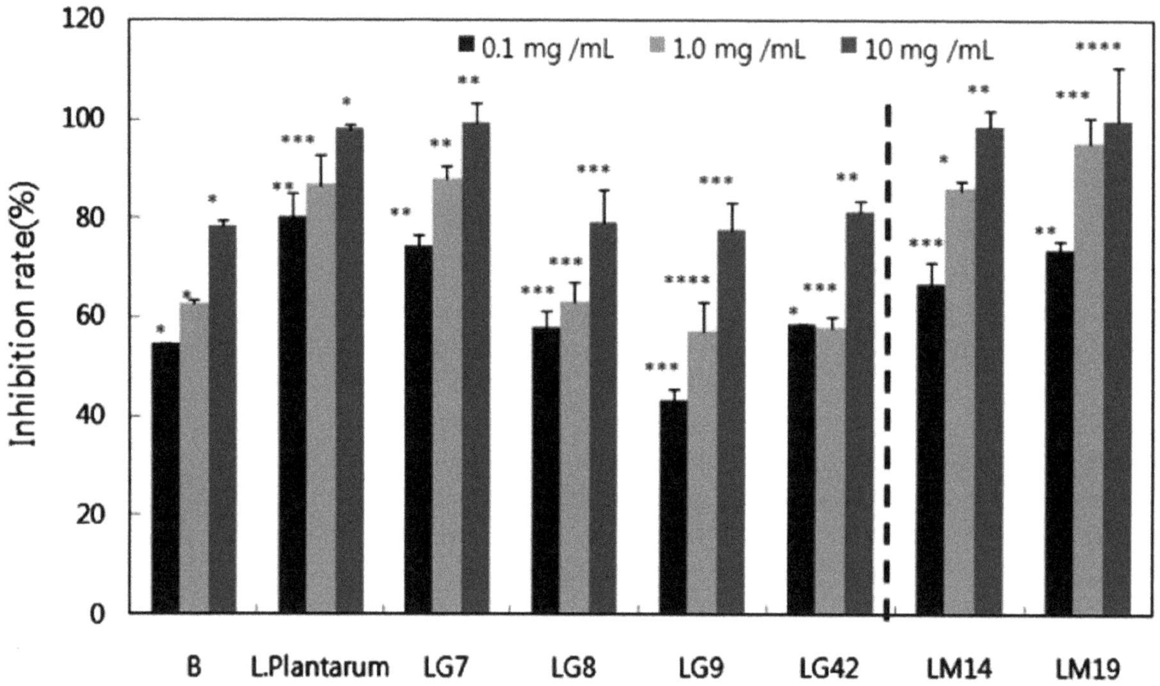

IMMUNE MODULATION EFFECTS

Anticancer Effects

The ingredients in kimchi contain antioxidants (vitamin C, carotin, flavonoids), digestible fiber, sulfurous compounds (glucosinolates, isothiocyanates, indoles, allyl compounds), capsaicin, and peptidoglucans. Because these compounds remove toxic substances from the body and suppress the activation of carcinogens, they have anticancer and antimutagenic effects. Cruciferous vegetables and some of the chemical compounds they contain are known to protect against carcinogens, and to stimulate the activity of phase I and phase II enzymes that act as detoxifying enzymes. In particular, sulforaphane (S-methylsulfinylbutyl isothiocyanate) is a type of isothiocyanate that activates phase II enzymes (glutathione S-transferase, GST), but does not activate some phase I enzymes that contribute to the activation of procarcinogens to carcinogens. Recently, there has been increasing interest in the chemoprotection of sulforaphane-containing cruciferous vegetables. These vegetables contain several types of isothiocyanate, including sulforaphane, and these isothiocyanates have anticancer and anticarcinogenic effects in numerous animal organs, such as the liver, kidneys, and small intestine.

The first stage in the development of cancer involves normal cells undergoing genetic mutations due to carcinogens. After making a methanol extract of cabbage kimchi and its fractions and applying them to the Ames test and SOS chromotest, which are tests of *in vitro* antimutagenic activity, a mutation-suppressing effect was observed for mutations caused by the carcinogens MNNG and AFB1. Also, when mouse embryo cells (C3H/10T1/2 cell) were exposed to the carcinogen MCA, foci of morphologically altered cells formed, but the extract reduced the total number of type II and type III foci (reduction rate 92%) and possible cancers in mice were considerably suppressed (Park, 1995, 2014).

There has recently been a lot of research on the anticancer effects of kimchi and kimchi extracts. *In vitro* anticancer tests, such as the SRB test, MTT test, and the growth inhibition test have shown Kimchi extracts to suppress the proliferation of human cancer cells such as AGS human gastric cancer cells, HT-29 human colon adenocarcinoma cells, MG 63 human osteosarcoma cells, HL-60 human leukemia cells, and Hep 3B human hepatoma cells. Kimchi fractions also inhibited DNA synthesis in cancer cells. When a sarcoma 180 cell was grafted into a particular mouse line (Balb/c mouse) and the mouse was administered with kimchi extract, measurements of the change in tumor weight showed that kimchi extract had a tumor growth-suppressing effect *in vivo*, as well (Lee et al., 1996; Oh et al., 1993).

Furthermore, colonic *Lactobacilli* from kimchi that have reached the colon via the stomach have been found to suppress the activity of enzymes like b-glucosidase and b-glucuronidase, which convert procarcinogens into carcinogens. This has been reported to be related to the low incidence of colon cancer in Korean individuals (Lee et al., 1996; Oh et al., 1993).

There are a large number of epidemiological survey results suggesting that the cabbage, garlic, and onions used in kimchi have a cancer suppressing effect in humans. When the Harvard Medical School in the United States surveyed the lifestyles of 47,909 bladder cancer patients between 1986 and 1996, they found that the incidence of bladder cancer was lower with increasing consumption of cabbage and other cruciferous vegetables, and cabbage and broccoli were particularly reported to reduce the risk of bladder cancer (Michaud et al., 1999). Also, when the lifestyles of 129 brain cancer patients were surveyed in China between 1993 and 1995, brain cancer incidence was reported to be lower in individuals who ate fresh vegetables, especially cabbage and onions, and people who ate fresh fish (Hu et al., 1999). There is an inverse correlation between the risk of lung cancer and intake of cabbage, cauliflower, and broccoli, and consumption of *Brassica* has also been reported to have an inverse correlation with gastric cancer (Vehoeven et al., 1996). At Austria's Wien University, cabbage and garlic were reported to have a protective effect against cancer (Frohlich et al., 1997). There are also reports that garlic can reduce the risk of cancer. The Unites States National Cancer Institute (NCI) discovered that the residents of Changshan County in China's Shandong Province had a low prevalence of stomach cancer and surveyed 214 residents. The results showed that garlic consumption was inversely correlated with *Helicobacter pylori* infection, and it was estimated that garlic could suppress the progression of early-stage gastric cancer (You et al., 1998). When a dietary survey was conducted on 223 colorectal cancer patients in Lausanne, Switzerland, from 1992 to 1997, garlic was concluded to have the highest protective effect against cancer (Levi et al., 1999). When 345 breast cancer patients were surveyed in France from 1986 to 1989, the risk of breast cancer was reported to decrease with increased fiber, garlic, and onion consumption (Challier et al., 1998).

Mutation Preventing Effects

Several ingredients and Lactobacilli in kimchi contribute to fermentation, and their immune activity-promoting action is recently becoming a subject of interest. Kimchi extracts lead to increased phagocytic activity by phagocytes *in vitro* and *in vivo*. Macrophages become active when they are simulated by exogenous infections, which leads to a process of proliferation involving spreading, phagocytic activity, pinocytosis, lysozymes, and cytoplasmic granules, and ultimately result in antibacterial and antitumoral activity. Among extracts, kimchi that has been fermented for 3 weeks showed higher activity (Choi et al., 1997). Also, kimchi solvent extracts show immune strengthening activity, increasing the production of interleukin-2 and the activity of natural killer (NK) cells (Kim et al., 1998), and they also have a positive effect on the immune system, including promoting the production of NO by macrophages, regulating transforming growth factor b1 (TGF-β1) in cancer cells, and production if interleukin-6 by spleen cells (Kim et al., 2001). Meanwhile, immune activity-strengthening action has also been demonstrated for kimchi *Lactobacilli*. When ascites tumor was induced in mice using sarcoma-180 cells before orally administering kimchi *Lactobacilli* homogenate, immune activity increased compared to the untreated group. Intestinally secreted IgA is a major index for protective action against infectious bacteria in the gut, and IgA was lowest in normal mice treated with *Lactobacilli*, followed by cholangiocarcinoma mice (ascites tumor induced with sarcoma-180) treated with *Lactobacilli*, untreated normal mice, and untreated cholangiocarcinoma mice. These results demonstrate that, even in cholangiocarcinoma mice, administration with *Lactobacilli* resulted in an increased in intestinal antibody secretion compared to the untreated group. Moreover, macrophages isolated from the *Lactobacilli*-treated group showed 66% increased NO production compared to macrophages isolated from the untreated group, and even for cholangiocarcinoma mice, NO production increased for the *Lactobacilli*-treated group by 12–27%, depending on the stimulator, compared to the untreated group. This shows that, when kimchi *Lactobacilli* are administered to cholangiocarcinoma mice, although there is a slight decrease in abdominal macrophages compared to healthy mice, there is an immune-activating effect and this effect can be seen to contribute to suppression of ascites tumors and solid tumors (Shin et al., 1998; Korea Food Research Institute, 1997; Yu, 1995). In conclusion, kimchi demonstrates various immune activity-promoting effects, such as partially increasing the proliferation speed of immune cells in the spleen and small intestine, increasing the production of NO by abdominal macrophages, increasing the production of IgA secreted in the colon, increasing the concentration of interleukin-2, and increasing the number of specific antibody cells. When the yeast

Candida albicans is administered to mice and they are fed appropriately matured kimchi (pH 4.3, acidity 0.6%), macrophage activity doubles. Kimchi consumption considerably increases the activity of NK cells, increasing anticancer function. Lactobacilli from Kimchi may modulate the Th1/Th2 balance via macrophage activation in the hypersensitive reaction caused by Th2 cells (Won et al., 2011).

Asthma Preventing Effects

Asthma is an inflammatory disease characterized by bronchial hyper-responsiveness that can proceed to life-threatening airway obstruction. The T helper 2 (Th2)-type cytokines interleukins-4 (IL-4), IL-5, and IL-13, produced by activated CD4+ T cells play a central role in the pathogenesis of asthma by controlling the key process of immunoglobulin E (IgE) production, growth of mast cells and the differentiation and activation of mast cells and eosinophils (Corrigan et al., 1993; Renz et al., 1993). In contrast, Th1 cytokines such as interferon-γ (IFN-γ) and IL-12, which down-regulate Th2 responses, inhibit the development of allergic lung inflammation [13,39]. Thus, interventions that inhibit Th2 cytokines by enhancing Th1 cytokine production, may be useful in the treatment of allergic asthma [36].

The relationship between dietary factors and asthma in a representative population-based sample of 19,659 men and women, aged 19-64 years, using data from the fourth and fifth Korean National Health and Nutrition Examination Survey (KNHANES), 2007-2011 was studied. The prevalence of asthma in Korean adults was 2.4%. Adults with asthma consumed fewer amounts of kimchi (P=.0444) and fish (P=.0175) but had a higher cereal intake than those without asthma (P=.0056). Multiple logistic regression analysis after controlling for confounding factors showed a significant inverse relationship between kimchi consumption and the prevalence of asthma [odds ratio (95% confidence interval) for subjects consuming 1 to <2 servings (40-79.9 g), 2 to <3 servings (80-119.9 g), and ≥3 servings (≥120 g), relative to those consuming <1 serving (<40 g): 0.726 (0.534-0.987), 0.506 (0.348-0.736), and 0.678 (0.502-0.916), respectively; P for trend=0.0131]. These results warrant future studies to explore the mechanisms responsible for the association between kimchi consumption and asthma (Kim et al., 2014). Probiotics have been shown to be effective in reducing symptoms. Three heat-killed lactobacilli, Lactobacillus plantarum, Lactobacillus curvatus and Lactobacillus sakei subsp sakei, isolated from kimchi, exerted inhibitory effects on airway hyper-responsiveness in a murine asthma model (Hong et al., 2010).

Anti-Viral Effects

Kimchi *Lactobacilli* have proven treatment effects against the influenza virus, bacterial diseases, and especially against avian influenza, and the reason that Korea suffered less loss from SARS or avian influenza has been revealed to be because of the immune function-strengthening effects of kimchi.

Influenza A viruses belong to the family Orthomyxoviridae and contain a genome composed of eight segments of single-stranded, negativesense RNA that each encodes one or two proteins (Neumann et al., 2009). 'Spanish influenza (H1N1). The pandemic of 1918-1919 killed as many as 50 million people worldwide, and remains unprecedented in its severity. The mortality pattern of the 'Spanish' influenza was unusual with high mortality rates for young adults. The typical mortality pattern observed with the Spanish influenza remains unexplained to date. 'Asian' influenza (H2N2). The 'Asian' influenza originated in Southern China in February 1957. From there, it spread to Singapore (March 1957), Hong Kong (April 1957), Japan (May 1957), and the United States and United Kingdom (October 1957). A second wave was detected in January 1958. In the United States, excess mortality was estimated to be

70,000. The pandemic was caused by a human/avian reassortant that introduced avian virus H2 HA and N2 NA genes into human populations. Furthermore, the Asian influenza virus also possessed a PB1 gene of avian virus origin (Gabriele Neumann et al., 2009).

Avian influenza (AI) is caused by viruses that are classified as members of the family Orthomyxoviridae and genus Influenzavirus A (Swayne & Suarez, 2000). These are pleomorphic RNA viruses with helical symmetry and glycoprotein projections from the envelope that have hemagglutinin (HA) and neuraminidase (NA) (Calnek et al., 1997). AI is classified into subtypes according to the combination of 16 HA and 9 NA molecules (Fouchier et al., 2005).

The antiviral efficacy of *L. plantarum* YML009 was compared with oseltamivir (Tamiflu). It was shown that YML009 proved tobemore effective than Tamiflu. Therefore, based on our results, it could be concluded that *L. plantarum* YML009 may be a novel probiotic candidate as anti-influenza prevention and infection. The study ends with the developmentofan anti-influenza probiotic candidate *L. plantarum* YML009 (Choi, 2014). Avian Influenza virus can be synergistically reduced in combination with probiotics therapy and there are resultant different mechanisms of action. *Leu. mesenteroides* YML003 has antiviral activities against LPAI H9N2 virus, after proper in vivo experiments; it may become a candidate to be applied to animals and humans (Seo, 2012a, 2012b).

Probiotics was first defined as "substances" produced by microorganisms that stimulate the growth of other microorganisms (Lilley et al., 1965). It was discovered that some bacteria were able to multiply and colonize an area more efficiently in the presence of "helpful" bacteria. This is particularly true for normal microflora residing in the gut of human and animals. It was observed that bacteria or their products commonly used for food preparations or food supplements were able to improve the growth of normal microflora in the gut of individuals as well as provide substantial protection against gastrointestinal diseases. Hence, it was proposed that the concept of probiotics be redefined as "viable microbial agents which, when used in animal or man, beneficially affects the host possibly by improving the balance of the indigenous microflora" (Salminen et al., 1999). Several lactic acid bacteria belonging to the *Lactobacillus*, *Leuconostoc*, *Lactococcus* species isolated from kimchi as well as *Enterococcus* isolated from Korean shrimp possess antiviral properties against porcine epidemic diarrhea virus (PEDV). The antiviral compounds are heat tolerant and showed moderate resistance to proteolytic digestion by trypsin (Cruz, 2006).

GUT MICROBIOTA IMPROVING EFFECTS

Obesity Preventing Effects

Kimchi has the ability to help prevent obesity, and it contains compounds with this functionality. In order to prevent obesity, there is a need for functions that promote energy metabolism, functions that promote burning of body fats, and functions that promote restriction and excretion of calorie intake. In other words, calorie intake must be restricted, energy metabolism must be promoted, and stored body fats must be broken down and burned off. Also, fecal excretion should be aided as a way of sending the energy and waste products in organs outside of the body (van der Klaauw, 2015).

The capsaicin in chili peppers that gives kimchi its spicy flavor displays several types of physiological activity, and of these, it plays an important role in obesity treatment and prevention. The capsaicin in chili peppers acts to promote energy metabolism, and in particular the burning of fats. Capsaicin stimulates the parasympathetic nervous system, increasing the secretion of adrenalin. This promotes the catalysis of white fat tissues and increases heat production by the body's energy-consuming brown fat cells, which results in the overall breakdown of body fats and a decrease in the amount of fat accumulated in the body (Lee et al., 2013). 3T3-L1 cells were treated with capsaicin with medium to observe the change in the expression of the obesity-related genes by using dot blot assay. As results, the treatment with capsaicin caused an up-regulation of the UCP-2 expression. And decrease body weight, serum triglyceride, serum total cholesterol and white adipose tissue (Lee, 2003). A group eating a high-fat diet with 5% added red pepper powder and a group eating a diet with 10% added kimchi (5% red pepper powder content) both showed a significant decrease in body weight compared to a group fed only a high-fat diet. Furthermore, body fat decrease even more in the group with added kimchi with red pepper powder and other kimchi ingredients, than in the group with the same amount of red pepper powder added by itself. Even when eating a high-fat diet, when kimchi was consumed at the same time, a similar body weight to the control group was maintained (Park, 1995). According to studies in humans, after eating 5g of red pepper powder (approximately the amount in 100g of kimchi) the increase in energy metabolism reached its peak within 60 minutes (approximately 40% increase), and after that, it gradually declined. Also, when the effect of capsaicin on heat production was investigated during a high-sugar, high-fat diet, it was reported to promote body heat production and increase burning of body fats, demonstrating a clear body fat-reducing effect, and suggesting that it would be capable of suppressing obesity (Galgani et al., 2010). Kimchi also acts to promote energy metabolism. Some of the functional, physiologically active substances in kimchi act to promote metabolism of energy-producing nutrients (especially lipids, sugars, etc.). Kimchi contains vitamin B complexes such as thiamine, riboflavin, niacin, and pantothenic acid, which act as coenzymes for various enzymes that participate directly in sugar and fat metabolism in the body. Kimchi also contains citric acid and acetic acid generated by *Lactobacillus* fermentation. Meanwhile, the most proactive method for preventing and treating obesity is the restriction of calories intake (especially sugars and fats), reducing the digestion and absorption of calories that have been consumed, and excretion outside of the body. The important substance that performs these roles is digestible fiber, and there it is contained in abundance in kimchi. The digestible fiber in kimchi helps to restrict calorie consumption, alleviate constipation, and promote excretion, which are important roles in the prevention and treatment of obesity. Soluble fiber has various types of physiological activity, but the most important actions are to give a feeling of satiety and the delay the absorption of glucose. Soluble fiber is easily dissolved in the gut, and during this process, it expands and becomes viscous, giving a sense of satiety. Accordingly, due to the feeling of fullness and the lack of appetite, food (calorie) consumption decreases. Soluble fiber also has the secondary function of making absorption and usage of digested glucose slower. Meanwhile, insoluble fiber cannot be digested by the human digestive system, and it is excreted without change. In particular, insoluble fiber increases the amount of feces, and so improves the speed of fecal excretion and aids the excretion of some waste substances and calories outside of the body. There are large amount of both soluble and insoluble fiber in kimchi (Cheigh & Park, 1994).

Kimchi has few calories compared to other foods, and because it contains large quantities of digestible fiber, it gives a sense of satiety, and it acts to remove waste substances from the gut to the outside of the body, helping regulation of body weight (Cheigh & Park, 1994). Moreover, when kimchi has been matured appropriately, its weight-loss effect increases (Kim et al., 2011). Also, when the effect of capsaicin on heat production was investigated during a high-sugar, high-fat diet, it was reported to promote the production of heat in the body, and to increase burning of body fats, providing a clear body fat-reducing effect and suggesting that it could help to suppress obesity (Kawada et al., 1986). In terms of its weight-loss, the capsaicin in red pepper powder promotes the breakdown of fats and increases heat production, raising energy consumption. According to a study in humans, following the consumption of 5g of red pepper powder (the amount in approximately 100g of kimchi), the increase in energy metabolism reached a peak within 60 minutes (approximately 40% increase) and then gradually declined. Also, when the effect of capsaicin on heat production was investigated during a high-sugar, high-fat diet, it was reported to promote the production of heat in the body, and to increase burning of body fats, providing a clear body fat-reducing effect and suggesting that it could help to suppress obesity (Kang, 2009). The intake of fermented red pepper during the weight control program decreased the body fat especially abdominal fat and prevent the decline of RMR during weight reduction period (Chang et al., 2003). Red pepper powder and kimchi stimulated the lipid metabolism of blood and adipose tissues (Choi, 2001).

There has also been a study on the effects of kimchi consumption and exercise on body composition and blood lipids in obese female middle school students. The subjects were divided into an exercise and kimchi consumption group (EKG), an exercise group (EG), a kimchi consumption group (KG), and a control group (CG). The experiment was conducted for 6 weeks, but during the experiment period, the average daily kimchi consumption in the EKG and KG was approximately 40g, which is less than the average daily consumption for the total Korean population. The results showed that the EKG and the KG demonstrated a significant decrease in body weight, BMI, obesity, total body fat, body fat percentage, and abdominal fat compared to the other groups. In particular, during the course of the experiment obesity changes were -5.82% for the EKG, -4.43% for the KG, and -3.16% for the EG, demonstrating a clear effect of kimchi consumption in the partial treatment of obesity across several parameters, including body weight and body composition, and confirming that the weight-loss effects are even greater when kimchi consumption is combined with exercise (Baek, 2001). W. koreensis OK1-6 supplementation has the potential antiobesity and glycemic control effect in mice fed a high-fat diet, which may be mediated by inhibiting body fat accumulations, altering lipid profile in liver and serum, down-regulating obesity related gene expressions in liver, and alleviating the insulin resistance. Kimch manufactured with the starter of the ornithine-producing lactic acid bacteria Weissella koreensis OK1-6 can be used as functional food in Korean diet and its health-promoting effect could be beneficial for preventing obesity and obesity-induced diabetes (Park et al., 2012). Twenty-two obese patients, who's BMI (basal metabolic index) was 25 kg/m2, did not have any fermented food including Kimchi for 2 weeks. The 22 patients then were randomly ordered two 4-week diet phases that were separated by a 4-week washout period (cross-over design). During each diet phase, the subjects consumed either fresh Kimchi or Kimchi ripened for 10 days (fermented Kimchi). In this 4-month-experiment, ingestion of Kimchi showed positive effects on various factors associated with metabolic syndrome (weight, BMI, waist to hip ratio, body fat percentage). Even more, positive effects including decreased systolic/diastolic BP, % body fat, fasting glucose, total cholesterol, and decreased trend of fasting insulin and leptin were shown after ingestion of fermented Kimchi compared to fresh Kimchi (Ahn, 2011).

Symbiotic Effects

Accumulating evidence suggests relationship of compositional changes of gut microbiota with onset of metabolic disorders and obesity. Kimchi, a traditional Korean side dish, is known for its beneficial impact on metabolic parameters and anti-obesity effects. Twenty-four obese women were randomly assigned to either fresh or fermented kimchi group for eight weeks of kimchi intervention. Pyrosequencing of fecal microbiota and microarray analyses of blood samples revealed that fresh and fermented kimchi interventions exerted differential effects on the obesity-related clinical parameters. Correlations of these effects with changes in blood gene expression and gut microbial population were more evident in the fermented kimchi group than the fresh kimchi group (Han et al., 2015, Figure 4).

ANTI-OXIDANT EFFECTS

Kimchi contains antioxidants (or free radical scavengers) that prevent lipid peroxidation and remove reactive oxygen species (ROS) and various free radicals (Cheigh, 1999).

Antioxidants in kimchi include polyphenols, such as carotenoids, flavonoids, and anthocyanins, as well as chlorophylls, and vitamin C and E. As kimchi's main ingredient, cabbage also contains antioxidant flavonols, such as hydroxybenzoic acid, hydroxycinnamic acid, kaempferol, and quercetin, as well as chlorophylls and carotenoids. In terms of spices, when the alcohol extracts of chili pepper seeds and chili pepper skin were added to soybeans and the ability to suppress peroxide formation was compared, chili pepper skin powder had a stronger antioxidant effect, and this was reported to result from tocopherols, carotenoids, and capsaicin (Cheigh & Park, 1994). Garlic contains substances such as allinin, garlic acid, and scorinin, and the ethanol fraction of garlic suppresses the production of lipoperoxide. The ethanol fraction of garlic contains sulfides, and it is probable that garlic's antioxidizing effect is related to the reducing nature of sulfide sulfhydryl (-SH) groups (Chan, 2013). Meanwhile, when the organic solvent extract of ginger was added to soybean oil in different concentrations to investigate its antioxidizing effect, all treatment groups showed an antioxidizing effect. The 3% solution was a superior antioxidant to tocopherol, and a similar level to butylated hydroxy anisol (BHA). Ginger's flavor components, such as gingerol, gingeron, and shogaol, are also known to act as antioxidants (Butt, 2011). Spring onion also contains antioxidant flavonoids, including quercetin 4'-O-b-D-glucoside, quercetin 3, 4'-O-bis-glucoside, and quercetin 7-4'-O-bis-glucoside, and has high levels of b-carotene and ascorbic acid (Jang et al., 1991; Han et al., 1995). The green parts of chives contain kaempferol 3-O-b-D-glucoside, kaempferol 3-O-b-xylosyl-D-glucoside, and quercetin 3-O-glucoside, which contribute to the antoxidizing effect (Jang et al., 1991; Jung et al., 1999; Lee et al., 1988).

Skin Care Effects

Kimchi contains antioxidants like vitamin C, polyphenol compounds, and chlorophyll, and so it inhibits the production of ROS within the body and eliminates them, suppressing aging and damage to skin cells in particular, while also protecting the skin from ultraviolet (UV) light. Kimchi solvent extracts have an effect of suppressing skin aging. When keratinocytes, the main epidermal cells, were artificially given an oxidizing stimulus by short-term exposure to hydrogen peroxide, and extracts from kimchi of different fermentation periods (1–5 weeks) were tested for detoxifying effect against hydrogen peroxide, 2-week fermented kimchi had by far the strongest effect. Inhibitory effects against oxidative stress from long-term exposure showed a similar tendency. When hydrogen peroxide was applied to fibroblasts, hypodermal cells in the skin, 2-week fermented kimchi showed the strongest cytotoxicity-suppressing effect among the different kimchi extracts (Ryu et al., 1997; Ryu et al., 1997). There are also results for kimchi's preventative effect against skin aging in hairless mice. Hairless mice that consumed cabbage kimchi, mustard lead kimchi, and chive kimchi had a thicker epidermis and thinner keratinized layer than the control group, as well as greater new collagen formation, demonstrating a preventative effect

Figure 4. Comparison of relative abundance of gut microbiota after eight weeks of kimchi intervention. Fecal samples were collected three times, before the initiation as well as after one and eight weeks of the intervention. (A) The compositions of phyla in the samples of a particular time-period were compared using bar plots. (B) The time-dependent compositional changes of major phylum are shown in line plots. (C) The compositions of genus in the samples of a particular time-period were compared using bar plots. (D) The time-dependent compositional changes of major genus are shown in line plots.
Source: (Han K et al., 2015).

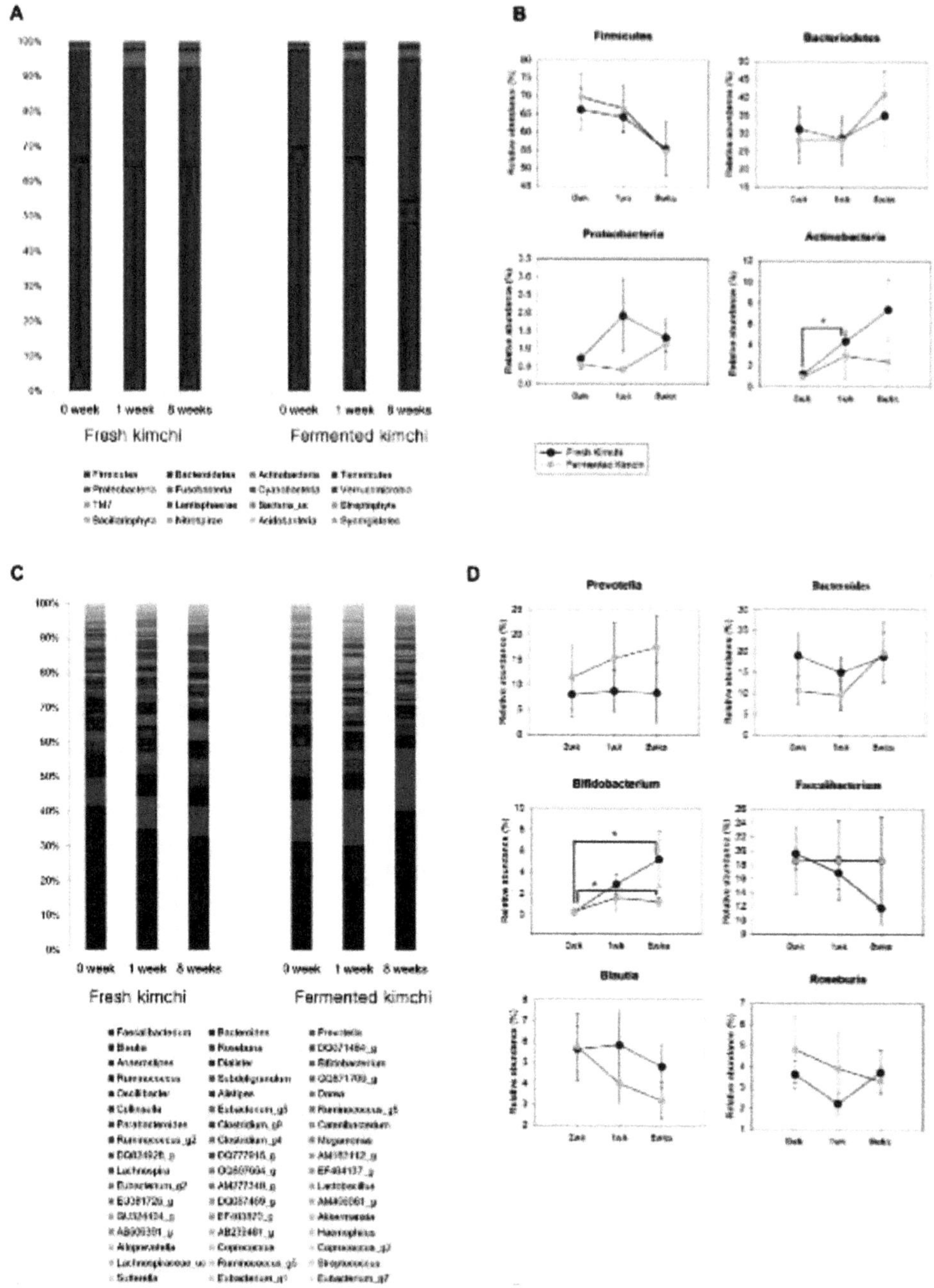

of kimchi consumption against skin aging. In a study looking at the cytotoxicity-suppressing effects of kimchi extract according to the method for inducing ROS, 2-week fermented kimchi had the greatest effect, while 0-week and 3-week fermented kimchi also showed an effect, but the effects were not as clear as they were in keratinocytes. The fermentation period-dependent difference in effect that was shown by this study is assumed to be due to changes in kimchi constituents according to fermentation time. As the skin ages, the thickness of the epidermis and the amount of collagen in the hypodermis decrease, while mucopolysaccharides increase. However, in the added kimchi group, the change in collagen content and the activity of fibroblasts were slower compared to the control group, and cytomorphological changes were observed in the mustard lead kimchi group in particular. In addition, the rate of keratinization of the skin was also slower in the kimchi group, and this trend of delayed skin aging was greater in the mustard leaf kimchi and chive kimchi groups compared to the cabbage kimchi group (Ryu et al. 2004). As physiological aging progresses, the epidermis becomes thinner and there is an increase in cytokeratine, which participates in skin keratinization. Furthermore, the activity of rough endoplasmic reticulum (RER) in hypodermal fibroblasts decreases, impairing collagen production (Gilchrest, 1984). However, in studies investigating the anti-skin aging activity of cabbage kimchi, mustard leaf kimchi, and chive kimchi, the hairless mice in the kimchi consumption groups had a thicker epidermis and thinner keratinized layer in their skin than the control group, and the mustard leaf kimchi and cabbage kimchi groups had far greater development of the hypodermal RER, demonstrating a preventative effect of kimchi consumption against skin aging. Also, there was an effect of reducing lipid oxidation in skin homogenate, and the cabbage kimchi group had low TBARS content in the EtOAc layer, as shown in Figure 5. The mustard leaf kimchi group had low TBARS in the EtOAc and CH_2Cl_2 layers, and this group in particular was found to have a ROS-eliminating effect as well. The fractions of these types of kimchi in different solvents were found to have hydrogen-donating activity, peroxide-inhibiting activity, and a protective effect against UV rays, but these effects were slightly different according to the kimchi type and extracted fraction (Gilchrest, 1984). When several kimchi solvent fractions were added to a cream and applied to the back of hairless mice before exposure to UV, there was less erythema for the CH_2Cl_2 layer for cabbage kimchi, the EtOAc layer for mustard lead kimchi, and the H_2O layer for chive kimchi, which shows that these fraction layers contain protective substances against UV radiation. Here, the protective effect differs according to the type of kimchi, with slightly more erythema occurring for chive kimchi than for cabbage kimchi or mustard leaf kimchi, and in particular, the hexane layer of chive kimchi had a weaker effect for suppressing erythema. This is thought to be because cabbage kimchi and mustard leaf kimchi, in addition to chlorophylls, also contain carotenoids, which have antioxidant and light-protective effects, but chive kimchi contains only chlorophylls (Ryu, 2000).

Anti-Aging Effect

There are also studies investigating the *in vivo* effects on senescence-accelerated mice (SAM) of types of kimchi that were found to have anti-aging functions *in vitro*. In groups that consumed kimchi, there was a blood lipid-reducing effect, and HMG-CoA reductase activity was lower than the control group. Also, in SAM that consumed kimchi, when looking at total ROS, antioxidant enzyme activity, and lipid concentration in various organs with age, although there were differences according to the kimchi ingredients, the organ, and the amount of aging, the kimchi consumption groups showed a clear anti-aging effect in terms of *in vivo* lipid composition, antioxidant enzyme activity, etc. Also, the concentration

*Figure 5. Antioxidant effect of solvent fractions of various kimchi on UV-irradiated mouse skin homogenate; Values are means ± SD (n=3). CH_2Cl_2, EtOAC, and BuOH were expressed dichloromethane, ethylacetate, and butanol respectively. *Significantly different from control at p<0.01. **Significantly different from control at p<0.05.*
Source: (Ryu BM et al., 2004).

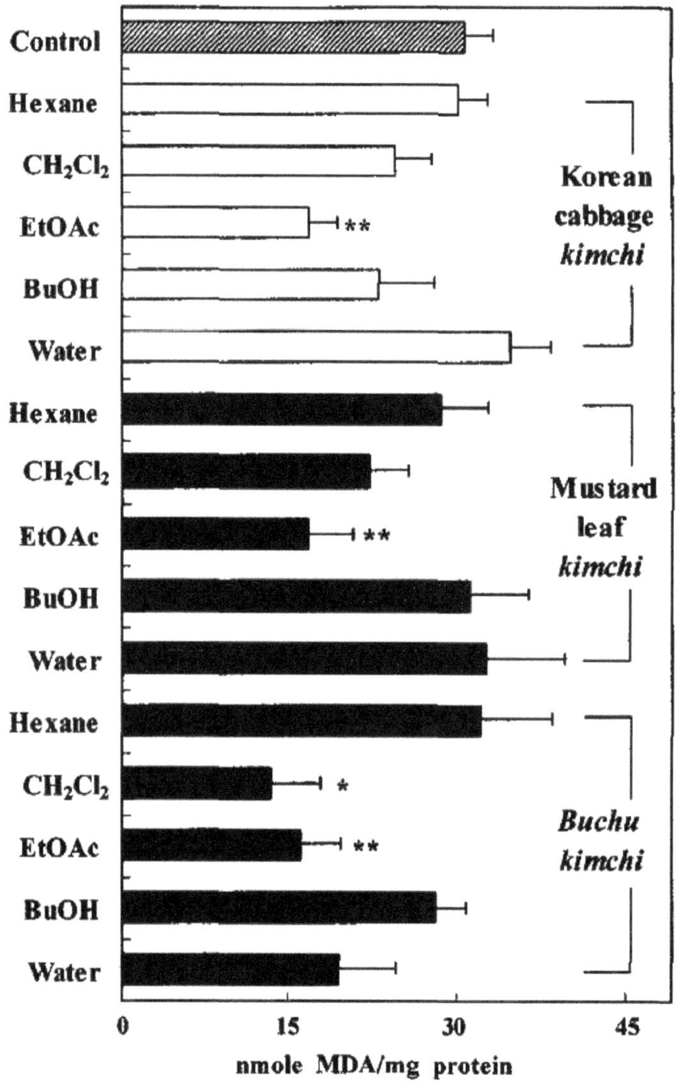

of lipofuscin, which is produced in the eye due to aging, was much lower in SAM that were fed kimchi (Lee, 2001). Exopolysaccharides produced by Bacillus Sp. Strains isolated from Korea fermented food, kimchi, has antioxidant and antiaging activity (Song, 2010).

In order to determine whether kimchi consumption has an anti-aging effect in humans, kimchi consumption was investigated in 20–29 year olds (n=93) and a 65-and-over elderly group (n=143) residing in the Gyeongsangnam-do region. After obtaining a blood sample, indices of aging such as total free radicals, OH radicals, GSH, GSSG, GSH/GSSG, and TBARS were measured, and the results are very interesting. When the surveyed subjects were divided into a high kimchi consumption and a low kimchi consumption group based on the average kimchi consumption of 112g, there was no significant difference within the 20–29 year old group, but in the elderly group, those subjects who consumed more than the average amount of kimchi had 21% and 26% lower total free radicals and OH radicals, respectively ($p<0.05$), while the antioxidant GSH and the GSH/GSSG ratio increased 8% an 12% ($p<0.05$), and there was no difference in GSSG concentration. This result provides one piece of evidence that kimchi consumption suppresses aging in humans. Also, a negative correlation between kimchi consumption and total free radicals ($r=-0.1862$) was established, while a positive correlation was established with GSH/GSSG ($r=0.1861$). Generally, in the human body, blood lipid concentration, TBARS, and free radical concentration increase with aging, and there is also a reduction in the antioxidation system GSH/GSSG, which acts to protect against aging, such that tissue damage due to oxidation cannot be suppressed, and this results in the progression of aging. In this study, there was little effect of kimchi consumption in 20–29 year olds, but in the elderly who consumed more than the average amount of kimchi, free radical production was suppressed, and the antioxidant system that responds to free radicals was enhanced (Kim et al., 2002a, b). As a result, we can expect that tissue damage due to oxidation would be inhibited and ultimately, kimchi consumption would suppress aging in the human body. The treatment of kimchi, especially optimally ripened kimchi (pH 4.1) attenuated cellular oxidative stress through increase in cell viability and inhibition of lipid peroxidation. In addition, the lifespan of young-, middle-, and old-aged WI-38 cell was extended, suggesting promising role of kimchi as an anti-aging agent. Kimchi during fermentation downregulated the age-related inflammatory gene expressions, NF-κB, COX-2, and iNOS. The present results indicate that anti-aging effect of kimchi against oxidative stress is related to extension of lifespan in HDFs as well as downregulations of mRNA and protein expressions of COX-2 and iNOS through NF-κB regulation. Therefore, this study suggests that kimchi, especially fermented kimchi, is a promising anti-aging functional food with protective activities against aging induced oxidative stress induced premature senescence (Kim et al., 2011).

OTHER HEALTH PROMOTING EFFECTS

Digestion Promoting Effects

Several investigators have observed that a high fiber diet causes a great fecal excretion and alter in vitro or in vivo digestibility of food proteins (Pantack et al., 1976). Reduction of in vitro digestibility by Godulbaegi was greater than that by fermented kimchi, but there was no a stepwise reduction in digestibility by the increased plant-to-protein weiht ratio. This indicates that the fiber constituents in raw Godulbaegi were more active in interfering with protein sources when compared to fermented plants (kimchi) (Hwang ct al., 1995). The amlyolytic enzymes (α-amlyase, β-amlyase, glucoamlyase) and protease of kimchi showed the highest activity at the 2nd day of fermentation at 20°C (Hahn et al., 2002, Figure 6).

Diabetes Alleviation Effects

Consumption of both fresh (1-day-old) and fermented (10-day-old) kimchi significantly decreased body weight, body mass index, and waist circumference. Fermented kimchi had additional effects on blood

Figure 6. Changes in pH, acicity, β-amlyase, α-amlyase and glucoamlyase activity of Kimchi during fermentation
Source: (Hahn YS et al., 2002).

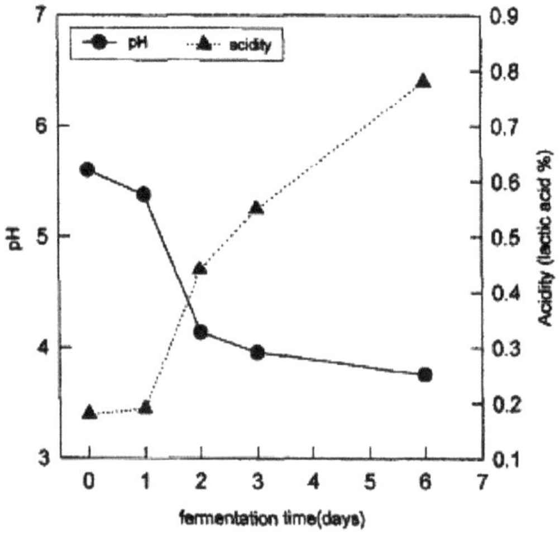

(A) Changes in pH and acidity of Kimchi during fermentation

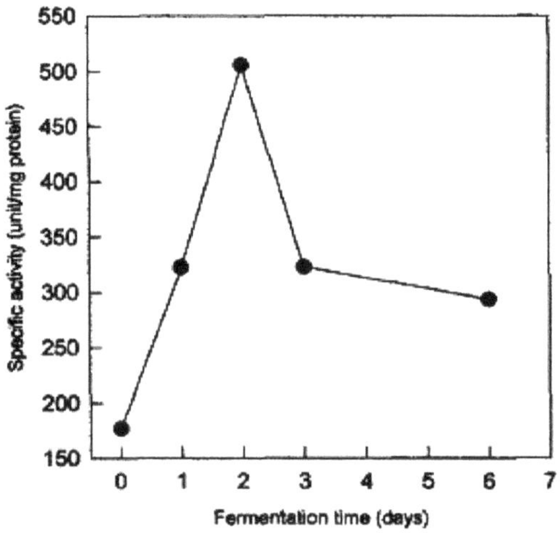

(B) Changes in β-amlyase activity of Kimchi during fermentation

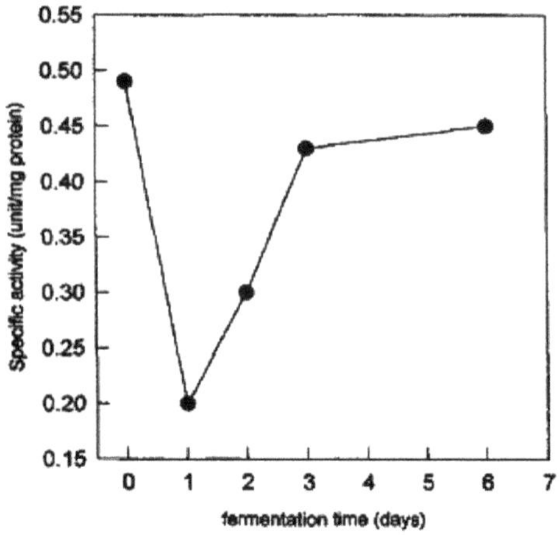

(C) Chanes in α-amlyase activity of Kimchi during fermentation

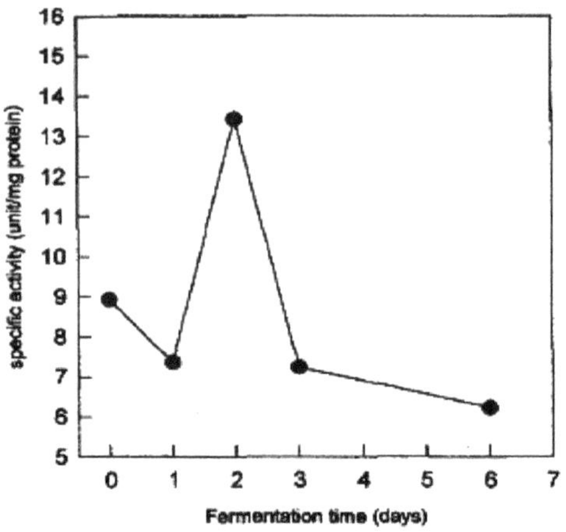

(D) Changes in glucoamlyase activity of Kimchi during fermentation

pressure and insulin resistance/sensitivity. The percentage of participants who showed improvement in glucose tolerance was high in the fermented kimchi group (An et al., 2013). Dietary Baechu kimchi has some antidiabetic effects even when fed with a high fat containing diet. Lower fasting blood glucose and better glucose tolerance were observed in the kimchi high (2.0% of freeze-dried Korean traditional Baechu kimchi) groups compared to the diabetic control groups and kimchi low (0.5% of freeze-dried Korean traditional Baechu kimchi) (Islam et al., 2009).

REFERENCES

An, S. Y., Lee, M. S., Jeon, J. Y., Ha, E. S., Kim, T. H., Ok, J. Y., & Lee, K. W. et al. (2013). Beneficial effects of fresh and fermented kimchi in prediabetic individuals. *Annals of Nutrition & Metabolism*, *63*(1-2), 111–119. doi:10.1159/000353583 PMID:23969321

Ariga, T., Oshiba, S., & Tamada, T. (1999). Platelet aggregation inhibitor in garlic. *Lancet*, *1*, 150–151. PMID:6109819

Baek, Y. H., Kwak, J. R., Kim, S. J., Han, S. S., & Song, Y. O. (2001). Effects of kimchi supplementation and/or exercise training on body composition and plasma lipids in obese middle school girls. *J. korean Soc. Food Sci. Nutr*, *30*, 906–912.

Butt, M. S., & Sultan, M. T. (2011). Ginger and its health claims: Molecular aspects. *Critical Reviews in Food Science and Nutrition*, *51*(5), 383–393. doi:10.1080/10408391003624848 PMID:21491265

Calnek, B. W., Luginbuhl, R. E., & Helmboldt, C. F. (1977). Disease of Poultry. Iowa State University.

Cha, S. D., Yu, J. W., Kim, T. W., Cho, H. S., & Lee, D. H. (2012). Effects of Lactobacillus plantarum CIB 001 on lipid metabolism of hypercholesterolemic rats. *Korean J. Food Sci. Technol*, *44*(3), 324–330. doi:10.9721/KJFST.2012.44.3.324

Challier, B., Perarnau, J. M., & Viel, J. F. (1998). Garlic, onion and cereal fiber as protective factors for breast cancer: French case-control study. *European Journal of Epidemiology*, *14*(8), 737–747. doi:10.1023/A:1007512825851 PMID:9928867

Chan, J. Y., Yuen, A. C., Chan, R. Y., & Chan, S. W. (2013). A review of the cardiovascular benefits and antioxidant properties of allicin. *Phytotherapy Research*, *27*(5), 637–646. doi:10.1002/ptr.4796 PMID:22888009

Chang, U. J., Kim, D. G., Kim, J. M., Suh, H. J., & Oh, S. H. (2003). Weight reduction effect of extract of fermented red pepper on female college students. *J. Korean Soc. Food Sci. Nutr*, *32*(3), 479–484. doi:10.3746/jkfn.2003.32.3.479

Cheigh, H. S., Park, K. Y., & Lee, C. Y. (1994). Biochemical, microbiological, and nutritional aspects of kimchi (Korean fermented vegetable products). *Critical Reviews in Food Science and Nutrition*, *34*(2), 175–203. doi:10.1080/10408399409527656 PMID:8011144

Cheigh, H. S., Song, E. S., & Jeon, Y. S. (1999). Changes of chemical and antioxidative characteristics of cholorophylls in the model system of mustard leaf kimchi during ferementation. *J. Korean Soc. Food Sci Nutr*, *28*(3), 520–525.

Choi, I. H., Noh, J. S., Han, J. S., Kim, H. J., Han, E. S., & Song, Y. O. (2013). Kimchi, a fermented vegetable, improves serum lipid profiles in healthy young adults: Randomized clinical trial. *Journal of Medicinal Food*, *16*(3), 223–229. doi:10.1089/jmf.2012.2563 PMID:23444963

Choi, K. H. (2014). *Antiviral effects of Lactobacillus plantarum YML009 isolated from Kimchi on influenza virus H1N1*. (MS Thesis). Youngnam University, Daegu, Korea.

Choi, M. W., Kim, K. H., & Park, K. Y. (1997). Effects of kimchi extracts on the growth of sarcoma-180 cells and phagocytic activity of mice. *J. Korean Soc. Food Sci Nutr*, *26*, 254–260.

Choi, S. H., Kim, H. J., Kwon, M. J., Baek, Y. H., & Song, Y. O. (2001). The effect of kimchi pill supplementation on plasma lipid concentration in healthy people. *J. Korean Soc. Food Sci. Nutr.*, *30*, 913–920.

Choi, S. M. (2001). *Antiobesity and anticancer effects of red pepper powder and kimchi*. (Ph.D Thesis). Pusan National University, Busan, Korea.

Corrigan, C. J., & Kay, A. B. (1992). T cells and eosinophils in the pathogenesis of asthma. *Immunology Today*, *13*(12), 501–507. doi:10.1016/0167-5699(92)90026-4 PMID:1361126

Deu John Mahandi Cruz. (2006). *Lactic acid bacteria isolated from kimchi and shrimp (Palaeomon macrodactylus) inhibit the infection of porcine epidemic diarrhea virus in vitro*. (Master Thesis). Chungnam National University, Gwangju, Korea.

Duan, L. P., Wang, H. H., & Wang, D. Q. H. (2004). Cholesterol absorption is mainly regulated by the jejunal and ileal ATP-binding cassette sterol efflux transporters Abcg5 and Abcg8 in mice. *Journal of Lipid Research*, *45*(7), 1312–233. doi:10.1194/jlr.M400030-JLR200 PMID:15102882

Fouchier, R. A., Munster, V., Wallensten, A., Bestebroer, T. M., Herfst, S., Smith, D., & Osterhaus, A. D. et al. (2005). Characterization of a novel influenza A virus hemagglutinin subtype (H16) obtained from black-headed gulls. *Journal of Virology*, *79*(5), 2814–2822. doi:10.1128/JVI.79.5.2814-2822.2005 PMID:15709000

Frohlich, R. H., Kunze, M., & Kiefer, I. (1997). Cancer preventive value of natural, non-nutritive food constituents. *Acta Medica Austriaca*, *23*, 108–113. PMID:9312973

Galgani, J. E., Ryan, D. H., & Ravussin, E. (2010). Effect of capsinoids on energy metabolism in human subjects. *The British Journal of Nutrition*, *103*(01), 38–42. doi:10.1017/S0007114509991358 PMID:19671203

Gilchrest, B. A. (1984). *Skin and Aging Process*. Boca Raton, FL: CRC Press. Inc.

Hahn, Y.S., & Oh, J.Y., & Song, J.E. (2002). The study on amylolytic enzyme and protease activities of kimchi. *Korean J. Food Sci. Technol.*, *34*, 269–273.

Han, J. S., Lee, S. H., Lee, K. I., & Park, K. Y. (1995). Standardizations of traditional special kimchi in Kyungsang province. *The East Asian Society of Dietary Life*, *5*(2), 27–38.

Han, K., Bose, S., Wang, J. H., Kim, B. S., Kim, M. J., Kim, E. J., & Kim, H. (2015). Contrasting effects of fresh and fermented kimchi consumption on gut microbiota composition and gene expression related to metabolic syndrome in obese Korean women. *Molecular Nutrition & Food Research*, *59*(5), 1004–1008. doi:10.1002/mnfr.201400780 PMID:25688926

Hong, H. J., Kim, E., Cho, D., & Kim, T. S. (2010). Differential suppression of heat-killed lactobacilli isolated from kimchi, a Korean traditional food, on airway hyperresponsiveness in mice. *Journal of Clinical Immunology*, *30*(3), 449–458. doi:10.1007/s10875-010-9375-8 PMID:20204477

Hu, J., La, V. C., Negri, E., Chatenoud, L., Bosetti, C., Jia, X., & Wang, C. et al. (1999). Diet and brain cancer in adults: A case-control study in northeast China. *International Journal of Cancer*, *81*(1), 20–23. doi:10.1002/(SICI)1097-0215(19990331)81:1<20::AID-IJC4>3.0.CO;2-2 PMID:10077146

Hwang, E. Y., Ryu, H. S., Chun, S. S., Park, K. Y., & Rhee, S. H. (1995). Effect of Godulbaegi (Korean Lettuce, *lxeris sonchifolia* H.) Kimchi on the in vitro digestibility of proteins. *J. Korean Soc. Food Nutr.*, *24*, 1010–1015.

Islam, M. S., & Choi, H. (2009). Antidiabetic effect of Korean traditional Baechu (Chinese cabbage) kimchi in a type 2 diabetes model of rats. *Journal of Medicinal Food*, *12*(2), 292–297. doi:10.1089/jmf.2008.0181 PMID:19459728

Jang, K. S., Kim, M. J., Oh, Y. A., Kang, M. S., & Kim, S. D. (1991). Changes in carotene content of Chinese cabbage kimchi containing various submaterials and lactic acid bacteria during fermention. *J. Food Sci. Nutr.*, *20*(1), 5–12.

Jang, Y. R., Kim, Y. K., Kwon, I. B., & Lee, H. Y. (1998). Screening and identification of the fibrinolytic bacterial strain from Jeot-gal, salt-fermented fish. *Korean J. Food Sci. Technol.*, *30*, 655–650.

Jiang, Z. Y., Parini, P., Eggertsem, G., Davis, M. A., Hu, H., Suo, G. J., & Einarsson, C. et al. (2008). Increased expression of LXR alpha, ABCG5, ABCG8, and SR-BI in the liver from normolipidemic, nonobese Chinese gallstone patients. *Journal of Lipid Research*, *49*(2), 464–472. doi:10.1194/jlr.M700295-JLR200 PMID:18007013

Jung, K. O., Lee, K. I., Suh, K. J., & Park, K. Y. (1999). Antimutagenic and anticancer effects of Buchu Kimchi. *J. Food Sci. Nutr.*, *4*, 33–37.

Jung, Y. K., Yang, Y. S., Kang, J. O., Kong, Y. S., & Kim, J. O. (1995). Fibrinolysis of fermented kimchi. *Korean Society of Life Science*, *5*(4), 203–210.

Kang, J. H. (2009). *Studies on the biofunctional properties of capsaicin in modulating obesity-induced inflammation and metabolic diseases*. (Ph.D Thesis). Ulsan University, Ulsan, Korea.

Kawada, T., Watanabe, T., Takaishi, T., Tanaka, T., & Iwai, K. (1986). Capsaicin induced b-adrenergic action on energy metabolism in rats: Influence of capsaicin on oxygen consumption, the respiratory quotient and substrate utilization. *Proceedings of the Society for Experimental Biology and Medicine*, *183*, 350–256. PMID:2876434

Kim, B. K., Park, K. Y., Kim, H. Y., Ahn, S. C., & Cho, E. J. (2011). Anti-aging effects and mechanisms of kimchi during fermentation under stress-induced premature senescence cellular system. *Food Science and Biotechnology*, *20*(3), 643–649. doi:10.1007/s10068-011-0091-9

Kim, E. K., An, S. Y., Lee, M. S., Kim, T. H., Lee, H. K., Hwang, W. S., & Lee, K. W. et al. (2011). Fermented kimchi reduces body weight and improves metabolic parameters in overweight and obese patients. *Nutrition Research (New York, N.Y.)*, *31*(6), 436–443. doi:10.1016/j.nutres.2011.05.011 PMID:21745625

Kim, H. (2012). *Selection of Lactobacillus strains for cholesterol reduction study and the mechanism through regulating ABCG5/8*. (Master Thesis). Handong Global University, Pohang, Korea.

Kim, H., Oh, S. Y., Kang, M. H., Kim, K. N., Kim, Y., & Chang, N. (2014). Association between kimchi intake and asthma in Korean adults: The fourth and fifth Korea National Health and Nutrition Examination Survey (2007-2011). *Journal of Medicinal Food*, *17*(1), 172–178. doi:10.1089/jmf.2013.3013 PMID:24456368

Kim, H. J., Lee, J. S., Chung, H. Y., Song, S. H., Suh, H., Noh, J. S., & Song, Y. O. (2007). 3-(4′-hydroxyl-3′, 5′-dimethoxyphenyl) propionic acid, an active principle of kimchi, inhibits development of atherosclerosis in rabbits. *Journal of Agricultural and Food Chemistry*, *55*(25), 10486–10492. doi:10.1021/jf072454m PMID:18004805

Kim, H. J., Sung, Y. B., Song, Y. O., Kang, M. R., Kim, T. W., Park, S. H., & Jang, J. Y. (2012). Kimchi suppresses 7-ketocholesterol-induced endoplasmic reticulum stress in macrophages. *Food Science and Biotechnology*, *21*(5), 1293–1299. doi:10.1007/s10068-012-0170-6

Kim, J. H., Ryu, J. D., Lee, H. G., Park, J. H., Moon, G. S., Cheigh, H. S., & Song, Y. O. (2002a). The effect of kimchi on production of free radicals and anti-oxidative enzyme activities in the brain of SAM. *Journal of the Korean Society of Food Science and Nutrition*, *31*(1), 117–123. doi:10.3746/jkfn.2002.31.1.117

Kim, J. H., Ryu, J. D., & Song, Y. O. (2002b). The effect of kimchi intake on free radical production and the inhibition of oxidation in young adults and the elderly people. *Korean Journal of Community Nutrition*, *7*, 257–265.

Kim, K. H., Kim, S. H., & Park, K. Y. (2001). Effects of kimchi extracts on production of nitric oxide by activated macrophages, transforming growth factor β1 of tumor cells and interleukin-6 in splenocytes. *J. Food Sci. Nutr.*, *6*, 126–132.

Kim, K. H., Kim, S. H., Rhee, S. H., & Park, K. Y. (1998). Effects of kimchi extracts on interleukin-2 production and natural killer cell activity in mice. *J. Food Sci. Nutr.*, *3*, 282–286.

Kim, M. J., Song, Y. S., & Song, Y. O. (1998). The Fibrinolytic activity of kimchi and its ingredients in *vivo* and in *vitro*. *J. Korean Soc. Food Sci. Nutr.*, *27*(4), 633–638.

Korea Food Research Institute. (1997). *Development of technology on production of commercial kimchi products with constant quality.* Research Report 389.

Kwon, M. J., Chun, J. H., Song, Y. S., & Song, Y. O. (1999). Daily kimchi consumption and its hypolipidemic effect in middle-aged men. *J. Korean Soc. Food Sci. Nutr.*, *28*, 1144–1150.

Kwon, M. J., Song, Y. S., Choi, M. S., Park, S. J., Jeong, K. S., & Song, Y. O. (2003a). Cholesteryl ester transfer protein activity and atherogenic parameters in rabbit supplemented with cholesterol and garlic powder. *Life Sciences*, *72*(26), 2953–2964. doi:10.1016/S0024-3205(03)00234-0 PMID:12706483

Kwon, M. J., Song, Y. S., Choi, M. S., & Song, Y. O. (2003b). Red pepper attenuates cholesteryl ester transfer protein activity and atherosclerosis in cholesterol-fed rabbits. *Clinica Chimica Acta*, *332*(1-2), 37–44. doi:10.1016/S0009-8981(03)00118-9 PMID:12763278

Kwon, M. J., Song, Y. S., & Song, Y. O. (1997). Effects of Kimchi on tissue and fecal lipid composition and apolipoprotein and thyroxine levels in rats. *J. Korean Food Sci. Nutr.*, *26*(3), 507–513.

Kwon, M. J., Song, Y. S., & Song, Y. O. (1998a). Antioxidative effect of kimchi ingredients on rabbits fed cholesterol diet. *Journal of the Korean Society of Food Science and Nutrition*, *27*, 1189–1196.

Law, M. R., Wald, N. J., & Thompson, S. G. (1994). By how much and how quickly does reduction in serum cholesterol concentration lower risk of ischaemic heart disease? *BMJ (Clinical Research Ed.)*, *308*(6925), 367–372. doi:10.1136/bmj.308.6925.367 PMID:8043072

Lee, G. R., Shin, M. K., Yoon, D. J., Kim, A. R., Yu, R., Park, N. H., & Han, I. S. (2013). Topical application of capsaicin reduces visceral adipose fat by affecting adipokine levels in high-fat diet-induced obese mice. *Obesity (Silver Spring, Md.)*, *21*(1), 115–122. doi:10.1002/oby.20246 PMID:23505175

Lee, J. J., Lee, Y. M., Kim, A. R., Chang, H. C., & Lee, M. Y. (2008). Effect of Leuconostoc kimchi GJ2 isolated from kimchi (fermented Korean Cabbage) on lipid metabolism in high cholesterol-fed rats. *Korean J. Food Preserv*, *15*, 760–768.

Lee, K. E., Choi, U. H., & Ji, G. E. (1996). Effect of kimchi intake on the composition of human large intestinal bacteria. *J. Korean Soc. Food Sci Tecbnol*, *28*, 981–986.

Lee, K. E., Choi, U. H., & Ji, G. E. (1996). Effect of kimchi intake on the composition of human large intestinal bacteria. *Korean J. Food Science and Technology (Campinas.)*, *28*, 981.

Lee, S. H., & Kim, S. D. (1988). Effect of various ingredients of kimchi on the kimchi fermentation. *J. Food Sci. Nutr.*, *17*(3), 249–254.

Lee, S. Y. (2001). *Anti-aging effects of kimchi diet in senescence accelerated mice (SAM P-8)*. (M. S. Thesis). Pusan National Univ, Korea.

Lee, W. J. (2003). *Effect of capsaicin on uncoupling protein-2 expression in 3T3-L1 cell line*. (M.S. Thesis). Inje University, Gimhae, Korea.

Lee, Y. M., Kwon, M. J., Kim, J. K., Suh, H. S., Chio, J. S., & Song, Y. O. (2004). Isolation and identification of active principle in Chinese cabbage kimchi responsible for antioxidant activity. *Korean Journal of Food Science and Technology*, *36*, 129–133.

Levi, F., Pasche, C., La Vecchia, C., Lucchini, F., & Franceschi, S. (1999). Food groups and colorectal cancer risk. *British Journal of Cancer*, *79*(7/8), 1283–1287. doi:10.1038/sj.bjc.6690206 PMID:10098773

Lilley, D. M., & Stillwell, R. H. (1965). Probiotics promoting factors produced by microorganisms. *Science*, *147*(3659), 747–748. doi:10.1126/science.147.3659.747 PMID:14242024

Michaud, D. S., Spiegelman, D., Clinton, S. K., Rimm, S. K., Willett, W. C., & Giovannucci, E. L. (1999). Fruit and vegetable intake and incidence of bladder cancer in a male prospective cohort. *Journal of the National Cancer Institute*, *7*(7), 605–613. doi:10.1093/jnci/91.7.605 PMID:10203279

Neumann, G., Noda, T., & Kawaoka, Y. (2009). Emergence and pandemic potential of swine-origin H1N1 influenza virus. *Nature*, *459*(7249), 931–939. doi:10.1038/nature08157 PMID:19525932

Noh, J. S., Choi, Y. H., & Song, Y. O. (2013). Beneficial effects of the active principle component of Korean cabbage kimchi via increasing nitric oxide production and suppressing inflammation in the aorta of aopE knockout mice. *The British Journal of Nutrition*, *109*(01), 17–24. doi:10.1017/S0007114512000633 PMID:22715945

Noh, K. A., Kim, D. H., Choi, N. S., & Kim, S. H. (1999). Isolation of fibrinolytic enzyme producing strains from kimchi. *Korean J. Food Sci. Technol*, *31*, 219–223.

Oh, Y. J., Hwang, I. J., & Leitzmann, C. (1993). Regular intake of kimchi prevent colon cancer. *Kimchi Sci Ind.*, *2*, 9.

Pantack, E. T., Hsiao, C. B., & Garland, W. A. (1976). Stimulatory effect of vegetable on intestinal drug metabolism in the rat. *The Journal of Pharmacology and Experimental Therapeutics*, *198*, 277.

Park, J. A., Tirupathi Pichiah, J. J., Yu, P. B., Oh, S. H., Daily, J. W. III, & Cha, Y. S. (2012). Anti-obesity effect of kimchi fermented with Weissella koreensis OK1-6 as starter in high-fat diet-induced obese C57BL/6J mice. *Journal of Applied Microbiology*, *113*(6), 1507–1516. doi:10.1111/jam.12017 PMID:22978326

Park, K. Y. (1995). The nutritional evaluation, and antimutagenic and anticancer effects of kimchi. *J. Korean Soc. Food Nutr*, *24*, 169.

Park, K. Y., Jeong, J. K., Lee, Y. E., & Daily, J. W. III. (2014). Health benefits of kimchi (Korean fermented vegetables) as a probiotic food. *Journal of Medicinal Food*, *17*(1), 6–20. doi:10.1089/jmf.2013.3083 PMID:24456350

Renz, H., Bradley, K., Saloga, J., Loader, J., Larsen, G. L., & Gelfand, E. W. (1993). T cells expressing specific V beta elements regulate immunoglobulin E production and airways responsiveness in vivo. *The Journal of Experimental Medicine*, *177*(4), 1175–1180. doi:10.1084/jem.177.4.1175 PMID:8459211

Ryu, B. M. (2000). *Effect of kimchi on inhibition of skin aging of hairless mouse, (PhD. Disseration)*. Busan, Korea: Pusan National Univ.

Ryu, B.M., Ryu, S.H., Yang, Y.C., Lee, Y.S., Jeon, Y.S., & Moon, G.S. (2004). Morphological changes in the skin of hairless mouse fed various kimchi diet. *J. Korean Soc. Food Sci. Nutr, 33*, 291-298.

Ryu, B. M., Ryu, S. H., Yang, Y. C., Lee, Y. S., Jeon, Y. S., & Moon, G. S. (2004). Morphological changes in the skin of hairless mouse fed various kimchi diet. *J Korean Soc Food Sci Nutr.*, *33*(9), 1469–1475. doi:10.3746/jkfn.2004.33.9.1469

Ryu, S. H., Jeon, Y. S., Kwon, M. J., Moon, J. W., Lee, Y. S., & Moon, G. S. (1997). Effect of kimchi ingaradients to reactive oxygen species in skin cell cytotoxicity. *J. korean Soc. Food Sci. Nutr.*, *26*(6), 998–1105.

Ryu, S. H., Jeon, Y. S., Kwon, M. J., Moon, J. W., Lee, Y. S., & Moon, G. S. (1997). Effect of kimchi ingredients to reactive oxygen species in skin cell cytotoxicity. *J. korean Soc. Food Sci. Nutr.*, *26*(5), 814–821.

Sainani, G. S., Desai, D. B., Gorhe, N. H., Natu, S. M., & Pise, D. V. (1979). Effects of dietary garlic on serum lipid prolic in Jain community. *The Indian Journal of Medical Research*, *69*, 776–779. PMID:511261

Salminen, S., Ouwehand, A. C., Benno, Y., & Lee, Y. K. (1999). Probiotics: How should they be defined? *Trends in Food Science & Technology*, *10*(3), 107–110. doi:10.1016/S0924-2244(99)00027-8

Seo, B. J. (2012). *Antiviral effects of Leuconostoc mesenteroides YML003 isolated from Kimchi on pathogenic Avian influenza (H9N2) virus*. (Ph.D Thesis). Youngnam University, Daegu, Korea.

Seo, B. J., Rather, I. A., Kumar, V. J. R., Choi, U. H., Moon, M. R., Lim, J. H., & Park, Y. H. (2012). Evaluation of Leuconostoc mesenteroides YML003 as a probiotic against low-pathogenic avian influenza (H9N2) virus in chickens. *Journal of Applied Microbiology*, *113*(1), 163–171. doi:10.1111/j.1365-2672.2012.05326.x PMID:22548634

Shin, K. S., Chae, O. W., Park, I. C., Hong, S. K., & Choe, T. B. (1998). Antitumor effects of mice fed with cell lysate of *Lactobacillus plantarum* isolated from kimchi. *Korean J. Biotechnol. Bioeng.*, *13*, 357–363.

Song, Y. R. (2010). *Study on exopolysaccharides with antioxidant and antiaging activity produced by Bacillus sp. Strains isolated from Korea fermented food, Kimchi*. (M.S. Thesis). Chunbuk National University, Jeonju, Korea.

Swayne, D. E., & Suarez, D. L. (2000). Highly pathogenic avian influenza. *Rev Sci Tech Off Inter Epiz*, *19*(2), 463–482. doi:10.20506/rst.19.2.1230 PMID:10935274

Van der Klaauw, A. A., & Farooqi, I. S. (2015). The hunger genes: Pathways to obesity. *Cell*, *161*(1), 119–132. doi:10.1016/j.cell.2015.03.008 PMID:25815990

Vehoeven, D. T., Goldbohn, R. A., van Poppel, G., Verhagen, H., & van den Brandt, P. A. (1996). Epidemiological studies on brassica vegetables and cancer risk. *Cancer Epidemiology, Biomarkers & Prevention*, *5*, 733–748. PMID:8877066

Won, T.J., Kim, B.J., Lim, Y.T., Song, D.S., & Oh, E.S., Lee Do, I., & Hwang, K.W. (2011). Modulation of Th1/Th2 balance by Lactobacillus strains isolated kimchi via stimulation of macrophage cell line J774A.1 in vitro. *Journal of Food Science*, *76*, H55–H61. PMID:21535768

You, W. C., Zhang, L., Gail, M. H., Ma, J. L., Chang, Y. S., Blot, W. J., & Xu, G. W. et al. (1998). Fraumeni JF Jr. *Helicobacter pylori* infection, garlic intake and precancerous lesions in a Chinese population at low risk of gastic cancer. *International Journal of Epidemiology*, *27*(6), 941–944. doi:10.1093/ije/27.6.941 PMID:10024185

Yu, E. J. (2004). *The cytotoxic, antioxidative, and antihypertensive activities in Dolsanleaf mustard and its kimchi. (Ph.D)*. Yosu, Korea: Yosu National University.

Yu, M. H., Im, H. G., Im, N. K., Hwang, E. Y., Choi, J. H., Lee, E. J., & Seo, H. J. et al. (2009). Antihypertensive activities of Lactobacillus isolated from Kimchi. *Korean J. Food Sci. Technol.*, *41*(4), 428–434.

Yun, Y. R., Kim, H. J., & Song, Y. O. (2014). Kimchi methanol extract and the kimchi active compound, 3'-(4'-hydroxyl-3',5'-dimethoxyphenyl)propionic acid, downregulate CD36 in THP-1 macrophages timulated by oxLDL. *Journal of Medicinal Food*, *8*(8), 886–893. doi:10.1089/jmf.2013.2943 PMID:25010893

Yusuf, S., Hawken, S., Ounpuu, S., Dans, T., Avezum, A., Lanas, F., & Lisheng, L. et al. (2004). Effect of potentially modifiable risk factors associated with myocardial infarction in 52 countries (the INTER-HEART study): Case-control study. *Lancet*, *364*(9438), 937–952. doi:10.1016/S0140-6736(04)17018-9 PMID:15364185

Chapter 5
Health Benefits of Tea:
Beneficial Effects of Tea on Human Health

Sumonto Mitra
Indian Institute of Toxicology Research, India

Shashi Khandelwal
Indian Institute of Toxicology Research, India

ABSTRACT

Tea is the second most widely consumed beverage throughout the world, after water. "Tea" is referred to the aromatic beverage prepared by incubating cured leaves of the plant Camellia sinensis *with hot or boiling water. The origin of tea has remained a mystery and has been associated with legends in the Chinese history. Under experimental conditions in laboratory, tea has been reported to act as an anti-cancer agent in various models of lung, pancreas, liver, breast, fore-stomach, oesophagus, duodenum, colon, and skin cancers induced by chemical carcinogens. Tea also contains a wide range of antioxidants and has been found to possess several others health benefits. This chapter summarizes the history behind its use, various health benefits, and current state of scientific literature and epidemiological evidence of its usefulness.*

SOURCE

Although tea in itself is presented in various forms throughout the world (white, yellow, green, Oolong and black) but there are other variants like "herbal tea" which does not contain any *C. sinensis* leaves and is usually referred to the various infusions of herbs or fruits. All the variants of tea essentially originate from the same botanical source but differ in the type of processing done to obtain specific flavour and properties.

The tea plant is an endemic evergreen shrub of the continent of Asia (east and southwest regions), which prefers tropical and sub-tropical climatic conditions with abundant rainfall and heights in the range of 2000-6500 feet above sea level. Although the quality of tea is directly related to greater heights at which they are grown, but several other popular tea variants are also grown at lower heights (near sea level). Supposedly it is the cool climate (at greater heights) which restricts growth of the leaves allowing

DOI: 10.4018/978-1-5225-0591-4.ch005

more flavours to get accumulated in them. An undisturbed tea plant can grow up to 30 feet in height, but usually they are pruned to a height to 3-5 feet to favour plucking of their tender leaves (which are then used for further processing). Pruning process also favours the growth of new leaves and this method is systematically used in commercial tea gardens to increase leaf harvesting. These tea bushes, if properly maintained, have a life span of over 100 years. The quality of tea plant gardens can be maintained by vegetative propagation of better quality plants for generations, thus allowing sustained supply of superior tasting tea.

Tea is primarily obtained from two variants of the *Camellia* plant- *Camellia sinensis var. sinensis* (used for most Chinese, Formosan, Japanese and Darjeeling tea), and *C. s. var. assamica*, (used in fermented Chinese tea and most Indian teas). The Assam tea type was characterized by large leaves and strong taste, while the Chinese variant is famous for its delicate flavour and smaller leaf size. The process of producing high quality tea starts right from the careful hand plucking of the tea leaves where "two leaves with a bud" is the usual norm. These leaves are then processed further, following different methods, to produce a variety of tea types. A summary of the various methods employed is given below and the final product obtained is depicted in Table 1.

- **Wilting:** Involves leaving the freshly harvested tea leaves on racks (whether under the sun or in indoor environment) for 12-24 hours during which the leaves loose much of their water content and become soft and pliable.
- **Bruising:** This method induces breakage of the tea leaves (either tossed in baskets or involves crushing of the leaves) which allows release of the natural enzymes.
- **Oxidation:** In this process, the tea leaves are maintained in a controlled environment (heat and moisture controlled) for the natural oxidation to take place. During this period, natural enzymes break down the tannins and/or transform them to yield the desired flavour and aroma. Most of the chlorophyll content is also broken down during this step. Different types of tea are prepared by controlling the duration of oxidation, such as 5-40% oxidation is used to make light oolong tea whereas 40-60% oxidation helps in making darker oolong variants. To produce black tea, a complete oxidation procedure is preferred.
- **Fixation:** This step is very important as it involves stopping the oxidation process and thus is used as a control point during tea production. Tea leaves are slightly heated or baked to stop the enzymatic oxidation process and to remove any undesirable aroma from the tea leaves, but care is taken so as to preserve the desired aroma and polyphenols which results in refined flavour.

Table 1. Processes involved in the production of various types of tea

Process	Wilting	Bruising	Oxidation	Fixation	Yellowing	Shaping	Drying	Curing	Final Product
Plucking of tea leaves	✓			✓		✓	✓	✓	Post fermented tea
				✓		✓	✓		Green tea
				✓	✓	✓	✓		Yellow tea
	✓			✓		✓	✓		White tea
	✓	✓	✓	✓		✓	✓	✓	Oolong tea
	✓	✓	✓			✓	✓		Black tea

- **Yellowing:** Performed only to produce yellow tea, the leaves are briskly heated inside a closed container which allows the transformation of green tea leaves to turn yellow mainly due to changes in the chlorophyll content.
- **Shaping:** This step is performed either manually or by employing rolling machines (for mass production) to provide different kind of shapes to the final product. Tea leaves can be rolled into stripes or knitted together to give various shapes to the product. Also during this process, several essential oils and other organic juices are released from the tea leaves which enhance the specific flavour of final product.
- **Drying:** The shaped leaves are dried by using a variety of methods involving panning, sun drying, air drying and baking. The most preferred method is baking which retains most of the original flavours of the leaves and is a better controlled process. This step marks the end of the processing of tea yielding specific types of tea which are ready for sale. This step is also very critical as several organic contents of the tea leaves are either retained or allowed to evaporate out so as to obtain a refined product.
- **Curing:** Although this step is very specific to fermented tea products, sometimes old oolong teas are also cured to invigorate flavour in them. This process is followed when prolonged oxidation of the tea leaves is desired (for which the oxidation process in the tea leaves were not entirely abolished in the fixation step). This process is used to manufacture Pu Erh tea and also in the production of flavoured tea types where specific flavours were added to the initial tea products and allowed to age for a certain period.

HISTORY

One legend states that the use of tea came into practice at around 2737 BC by the famous Chinese emperor and herbalist Shennong (also pronounced as Shen Nung) (Helen, 2010). The legend states that one day while boiling water for consumption, some leaves from a neighbouring tree fell into the pot of hot water. Shennong wanted to try the infusion to understand its effects and soon realised that this infusion invigorated his body with energy and was also pleased with its aesthetic taste. Thus he recommended the use of these leaves (which turned out to be coming from "tea tree") to be used as an infusion. Till date, the oldest cultivated tea tree has been documented to be present in the Fengqing County in the Lincang city of Yunnan province in China, which is approximately 3200 years old (Urchin, 2012).

For the next few hundred years, people in China used to drink tea probably due to its medicinal qualities. This explanation is well supported by the fact that Laozi (ca. 600-517 BC), the classical Chinese philosopher, designated tea as "the froth of liquid jade" and termed it as an indispensible ingredient to the "elixir of life" (Jane, 2004). Another book termed as "the Divine Farmer's herb-Root Classic" which was written in the era of the western Han dynasty (around 1st century BC) and was attributed to Shennong, illustrates a reference about tea. The first known book which demonstrates the instructions on preparing and buying was written by Wang Bao in 59 BC and was entitled "A Contract with a Servant". This book signifies the knowledge acquired about tea by this time and also establishes that tea was used not only for consumption but was also used as a commodity for business purpose.

Even at this juncture in Chinese history, where tea had been in use for several decades, not everyone had the opportunity to drink tea. This was primarily due to the limited source of tea plants which prevailed until the Han dynasty (206 BC – 220 AD), wherein only the royal family and the rich society could afford this delicacy. Due to the medicinal benefits of tea infusion, it was used in various rituals and was considered a part of religious offering. One proof of the medicinal use of tea can be found in the written text of the famous physician named Hua Tuo, who during 3rd century AD described the ability of tea to improve mental conditions (Laura, 2007).

As tea plantations were discovered with time during the Shang dynasty (618 – 907 AD), its consumption also became popular among the lower classes. By this time, tea production was given enough importance so as to start tea plantations across the Chinese kingdom. It was also during the era of the Sui dynasty (589-618 AD) that tea was introduced in Japan by Buddhist monks who studied/travelled across China and brought back tea while returning. But until this time, the method of producing tea was rather discrete and the knowledge was passed on from generations to generations verbally in certain specified groups in the country. It was only in the 8th century by the publication of "Cha Ching, a definitive tea production manual" by Lu Yu that brought in uniformity in the different ways of tea production (cultivation and manufacturing) and consumption (preparation of tea infusion). It was with this collection of information that tea production flourished in different parts within China and uniformity was brought in among various sections of the people who could now enjoy tea consumption equivalently.

Following the customs in China, tea was initially consumed by the Japanese priests and the rich people, upon its introduction in the country due to its medicinal properties. Initially tea was associated with Zen Buddhism since it was consumed by the priests during meditation rituals. Very soon the Japanese priests started the "Japanese tea ceremony" wherein tea was shared as a customary ritual in sacred and spiritual manner. According to the ancient scriptures, tea seeds were first introduced in Japan by a priest named Saicho in 805 AD and then followed by another named Kukai in 806 AD. Uji tea was sequentially developed by another priest named Myoe Shonin and subsequently Eisai formulated the oldest tea speciality book in Japan termed Kissa Yojoki (meaning: how to stay healthy by drinking tea). The Japanese emperor Shomu took up the tea drinking tradition to the royal family and was followed by emperor Kiasung who started to divide various types of tea according to its individual taste.

Apart from Japan, tea also started to be consumed in Korea where historical documents record the first offering of tea in various spiritual ceremonies in the year 661 AD. During Goryeo dynasty (918-1392 AD), tea offerings were made in Buddhist temples to the spirits of revered monks. Till this period, tea was popularly consumed in China and Japan but things started to change during the Ming dynasty (1368-1644 AD) by the introduction of foreign trade. To meet the demands of trade, the Chinese started to experiment with the processing of tea and developed the method of fermentation which gave rise to Oolong and black tea variants which were found to last longer. They also started producing flavoured tea types.

The global expansion of tea started in 16th century when the Portuguese established a trading port in Macau. The Portuguese priests were initially thought to bring back tea from China to their homeland, where tea became popular. Tea finally arrived in England during the 17th century following the marriage of King Charles II with a Portuguese princess, Catherine of Braganza. The queen introduced tea to the royal family of England which soon became popular in the aristocratic society. Tea for the first time in England was introduced to common public in 1650 through the establishment of coffee houses. It was during the same era that tea enjoyed worldwide popularity which is indicated by its presence in various countries like France, Germany and the Netherlands. Although the British East India Company is credited for the introduction of tea in India somewhere in the 18th century, but indigenous tribes like the Singpho (inhabitants of the Indian state of Assam and Arunachal Pradesh) and Khamti (resides in Arunachal Pradesh) verify that they have been using tea since the 12th century. Interestingly, the Assam variety of tea is also found in plenty in these regions within India. Tea was introduced in India by the British as a tactical move to break the monopoly of China in the tea industry (Sen, 2005). Tea was also introduced to the British colonies in America during the same time.

Apart from its health benefits, tea has also enjoyed its share of political importance. Tea played a very important role in two of the famous revolutions of significant historical importance. They are the Boston Tea Party in America and the first Opium war in China (involving Britain in both the cases).

FUNCTIONALITY

Tea has been found to be beneficial in conditions like high blood pressure and cholesterol, atherosclerosis and coronary heart disease, and metabolism of xenobiotic compounds. Apart from having beneficial effects during altered physiological conditions, tea is also found to positively regulate glucose metabolism, fatty acid oxidation, insulin sensitivity and also confer protection against neuro-damage (brain damage) and ageing.

Scientific evidence has shown that green tea polyphenols can protect the heart from tissue injury under conditions of oxidative injury and also during hypoxia/re-oxygenation damage (Bordoni et al., 2002). This ability was found to be due to its ability to reduce hydrogen peroxide (H_2O_2) induced cell damage and likely by the inhibition of Akt and GSk-3ß signalling cascades (Chen, Hsieh, Chiu, Hsu, & Liou, 2014). Even when consumed occasionally, tea can protect against ultra-violet radiation induced genotoxity (DNA damage) in humans (Malhomme et al., 2010). Since oxidative injury is a common factor in initiating cell damage in various body organs, tea polyphenols were found to have potential anti-oxidant effect; their protective ability was observed in various animal models. Green tea extract administration was reported to rescue experimental animals from ischemia induced injury of the gut (Muià et al., 2005). Similarly, cigarette smoke induced lung damage as evidenced by inflammation and cell death is also found to be significantly recovered by black tea consumption in animal models (Banerjee et al., 2007).

Tea polyphenols were also found to be beneficial in muscle dystrophy where they increase glutathione levels in cells via interaction of EGCG with its receptor 67LR (Dorchies, Wagner, Buetler, & Ruegg, 2009). Significant reduction of peroxidative content and restoration of antioxidant enzymes were also reported to rescue renal cells from cyclosporine induced toxicity following green tea extract administration (Samy, Omayma, & Mohammed, 2014), which was primarily mediated by its regulation of Renin-angiotensin-aldosterone system (RAAS) (Ryu et al., 2010). Tea polyphenols have also the ability to rescue kidneys from ischemia/reperfusion injury by modulating TLR4/NF-κB p65 signal pathway (Li et al., 2014).

Along with its anti-oxidant and anti-inflammatory potential, tea was found to possess neuro-protective property. Among others, theanine is the most powerful neuro-protective compound present in tea. It was found to reduce glutamate induced excitotoxic cell death and has an overall beneficial effect under ischemic conditions (Kakuda, 2002). Structurally, theanine resembles glutamate and is supposed to interact with NMDA as well as AMPA receptors, thereby mediating its neuro-protective ability (Kakuda, Nozawa, Sugimoto, & Niino, 2002). Theanine was found to possess neuro-protective ability under both in-vitro as well as in-vivo conditions. Simultaneously, tea catechins were reported to reduce arteriosclerosis (a major factor in ischemic cerebrovascular disease) by mitigating reactive oxygen species induced oxidation of low-density lipoprotein which is directly related to its free oxygen radical scavenging ability (Kakuda, 2002). Tea polyphenols were also reported to inhibit neurological impairments induced by cerebral hypoperfusion (Xu et al., 2010). Apart from imparting a positive effect on the physiological function of the neurological system, tea was also found to protect against environmental toxins induced neurological alterations (Cho et al., 2008) which indicate towards one of its most important role as a functional food which can be used as a preventive medicine rather than as a therapeutic agent.

CHEMICAL, PHYSICAL, AND PHYSIOLOGICAL PROPERTIES

Apart from its invigorating taste and aroma, tea has often been used for its medicinal properties from its initial days till date. Tea is a rich source of various substances including polyphenols (phenols, tannins, catechin, flavonols, anthocyanidins, and phenol-acids), organic acids, essential oils, vitamins and various other saccharides, lipids, pigments, vitamins and inorganic compounds. It is a rich source of manganese (0.5 mg/cup) and caffeine (30-90 mg/cup).

An estimated composition of fresh tea leaves (Var. assamica) is given in Table 2 (International Agency for Research on Cancer, n.d).

Table 2. Composition of fresh tea leaf

Substance	% Dry Weight
Polyphenols	25
Epi-gallocatechin gallate	9-13
Epi-catechin gallate Epi-gallocatechin	3-6 3-6
Epi-catechin	1-3
Others	1-2
Flavonols and flavonol glycosides	3-4
Flavanediols	2-3
Polyphenolic acids and depsides	5
Other polyphenols	3
Caffeine	3-4
Theobromine	0.2
Theophylline	0.04
Amino acids	4
Organic acids	0.5
Monosaccharides	4
Polysaccharides	13-14
Protein	15
Cellulose	7
Lignin	6
Lipids	3
Chlorophyll and other pigments	0.5
Ash	5
Volatiles	0.01-0.02

Although tea is a rich source of several essential amino acids including valine, leucine, threonine and phenylalanine; theanine alone accounts for almost 40% of its total amino acid content. Tea also serves as a source of alkaloids like caffeine, theobromine and theophylline. Caffeine in tea is bound to tannin (collectively termed "theine") which is why caffeine from tea is less toxic to human health when compared to coffee. Among the polyphenols, catechins are by far the most bio-active compounds in which epigallocatechine (EGCG) makes up to almost 50-60% of all catechins. Flavonols are widespread pigments found in vegetables and are resistant to processing. Anthocyanidins are produced by the hydrolysis of anthocyanins (vegetable pigments) under the influence of enzymes and acids, and are responsible for the astringent taste of tea.

Tea also contains a variety of phenolic compounds primarily gallic acid, theogalline, chlorogenic acid, ellagic acid, coumaric acid and caffeic acid. The total carbohydrate (saccharide) content of tea

Figure 1. Major types of tea polyphenols

The major green tea polyphenols are;

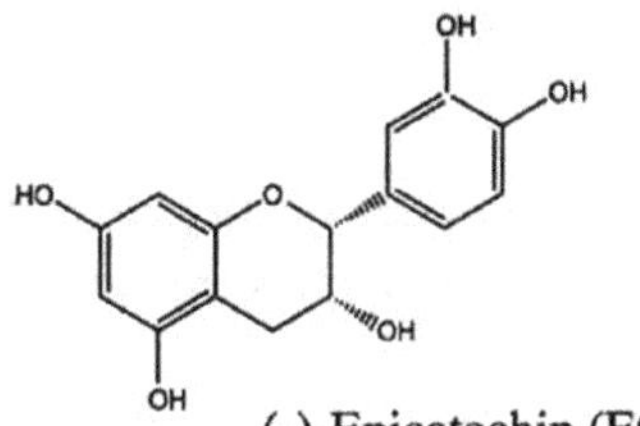

(-)-Epicatechin (EC)

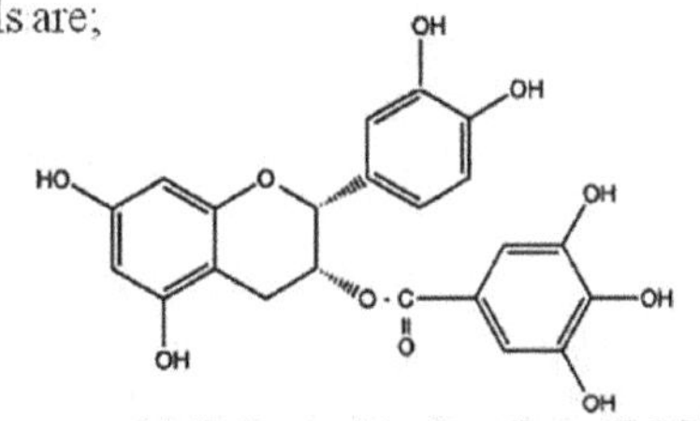

(-)-Epicatechin-3-gallate (ECG)

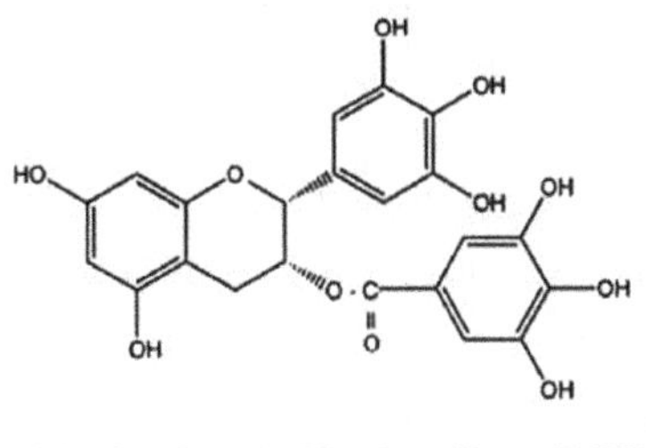

(-)-Epigallocatechin-3-gallate (EGCG)

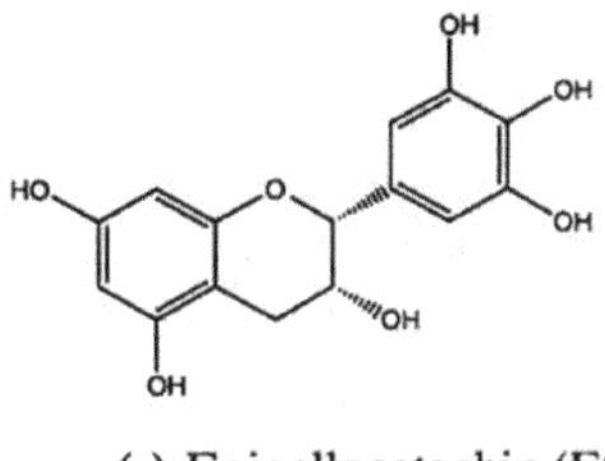

(-)-Epigallocatechin (EGC)

And the major black tea polyphenols are;

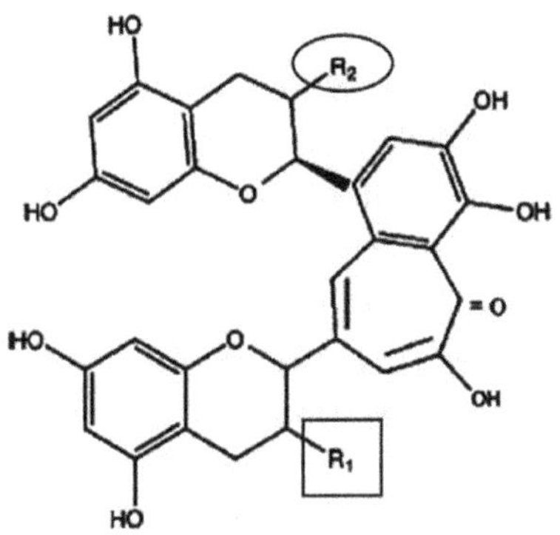

	R_1	R_2
Theaflavin	OH	OH
Theaflavin-3-gallate	Gallate	OH
Theaflavin-3'-gallate	OH	Gallate
Theaflavin-3,3'-digallate	Gallate	Gallate

is estimated to be around 15-20% of dry weight and is the critical component to develop the taste and flavour. Along with taste, the organic acids present in tea attribute specific aroma to the beverage. An estimated 25 different types of organic acids present in tea are the products of various metabolic pathways (biosynthesis of alkaloids, glycosides and amino acids, etc). Some of the organic acids present in tea are: malic acid, citric acid, succinic acid, oxalic acid, palmitic acid, linoleic acid, etc. The amount of essential oils in tea is very low (0.02% in fresh fleches) which contains nearly 300 different aromatic compounds. Although most of them (70-80%) are lost during the processing of tea required while giving its final form, but several others are produced within them during these processing steps which gives them their characteristic aroma. Tea also contains an array of vitamins which comprise the fat-soluble (A, D, E, and K) and water-soluble (C, B1, B2, B3, B5, B11, C, P and inosite). Apart from all of the above mentioned components, tea also serves as a reservoir of various inorganic compounds. There are around 27 different minerals including potassium (K), magnesium (Mg), manganese (Mn), fluorine (F), calcium (Ca), sodium (Na), sulphur (S), iron (Fe), copper (Cu), nickel (Ni), silicon (Si), zinc (Zn), selenium (Se), etc.

HEALTH BENEFITS

Theanine is very important for the proper functioning of T-cell mediated immune system, where it helps to maintain their activation status. Theine, a biologically active compound is found to stimulate the central nervous and cardiovascular system, relax blood vessels, improve digestion, improve circulation and prevent aggregation of platelets. Theobromine also stimulates the activity of heart, acts as a vasodilator, dilates bronchi and has diuretic effects. Though theophyllin is much similar to theobromine, it is a more potent diuretic. EGCG is the most potent anti-oxidant found in tea and is comparatively 25-100 times more active than vitamin C and E, respectively. This antioxidant activity of EGCG is primarily attributed to its ability to absorb free radicals and is thus related to the cancer preventing ability of tea. Apart from EGCG, another catechin called epigallocatechine-3-gallate (ECG) strengthens the immune system by interacting with lymphocyte cells. Catechins were also found to have vascular modulating properties and have been used in treating capillaropathies especially in cases of vascular oedema. Catechins also possess anti-bacterial properties and have been used in treating dysentery. Flavonols possessing P-vitamin properties were found to increase the durability of capillaries, facilitate vitamin C assimilation and regulate thyroid gland activity. Anthocyanidins help to strengthen capillaries and joints, enhance vision and prevent atherosclerosis, cancer and arterial hypertension. Phenolic acid attributes astringent, cholagogic and anti-inflammatory properties to tea. They also regulate thyroid gland function and stimulate the anti-toxic function of liver.

Flavonoids also exhibit anti-allergic and anti-carcinogenic properties apart from being potent antioxidants. Although the carbohydrate content in tea is less important in serving as a source of energy, but it helps to stabilize the vitamin B content. The organic acids facilitate digestion by stimulating the release of gastric juices, regulate intestinal flora thereby reducing chances of gastro-intestinal diseases and also activate peristaltic movements. Malic acid catalyzes ATP formation, has anti-inflammatory property and it improves iron absorption from food. Citric acid regulates the acid-base balance and has anti-oxidant property. Succinic acid enhances energetic metabolism and protects against damage caused by radiations. Oxalic acid helps in calcium assimilation, whereas palmitic acid serves as a source of energy. Linoleic acid is an important constituent which helps in the assimilation of vitamin A, D, E and K and also prevents their oxidation. The pigments present in tea add up to its anti-oxidant property. The healing and prophylactic properties of tea are attributed to the presence of essential oils, and their most important property is to affect the CNS. These substances help to reduce stress, have beneficial effects during emotional excitability and also enhance the work capacity. While brewing, the fat-soluble vitamins do not make it to the solution and thus only water-soluble vitamins are consumed. These water-soluble vitamins provide a wide array of beneficial effects which are not limited to the following functions- metabolism, endocrine gland activity, antibody production, liver function, CNS activity, anti-ageing, and anti-allergic. The mineral components of tea are beneficial in various aspects, like in regulation of water-salt balance, muscle contraction, metabolism, endocrine activity, immunity, structural regulation, oxido-reduction reactions, haematogenesises and hematopoesis.

MECHANISMS OF ANTIOXIDANT ACTION

Since tea undergoes different types of processing resulting in varied compositions of the final product, the oxidant activity of tea may vary. Tea polyphenols can behave both as an anti-oxidant as well as pro-oxidant which is governed by the type of polyphenol present and also on redox status of the cell. Presence of redox active proteins within the cells like oxidant scavenging proteins (catalase, superoxide dismutase, glutathione peroxidise, etc) and/or levels of oxidized proteins and lipids can also affect the oxidant property of tea polyphenols. For example, EGCG has been reported to reduce mitochondrial damage by acting as an anti-oxidant molecule and can reduce lipid-infusion mediated insulin resistance by inducing the activities of oxidant responsive enzymes (Meng, Velalar, & Ruan, 2008; Li et al., 2011). On the contrary, EGCG is found to induce free radical generation in cancer cells by producing hydrogen peroxide mediated by its pyrogallol moiety and also through the reduction of iron (from Fe^{3+} to Fe^{2+}) which triggers the production of reactive oxygen species (ROS) by initiating Fenton reaction (Nakagawa, Hasumi, Woo, Nagai, & Wachi, 2004; Nakagawa et al., 2002). Due to high biological prevalence of EGCG content in tea, focused research on its oxidant activity revealed that the galloyl group on ring B and D is primarily responsible for its radical scavenging ability. Electron paramagnetic resonance (EPR) spectroscopy studies have been used to demonstrate the activity of these groups and its effectiveness in scavenging OH and O_2^- radicals (Severino et al., 2009). In similar studies using 2,2'-azobis (2, 4-di-methylvaleronitrile) (AMVN) to produce peroxyl radicals, the B-ring structure was found to be more vital for the antioxidant activity of EGCG and EGC, irrespective of the presence of the 3-galloyl moiety (Valcic, Burr, Timmermann, & Liebler, 2000). Other reports employing 1D or 2D NMR technique to study the reaction between epicatechin with peroxyl radicals generated by thermolysis of the azo initiator azo-bisisobutyrylnitrile (AIBN) also found that the B-ring to be the initial reaction site (Sang et al., 2003). The basic chemistry behind these anti-oxidant activities of tea polyphenols (designated as PhOH) is proposed to be of two kinds: hydrogen atom transfer (HAT) or single electron transfer reactions (SET) or sometimes both. Lambert and Elias (2010) proposed the following mechanisms for each of these chemical reactions as follows; where L_1H is unsaturated fatty acid, $L_1\bullet$ is the alkyl radical, $L_1O_2\bullet$ is hydroperoxyl radical, and L_1OOH are lipid peroxides.

Hydrogen atom transfer:

$L_1H \rightarrow L_1\bullet$ (initiation)

$L_1\bullet + O_2 \rightarrow L_1O_2\bullet$ (formation of peroxylradical, $\sim 10^9\ M^{-1}s^{-1}$)

$L_1O_2\bullet + L_2H \rightarrow L_1OOH + L_2\bullet$ (chain propagation, $\sim 10^1\ M^{-1}s^{-1}$)

$L_1O_2\bullet + PhOH \rightarrow L_1OOH + PhO\bullet$ (chain interruption)

Since reaction kinetics of the chain interruption step is faster than the chain propagation reactions, tea polyphenols can effectively restrict the chain propagation of lipid peroxidation reactions, thereby reducing reactive oxygen species mediated cellular damage.

Single electron transfer:

$PhOH + LO_2\bullet \rightarrow PhOH^+ + LO_2^-$

$PhOH^+ + H_2O \leftrightarrow PhO\bullet + H_3O^+$

$LO_2^- + H_3O^+ \leftrightarrow LOOH + H_2O$

In another set of circumstances, tea polyphenols were reported to get oxidized by transition metals under elevated pH thereby producing different oxygen radicals like superoxide ($O^{2-}\bullet$), hydroperoxyl radical ($HO_2\bullet$) and hydrogen peroxide (H_2O_2). Under cellular availability of oxidant responsive enzymes, these radicals are easily broken down to neutralize the effect (cancer cells have less of these enzymes and thus this is one of the mechanisms of tea polyphenols affecting them). Apart from direct interactions with free radicals, several other indirect mechanisms exist through which tea polyphenols can exert their antioxidant action which includes inhibition of Nf-kB and AP1 (redox-sensitive transcription factors), inhibition of iNOS, lipoxygenases, cyclooxygenases and xanthine oxidase (pro-oxidant enzymes) and induction of GST and SOD enzymes (phase II antioxidant enzymes).

ANTICANCER EFFECTS

Green tea polyphenols have been widely studied and reported to possess anti-cancer properties. EGCG has been found to induce differential levels of reactive oxygen species in normal (reduces) and oral carcinoma cells (increases) which can kill cancerous cells specifically (Yamamoto et al., 2003). Apart from modulating the oxidant-antioxidant balance, various green tea polyphenols (catechins, 2-epigallocatechin-3-gallate (EGCG), 2-epigallocatechin, 2-epicatechin-3-gallate, 2-epicatechin) and black tea polyphenols (theaflavin, theaflavin-3-gallate, and theaflavin-3,3-digallate) were reported to inhibit the mitogen activated protein kinase (MAPK) activities which are responsible for Ras-dependent cancer activity (Chung, Huang, Meng, Dong, & Yang, 1999). One of the possible reasons for this observation is that both green tea and black tea polyphenols were found to inhibit the activity of epidermal growth factor receptor (EGFR) (Liang et al., 1999), which is often found involved in the development of cancer.

Both green and black tea polyphenols were not only capable of inducing cell death, but they also have the ability to inhibit cell growth through the inhibition of a key protein called activator protein 1 (AP1) (Yang et al., 2000). A thorough characterization of various tea polyphenols depicted that the sensitivity of oral carcinoma cells are as follows: (−)-catechin gallate (CG) = epicatechin gallate (ECG) > epigallocatechin gallate (EGCG) > epigallocatechin (EGC) >> epicatechin (EC), catechin (C). Similarly, the cytotoxicity of CG is in the following order immortalized epithelioid gingival S-G cells > tongue squamous carcinoma CAL27 cells > salivary gland squamous carcinoma HSG cells >> normal gingival HGF-1 fibroblasts (Babich, Zuckerbraun, & Weinerman, 2007). One of the primary targets of green tea polyphenols was found to be the protein tumour necrosis factor-alpha (TNF-α), which is an important factor for the initiation and progression of tumour development and metastasis (Fujiki et al., 2000). The implications of tea polyphenols has also been reported on several other important enzymes like urokinase, Ornithine decarboxylase, NADPH-cytochrome P450 reductase, protein kinase C, steroid 5-alpha reductase and nitric oxide synthase. Tea extract was also found to possess anti-angiogenic property and can also inhibit telomerase activity (Ramshankar & Krishnamurthy, 2014). The anti-angiogenic effect was found to be due to the inhibition of STAT1 and STAT3 (signal transducers and activators of transcription 1 & 3 respectively) molecules and is mediated through inhibition of the extracellular matrix remodelling enzyme MMP9 (matrix metalloproteinase 9) (Leong, Mathur, & Greene, 2008). Simultaneously, EGCG was reported to inhibit alternative EGFR mediated pathways and reduce the phosphorylation of another receptor called HER-2/neu receptor (HER-2) which is associated with poor prognosis of breast and head & neck cancer (Masuda, Suzui, Lim, & Weinstein, 2003). The same study reported the ability of physiologically relevant levels of EGCG to sensitize the cancer cell lines to the drug "Taxol" which is frequently used to treat these two types of cancer cases. In line with this report, and also due to its antioxidant property which might be helpful in reducing collateral damage to normal cells, green tea was proposed to be used as an adjuvant in cancer therapy (especially in chemo/radio-therapy) (Lecumberri, Dupertuis, Miralbell, & Pichard, 2013). Consequently, since DNA damage is one of the primary initial factors for the development of cancer of various organs, green tea extract was tested and found to reduce the extent of DNA damage induced by Benzo(a)pyrene diolepoxide (BPDE), a chemical from cigarette smoke known to induce DNA-adduct in lung tissue (Zhang et al., 2002).

ANTI-AGING PROPERTIES

The physiological process of ageing is conserved in all forms of animal life. The primary factors underlying this process were suspected to be reactive oxygen species (ROS) and mitochondrial dysfunction associated with increased ROS generation (Cui, Kong, & Zhang, 2012). As already mentioned above, due to the anti-oxidant property of tea polyphenols and also due to its ability to protect mitochondrial damage, it can serve as a potential dietary source possessing anti-ageing property. In line with this speculation, another theory of ageing states that progressive loss of the distal ends of chromosomes (termed "telomeres") due to the activity of the enzyme telomerase is a contributing factor in accelerating ageing and its associated risk of cancer development (Garber, 2012). Since tea polyphenols were also found to possess the ability to inhibit telomerase activity (Ramshankar & Krishnamurthy, 2014), it delays the ageing process. Under normal physiological conditions, sunlight exposure (mainly UV radiations) induced skin inflammation → immune reaction → cellular destruction due to collagenase degradation enzymes → wrinkle formations plays a significant process in inducing skin alterations resulting in first visible signs of ageing. Application of the water extract of various kinds of tea (white, black and green) were demonstrated to reduce skin inflammation, inhibit matrix metalloproteinase enzyme mediated collagenase degradation and also delay the appearance of wrinkles (Lee, Kim, & Kim, 2014; Roh et al., 2015). Green tea polyphenols were found to induce anti-ageing effects through its restorative effects on the metabonomic profile on d-galactose (d-gal) induced ageing rats (Fu et al., 2011). Tea polyphenols were primarily found to affect the profiles of lecithin metabolism, amino acid metabolism and phospholipids metabolism. Tea catechins (EGCG, ECG, EGC, and EC) were also reported to reduce erythrocyte malondialdehyde (MDA) levels and restore glutathione levels which were found to be otherwise affected under normal ageing process (Maurya & Rizvi, 2009). Since ageing is associated with declining cognitive abilities, various extracts were found to restore the cognitive function in aged rats, reduce beta amyloid induced neuro-damage and also recover the cognitive functions in aged animals (Wei et al., 2014; Rodrigues et al., 2013). This neuro-protective ability was attributed to its protective ability of the brain mitochondria which is empirically known to be the cellular target of free radicals and associated with almost all the neurodegenerative states including Alzheimer's, Parkinson's, Huntington's disease and others (Assuncao, & Andrade, 2015; Mandel, Amit, Weinreb, & Youdim, 2011). Emerging studies also indicate a positive regulation of the epigenetic changes by EGCG which can contribute to delayed ageing and the improve quality of health (Daniel & Tollefsbol, 2015).

CLINICAL AND EPIDEMIOLOGICAL EVIDENCES

After its huge success as an anti-cancer agent under laboratory conditions, tea polyphenols have enjoyed comparably limited application as a chemo-preventive or therapeutic compound in clinical studies. Epidemiological studies also report contradictory efficacy of tea polyphenols in humans against cancers of various origins. Few initial studies indicated towards the possibility of tea being a chemo-preventive agent whose regular intake may reduce the possibility of cancer risk among Japanese population (Imai, Suga, & Nakachi, 1997). On the contrary, green tea consumption was also found to be associated with increased risk of developing oesophageal cancer in the Japanese population by 22.1% (Ishikawa et al., 2006). Interestingly, in the above two cases, one study showing cancer preventive action of tea does not indicate the temperature of tea which was consumed whereas the latter study clearly indicates that it is hot tea which increases the chance of developing oesophageal cancer, which can also relate to the thermal effect of hot tea responsible for damage of oesophageal cells thereby inducing their cancerous transformation.

Recent reports on the effect of tea consumption and the risk of gastric cancer indicates that in seven of such studies, no correlation exists whereas in another eight case-control studies an inverse correlation was found which indicate towards an positive effect of tea consumption against cancer development/ progression. Concurrently a single study states a negative association between tea consumption and cancer. Meta-analysis of such varied reports warrants further clinical studies before the establishment of tea and its associated molecules to be used as a preventive/therapeutic agent (Hou, Amarnani, Chong, & Bishayee, 2013). Interestingly, most of such studies indicated a statistically significant protective effect of tea consumption against gastric cancer in women population when compared to their male counterparts involved in the same study.

In females, consumption of >= 5 cups of tea has been associated with a preventive trend towards the development of breast cancer development which was primarily related to its anti-cancer property rather than any therapeutic effect (Seely, Mills, Wu, Verma, & Guyatt, 2005). Another meta-analysis study indicated potential effect of tea consumption towards reduction in breast cancer recurrence with mild protection in cancer induction (Ogunleye, Xue, & Michels, 2010). However, it should be emphasized that the protective effects of tea were found when concentrations used was high which is difficult to achieve under normal circumstances. Alternatively, this problem can be bypassed by engineering tea catechins which may possess better absorption and bioavailability following consumption.

Among others, increased green tea but not black tea consumption was associated with significantly reduced incidence of lung cancer (Tang, Wu, Zhou, Wang, & Yu, 2009). Green tea was also protective against adult leukaemia in Chinese population (Zhang et al., 2008). In cases of oral cancer, phase I clinical trial showed improved reduction of lesion in golden Syrian hamsters induced by DMBA (7,12-dimethyl-benz[a]anthracene) injection with significant reduction of epidermal growth factor receptor (a bio-marker used in cancer studies) (Li, Han, & Chen, 1999). Similarly, a phase II case-control matched study also indicated a positive effect of green tea extract on reducing oral pre-malignant carcinogenesis conditions (Tsao et al., 2009). Another study reports that consumption of 10 Japanese-size cups of green tea per day significantly reduces primary cancer occurrence in the general population, and prevents recurrence of colorectal adenomas in patients with tertiary cancer (Fujiki et al., 2012). On the contrary, there are several reports which indicate that there are no significant positive effects of tea consumption towards cancer prevention (Baker et al., 2005; Laurie, Miller, Grant, Kris, & Ng, 2005; Fritz et al., 2013). Whereas, it has also been found that in certain cases, tea consumption can hamper the efficacy of anti-cancer drugs such as bortezomib and other boronic acid-based proteasome inhibitors (Golden et al., 2009). Apart from its clinical evidences, epidemiological studies demonstrate that drinking tea may be beneficial in delaying the ageing process (Zeng et al., 2015; Arab, Khan, & Lam, 2013).

CONCLUSION

Due to the presence of such wide range of bio-active molecules in a "cup" of tea, it makes tea an attractive and compelling example of a functional food. The relative ease of purchase and hassle free consumption makes it a preferred beverage throughout the world. This makes tea a relevant model of understanding and empowering the health benefits of functional foods in human life.

REFERENCES

Arab, L., Khan, F., & Lam, H. (2013). Epidemiologic evidence of a relationship between tea, coffee, or caffeine consumption and cognitive decline. *Advances in Nutrition*, *4*(1), 115–122. doi:10.3945/an.112.002717 PMID:23319129

Assuncao, M., & Andrade, J. P. (2015). Protective action of green tea catechins in neuronal mitochondria during aging. *Frontiers in Bioscience*, *20*(2), 247–262. doi:10.2741/4307 PMID:25553449

Babich, H., Zuckerbraun, H. L., & Weinerman, S. M. (2007). In vitro cytotoxicity of (-)-catechin gallate, a minor polyphenol in green tea. *Toxicology Letters*, *171*(3), 171–180. doi:10.1016/j.toxlet.2007.05.125 PMID:17606338

Baker, J. A., McCann, S. E., Reid, M. E., Nowell, S., Beehler, G. P., & Moysich, K. B. (2005). Associations between black tea and coffee consumption and risk of lung cancer among current and former smokers. *Nutrition and Cancer*, *52*(1), 15–21. doi:10.1207/s15327914nc5201_2 PMID:16090999

Banerjee, S., Maity, P., Mukherjee, S., Sil, A. K., Panda, K., Chattopadhyay, D., & Chatterjee, I. B. (2007). Black tea prevents cigarette smoke-induced apoptosis and lung damage. *Journal of Inflammation*, *4*(3). PMID:17300721

Bordoni, A., Hrelia, S., Angeloni, C., Giordano, E., Guarnieri, C., Caldarera, C. M., & Biagi, P. L. (2002). Green tea protection of hypoxia/reoxygenation injury in cultured cardiac cells. *The Journal of Nutritional Biochemistry*, *13*(2), 103–111. doi:10.1016/S0955-2863(01)00203-0 PMID:11834226

Chen, W. C., Hsieh, S. R., Chiu, C. H., Hsu, B. D., & Liou, Y. M. (2014). Molecular identification for epigallocatechin-3-gallate-mediated antioxidant intervention on the H2O2-induced oxidative stress in H9c2 rat cardiomyoblasts. *Journal of Biomedical Science*, *21*, 56. PMID:24913014

Cho, H. S., Kim, S., Lee, S. Y., Park, J. A., Kim, S. J., & Chun, H. S. (2008). Protective effect of the green tea component, L-theanine on environmental toxins-induced neuronal cell death. *Neurotoxicology*, *29*(4), 656–662. doi:10.1016/j.neuro.2008.03.004 PMID:18452993

Chung, J. Y., Huang, C., Meng, X., Dong, Z., & Yang, C. S. (1999). Inhibition of activator protein 1 activity and cell growth by purified green tea and black tea polyphenols in H-ras-transformed cells: Structure-activity relationship and mechanisms involved. *Cancer Research*, *59*(18), 4610–4617. PMID:10493515

Cui, H., Kong, Y., & Zhang, H. (2012). Oxidative stress, mitochondrial dysfunction, and aging. *Journal of Signal Transduction*, 646354. PMID:21977319

Daniel, M., & Tollefsbol, T. O. (2015). Epigenetic linkage of aging, cancer and nutrition. *The Journal of Experimental Biology*, *218*(Pt 1), 59–70. doi:10.1242/jeb.107110 PMID:25568452

Dorchies, O. M., Wagner, S., Buetler, T. M., & Ruegg, U. T. (2009). Protection of dystrophic muscle cells with polyphenols from green tea correlates with improved glutathione balance and increased expression of 67LR, a receptor for (-)-epigallocatechin gallate. *BioFactors (Oxford, England)*, *35*(3), 279–294. doi:10.1002/biof.34 PMID:19322813

Fritz, H., Seely, D., Kennedy, D. A., Fernandes, R., Cooley, K., & Fergusson, D. (2013). Green tea and lung cancer: A systematic review. *Integrative Cancer Therapies*, *12*(1), 7–24. doi:10.1177/1534735412442378 PMID:22532034

Fu, C., Wang, T., Wang, Y., Chen, X., Jiao, J., Ma, F., & Bi, K. et al. (2011). Metabonomics study of the protective effects of green tea polyphenols on aging rats induced by d-galactose. *Journal of Pharmaceutical and Biomedical Analysis*, *55*(5), 1067–1074. doi:10.1016/j.jpba.2011.03.011 PMID:21444175

Fujiki, H., Imai, K., Nakachi, K., Shimizu, M., Moriwaki, H., & Suganuma, M. (2012). Challenging the effectiveness of green tea in primary and tertiary cancer prevention. *Journal of Cancer Research and Clinical Oncology*, *138*(8), 1259–1270. doi:10.1007/s00432-012-1250-y PMID:22699930

Fujiki, H., Suganuma, M., Okabe, S., Sueoka, E., Suga, K., Imai, K., & Nakachi, K. (2000). A new concept of tumor promotion by tumor necrosis factor-alpha, and cancer preventive agents (-)-epigallocatechin gallate and green tea--a review. *Cancer Detection and Prevention*, *24*(1), 91–99. PMID:10757128

Garber, K. (2012). At loose ends: Telomere theories of aging and cancer begin to converge. *Journal of the National Cancer Institute*, *104*(11), 803–806. doi:10.1093/jnci/djs271 PMID:22673587

Golden, E. B., Lam, P. Y., Kardosh, A., Gaffney, K. J., Cadenas, E., Louie, S. G., & Schönthal, A. H. et al. (2009). Green tea polyphenols block the anticancer effects of bortezomib and other boronic acid-based proteasome inhibitors. *Blood*, *113*(23), 5927–5937. doi:10.1182/blood-2008-07-171389 PMID:19190249

Helen, S. (2010). *Tea, a global history*. Reaktion Books Ltd.

Hou, I. C., Amarnani, S., Chong, M. T., & Bishayee, A. (2013). Green tea and the risk of gastric cancer: Epidemiological evidence. *World Journal of Gastroenterology*, *19*(24), 3713–3722. doi:10.3748/wjg.v19.i24.3713 PMID:23840110

Imai, K., Suga, K., & Nakachi, K. (1997). Cancer-preventive effects of drinking green tea among a Japanese population. *Preventive Medicine*, *26*(6), 769–775. doi:10.1006/pmed.1997.0242 PMID:9388788

International Agency for Research on Cancer (IARC) Monograph. (n.d.). *Chemical composition of tea*. Retrieved July 27, 2015 from http://monographs.iarc.fr/ENG/Monographs/vol51/mono51-8B.pdf

Ishikawa, A., Kuriyama, S., Tsubono, Y., Fukao, A., Takahashi, H., Tachiya, H., & Tsuji, I. (2006). Smoking, alcohol drinking, green tea consumption and the risk of esophageal cancer in Japanese men. *Journal of Epidemiology*, *16*(5), 185–192. doi:10.2188/jea.16.185 PMID:16951537

Jane, P. (2004). The discovery of Tea. In *Afternoon tea* (p. 10). The Jarrold Group.

Kakuda, T. (2002). Neuroprotective effects of the green tea components theanine and catechins. *Biological & Pharmaceutical Bulletin*, *25*(12), 1513–1518. doi:10.1248/bpb.25.1513 PMID:12499631

Kakuda, T., Nozawa, A., Sugimoto, A., & Niino, H. (2002). Inhibition by theanine of binding of [3H]AMPA, [3H]kainate, and [3H]MDL 105,519 to glutamate receptors. *Bioscience, Biotechnology, and Biochemistry*, *66*(12), 2683–2686. doi:10.1271/bbb.66.2683 PMID:12596867

Lambert, J. D., & Elias, R. J. (2010). The antioxidant and pro-oxidant activities of green tea polyphenols: A role in cancer prevention. *Archives of Biochemistry and Biophysics*, *501*(1), 65–72. doi:10.1016/j.abb.2010.06.013 PMID:20558130

Laura, M. (2007). *Tea: The Drink that Changed the World*. Tuttle Publishing.

Laurie, S. A., Miller, V. A., Grant, S. C., Kris, M. G., & Ng, K. K. (2005). Phase I study of green tea extract in patients with advanced lung cancer. *Cancer Chemotherapy and Pharmacology*, *55*(1), 33–38. doi:10.1007/s00280-004-0859-1 PMID:15309507

Lecumberri, E., Dupertuis, Y. M., Miralbell, R., & Pichard, C. (2013). Green tea polyphenol epigallocatechin-3-gallate (EGCG) as adjuvant in cancer therapy. *Clinical Nutrition (Edinburgh, Lothian)*, *32*(6), 894–903. doi:10.1016/j.clnu.2013.03.008 PMID:23582951

Lee, K. O., Kim, S. N., & Kim, Y. C. (2014). Anti-wrinkle Effects of Water Extracts of Teas in Hairless Mouse. *Toxicological Reviews*, *30*(4), 283–289. doi:10.5487/TR.2014.30.4.283 PMID:25584148

Leong, H., Mathur, P. S., & Greene, G. L. (2008). Green tea catechins inhibit angiogenesis through suppression of STAT3 activation. *Breast Cancer Research and Treatment*, *117*(3), 505–515. doi:10.1007/s10549-008-0196-x PMID:18821062

Li, N., Han, C., & Chen, J. (1999). Tea preparations protect against DMBA-induced oral carcinogenesis in hamsters. *Nutrition and Cancer*, *35*(1), 73–79. doi:10.1207/S1532791473-79 PMID:10624709

Li, Y., Zhao, S., Zhang, W., Zhao, P., He, B., Wu, N., & Han, P. (2011). Epigallocatechin-3-O-gallate (EGCG) attenuates FFAs-induced peripheral insulin resistance through AMPK pathway and insulin signaling pathway in vivo. *Diabetes Research and Clinical Practice*, *93*(2), 205–214. doi:10.1016/j.diabres.2011.03.036 PMID:21514684

Li, Y. W., Zhang, Y., Zhang, L., Li, X., Yu, J. B., Zhang, H. T., & Liu, H. G. et al. (2014). Protective effect of tea polyphenols on renal ischemia/reperfusion injury via suppressing the activation of TLR4/NF-κB p65 signal pathway. *Gene*, *542*(1), 46–51. doi:10.1016/j.gene.2014.03.021 PMID:24630969

Liang, Y. C., Chen, Y. C., Lin, Y. L., Lin-Shiau, S. Y., Ho, C. T., & Lin, J. K. (1999). Suppression of extracellular signals and cell proliferation by the black tea polyphenol, theaflavin-3,3'-digallate. *Carcinogenesis*, *20*(4), 733–736. doi:10.1093/carcin/20.4.733 PMID:10223207

Malhomme, H., Seagrove, S., Mehta, A., Divekar, P., Campbell, S., & Curnow, A. (2010). Using natural dietary sources of antioxidants to protect against ultraviolet and visible radiation-induced DNA damage: an investigation of human green tea ingestion. *Journal of Photochemistry and Photobiology B*, *101*(2), 169-173.

Mandel, S. A., Amit, T., Weinreb, O., & Youdim, M. B. (2011). Understanding the broad-spectrum neuroprotective action profile of green tea polyphenols in aging and neurodegenerative diseases. *Journal of Alzheimer's Disease*, *25*(2), 187–208. PMID:21368374

Masuda, M., Suzui, M., Lim, J. T., & Weinstein, I. B. (2003). Epigallocatechin-3-gallate inhibits activation of HER-2/neu and downstream signaling pathways in human head and neck and breast carcinoma cells. *Clinical Cancer Research*, *9*(9), 3486–3491. PMID:12960141

Maurya, P. K., & Rizvi, S. I. (2009). Protective role of tea catechins on erythrocytes subjected to oxidative stress during human aging. *Natural Product Research*, *23*(12), 1072–1079. doi:10.1080/14786410802267643 PMID:18846469

Meng, Q., Velalar, C. N., & Ruan, R. (2008). Regulating the age-related oxidative damage, mitochondrial integrity, and antioxidative enzyme activity in Fischer 344 rats by supplementation of the antioxidant epigallocatechin-3-gallate. *Rejuvenation Research*, *11*(3), 649–660. doi:10.1089/rej.2007.0645 PMID:18593283

Muià, C., Mazzon, E., Di Paola, R., Genovese, T., Menegazzi, M., Caputi, A. P., & Cuzzocrea, S. et al. (2005). Green tea polyphenol extract attenuates ischemia/reperfusion injury of the gut. *Naunyn-Schmiedeberg's Archives of Pharmacology*, *371*(5), 364–374. doi:10.1007/s00210-005-1076-0 PMID:15997392

Nakagawa, H., Hasumi, K., Woo, J. T., Nagai, K., & Wachi, M. (2004). Generation of hydrogen peroxide primarily contributes to the induction of Fe(II)-dependent apoptosis in Jurkat cells by (-)-epigallocatechin gallate. *Carcinogenesis*, *25*(9), 1567–1574. doi:10.1093/carcin/bgh168 PMID:15090467

Nakagawa, H., Wachi, M., Woo, J. T., Kato, M., Kasai, S., Takahashi, F., & Nagai, K. et al. (2002). Fenton reaction is primarily involved in a mechanism of (-)-epigallocatechin-3-gallate to induce osteoclastic cell death. *Biochemical and Biophysical Research Communications*, *292*(1), 94–101. doi:10.1006/bbrc.2002.6622 PMID:11890677

Ogunleye, A. A., Xue, F., & Michels, K. B. (2010). Green tea consumption and breast cancer risk or recurrence: A meta-analysis. *Breast Cancer Research and Treatment*, *119*(2), 477–484. doi:10.1007/s10549-009-0415-0 PMID:19437116

Ramshankar, V., & Krishnamurthy, A. (2014). Chemoprevention of oral cancer: Green tea experience. Journal of Natural Science. *Biologie Medicale*, *5*(1), 3–7.

Rodrigues, J., Assunção, M., Lukoyanov, N., Cardoso, A., Carvalho, F., & Andrade, J. P. (2013). Protective effects of a catechin-rich extract on the hippocampal formation and spatial memory in aging rats. *Behavioural Brain Research*, *246*, 94–102. doi:10.1016/j.bbr.2013.02.040 PMID:23473881

Roh, E., Kim, J. E., Kwon, J. Y., Park, J. S., Bode, A. M., Dong, Z., & Lee, K. W. (2015). Molecular Mechanisms of Green Tea Polyphenols with Protective Effects against Skin Photoaging.[Epub ahead of print]. *Critical Reviews in Food Science and Nutrition*, 00. doi:10.1080/10408398.2014.1003365 PMID:26114360

Ryu, H. H., Kim, H. L., Chung, J. H., Lee, B. R., Kim, T. H., & Shin, B. C. (2010). Renoprotective effects of green tea extract on renin-angiotensin-aldosterone system in chronic cyclosporine-treated rats. *Nephrology, Dialysis, Transplantation*, *26*(4), 1188–1193. doi:10.1093/ndt/gfq616 PMID:20947539

Samy, A. H., Omayma, A. R., & Mohammed, A. E. (2014). Protective Effect of Green Tea Extract on Cyclosporine A: Induced Nephrotoxicity in Rats. *The Journal of Biological Sciences*, *14*(4), 248–257. doi:10.3923/jbs.2014.248.257

Sang, S., Tian, S., Wang, H., Stark, R. E., Rosen, R. T., Yang, C. S., & Ho, C. T. (2003). Chemical studies of the antioxidant mechanism of tea catechins: Radical reaction products of epicatechin with peroxyl radicals. *Bioorganic & Medicinal Chemistry*, *11*(16), 3371–3378. doi:10.1016/S0968-0896(03)00367-5 PMID:12878131

Seely, D., Mills, E. J., Wu, P., Verma, S., & Guyatt, G. H. (2005). The effects of green tea consumption on incidence of breast cancer and recurrence of breast cancer: A systematic review and meta-analysis. *Integrative Cancer Therapies*, *4*(2), 144–155. doi:10.1177/1534735405276420 PMID:15911927

Sen, C. T. (2004). *Food Culture in India*. Greenwood Publishing Group.

Severino, J. F., Goodman, B. A., Kay, C. W., Stolze, K., Tunega, D., Reichenauer, T. G., & Pirker, K. F. (2009). Free radicals generated during oxidation of green tea polyphenols: Electron paramagnetic resonance spectroscopy combined with density functional theory calculations. *Free Radical Biology & Medicine*, *46*(8), 1076–1088. doi:10.1016/j.freeradbiomed.2009.01.004 PMID:19439236

Tang, N., Wu, Y., Zhou, B., Wang, B., & Yu, R. (2009). Green tea, black tea consumption and risk of lung cancer: A meta-analysis. *Lung Cancer (Amsterdam, Netherlands)*, *65*(3), 274–283. doi:10.1016/j.lungcan.2008.12.002 PMID:19128856

Tsao, A. S., Liu, D., Martin, J., Tang, X. M., Lee, J. J., El-Naggar, A. K., & Papadimitrakopoulou, V. et al. (2009). Phase II randomized, placebo-controlled trial of green tea extract in patients with high-risk oral premalignant lesions. *Cancer Prevention Research (Philadelphia, Pa.)*, *2*(11), 931–941. doi:10.1158/1940-6207.CAPR-09-0121 PMID:19892663

Urchin Tea. (2012, December 11). *The Oldest Tea Tree on the Earth*. Retrieved from http://teaurchin.blogspot.com/2012/12/the-worlds-oldest-tea-tree.html

Valcic, S., Burr, J. A., Timmermann, B. N., & Liebler, D. C. (2000). Antioxidant chemistry of green tea catechins. New oxidation products of (-)-epigallocatechin gallate and (-)-epigallocatechin from their reactions with peroxyl radicals. *Chemical Research in Toxicology*, *13*(9), 801–810. doi:10.1021/tx000080k PMID:10995252

Wei, C. C., Yu, C. W., Yen, P. L., Lin, H. Y., Chang, S. T., Hsu, F. L., & Liao, V. H. (2014). Antioxidant activity, delayed aging, and reduced amyloid-β toxicity of methanol extracts of tea seed pomace from Camellia tenuifolia. *Journal of Agricultural and Food Chemistry*, *62*(44), 10701–10707. doi:10.1021/jf503192x PMID:25295856

Xu, Y., Zhang, J. J., Xiong, L., Zhang, L., Sun, D., & Liu, H. (2010). Green tea polyphenols inhibit cognitive impairment induced by chronic cerebral hypoperfusion via modulating oxidative stress. *The Journal of Nutritional Biochemistry*, *21*(8), 741–748. doi:10.1016/j.jnutbio.2009.05.002 PMID:19615878

Yamamoto, T., Hsu, S., Lewis, J., Wataha, J., Dickinson, D., Singh, B., & Schuster, G. et al. (2003). Green tea polyphenol causes differential oxidative environments in tumor versus normal epithelial cells. *The Journal of Pharmacology and Experimental Therapeutics*, *307*(1), 230–236. doi:10.1124/jpet.103.054676 PMID:12954803

Yang, G. Y., Liao, J., Li, C., Chung, J., Yurkow, E. J., Ho, C. T., & Yang, C. S. (2000). Effect of black and green tea polyphenols on c-jun phosphorylation and H(2)O(2) production in transformed and non-transformed human bronchial cell lines: Possible mechanisms of cell growth inhibition and apoptosis induction. *Carcinogenesis*, *21*(11), 2035–2039. doi:10.1093/carcin/21.11.2035 PMID:11062165

Zeng, Y., Chen, H., Ni, T., Ruan, R., Feng, L., Nie, C., & …, Vaupel, J.W. (2015). GxE interactions between FOXO genotypes and drinking tea are significantly associated with prevention of cognitive decline in advanced age in China. *The Journals of Gerontology. Series A, Biological Sciences and Medical Sciences*, *70*(4), 426–433. doi:10.1093/gerona/glu060 PMID:24895270

Zhang, H., Spitz, M. R., Tomlinson, G. E., Schabath, M. B., Minna, J. D., & Wu, X. (2002). Modification of lung cancer susceptibility by green tea extract as measured by the comet assay. *Cancer Detection and Prevention*, *26*(6), 411–418. doi:10.1016/S0361-090X(02)00127-7 PMID:12507225

Zhang, X. D., Zhao, X. Y., Zhang, M., Liang, Y., Xu, X. H., D'Arcy, C., & Holman, J. (2008). A case-control study on green tea consumption and the risk of adult leukemia. *Zhonghua Liu Xing Bing Xue Za Zhi*, *29*(3), 290–293. PMID:18788532

Chapter 6
Herbal Benefits of Tea

Etetor Roland Eshiet
Sustainable Energy Environmental and Educational Development (SEEED), USA

Ernest E. Smith
Texas Tech University, USA

ABSTRACT

This chapter per the authors will introduce the reader to Complementary and Alternative Medicine (CAM) and shall discuss herbalism as a subset of CAM. Particular emphasis will be placed on herbal teas or rather infusions and decoctions used in disease therapy. This chapter will enumerate the different types of teas and shall use maps, graphs, and other tools to illustrate location, consumption, use and availability. Furthermore, the authors will highlight potential health benefits, recent studies (in vitro, in vivo) undertaken by research scientists to validate efficacy, and shall call for more research (clinical data management, clinical trials, etc.) and support for ongoing work in this area of expertise. The authors shall place a spotlight on the plant family, Asteraceae, and their herbal plants of interest, Artemisia annua and Brickellia cavanillesii. Extensive studies have been performed to determine the therapeutic potential of Brickellia cavanillesii plant at Ernest E. Smith laboratory, The Institute of Environmental and Human Health (TIEHH), Texas Tech University, Lubbock, USA.

INTRODUCTION

Complementary and Alternative Medicine (CAM)

The use of complementary and alternative medicine (CAM) in disease therapy dates back to prehistoric man, and has increased exponentially over time. Before the advent of modern science, early humans employed the use of alternative remedies as therapy for disease. Archeological records indicate that during the Stone Age, treatment of biologic disorders involved certain practices. The methods utilized involved a broad spectrum of approaches that is termed CAM by scientists today. Early civilizations embraced these practices as is evidenced in Persian, Greek, Egyptian and Chinese cultures amongst others. CAM continues to grow with concomitant recognition by scientific researchers and healthcare professionals

DOI: 10.4018/978-1-5225-0591-4.ch006

around the globe. The motives for using CAM are variant and may include: to fight disease, to increase the body's ability to fight disease, to improve physical and emotional well-being, to counteract ill effect from disease, and as advised by healthcare professionals (Molassiotis, 2005). CAM, as the name connotes, is comprised of diverse medicinal and health care systems, practices, and products that are not typically considered to be a part of conventional medicine. Complementary medicine is used together with conventional medicine whereas alternative medicine is utilized in place of conventional medicine; CAM encapsulates traditional (conventional), alternative and integrative remedies. Treatment may be considered 'complementary' when non-orthodox methods are utilized simultaneously with conventional medicine. When non-orthodox methods are used in place of conventional medicine, it is considered 'alternative.' Approaches that utilize the systematic use of conventional and alternative treatment are termed 'integrative.' The National Center for Complementary and Alternative Medicine (NCCAM) classifies CAM into four distinct categories:

1. Whole medical systems;
2. Mind-body medicine;
3. Biologically based practices; and
4. Manipulative and body based practices (NCCIH, 2015).

Whole medical systems are built upon complete systems of theory and practice which evolved earlier than and apart from the conventional medical approach used by western cultures. Mind-body medicine employs a variety of techniques designed to enhance the mind's capacity to affect body function and symptoms. Techniques such as meditation, prayer, mental healing and therapies that involve art, music and dance are usually applied by CAM practitioners. Biologically- based practices use substances found in nature such as herbs, foods and vitamin. Manipulative and body based practices involve the manipulation and/or movement of one or more parts of the body and includes chiropractic and osteopathic manipulation and massage therapy (NCCIH, 2015; Eshiet, 2010; Eshiet et al., 2014a, 2014b). This chapter focuses on biological-based practices as is demonstrated in the herbal benefits of tea (herbalism).

Herbalism

Herbalism also known as phytotherapy is an integral component of CAM, and is a veritable source of alternative medicine. The practice of herbalism dates back to primordial periods. Herbalism is a biologically-based practice whereby plants and plant extracts are used in traditional medicine. Plants synthesize many secondary metabolites which are useful for the maintenance of health in humans and other animals. Of these secondary metabolites, less than 10% (~ 12,000) have been isolated (Lai 2004; Tapsell 2006). Herbal plants have been used by all cultures throughout history. Records show that marshmallow root, hyacinth and yarrow were found placed around the bones of a Stone Age man in Iraq (Zand et al., 2003). Marshmallow is a demulcent herb which is soothing to inflamed or irritated mucous membranes such as sore throat. Hyacinth is a diuretic that facilitates the excretion of excess water from the body while yarrow is a renowned cold and fever remedy. Other records show that in 2735 B.C., Sheng Nong, a Chinese emperor, wrote an authoritative exposition that continues to find use today. In his exposition, Sheng Nong suggested the use of Ma Huang (ephedra) against respiratory distress. Ephinedrine, extracted from ephedra, is used extensively as a decongestant and can be found in its synthetic form, pseudoephinedrine, in many allergy, sinus, and cold relief medications manufactured by pharmaceutical companies (Zand et al., 2003). Texts from the ancient cultures of Mesopotamia, Egypt and India describe and illustrate the therapeutic properties of castor oil, linseed oil, white poppies and others. In 1649, one of the first manuals that the layperson could use for health care was written in Europe. It was authored by Nicholas Culpeper and titled "A Physical Directory." A few years later Culpeper wrote "The English Physician." Both manuals enjoyed remarkable respectability and are widely referred to and quoted (Herb Palace 2004). The first U.S. pharmacopeia was published in 1820. It included a compendium of herbal drugs: their properties, uses, dosages, and testing purity. This publication was revised periodically and by the year 1906 it had become the legal standard for medical compounds. However, as western medicine evolved from an art to a science in the nineteenth century, herbalism began to lose its popularity. As scientific methods were developed to extract and synthesize the active ingredients in plants, pharmaceutical laboratories became the producers of drugs. Consequently, in the industrialized parts of the world, herbalism as a customary approach to medicine suffered a significant decline. It is estimated that about 80% of the world population use herbal medicine as primary health care (WHO, 2003; Ekor, 2014). WHO observes that of 119 plant-derived pharmaceutical medicines, approximately 74% are used in modern medicine in ways that relate directly with their native usage. Of over 750,000 plants on earth, only a few have been scientifically studied. Modern pharmacology places emphasis on the active ingredients of herbal plants. Scientists perform research which focuses on identifying and isolating these active ingredients. Herbalism, on the other hand, considers the synergistic interaction of all the components of the whole plant for the treatment of acute and chronic conditions. Examples of herbalistic treatments include Aloe vera which is used traditionally in the healing of burns and wounds (Maenthaisong et al., 2007) and; cranberry (*Vaccinium oxycoccos*) used in treating urinary tract infections in women with recurrent symptoms (Jepson & Craig, 2008).

A study exploring the use of CAM in a subset of patients resident in Kuching, Sarawak, Malaysia may be indicative of the consistent popularity of herbalism as a component of CAM (Lee et al., 2004). This investigation revealed that herbal remedies may be the second mode of therapy after massage (Figure 1). A series of studies performed to determine CAM in the United States of America showed that in 1990 about 33.8% of Americans used alternative remedies which included oral supplements, chiropractic and acupuncture. This percentage rose to 42.1% in 1997. Fifteen million adults took CAM products and prescription drugs simultaneously; approximately 12.1% of patients took herbal supplements while 5.5% took megavitamins. A 2002 medication use in America report indicated that about 14% of the surveyed population used herbal remedies or supplements (Eisenberg et al., 1993; Eisenberg et al., 1998; Kaufman et al. 2002, Shane-McWhorter 2007). Unfortunately, many patients do not inform their physicians of their use of phytotherapies which may lead to potentially dangerous adverse interactions with pharmacotherapies. It cannot be overemphasized that healthcare professionals need to be better informed about herbal products that patients take singularly, or in combination with conventional medications. This invariably will afford clinicians ability to provide patients with excellent advice, and relevant complimentary information for safe administration and monitoring. There is a compelling need to comprehend the potential use, adverse effects, and drug-drug or drug-disease interactions triggered by herbal plants (Shane-McWhorter, 2007). Tea preparations are arguably the most prevalent form of administering herbal extracts. The benefits therein is the subject of this chapter.

Figure 1. Comparative use of complementary and alternative medicine (CAM) amongst Malaysians
Adapted from Lee et al, 2014.

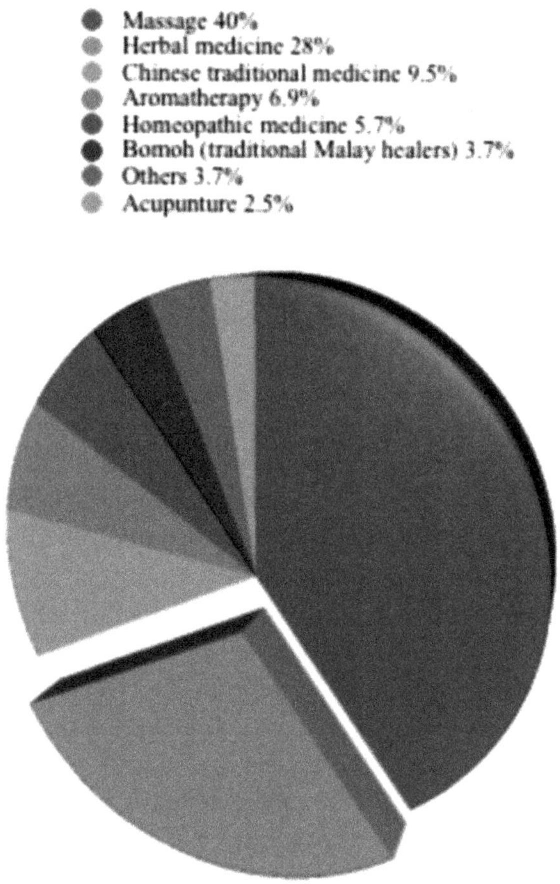

TEA

All definitions agree that the word "tea" is used to refer to an aromatic beverage prepared by either pouring hot or boiling water over cured leaves of the *Camellia sinensis* plant, or from leaves and twigs of certain herbal plants.

Types of Tea

For the purpose of clarity, the authors shall divide tea into two distinct categories; a) conventional tea and; b) medicinal herbal tea.

Conventional Tea

Tea, otherwise known for present purposes as "conventional tea," is a riveting, soothing, gentle, relaxing, mild-mannered drink prepared from the leaves of one of three species – China bush, Assam bush, Java bush - of the plant, *Camellia sinensis* (Theaceae). *C. sinensis*, a sturdy evergreen shrub featuring dark, glossy-green, serrated leaves is originally native to Eastern Asia, an area between North Burma and Southwest China (latitude 29°N and longitude 98°E) (Heiss & Heiss, 2007; Martin, 2007). Flowers are yellowish white, diameter 0.98 – 1.87 inches (2.5 – 4 cm); with 7 to 8 petals. Leaves are 1.6 – 5.9 inches (4 – 15 cm) in length and 0.79 – 1.97 inches (2 – 5 cm) in breadth. Tea is largely consumed for its stimulating, refreshing and medicinal properties. Over time a multitude of methodologies have been developed to process tea for human consumption. Historical records show that tea leaves were steamed, pounded, and shaped into cake form during the Tang dynasty (618-907 AD). Loose-leaf tea was cultivated and enjoyed a surge in popularity during the Song dynasty (960-1279 AD). A technique that allowed tea leaves to remain green was developed during the Yuan (1279-1368 AD) and Ming (1368-1644 AD) dynasties. Unfermented tea leaves were initially pan-fried, and subsequently rolled and dried to interrupt the oxidation process which darkens the leaves. "Black dragon (Oolong) tea," where leaves are allowed to ferment partially (8-85%) before pan-frying, was developed in the 15th Century. Presently, western cultures have a preference for the fully oxidized black tea.

After water, tea is the most widely drunk beverage in the world (Figure 2; Macfarlane & Macfarlane, 2004; Lewis, 2012). *Camellia sinensis* is cultivated in over 30 countries of the world (~ 78% black, ~

Figure 2. Annual per capita tea consumption of 2009
Adapted from Lewis, 2012.

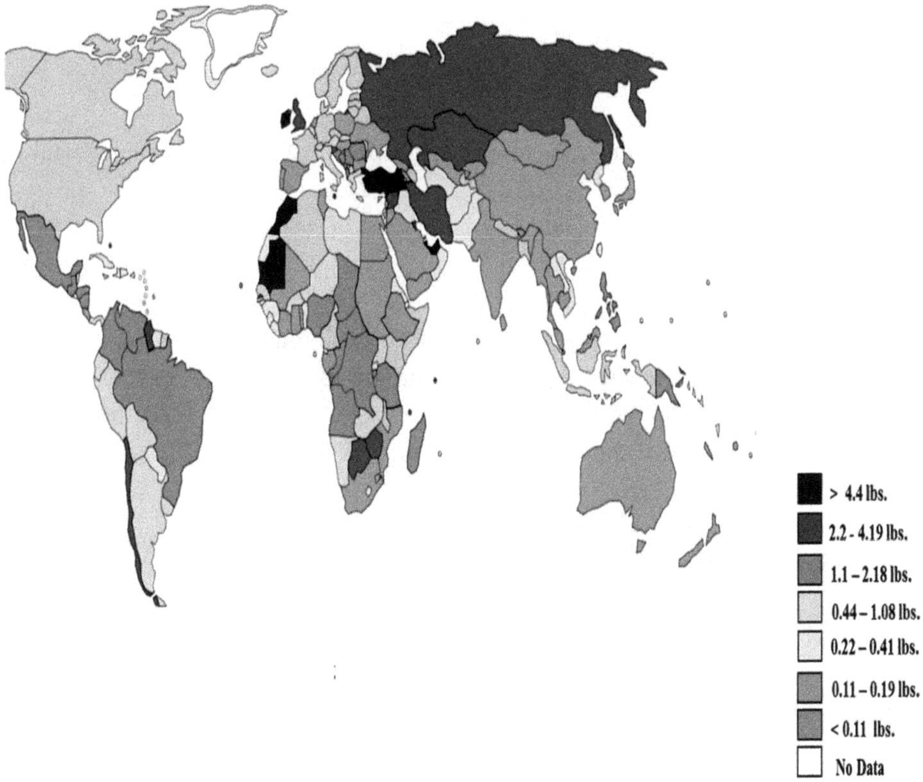

20% green, ~ 2% oolong) (Graham, 1992; Mukta & Ahmad, 2000). About 50 - 60 billion cups of tea is drunk respectively in the United Kingdom and the United States of America every year; in the United Kingdom a per capita intake of approximately 3.5 – 4 cups/person/day is consumed (Ashenef, 2014). Tea's rich, distinct taste characterized by a unique balance of flavor and aroma ranges from the fresh tasting, sweet, delicate green tea (Chinese), the aromatic, flavorful, bracing black tea (Indian), to the carefully tended, fresh, astringent tea (Java). Each tea preparation bears the singular stamp of the culture that produced it. Factors such as soil type, growing conditions, weather conditions, leaf style, pruning, timing of the pickings, skill and experience etc., combine with tradition, culture and terroir to produce the spectacular teas renown all over the world.

Medicinal Herbal Tea

The use of the word "tea" has been expanded to include infusions and decoctions prepared from the leaves and twigs of herbal plants believed to possess ameliorative or therapeutic properties. Medicinal herbal tea may be defined as a beverage prepared by infusion or decoction of herbal plant materials, and served either hot or cold, for the singular purpose of providing relief or healing to the consumer. The plant material used usually determines the mode of preparation. Infusions are made by steeping the plant material i.e. seeds, flowers and leaves in hot (boiling) water. Decoctions are made by gently simmering the plant material i.e. dried seeds, roots and barks in water.

Generic recipe for preparing infusions:

1. Pour a quart of boiling water over 4 tablespoons of dried plant material (~8 tablespoons of fresh).
2. Cover and steep for 30 – 45 minutes.

Generic recipe for preparing decoctions:

1. Place 4 tablespoons of dried plant material (~8 tablespoons of fresh) in a pot of water (1 quart).
2. Slowly bring to a boil.
3. Cover and simmer for 30 – 45 minutes.
4. Strain (Vinskofski, 2015).

Medicinal herbal tea, consumed largely for its beneficial and remediative properties, is believed to provide therapy for a plethora of health anomalies including the leading causes of mortality such as ischemic heart disease, stroke, chronic obstructive pulmonary disease (COPD), lower respiratory infections, lung cancer (plus trachea and bronchus cancers), HIV/AIDS, diarrhea, diabetes mellitus, and hypertension (Figure 3, WHO, 2014).

Potential Health Benefits

Health Benefits of Conventional Tea

Although tea lovers all over the world drink tea for its invigorating properties and distinctive, distinguished taste, mythology of many races, especially that of the Indochinese, suggest that *Camellia sinensis* may possess a number of remediative characteristics. Literature obtained from scientific investigations reveal

Figure 3. The top ten causes of mortality
Adapted from WHO, 2014.

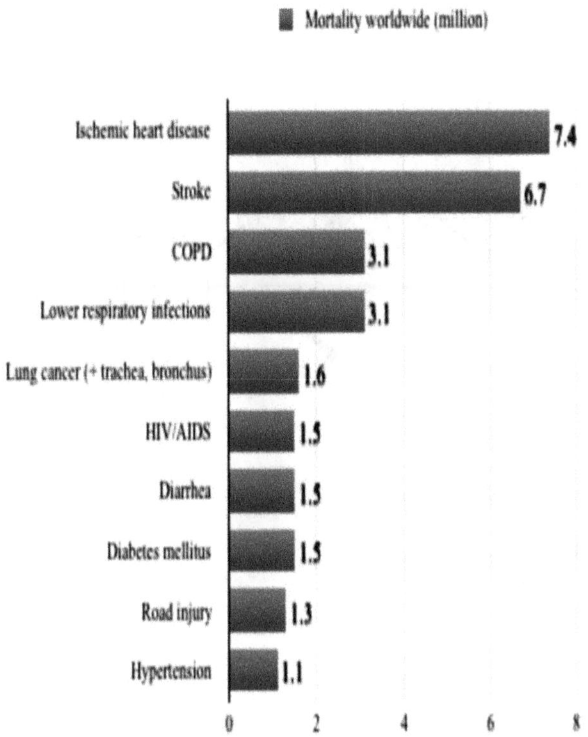

that tea may have efficacy in disease therapy. Tea is believed to be rich in certain nutrients, particularly minerals. Volatile compounds, polyphenols, amino acids, proteins, glucides, and alkaloids also make up the complex chemistry of tea. Polyphenols, the most biologically active component of tea, is acclaimed for its anti-carcinogenic, anti-mutagenic and anti-oxidative attributes. Compounds such as fluoride, caffeine, chromium and manganese enable humans meet their daily dietary requirements (Reto et al. 2007). The major constituents of green tea are flavanols, or catechins of epigallocatechin gallate (EGCG), epigallocatechin (EGC), epicatechin gallate (ECG), and epicatechin (EC). The primary polyphenols in oolong and black tea are theaflavins (i.e. theaflavins, theaflavin 3-gallate,theaflavin 3'-gallate, theaflavin 3, 3'-gallate) and thearubigins (Figure 4-10) (Chan et al., 2011; NBCI, 2015a-f; Chemfaces, 2015). Tea contains the flavonols, quercetin, myricetin and kaempferol (Higdon, 2002; NBCI, 2015g-i, Figure 11-13).

However, an analysis of several studies performed to chemically characterize *Camellia sinensis* indicates that variability exists amongst tea plants grown in disparate locations. This may be due, in part, to localized environmental conditions and soil composition. Crude aqueous extracts taken from different parts of *Camellia sinensis* plant, cultivated in Iran, exhibited significant antiviral activity when exposed to human herpesvirus 1 (HSV-1) *in vitro* (Farahani, 2012). The plentiful content of flavonoids, saponins and terpenes in *Camellia sinensis* may be responsible for its use singly, or in combination, to treat various forms of arthritic and inflammatory disorders. A study performed to assess the anti-inflammatory activity of *Camellia sinensis* in rats implanted with cotton pellet granuloma showed a significant reduction ($P \leq 0.01$) in total leukocyte number, ESR and spleen weight. Inflammation is characterized by tumor, calor, rubor, and function laesia (Mishra, 2014). Experimentation conducted by Chan et al., supports

Figure 4. 2D structure of Epigallocatechin gallate (ECGC)

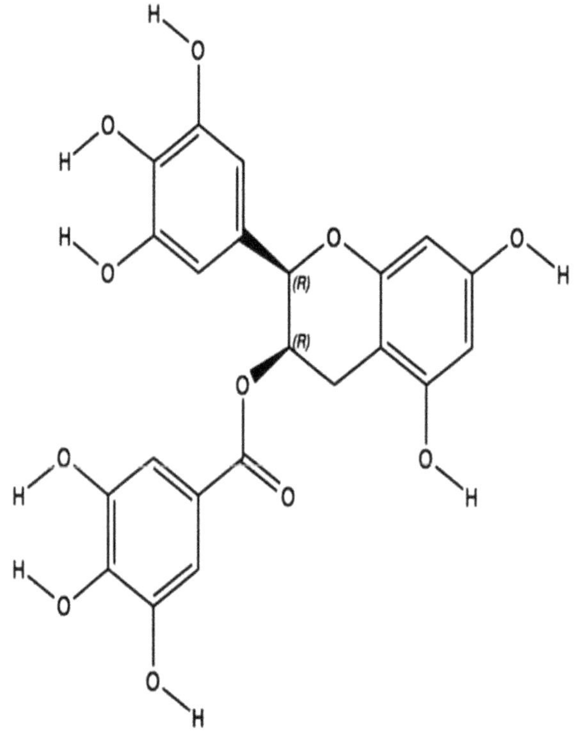

Figure 5. 2D structure of Epigallocatechin (EGC)

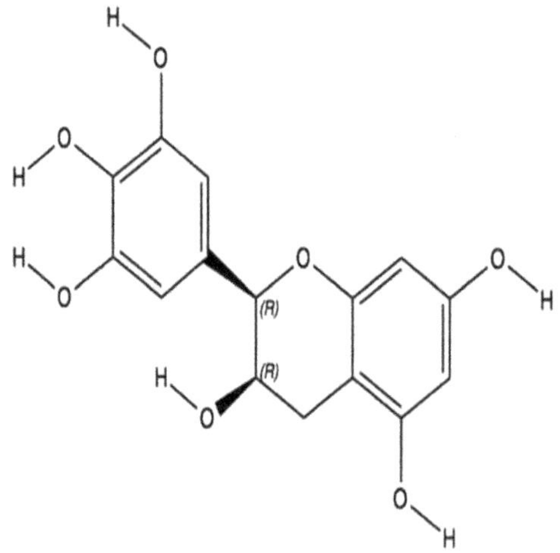

the antioxidant and antibacterial activity of *Camellia sinensis*. Extracts and fractions of variations of *C. sinensis* inhibited the growth of *M. luteus*. *B. cereus*, and *S. aureus* disproportionately (Chan et al., 2011). Human observational studies show that consuming three (24 oz.) or more cups of tea everyday may lead to a reduction (~ 11%) in cardiovascular disease especially myocardial infarction and stroke. *In vivo* studies involving green and black tea is suspected to inhibit the incidence of prostrate, stomach,

Figure 6. 2D structure of Epicatechin gallate (ECG)

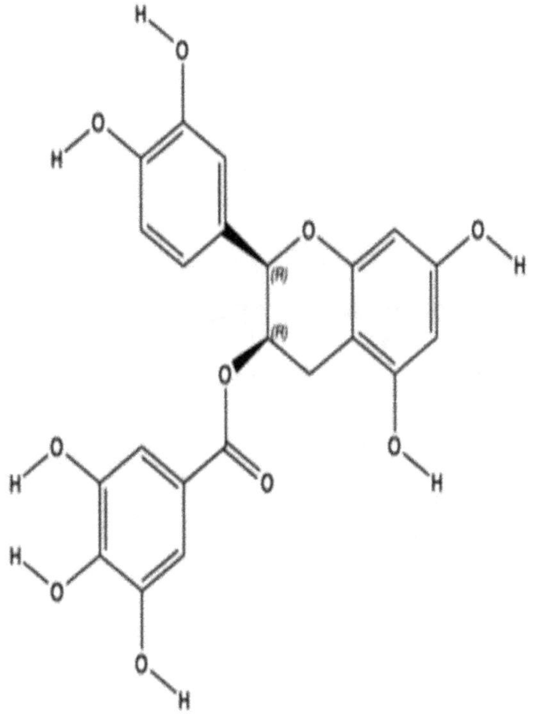

Figure 7. 2D structure of Epicatechin (EC)

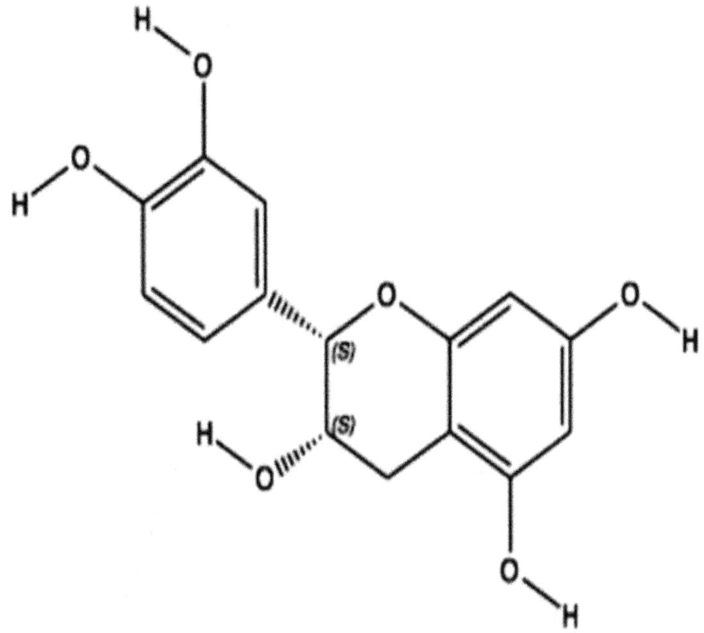

Figure 8. 2D structure of Theaflavin

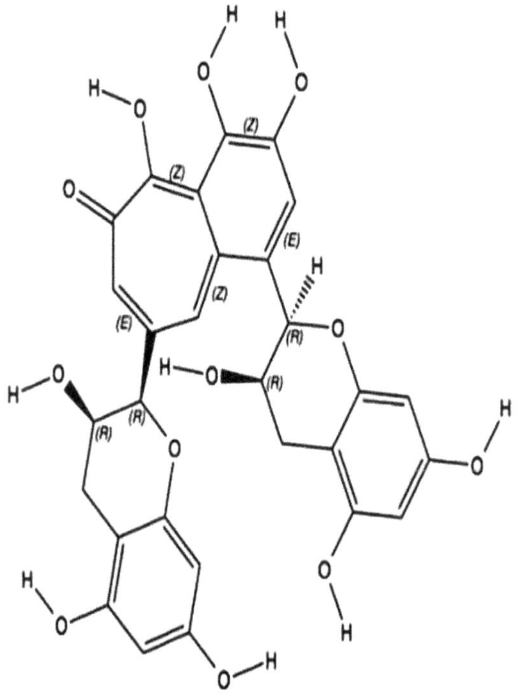

Figure 9. 2D structure of Theaflavin 3 gallate

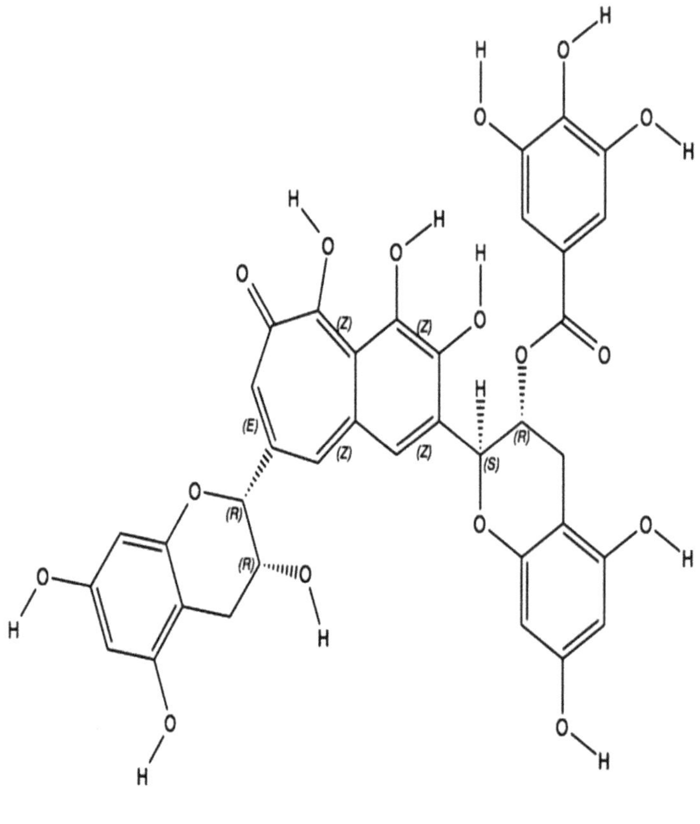

Figure 10. 2D structure of Theaflavin gallate

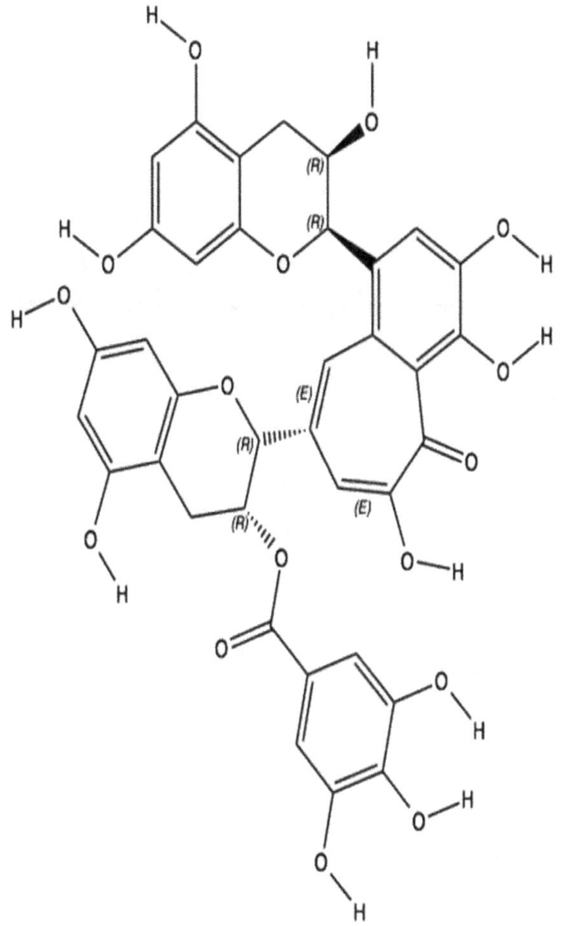

Figure 11. 2D structure of Quercetin

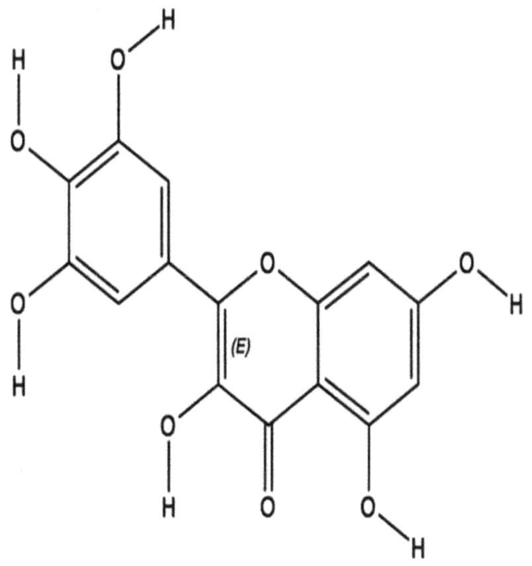

Figure 12. 2D structure of Myricetin

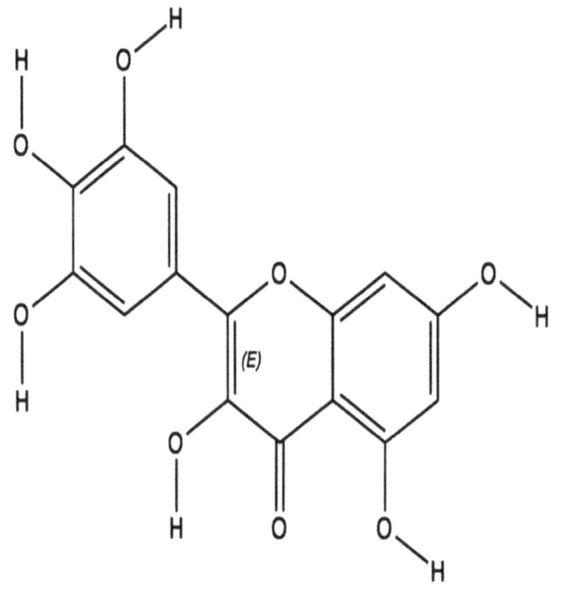

Figure 13. 2D structure of Kaemferol

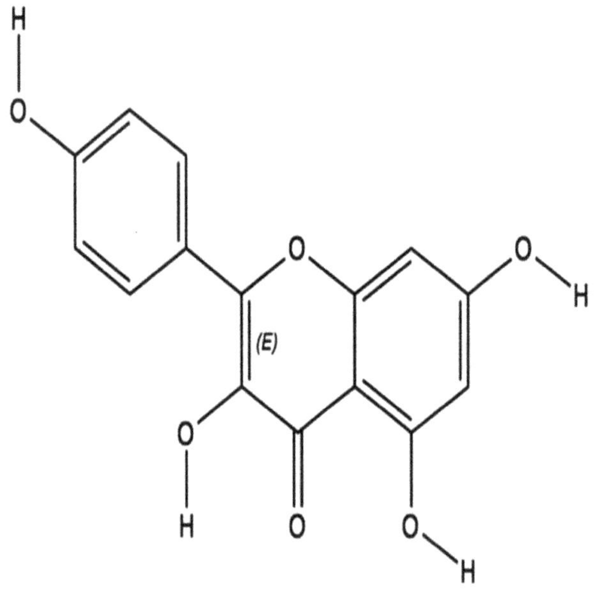

pancreas, mouth, bladder, skin, esophagus, lung, and colon cancer (Higdon 2002). Further investigations suggest that incorporating tea extracts in dental products i.e. chewing gum, mouthwash, dental floss and denitrification may inhibit the development of dental caries (Geonka, 2013). Other interesting laboratory investigations include a study that shows that the frequent drinking of hot tea lowered body mass index (BMI) and reduced mean waist circumference when compared with non-drinkers (men: 25 vs. 28 kg/m^2;

women: 26 vs. 29 kg/m^2; both $p < 0.01$) after controlling for cofounders such as age, physical activity, total energy intake etc. (Vernarelli & Lambert, 2012).

Health Benefits of Medicinal Herbal Tea

As previously stated, medicinal herbal tea is a terminology used to describe infusions and decoctions of plants, not including *Camelia sinensis*, consumed primarily for their presumed therapeutic potential in the treatment of a myriad of physiological abnormalities. There are close to a million plants that exist globally. It can be argued that preparations from many of these plants have remediative capabilities. However, it would be daunting to discuss the properties of each plant in this discourse. While some herbal teas have been determined to have promise and are consumed widely, several are yet to undergo scientific determination. This discussion is therefore constrained to focus on plants that have piqued academic curiosity and have demonstrated some benefit in disease treatment. Plants of primary interest in the present discussion are *Artemisia annua* (Asteraceae), and *Brickellia cavanillesii* (Asteraceae). Plants of the Asteraceae family have been strenuously investigated for their acclaimed medicinal properties. *A. annua*, consumed in the tropical developing countries of South Asia, Africa, and South America for its anti-malarial activity, has been the object of outstanding international recognition leading to the award of one-half of the 2015 Nobel Peace Prize in Medicine or Physiology to Tu Youyou ; *B. cavanillesii*, consumed extensively in neotropical Americas for its hypoglycemic properties, is a subject of vigorous exploratory, investigative research at Ernest Smith laboratory, The Institute of Environmental and Human Health (TIEHH), Texas Tech University, Lubbock, Texas, USA.

Artemisia Annua (Asteraceae)

Artemisia annua (English name: Sweet wormwood, Chinese wormwood, Sweet annua) is a weed, native to Asia, predominantly China, but now cultivated and naturalized in many countries of the world. *A. annua* is typically about 2 m tall with single stem, alternate branches. Leaves: fern-like, alternating, 2.5 – 5 cm in length, 1-3 cm in width, aromatic odor, deeply dissected. Flowers: tiny, bright yellow, core panicles with capitula 2 -3 mm across. Tea preparations are made using the dried aerial parts of the flowers which are usually collected before full bloom. (Ferreira & Jannick, 1996). The anti-pyretic (fever-reducing) properties of *A. annua* was recognized as early as the 4th century AD (Hsu, 2006). Studies performed show that *A. annua* contains sesquiterpene lactones, flavonoids and essential oils (Klayman et al. 1984). In 1971, Tu Youyou et al., isolated the sesquiterpene lactone compound Artemisinin (qinghaosu) ($C_{15}H_{22}O_5$, MW: 282.33218 g/mol, Figure 14), distilled from the dried leaves and flower clusters of *A. annua*. It is believed that Artemisinin may inhibit the malaria-triggering protozoal organisms in the genus Plasmodium. Artemisinin targets Plasmodium organisms that contain hemozoin, producing radicals that attack the parasite proteins, and ultimately eradicating the organisms. Presently, there are several derivatives of Artemisinin including Artesanate and Artemethen employed in malaria treatment. WHO recommends Artemisinin combination therapy (ACT) as the first-line treatment for uncomplicated malaria (WHO, 2015). Unfortunately, ACT's relatively high cost and inconsistent availability in areas plagued with malaria has led to a call by non-governmental organizations (NGOs) for the use of *A. annua* teas as an alternative therapy in communities where conventional medication is not readily obtained (Wilcox et al. 2011). Because the concentration of Artemisinin in infusions are considered inadequate, the medicinal value of tea preparations of *A. annua* in the treatment of malaria is debatable. However, studies

Figure 14. 3D structure of Artemisinin

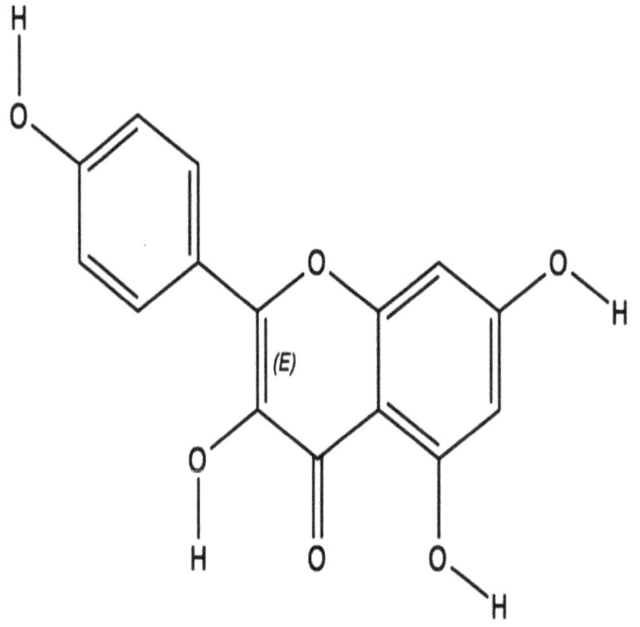

involving clinical trials may suggest otherwise (Mueller et al. 2000; Mueller et al. 2004). Furthermore, in an extensive study ($\geq$ 3,000 patients), infusions of *A. annua* was found to be widely accepted, and well tolerated with few side effects; perhaps, better tolerated than quinine. Participants also had highly encouraging recovery rates (Wilcox et al. 2011).

Brickellia Cavanillesii (Asteraceae)

Brickellia cavanillesii (Asteraceae), is one of the more popular herbal plants consumed in Central America, Mexico, and the southwestern parts of the U.S.A. for the treatment of Type 2 diabetes mellitus (T2DM), stomach ulcers, gastritis, dyspepsia, and pain (Figure 15) . *B. cavanillesii* is a bitter tasting shrub known in many Latin American countries by its Spanish name "prodigiosa," "hamula," or "atanasia amarga" (Figure 16). Prior investigations indicate that *Brickellia cavanillesii* may possess anti-carcinogenic, antioxidative, antispasmodic, antihypertensive, and hypoglycemic abilities (Navarrete et al., 2011; Escandón-Rivera et al., 2012; Mata & Escandón, 2012; Vinas & Smith, 2013; Villarreal et al., 2014; Eshiet et al., 2014a, 2014b; Pérez-Vásquez et al, 2014a, 2014b). It is available commercially in herbal stores and is presently and commonly used by diabetics as a cheaper alternative to insulin. Extant literature states that the chemical composition of *B. cavanillesii* consists of Brickelin, resin, essential oil, fat, tannin, coloring material, gum, starch, chlorophyll, and mineral salts (HHS, 1997). Other characterization investigations reiterate that Brickellin, an O-methylated flavonol, is a major component of *B. cavanillesii*. Proton Nuclear Magnetic Resonance (^{1}HNMR), Carbon-13 Nuclear Magnetic Resonance (^{13}CNMR), and Electron Impact Mass Resonance (EIM) spectra were used to revise and confirm the structure of Brickellin ($C_{20}H_{20}O_9$), 2' 5-dihydroxy-3, 6, 7, 4', 5'-pentamethoxyflavone (Iinuma et al., 1985) (Figure 17). In another study performed on *Brickellia cavanillesii* (Rodriguez-Lopez et al. 2006) a natural

Figure 15. Distribution of Brickellia cavanillesii

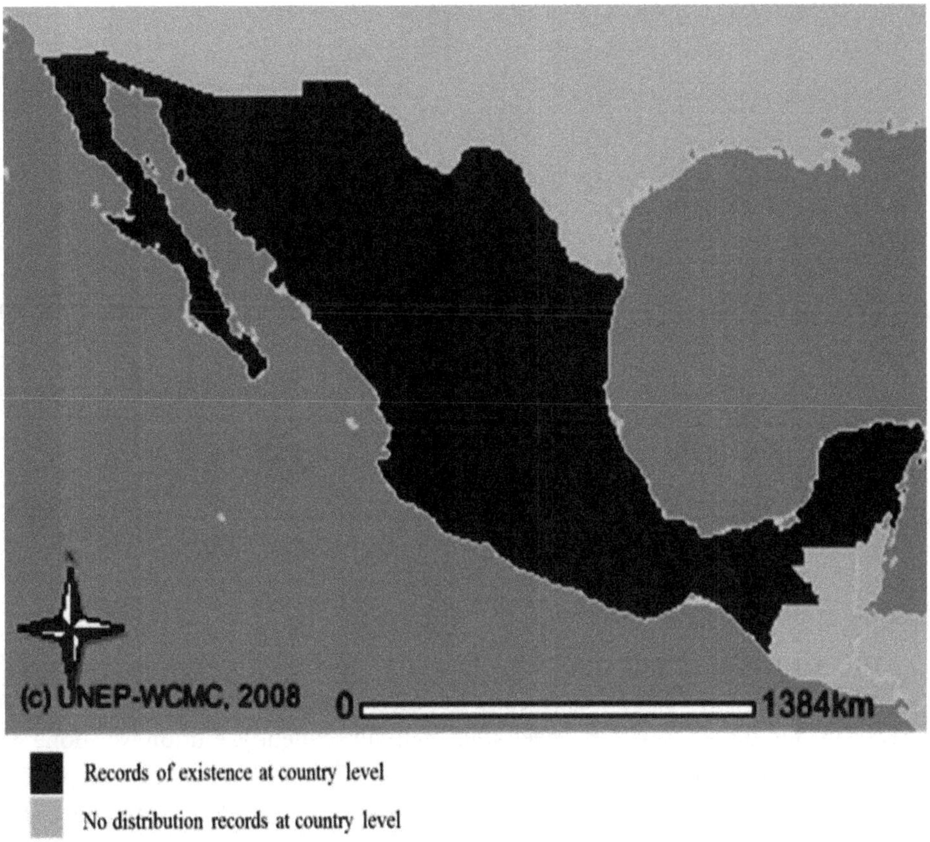

Figure 16. Brickellia cavanillesii (Asteraceae) plant

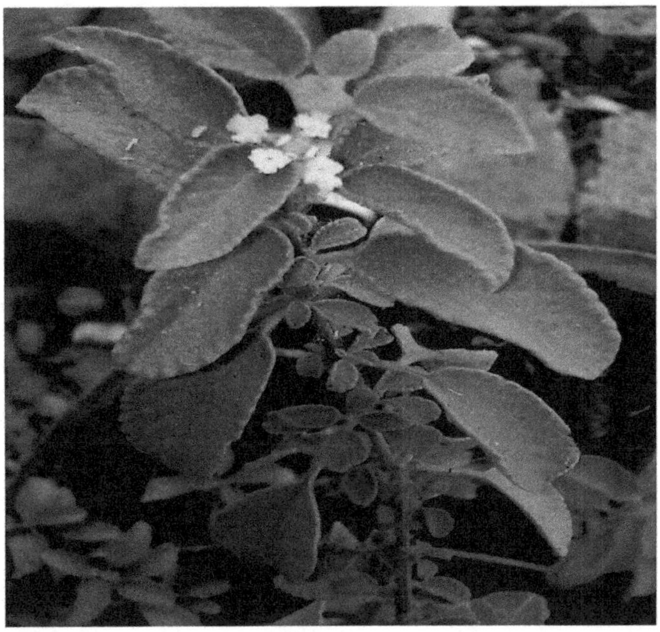

Figure 17. Pentamethoxyflavone

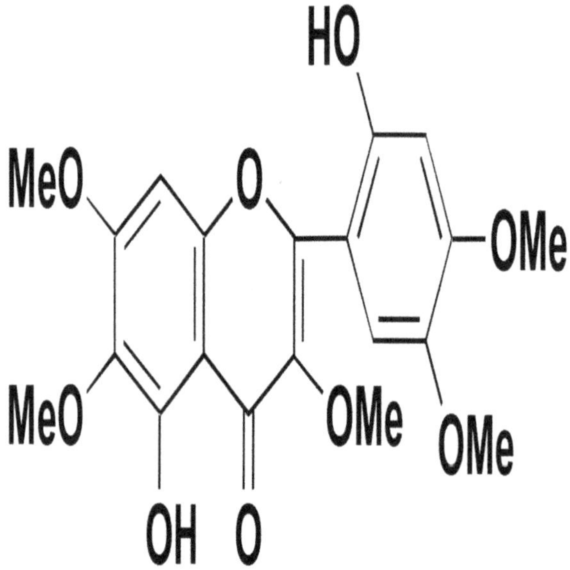

product, 6-Acetyl-5-hydroxy-2, 2-dimethyl - 2H – chromene ($C_{13}H_{14}O_{3,}$ MW: 218.252 g/mol Figure 18) was isolated. Chromene was isolated by subjecting the methanolic extract of *Brickellia cavanillesii* to vacuum liquid chromatography (11 x 3 cm) over silica gel. Subsequently, elution was done with hexane to isolate chromene. Recrystallization from hexane CH_2Cl_2 (75:25) by slow evaporation produced yellow plates (m.p.376.6K) (Rodriguez-Lopez et al., 2006). Literature indicates that chromene is an intermediate in the synthesis of isoencecalin (Ahluwalia & Arora, 1981). Chromene has also been isolated from *Blepharispermun subsessile* (Kulkarni et al., 1987). Chromene belongs to the class of plant secondary

Figure 18. Acetyl-5 hydroxy+ 2-dimethyl-2H-chromene

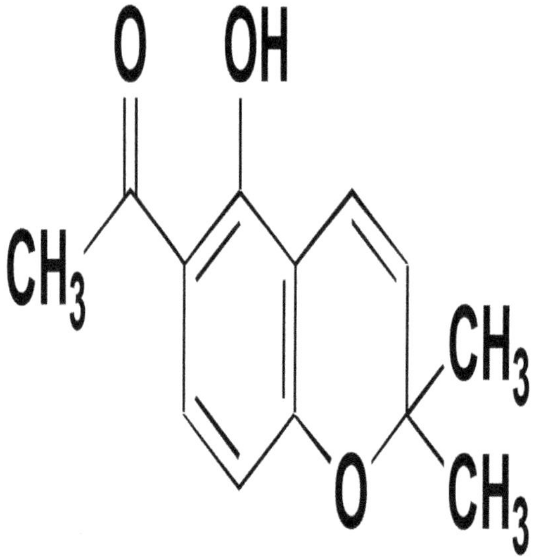

metabolites called flavanoids (bioflavonoids) or vitamin P and citrin. Studies done on chromene show that it has anti-fungal activity against *Candida albicans* and *Cryptococcus neoformans*. (Agarwal et al., 2000). Bioassay-guided fractionation of active aerial extracts of *B. cavanillesii* resulted in the isolation of:

1. **Chromenes:** 6-acetyl-5-hydroxy-2,2-dimethyl- 2H-chromene and 6-hydroxyacetyl-5-hydroxy-2,2-dimethyl-2H-chromene;
2. **Sesquiterpene Lactone:** Caleins B and caleins C; and
3. **Flavonoids:** Acacetin, genkwanin, isorhamnetin, kaempferol, quercetin, and 3,5-di-O-caffeoylquinic acid (Escandón-Rivera et al., 2012).

High performance liquid chromatography with diode-array detection (HPLC-DAD) methods have also been utilized to confirm the presence of the chromenes: 6-acetyl-5-hydroxy-2, 2-dimethyl- 2H-chromene, and 6-hydroxyacetyl-5-hydroxy-2, 2-dimethyl-2H-chromene, in the infusion of *Brickellia cavanillesii* plant (Perez-Vasquez, 2014).

Quantitative analysis of a methanol extract of lyophilized *B. cavanillesii* using gas chromatography (GC) techniques: a) GC-flame ionization detector (GC-FID); b) GC-Mass spectrometry (GC-MS); c) Purge and Trap GC-MS (P & T GC-MS) resulted in the identification of twenty-one (21) bioactive compounds. The compounds were:

1. Cyclohexene, 6-ethenyl-6-methyl-1-(1-methylethyl)-3-(1-methylethylidene)-, (S)-;
2. Bicyclo (2.2.1) heptan-2-one, 1, 7, 7-trimethyl-(1S, 4S)-;
3. Phenol, 2-methoxy-4-(1-propenyl)-;
4. Benzene, 1-(1, 5-dimethyl-4-hexenyl)-4-methyl-;
5. Naphthalene, 1, 2, 3, 5, 6, 8a-hexa- hydro4, 7-dimethyl-1-1-(1-methylethyl)-, (1S-cis)-;
6. Phenol, 2-methoxy-;
7. Benzaldehyde, 3-hydroxy-4-methoxy-;
8. 11, 13-Eicosadienoic acid, methyl ester;
9. 2-Furancarboxaldehyde, 5-methyl-;
10. Maltol;
11. Phenol;
12. Hydroquinone;
13. 1H-Indene, 1-ethylideneoctahydro-7a-methyl-, (1E, 3a.alpha, 7a.beta.);
14. 3-mcthyl butanal;
15. (D)-Limonene;
16. 1-methyl-4-(1-methyl ethyl) benzene;
17. Butanoic acid methyl ester;
18. 2-methyl propanal;
19. 2-butanone;
20. 2-pentanone; and
21. 2-methyl butanal (Figures 19-44) (Eshiet et al. 2010; Eshiet et al., 2014a, 2014b).

These compounds, terpenes, derivatives of terpenes, esters, ketones, aldehydes, and phenol-derived aromatic compounds are the primary constituents of the essential oils of many plants and flowers. Several research findings suggest that the identified compounds (**1**-**21**) have measurable medicinal value.

Figure 19. Packet containing Brickellia cavanillesii leaves and twigs (front)

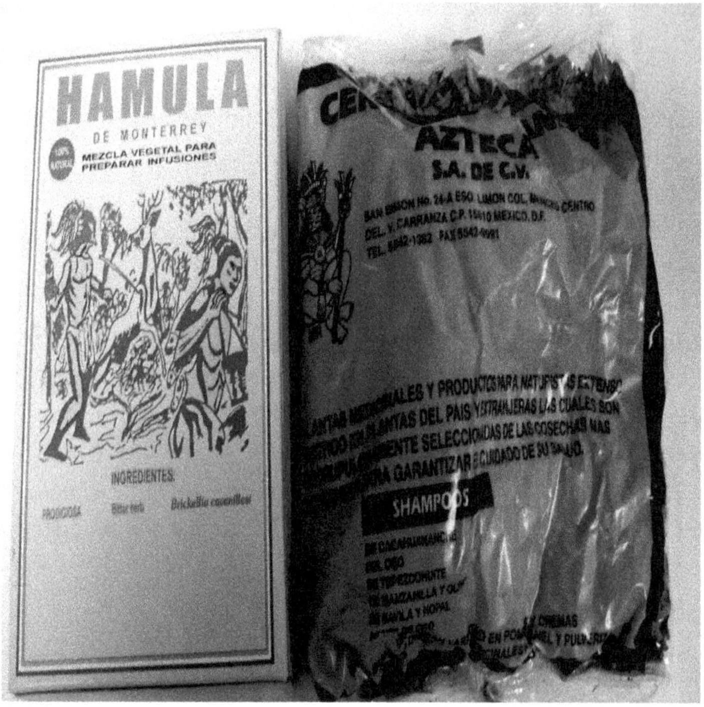

Figure 20. Packet containing Brickellia cavanillesii dried leaves and twigs (back)

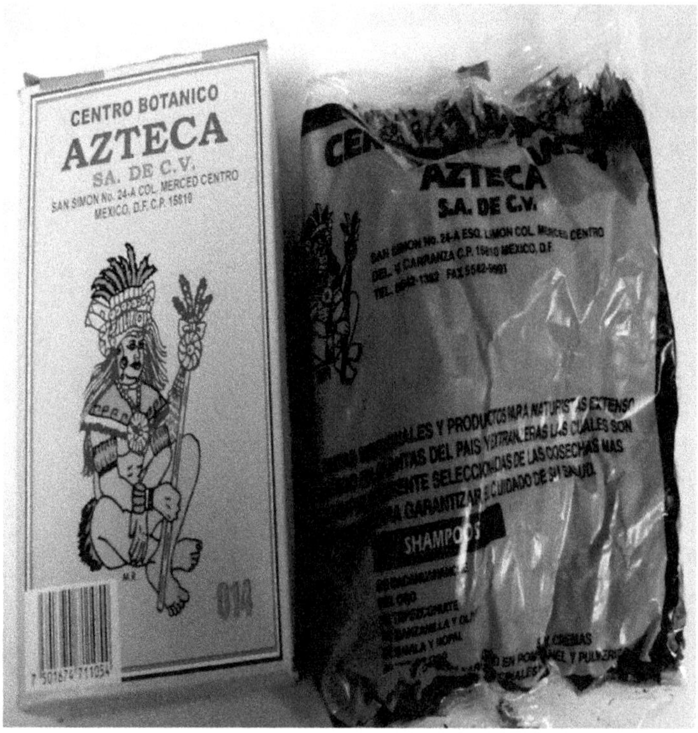

Figure 21. Twigs of Brickellia cavanillesii (Asteraceae)

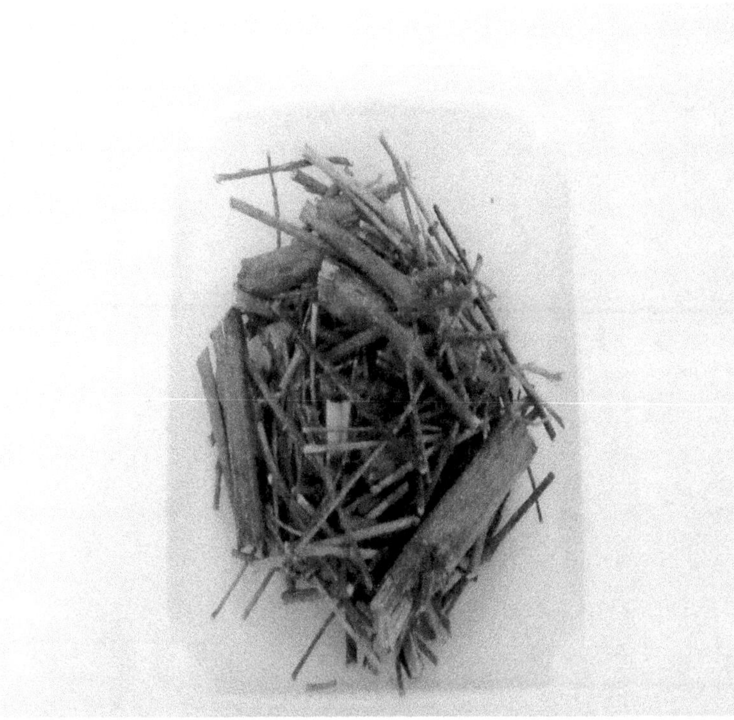

Figure 22. Powder of Brickellia cavanillesii (Asteraceae) dried leaves and twigs

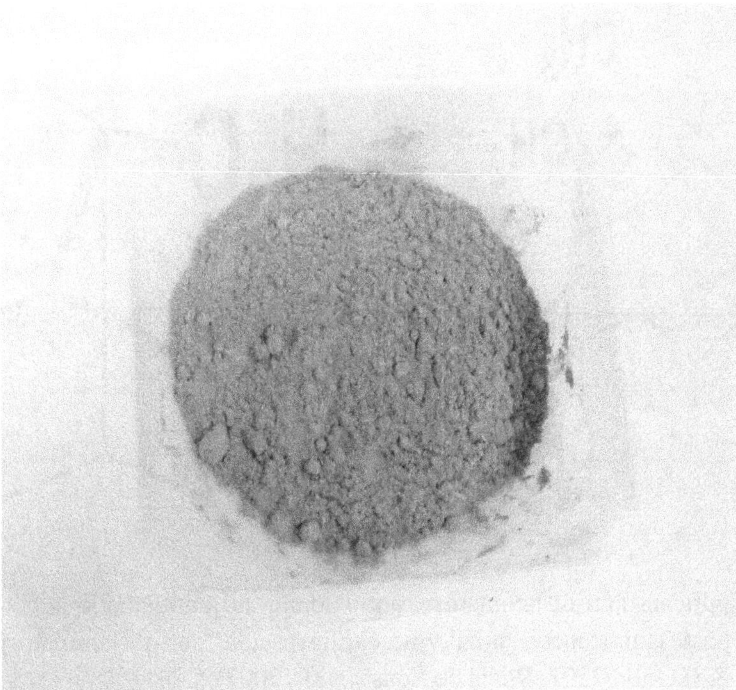

Figure 23. Lyophilized extracts of Brickellia cavanillesii (Asteraceae) dried leaves and twigs

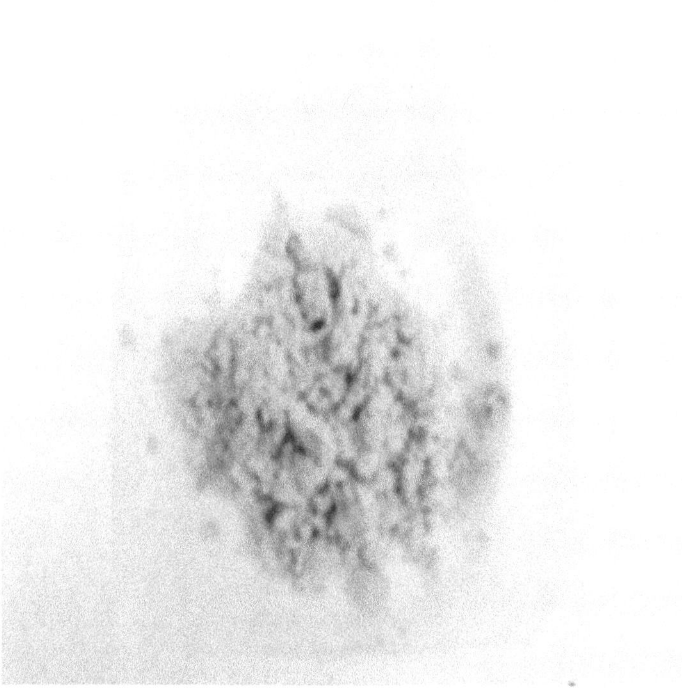

Figure 24. Cyclohexane, 6-ethenyl-6-methyl-1-(1-methylethyl)-3-(1-methylethylidene)-, (S)

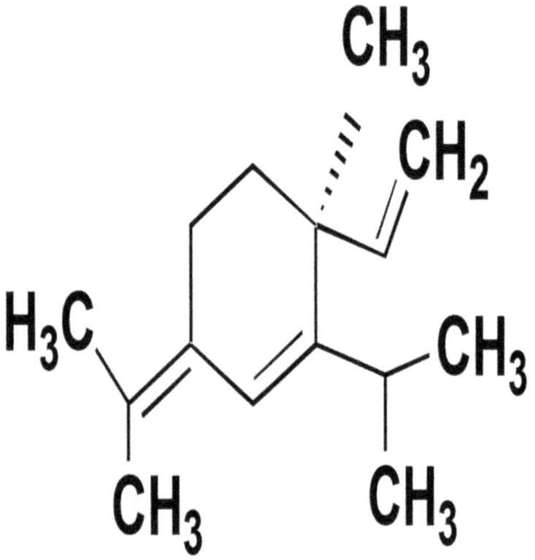

Figure 25. Bicyclo (2.2.1) heptan-2-one, 1, 7, 7-trimethyl-, (1S, 4S)

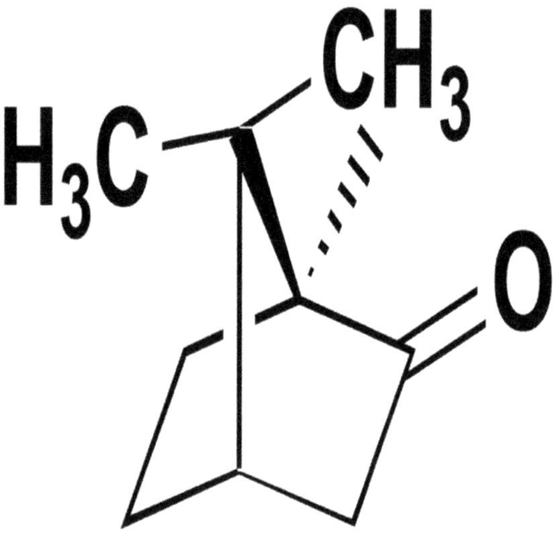

Flavonoids have significant anti-inflammatory, antioxidant and antidiabetic attributes (Fawzy et al. 2008); essential oils possess anticancer, antiallergic, cardiovascular, anti-inflammatory and antimicrobial properties (Yamoto & Gaynor, 2001; Ruela de Sousa et al., 2007).

Exploratory *in vitro* toxicological/biological assays investigating therapeutic potential, proteomics and genomics indicate that there may be considerable biological benefit in the lyophilized extracts of

Figure 26. Phenol, 2-methoxy-4-(1-propenyl)-

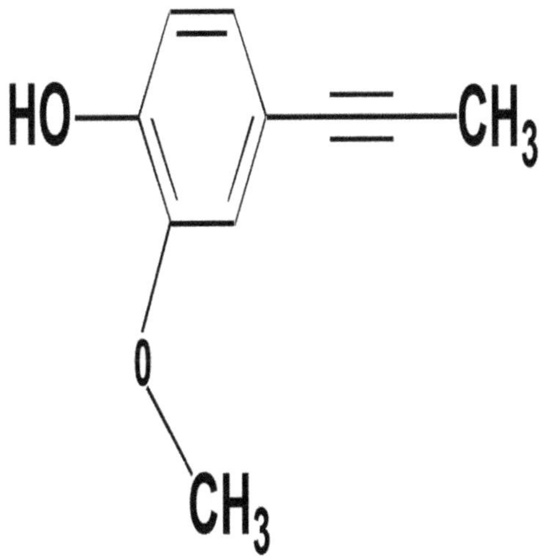

Figure 27. Benzene, 1 - (1, 5 - dimethyl -4- hexenyl) –methyl –

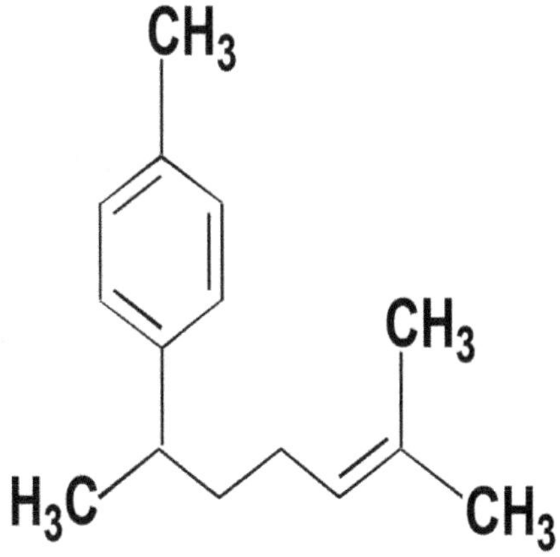

Figure 28. Naphthalene, 1, 2, 3, 5, 6, 8a-hexahydro-4, 7-dimethyl-1-(1-methylethyl)-, (IS-cis) –

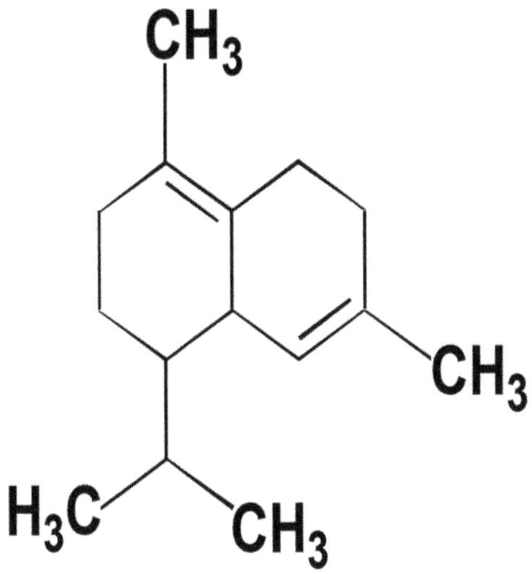

Figure 29. Phenol, 2–methoxy –

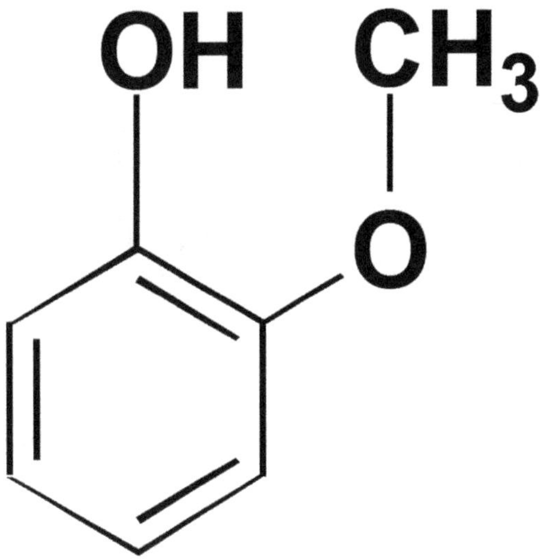

B. cavanillesii (LBC) (Eshiet et al. 2010; Eshiet et al. 2014b) in the therapy of Type 2 diabetes mellitus (T2DM). Possible therapeutic effects of LBC were concentration dependent with and without fetal bovine serum (FBS). Western blot analysis of glucose facilitated transporter protein 2 (GLUT 2) expression of human carcinoma liver (HepG2) cells exposed to 0 mg/mL (control) and 0.2 mg/mL LBC for 2, 4, 6, and 24 h suggest that GLUT 2 was increased. Increase in GLUT 2 expression in the absence of FBS was statistically significant with time of exposure. Significant difference was observed for GLUT 2 expression between 6 and 24 h and also between 4 and 24 h at 0.2 mg/mL LBC. Gene expression analysis conducted attempted to elucidate a mechanism of action using apoptosis and GLUT 2 gene expression as biomarkers. Observed findings show that several antiapoptotic genes were significantly up-regulated whereas some apoptotic genes were significantly down-regulated. The most significant up-regulation

Figure 30. Benzaldehyde, 3-hydroxy-4-methoxy

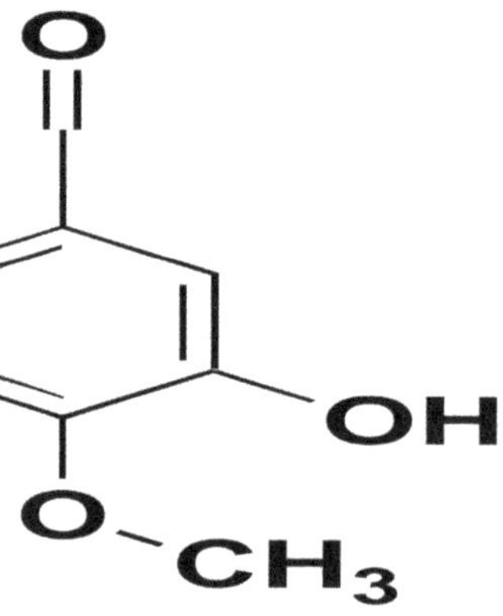

Figure 31. 11, 13-Eicosadienoic acid, methyl ester

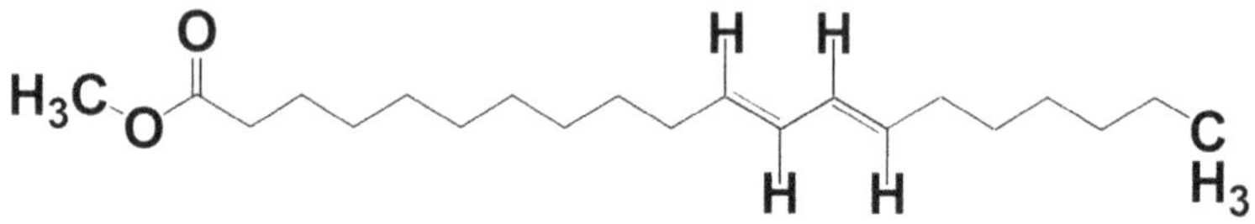

Figure 32. 2-Furancarboxaldehyde, 5-methyl –

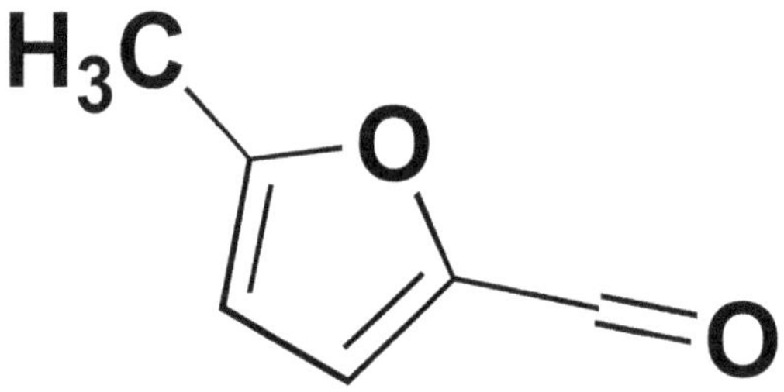

Figure 33. Maltol

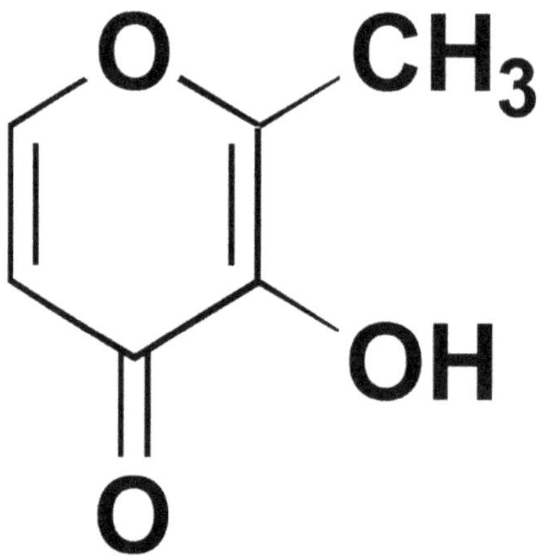

Figure 34. Phenol

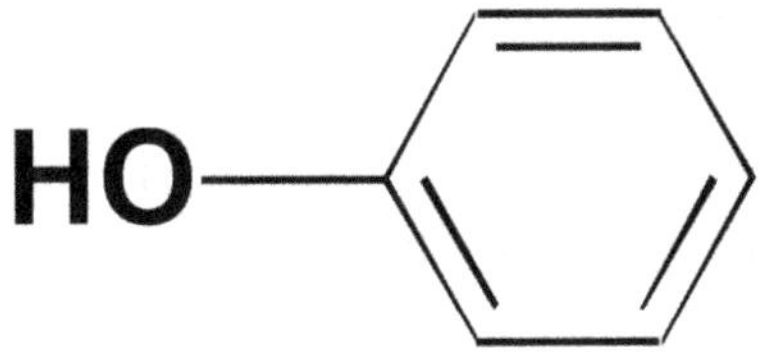

Figure 35. Hydroquinone

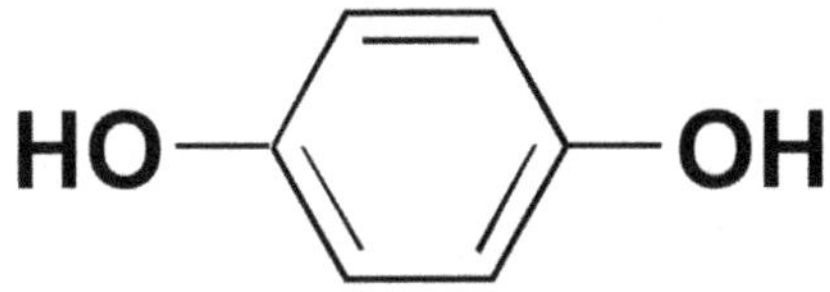

Figure 36. 1 H-Indene, 1-ethylideneoctahydro-7a-methyl-, (1E, 3a.alpha, 7a.beta.)

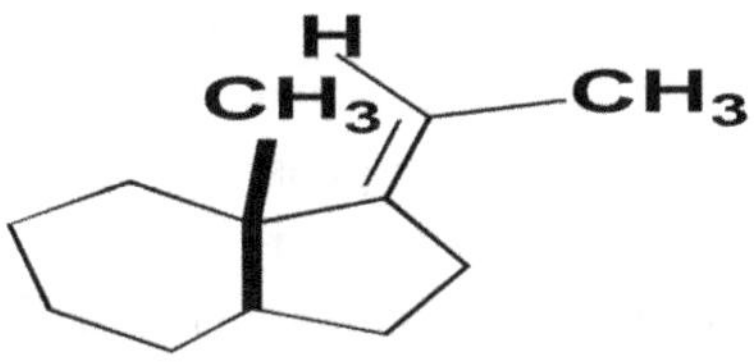

Figure 37. 3-Methyl butanal

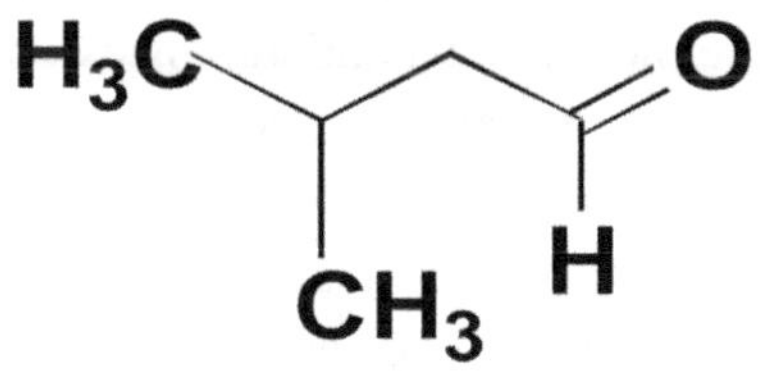

Figure 38. (D)-Limonene

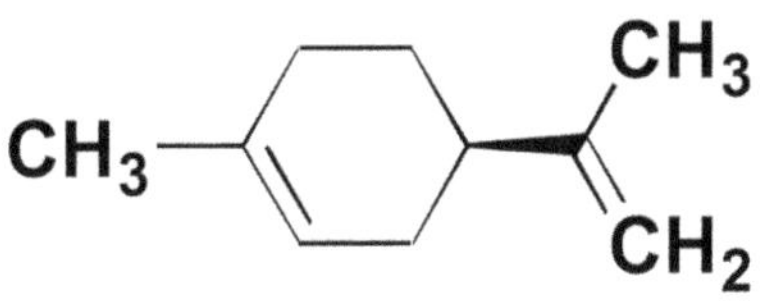

Figure 39. 1-Methyl-4-(1-methyl ethyl) benzene

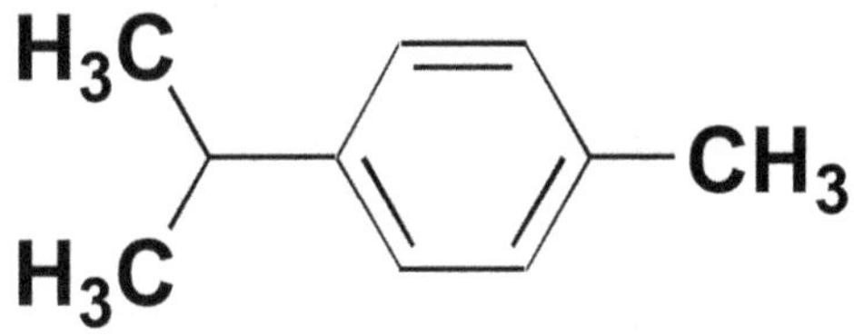

Figure 40. Butanoic acid methyl ester

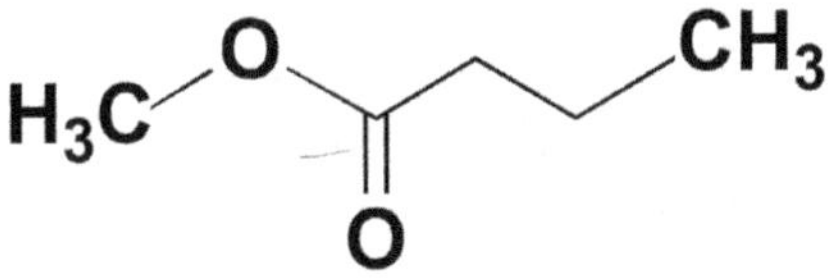

Figure 41. 2-Methyl propanal

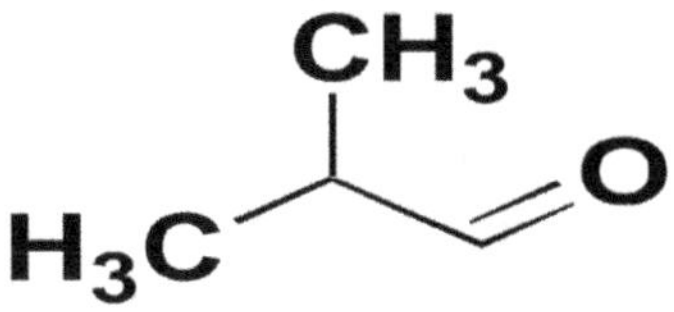

Figure 42. 2-Butanone

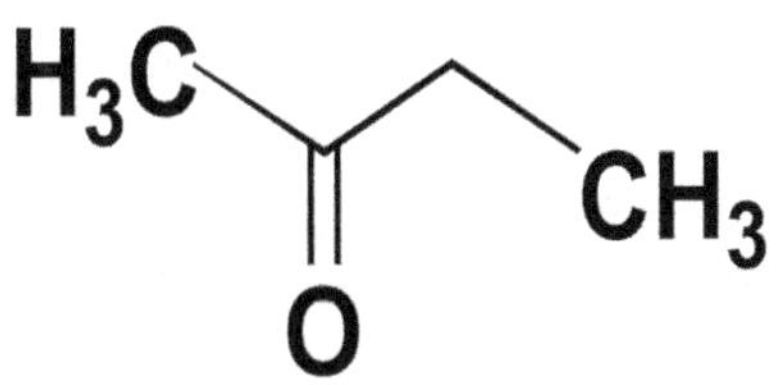

Figure 43. 2-Pentanone

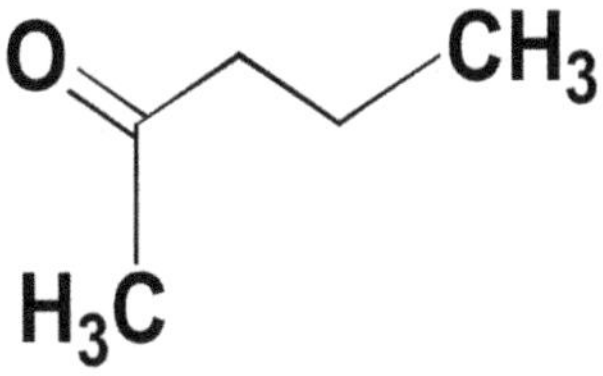

Figure 44. 2-Methyl butanal

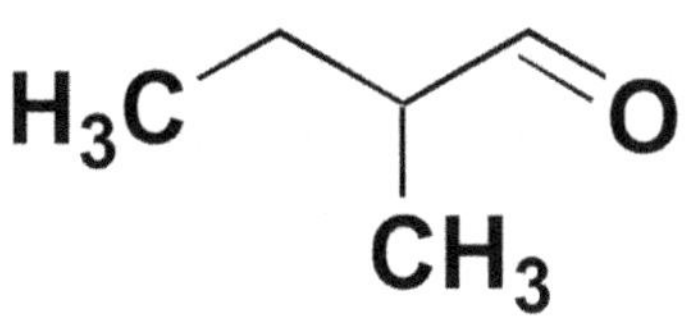

was by BCL2L1; BCL2L1 is reputed to be an apoptosis inhibitor. Data acquired from the GLUT 2 gene expression study suggest that LBC may induce GLUT 2 gene expression and supports claims that *B. cavanillesii* exhibits antidiabetic activity (Eshiet 2010; Eshiet et al. 2014a, 2014b, 2015). Investigative *in vivo* assays demonstrated that dichloromethane-methanol extracts (10-300 mg/kg) obtained from the leaves of *Brickellia cavanillesii* triggered a dose-dependent reduction of ethanol-induced gastric lesions in rats (ED50 = 30 mg/kg); gastro-protective effect of *B. cavanillesii* was demonstrated to be the same as that induced by carbenoxolene. Furthermore, aerial aqueous extracts of *Brickellia cavanillesii* reduced postprandial hyperglycemia in diabetic mice throughout the course of oral glucose and sucrose tolerance testing (Escandion-Rivera et al. 2012; Mata & Escandion, 2012; Perez-Vasquez et al., 2014).

Another herbal plant undergoing extensive experimentation is *Tecoma stans* (Bignoniaceae). *T. stans* is consumed for its presumed antidiabetic properties. Gas chromatographic characterization of methanol extracts of lyophilized *Tecoma stans* (LTS) support other characterization studies that show that *T. stans* contains two major compounds, Tecomine and Tecostamine, believed to be responsible for decreasing blood glucose levels (Zhu et al., 2008). Presently, complimentary and supplementary studies are being conducted, at Ernest E. Smith laboratory, The Institute of Environmental and Human Health (TIEHH), Texas Tech University, Lubbock USA, to isolate bioactive components of LBC and LTS using Liquid Chromatography Mass Spectroscopy (LCMS) methodologies; definitive, integrative *in vivo* and *in vitro* biological assays employing a broad spectrum of biomarkers are also being performed to elucidate mechanism of action. It is hoped that these studies will provide further clarity in determining the efficacy of LBC and LTS as therapeutic agents.

CONCERNS

The growing trend of using tea preparations, and CAM to a larger extent, as ameliorative therapy has elicited a number of troubling concerns. Of particular interest are potential drug interactions and side effects. Herbal tea variability, contamination, standardization, and identification are a few other concerns generated by CAM usage. Complications arising from interactions between CAM remedies and prescribed medication are prevalent. Less than forty percent of patients are believed to share their usage of CAM products with their healthcare professional leading to improper diagnosis (Eisenberg et al. 1998; Shane-McWhorter, 2007). Patients taking CAM remedies have been known to experience serious side effects (Shaw et al. 1997; Boullata & Nace, 2000). Unfortunately, the Food and Drug Administration (FDA) considers herbal plants and its supplements foods, not drugs. This puts this category of products outside the ambit of the strict testing, manufacturing, labeling standards and regulations that pharmaceutical drugs are typically subjected to. Although, many prescription drugs and over-the-counter medications are prepared from plants, these products are purified ingredients that are FDA regulated. Conversely, herbal plants, and its supplements, may contain entire plant materials that have not undergone FDA approved clinical trials to assure efficacy in the treatment or management of disorders (JHM, 2015). In 1999, the United States government initiated a program designed to determine the effectiveness of herbal plants, and other CAM remedies, in disease therapy. In excess of $2.5 billion was expended on this exercise. Results obtained were at best inconclusive. Herbal derivatives involved in this investigation failed to show any significant difference with control (dummy pills). However, more studies are presently being conducted, and grants have been awarded towards studies further exploring the use of CAM treatments (Marchione, 2009).

CONCLUSION

The efficacy, or otherwise, of plant extracts (~herbal teas) in disease therapy remains a primary concern to healthcare professionals and the international scientific community. Although an enormous number of plants used in disease therapy have been reported in literature and may in fact represent alternatives to developing new oral agents, valid ethnobotanical information about them is limited, doubtful and ambiguous (Martinez, 1954; Bailey & Day, 1989; Marles & Farnsworth, 1994; Aguilar et al. 1994). The result of our investigations leads us to suggest that concerted effort must be sustained in the pursuance of scientific investigation of traditional tea preparations as it may present valuable leads and potential for the development of alternative drugs and therapeutic remedies. Tea preparations constitute a tremendous resource for alternative remedy especially at disease onset. Consequently, it is imperative that studies are undertaken to assure the quality, efficacy, and safety of plants. The lyophilization of plant extracts typically ensures durability and standardization. These are critical ingredients necessary in determining the dosage of therapeutic agents. Performing experimental procedures utilizing lyophilized plant extracts may perhaps provide data sets that are truly measurable and reproducible.

REFERENCES

Agarwal, S. K., Verma, S., Singh, S. S., Tripathy, A. K., Khan, Z. K., & Kumar, S. (2000). Antifeedant and antifungal activity of chromene compounds isolated from Blepharispermum subsessile. *Journal of Ethnopharmacology*, *71*(1-2), 231–234. doi:10.1016/S0378-8741(00)00158-6 PMID:10904167

Aguilar, A., Camacho, J. R., Chino, S., Jaquez, P., & Lopez, M. E. (1994). *Herbario Medicinal del Instituto Mexicano del Seguro Social*. Instituto Mexicano del Seguro Social Informacion Ethnobotanica. Mexico.

Ahluwalia, V. K., & Arora, K. K. (1981). Nuclear Iso Prenylation of Poly Hydroxy Acetophenones Acid Catalyzed Condensation with Isoprene. *Tetrahedon*, *37*, 1437–1439. doi:10.1016/S0040-4020(01)92463-9

Ashenef, A. (2014). Essential and toxic metals in tea (Camellia sinensis) imported and produced in Ethiopia. *Food Additives & Contaminants: Part B, 7*(1), 30-6. Doi:10.1080/19393210.2013.831951

Bailey, J., & Day, C. (1989). Traditional Plant Medicines as Treatments for Diabetes. *Diabetes Care*, *12*(8), 553–564. doi:10.2337/diacare.12.8.553 PMID:2673695

Boullata, J. I., & Nace, A. M. (2000). Safety issues with herbal medicine. *Pharmacotherapy*, *20*(3), 257–356. doi:10.1592/phco.20.4.257.34886 PMID:10730682

Chan, E. W. C., Soh, E. Y., Tie, P. P., & Law, Y. P. (2011). Antioxidant and antibacterial properties of green, black and herbal teas of Camellia sinensis. *Pharmacognosy Research, 3*(4), 266-72.

Department of Health and Human Services (HHS). (1997). *New dietary ingredients: Brickellia cavanillesii*. Retrieved November 14, 2015 from: http://www.fda.gov/OHRMS/DOCKETS/95s0316/rpt0010_.pdf

Eisenberg, D. M., Davis, R. B., Erner, S. L., Appel, S., Wilkey, S., Van Rompay, M., & Kessler, R. C. (1998). Trends in alternative medicine use in the United States, 1990-1997: Results of a follow-up national survey. *Journal of the American Medical Association*, *280*(18), 1569–1575. doi:10.1001/jama.280.18.1569 PMID:9820257

Eisenberg, D. M., Kessler, R. C., Foster, C., Norlock, F. E., Calkins, D. R., & Delbanco, T. L. (1993). Unconventional medicine in the United States: Prevalence, costs, and patterns of use. *The New England Journal of Medicine*, *328*(4), 246–252. doi:10.1056/NEJM199301283280406 PMID:8418405

Ekor, M. (2014). The growing use of herbal medicines: issues relating to adverse reactions and challenges in monitoring safety. *Frontiers in Pharmacology, 4*(177), 1-10. Doi: 10.3389/fphar.2013.00177

Escandón-Rivera, S., González-Andrade, M., Bye, R., Linares, E., Navarrete, A., & Mata, R. (2012). α-glucosidase inhibitors from Brickellia cavanillesii. *Journal of Natural Products*, *75*(5), 968–974. doi:10.1021/np300204p PMID:22587572

Eshiet, E. R. (2010). *Chemical characterization of diabetic herbal tea and in vitro evaluation of glucose transport and metabolism gene expression profile.* (Unpublished Doctoral Dissertation). Texas Tech University, Lubbock, TX.

Eshiet, E. R., Zhu, J., Anderson, T. A., & Smith, E. E. (2014a). Chemical characterization of Brickellia cavanillesii (Asteraceae) using gas chromatographic methods. *Food Sci Nutr*, *2*(2), 105–113. doi:10.1002/fsn3.52 PMID:24804069

Eshiet, E. R., Zhu, J., & Smith, E. E. (2014b). Lyophilized tea extracts of Brickellia cavanillesii (Asteraceae): In vitro characterization of biological activity. *Journal of Food Science*, *79*(7), T1454–T1461. doi:10.1111/1750-3841.12519 PMID:24962327

Eshiet, E. R., Zhu, J., & Smith, E. E. (2015). The biologic potential of lyophilized extracts of Brickellia cavanillesii (Asteraceae): Apoptosis and glut 2 gene expression. *Journal of Food Processing & Technology*, *7*(1). doi:10.4172/2157-7110.1000541

Farahani, M. (2012). Assessment of antiherpetic effect of Camellia sinensis against herpes simplex virus type 1. *Journal of Isfahan Medical School, 30*(207).

Fawzy, A. G., Abdallah, H. M., Marzonk, M. S. A., Soliman, F. M., & Sleem, A. (2008). Antidiabetic and antioxidant activities of major flavonoids of Cynanchum acutum L. (Asclepiadaceae) growing in Egypt. *Z. Naturforsch.*, *63c*, 658–662. PMID:19040103

Ferreira, J. F. S., & Jannick, J. (Eds.). (1996). *Progress in new crops*. Arlington, VA: ASHS press.

Goenka, P., Sarawgi, A., Karun, V., Nigan, A., Dutta, S., & Marwah, N. (2013). Camellia sinensis (tea): implications and role in preventing dental decay. *Pharmacognosy Reviews, 7*(14), 152-6.

Graham, H. W. (1992). Green tea composition, consumption, and polyphenol chemistry. *Preventive Medicine*, *21*(3), 334–350. doi:10.1016/0091-7435(92)90041-F PMID:1614995

Heiss, M. L., & Heiss, R. J. (2007). *The story of tea: a cultural history and drinking guide*. New York: Ten Speed Press.

Herb Palace. (2004). *History of Herbal Medicine.* Retrieved November 9, 2015 from, http://www.herb-palace.com/alternative-medicine/herbal-medicine.html

Higdon, J. (2002). *Tea.* Linus Pauling Institute. Retrieved November 2, 2015 from http://lpi.oregonstate.edu/book/export/html/435

Hsu, E. (2006). Reflections on the discovery of the antimalarial qinghao. *British Journal of Clinical Pharmacology*, *61*(6), 666–670. doi:10.1111/j.1365-2125.2006.02673.x PMID:16722826

Iinuma, M., Roberts, M. F., Matlin, S. A., Stacey, V. E., Timmermann, B. N., Mabryd, T. J., & Browne, R. (1985). Synthesis and revised structure of the flavone Brickellin. *Phytochemistry*, *24*(6), 1367–1368. doi:10.1016/S0031-9422(00)81135-8

Jepson, R. G. I., & Craig, J. C. (2008). Cranberries for preventing urinary tract infections. *Cochrane Database Syst Rev, 23*(1). 10.1002/14651858.CD001321.pub4

John Hopkins Medicine. (2015). *Herbal medicine*. Retrieved November 14, 2015 from: http://www.hopkinsmedicine.org/healthlibrary/conditions/complementary_and_alternative_medicine/herbal_medicine_85,P00181/

Kaufman, D. W., Kelly, J. P., Rosemberg, L., Anderson, T. E., & Mitchell, A. A. (2002). Recent patterns of medication use in the ambulatory adult population of the United States. *Journal of the American Medical Association*, *287*(3), 337–344. doi:10.1001/jama.287.3.337 PMID:11790213

Klayman, D. L., Lin, A. J., Acton, N., Scovill, J. P., Hotch, J. M., Millous, W. K., & Dobek, A. S. et al. (1984). Isolation of artemisinin (qinghaosu) from Artemisia annua growing in the United States. *Journal of Natural Products*, *47*(4), 715–717. doi:10.1021/np50034a027 PMID:6387056

Kulkarni, M., Nagasampagi, B. A., Deshpande, S. G., & Sharma, R. N. (1987). Five chromenes from Blepharispermum subsessile. *Phytochemistry*, *26*(11), 2969–2971. doi:10.1016/S0031-9422(00)84573-2

Lai, P. K., & Roy, J. (2004). Antimicrobial and chemopreventive properties of herbs and spices. *Current Medicinal Chemistry*, *11*(11), 1451–1460. doi:10.2174/0929867043365107 PMID:15180577

Lee, P. Y., Taha, A. B. A., Lin, K., Ghazali, S. R., & Almashoor, S. H. S. A. (2007). Usage of complimentary and alternative medicine among primary care clinic attendees, Kuching, Sarawak, Malaysia, January – April, 2004. *Asia Pacific Journal of Family Medicine, 6*(1).

Lewis, M. W. (2012). Hot, caffeinated, and expanding: the global geography of coffee, tea, and yerba mate. *GeoCurrents*. Retrieved October 26, 2015 from http://www.geocurrents.info/economic-geography/hot-caffeinated-and-expanding-the-global-geography-of-coffee-tea-and-yerba-mate

Macfarlane, A., & Macfarlane, I. (2004). The empire of tea. The Overlook Press.

Maenthaisong, R., Chaiyakunapruk, N., Niruntrapom, S., & Kongkaew, C. (2007). The efficacy of Aloe vera used for burn wound healing: A systematic review. *Burns*, *33*(6), 713–718. doi:10.1016/j.burns.2006.10.384 PMID:17499928

Marchione, M. (2009). Two billion, five hundred million dollars spent, no alternative cures. *Phys.org*. Retrieved November 13, 2015 from http://phys.org/news/2009-06-25b-spent-alternative-med.html

Marles, R. J., & Farnsworth, N. R. (1994). Plants as Sources of Antidiabetic Agents. *Economic and Medicinal Plant Research*, *6*, 149–187.

Martin, L. C. (2007). Tea: the drink that changed the world. Turtle Publishing.

Martinez, M. (1954). Plantas utiles de la flora Mexico. Mexico. *Ediciones Botas, 400*.

Mata, R., & Escandón, S. (2012). Calein C, an Alpha-Glucosidase Inhibitor from Brickellia cavanillesii. *Planta Medica*, *78*(05), 96. doi:10.1055/s-0032-1307604

Mishra, N. K., Chandini, D., Saijyothi, G., Divya, G., & Venkatalakshmi, I. (2014). Anti-inflammatory activity of Camellia sinensis by using cotton pellet granuloma in rat. *Pharma Science Monitor, 5*(2), 108-17.

Molassiotis, A., Fernadez-Ortega, P., Pud, D., Scott, J. A., Panteli, V., Margulies, A., & Patiraki, E. et al. (2005). Use of complementary and alternative medicine in cancer patients: A European survey. *Annals of Oncology*, *16*(4), 655–663. doi:10.1093/annonc/mdi110 PMID:15699021

Mueller, M. S., Karhagomba, I. B., Hirt, H. M., & Wemakor, E. (2000). The potential of Artemisia annua L. as a locally produced remedy for malaria in the tropics: Agricultural, chemical and chemical aspects. *Journal of Ethnopharmacology*, *73*(3), 487–493. doi:10.1016/S0378-8741(00)00289-0 PMID:11091003

Mueller, M. S., Runyambo, N., Wagner, I., Bormann, S., Dietz, K., & Heide, L. (2004). Randomized controlled trial of a traditional preparation of Artemisia annua L. (Annual wormwood). *Trop Med Hyg*, *98*(5), 318–321. doi:10.1016/j.trstmh.2003.09.001 PMID:15109558

Muktar, H., & Ahmad, N. (2000). Tea polyphenols: Prevention pf cancer and optimizing health. *The American Journal of Clinical Nutrition*, *71*, 1698–1702.

National Center for Biotechnology Information. (2015a). *PubChem compound database; CID=65064*. Retrieved November 9, 2015 from https://pubchem.ncbi.nlm.nih.gov/compound/65064

National Center for Biotechnology Information. (2015b). *PubChem compound database; CID=72277*. Retrieved November 9, 2015 from https://pubchem.ncbi.nlm.nih.gov/compound/72277

National Center for Biotechnology Information. (2015c). *PubChem compound database; CID=107905*. Retrieved November 9, 2015 from https://pubchem.ncbi.nlm.nih.gov/compound/107905

National Center for Biotechnology Information. (2015d). *PubChem compound database; CID=182232*. Retrieved November 9, 2015 from https://pubchem.ncbi.nlm.nih.gov/compound/182232

National Center for Biotechnology Information. (2015e). *PubChem compound database; CID=114777*. Retrieved November 9, 2015 from https://pubchem.ncbi.nlm.nih.gov/compound/114777

National Center for Biotechnology Information. (2015f). *PubChem compound database; CID=22833650*. Retrieved November 9, 2015 from https://pubchem.ncbi.nlm.nih.gov/compound/22833650

National Center for Biotechnology Information. (2015g). *PubChem compound database; CID=5280343*. Retrieved November 2, 2015 from https://pubchem.ncbi.nlm.nih.gov/compound/5280343

National Center for Biotechnology Information. (2015h). *PubChem compound database; CID=5281672*. Retrieved November 2, 2015 from https://pubchem.ncbi.nlm.nih.gov/compound/5281672

National Center for Biotechnology Information. (2015i). *PubChem compound database; CID=5280863*. Retrieved November 2, 2015 from https://pubchem.ncbi.nlm.nih.gov/compound/5280863

National Center for Complementary and Integrative Health. (2015). *Complementary, alternative, or integrative health. What's in a name?* Retrieved November 9, 2015 from, https://nccih.nih.gov/sites/nccam.nih.gov/files/CAM_Basics_Whats_In_A_Name_03-26-2015.pdf

Navarrate, A., Palacios-Espinosa, F., & Mata, R. (2011). Gastroprotective effect of Brickellia cavanillesii (Cav) B. L. Robinson (Asteraceae) in rats. *Planta Medica, 77*, 52. doi:10.1055/s-0031-1273581 PMID:20560115

Chemfaces. (2015). *Theaflavin-3'-gallate:Number, C. A. S.28543-07-9.* Retrieved November 9, 2015 from http://www.chemfaces.com/natural/Theaflavin-3-gallate-CFN98599.html

Pérez-Vásquez, A., García-Nolck, C., Linares, E., Bye, R., & Mata, R. (2014a). Antidiabetic activity and chemical composition of essential oil from Brickellia cavanillesii. *Planta Medica, 80*(10), PD58. doi:10.1055/s-0034-1382479

Pérez-Vásquez, A., Hernadez-Arámburo, M., Linares, E., Bye, R., & Mata, R. (2014b). Validation of a HPLC-DAD method for chromenes markers in Brickellia cavanillesii. *Planta Medica, 80*(10), PPL13. doi:10.1055/s-0034-1382649

Reto, M., Figueria, M. E., Filipe, H. M., & Almedia, C. M. M. (2007). Chemical composition of green tea (Camellia sinensis) infusions commercialized in Portugal. *Plant Foods for Human Nutrition (Dordrecht, Netherlands), 62*(4), 139–144. doi:10.1007/s11130-007-0054-8 PMID:17899383

Rodriguez-Lopez, V., Moreno-Escobar, J. A., Avila-Torres, O., & Tlahuext, H. (2006). 6-Acetyl-5-hydroxy-2, 2-dimethyl-2H- Chromene. *Acta Crystallographica. Section E, Structure Reports Online, 62*(9), 03616–03617. doi:10.1107/S1600536806028947

Ruela de Sousa, R. R., Queiroz, K. C. S., Souza, A. C. S., Gurgueira, S. A., August, A. C., Miranda, M. A., & Aoyama, H. et al. (2007). Phosphoprotein levels, IMAPK activities and NFjB expression are affected by fisetin. *Journal of Enzyme Inhibition and Medicinal Chemistry, 22*(4), 439–444. doi:10.1080/14756360601162063 PMID:17847710

Shane-McWhorter, L. (2007). Complimentary & alternative medicine (CAM) supplement use in people with diabetes: a clinician's guide. Alexandria, VA: American Diabetes Association (ADA).

Shaw, D., Leon, C., Koley, S., & Murray, V. (1997). Traditional remedies and food supplements: A 5-year toxicology study (1991-1995). *Drug Safety, 17*(5), 342–356. doi:10.2165/00002018-199717050-00006 PMID:9391777

Tapsell, L.C. (2006). Health benefits of herbs and spices: The past, the present, the future. *Medical Journal of Australia, 185*(4 suppl), S2-S4.

Vernarelli, J. A., & Lambert, J. D. (2012). Tea consumption is inversely associated with weight status, and other markers for metabolic syndrome in US adults. *European Journal of Nutrition, 52*(3), 1039–1048. doi:10.1007/s00394-012-0410-9 PMID:22777108

Villarreal G. M. A., Estrada, S. S., Guadarrama, A. B. A., & Molina, R. V. (2014). Antidiabetic and antihypertensive effect of Brickellia cavanillesii. *Planta Med, 80*, P2B3. Doi: 10.1055/s-0034-1394880

Vinas, R., & Smith, E. E. (2013). Preliminary evaluation of Prodigiosia herbal tea in cytotoxicity and Glut 2 expression of HepG2 cells. *Toxicological and Environmental Chemistry*, *90*(4), 669–678. doi:10.1080/02772248.2013.801977

Vinskofski, S. (2015). Medicinal herbal tea: infusions and decoctions. *Learning and Yearning*. Retrieved October 23, 2015 from http://learningandyearning.com/infusions-and-decoctions

Wilcox, M. L., Burton, S., Oyweka, R., Namyalo, R., Challand, S., & Lindsey, K. (2011). Evaluation and pharmacovigilance of projects promoting cultivation and local use of Artemisia annua for malaria. *Malaria Journal*, *10*(84), 1–6. PMID:21214892

World Health Organization (WHO). (2003). *Traditional Medicine*. Retrieved November 9, 2015 from, http://www.who.int/mediacentre/factsheets/2003/fs134/en/

World Health Organization. (2014). *The top ten causes of death. Fact sheet no. 310*. Retrieved October 23, 2015 from http://www.who.int/mediacentre/factsheets/fs310/en/

World Health Organization. (2015). *Guidelines for the treatment of malaria* (3rd ed.). Retrieved November, 7 2015 from http://apps.who.int/iris/bitstream/10665/162441/1/9789241549127_eng.pdf?ua=1

Yamamoto, Y., & Gaynor, R. (2001). Therapeutic potential of inhibition of NF-kB pathway in the treatment of inflammation and cancer. *The Journal of Clinical Investigation*, *107*(2), 135–142. doi:10.1172/JCI11914 PMID:11160126

Zand, J., Rountree, R., Rountree, B., & Walton, R. (2003). *Smart medicine for a healthier child: A practical A-to-Z to natural and conventional treatments for infants and children*. New York: Pengium.

Zhu, J., Vinas, R., & Smith, E. E. (2008). In vitro evaluation of human liver cancer cells and the potential cytotoxicity of Tecoma stans (Bignoniaceae) and Brickellia cavanillesii (Asteraceae) both single and in combination. *Toxicological and Environmental Chemistry*, *90*(4), 801–808. doi:10.1080/02772240701740387

Chapter 7
Functional Properties of Camel Milk

Omar Amin Alhaj
King Saud University, Saudi Arabia

ABSTRACT

This chapter focuses on the potential health benefits of camel milk including angiotension I-converting enzyme-inhibitory, anti-cancer and antioxidant activities, antidiabetic, antimicrobial and hypoallergenicity effects. The bioactivity of oligosaccharide, conjugated linoleic acid and D-amino acid in camel milk is provided. The proposed mechanisms behind these bioactive components and potential health claims are explained. This chapter also describes camel milk composition, nutritional value, production and population. The current available information in the literature on camel milk is not abundant. More research is needed to give better understanding on functional properties of camel milk.

INTRODUCTION

The primary purpose of food including dairy products is to provide nutrients to fulfil the body's traditional requirements and other functions including cultural and social wellbeing. Although, in the recent decades life style has changed and become more complicated regarding life standard, hygiene, diet, use of antibiotics and other antimicrobial substances, hence a new concept of food need to be introduced. It has long been recognized that some non-traditional foods, for example camel milk, fortified food and beverages that provide particular health benefits and interestingly, in recent decades they have been modified to provide disease-preventive attributes, in addition to their particular functional health benefits. The concept of functional foods has also been developed and their types have been expanded to become one of the popular foods worldwide. The estimated growth rate of functional food in the global market is 15-20% per year, and the industry is claimed to be worth up to US$168 billion of the annual share (Euromonitor, 2010; Hilliam, 2003). However, there is no internationally accepted definition of functional foods exist, because it is a more of a concept rather than a well-defined group of food products (ILSI, 1999). So far, various definitions have been proposed by a number of researchers and/or foundations including International Food Information Council (IFIC) in 2011 as "food thought to provide benefits

DOI: 10.4018/978-1-5225-0591-4.ch007

beyond basic nutrition and may play a role in reducing or minimizing the risk of certain diseases and other health conditions". The EU official directives have not given functional foods a firm definition, but the International Life Science Institute (ILSI) Europe in 1999 has proposed a working definition as food can be considered as 'functional' if it is "satisfactorily demonstrated to affect beneficially one or more target functions in the body, beyond adequate nutritional effects, in a way that is relevant to either an improved state of health and well-being and/or reduction of risk of disease".

Consumers are now more aware of functional foods than before, in 2013, 46% of consumers strongly agree that certain foods have health benefits beyond basic nutrition (IFIC, 2013). The recent information by IFIC showed that 91% of consumers are aware about the healthfulness of their food and beverages, furthermore, 88% knowledge a lot about food ingredients (IFIC, 2015).

According to the latest statistics of the Food and Agriculture Organization (FAO), the total heads of camels worldwide is estimated to be about 27 million, which mainly live in Africa (82.5%) and Asia (17.5%) (FAOSTAT, 2013). Camels are mainly classified into two species belonging to the genus *Camelus*; Dromedary camels having one- humped (*Camelus dromedarius*) are the dominant species which tend to live in the arid regions, whereas Bactrian camel having two-humped (*Camelus bactrianus*) mainly prefer living in the cooler regions (Al haj & Al Kanhal, 2010).The dairy camels in the world produce about 3 million ton of whole fresh milk per year distributed between Asia (8.7%) and Africa (91.3%), whereas Somalia is the biggest producer worldwide followed by Kenya, Mali, Ethiopia, and Saudi Arabia, respectively (FAOSTAT, 2013). Humans consume only 1.3 million tons per year while remaining amount are fed to calves (FAO, 2008). This is because most of the camel herds are located in the arid and desert regions which are far from the commercial markets. Recently very few camel milk products are available in the urban markets. Nowadays, there is a general need to launch a number of camel milk based functional products to the commercial market due to increasing demand in recent years (Al haj & Al Kanhal, 2010). These products have to be clinically proven and scientifically evident supported (Ghosh, 2009). This chapter focuses on the functional properties of camel milk components as well as proposed mechanism behind each health claim. The compositional and nutritional aspects of camel milk are also highlighted.

BACKGROUND

Camel Milk Composition

Camel milk has an important role in human nutrition in the arid regions; however camel milk is generally described as opaque-white, frothy, sweet and sharp but sometimes salty in taste (Al haj & Al Kanhal, 2010). These variations in taste are due to the type of fodder and unavailability of water (Farah, 1996). Although camel milk shows convergent gross chemical composition compared to other mammalian milks, on the other hand few differences were found in some sub-constituents for example absence of β-Lactoglobulin, high β-casein, and low αs-casein content (Table 1). These differences provide camel milk with some additional functional properties, for example, hypoallergenicity and higher digestibility in the gut of infants (El-Agamy *et al.*, 2009; Abou-Soliman, 2005). Nevertheless, references data (Claeys *et al.*, 2014; Al haj & Al Kanhal, 2010; Konuspayeva *et al.*, 2009) have exhibited wide ranges of variation in camel milk composition. Since these variations was due to several factors such as analytical measurement procedures, regional locations, stage of lactation, age, nutrient conditions and breeds (Khaskheli *et al.*, 2005; Al haj & Al Kanhal, 2010). The mean values of camel milk composition and range of variation are shown in Table 1.

CAMEL MILK BIOACTIVITY

Camel milk is an important nutritional and functional source that consist a complex mixture of high quality proteins, carbohydrates, fats, minerals, and vitamins; which deliver human health with several key bioactive properties (Al haj & Al Kanhal, 2010). Early reports (Abdelgadir *et al.*, 1998; Shalash, 1984) showed that non-fermented or fermented camel milk were used worldwide as a potential treatment for a number of diseases including tuberculosis, dropsy, asthma jaundice and leishmaniasis. Furthermore, children having biliary atresia and postpartum respiratory insufficiency were given camel milk until their liver transplant and lungs developed and function well (Yagil, 1987). These potential health claims were due to a number of bioactive components, which either exist naturally in camel milk (Agrawal *et al.*, 2007; El-Agamy*et al.*, 1992); or encrypted in the primary structure of camel milk constitutes and could be released *in vivo* by gastrointestinal digests or *in vitro* by digestive or microbial proteolytic enzymes (Alhaj *et al.*, 2016; Moslehishad *et al.*, 2013; Salami *et al.*, 2011; Alhaj *et al.*, 2010; Salami *et al.*, 2010; Korhonen & Pihlanto, 2003). Bioactive components are defined by Park (2009) as "compounds either naturally existing in food or ones formed and/or formulated during food processing that may have physiological and biochemical functions when consumed by humans". Bioactive components derived from camel milk were found to be stable even after sterilization process and provide potential health benefits including ACE-inhibitory activity, antimicrobial, anticancer and antioxidant effect (Alhaj *et al.*, 2016; Amr *et al.,* 2015; Al-Saleh *et al.,* 2014; Alhaj *et al.*, 2011). In contrast, lactoferrin were completely inactivated after pasteurization (Claeys *et al.*, 2014). Several studies have shown that bioactive components in camel milk could provide a number of health benefits (Abd El-Salam & El-Shibiny, 2013; Al-Juboori, 2013; Al haj & Al Kanhal, 2010; Shamsia, 2009).

BIOACTIVITY OF CAMEL MILK PROTEINS

Many food proteins including egg, corn, dairy products, wheat gluten, rice, fish and soybean proteins were found to encrypt bioactive peptides in their primary structures (Kitts & Weiler, 2003). Milk and dairy products have developed a high reputation as the most significant home of bioactivities because most of the well-known bioactive peptides are derived from milk proteins (Meisel, 2004). Furthermore, milk proteins, in addition to their high nutritional value, are available in the market in large amounts at moderate cost (Léonil *et al.*, 2000). The protein content in bovine milk is 3.3% compared to 3.1% in camel milk which is made up of amino acids. The range of health claims is usually depending of the amino acid sequence of bioactive peptides. It has been reported that most of the milk protein derived bioactive peptides contain up to 23 amino acid residues per molecule (Otte *et al.*, 2007; Korhonen & Pihlanto, 2003). Kitts & Weiler (2003) have defined bioactive peptides as "specific protein fragments

Table 1. Mean values, standard deviation (SD), and range of variation of camel milk components

Components	Mean Value (SD)	Range of Variation
Total solids	11.9% (±1.5)	8.64 - 15.06%
Proteins	3.1% (±0.5)	2.15 - 4.90%
Casein/whey ratio	N/A	2.7 – 3.2
Casein (CN)	N/A	1.63-2.76% or 22.1 – 26 g/l*
β- CN	65%	N/A
α_{s1}- CN	21%	N/A
κ- CN	3.47%	N/A
Whey proteins	N/A	0.63 - 0.80% or 5.9 - 8.1 g/l*
β-Lactoglobulin	absent*	absent
α-Lactalbumin	N/A	0.8 - 3.5 g/l*
Lactoferrin	N/A	0.02 - 7.28 g/l*
Lysozyme	N/A	(60 - 1350) x 10^{-6}*
Immunoglobulins (Ig)	N/A	1.5 – 19.6 g/l*
NPN	0.68 g/l*	N/A
Lactose	4.4% (±0.7)	2.40 - 5.80%
Fat	3.5% (±1.0)	1.2 - 6.4%
Cholesterol	34.5 mg / 100g	31.3 – 37.1 mg / 100 ml*
Conjugated linoleic acid (CLA)	0.4%*	N/A
Mineral	0.79% (±0.07)	0.60 - 0.90%
Potassium (K)	155.66 mg / 100 g (±37.88)	58 - 104 mg / 100 ml*
Calcium (Ca)	114.34 mg / 100 g (±13.35)	105 – 157 mg / 100 ml*
Sodium (Na)	58.87 mg / 100 g (±16.22)	36 – 73 mg / 100 ml*
Magnesium (Mg)	10.45 mg / 100 g (±1.78)	8 – 16 mg / 100 ml*
Zinc (Zn)	0.53 mg / 100 g (±0.08)	0.19 – 0.6 mg / 100 ml*
Iron (Fe)	0.29 mg / 100 g (±0.09)	0.7 – 0.37 mg / 100 ml*
Manganese (Mn)	0.05 mg / 100 g (±0.03)	N/A
Vitamin	N/A	N/A
A	N/A	5 - 97μg / 100 ml*
D	N/A	0.3 – 1.6 μg / 100 ml*
E	N/A	21 – 150 μg / 100 ml*
C	N/A	2400 – 18,400 μg / 100 ml*
B1	N/A	10 – 60 μg / 100 ml*
B2	N/A	42 – 168 μg / 100 ml*
B3	N/A	400 – 770 μg / 100 ml*
B5	N/A	88 – 368 μg / 100 ml*
B6	N/A	50 – 55 μg / 100 ml*
B12	0.2 μg / 100 ml*	N/A

Mean values, standard deviation (SD) and range of variation were adapted from Al haj & Al Kanhal, (2010); *adopted from Claeys *et al.* (2014). N/A stands not available.

that have a positive impact on body functions or conditions and may ultimately influence health". Bioactive peptides in milk could be generated or enriched by adding starter or non-starter cultures due to their metabolic products required for their growth (Alhaj *et al.*, 2007). Thence, milk cultured with combination of two or more type of strains exhibited a wider variety of functional components (Kuwabara *et al.*, 1995). However, the addition of *Lactobacillus helveticus* or/and *Lactobacillus acidophilus* solely or in combination to camel milk was reported to release ACE-inhibitory peptides (Alhaj, 2012); antioxidant peptides (Al-Saleh *et al.*, 2014); antimicrobial peptides (Alhaj, 2015). Likewise, the ACE-inhibitory, antimicrobial and antioxidant activities of camel whey proteins were found to improve after treatment with proteolytic enzymes such as trypsin, chymotrypsin and pepsin (Salami *et al.*, 2011; 2010). The potential health claims and activities of camel milk will be discussed individually in the following sections.

Angiotension Converting Enzyme (Ace) Inhibitory Activity

ACE-inhibitory peptides are one of the most favored bioactive peptides applied in foodstuff formula to provide health benefits (Meisel & Bockelmann, 1999). The inhibition of angiotension converting enzyme using milk bioactive peptides is the most intensive studied mechanism internationally. As one of the major blood pressure regulators, the angiotensin-I-converting enzyme (ACE) was defined by Pan *et al.* (2005) as "an exopeptidase that cleaves dipeptides from the C-terminal ends of various peptide substrates and regulates the activity of several endogenous bioactive peptides" (P. 123). ACE acts on angiotensin-I in renin angiotensin system to hydrolyze the dipeptide; His-Leu from its C-terminal lead to producing a potent vasopressor angiotensin-II (Skeggs *et al.*, 1956). Thus, a small decrease of 5-mm Hg in diastolic blood pressure (DBP) can reduce 15% of the risk of developing cardiovascular diseases (Meisel *et al.*, 2006).

ACE-inhibitory peptides are present in the primary structure of various food proteins sources including milk protein (Meisel *et al.*, 2006; Jang & Lee, 2005; Li *et al.*, 2004). The level of ACE-inhibitory activity was found to essentially depend on the strain and degree of hydrolysis of protein (Alhaj *et al.*, 2016), type of proteolytic enzyme and molecular weight (Salami *et al.*, 2011). ACE-inhibitory bioactive peptides are produced using individual or combined cultures. The addition of *L. rhamnosus* to camel milk was recently studied and exhibited ACE-I activity (Moslehishad *et al.*, 2013). Furthermore, Quan *et al.* (2008) identified ACE-inhibitory peptides (Ala-Ile-Pro-Pro-Lys-Lys-Asn-Gln-Asp) from Mongolia camel milk proteins using *Lactobacillus helveticus* 130B4. In another study, Alhaj *et al.,* (2012) identified two ACE-inhibitory peptides corresponding to β-casein from water soluble permeates (WSP) of dromedary camel milk using *Lactobacillus acidophilus* solely. The identified ACE- inhibitory peptides were FQEPFPDPVR and VLPFQEPVPDPVRG. Donker *et al.* (2007) pointed out that most effective ACE-inhibitory peptides were originated from β-casein which represents about 65% of the total camel milk caseins (Kappeler *et al.*, 2003). Furthermore, Seven ACE-inhibitory peptides were identified from WSP of dromedary camel milk incubated with *Lactobacillus helveticus* solely (Alhaj *et al.*, 2012). Three peptides were released from sequences 1 (LSLSQF, SLSQF, or SQF) KVLPVPQ, three peptides of the sequences 2 (TDLEN, DLEN, or LEN) LHLPLPL, and one peptide of the sequence 3 KVLPVVPQQMVPYPQ. All identified ACE-inhibitory peptides were corresponding to β-casein of *Camelus dromedarius* milk and some contain at least one proline (P) residue at their C-terminal position. The C-terminal sequence of ACE-inhibitory peptides play important role in the binding to the ACE (López-Fandiño *et al.*, 2006). Thus, amino acids having hydrophobic properties such as tryptophan (W), phenylalanine (F), tyrosine

(Y) and especially proline (P) are appeared to contribute substantially to inhibitory potency (López-Fandiño *et al.*, 2006; Li *et al.*, 2004).

Antidiabetic Activity

It has been early reported that camel milk has good results for stabilization of juvenile diabetes (Yagil, 1987). Camel milk supplementation can improve the glycemic control and reduce the doses of insulin for type 1 diabetes patients (Khan *et al.*, 2012; Agrawal *et al.*, 2011; Agrawal *et al.*, 2003). In another study, the consumption of camel milk in India has lowered the prevalence of diabetes in the Raica community (Agrawal *et al.*, 2007; Singh *et al.*, 2008). In animal study, the supplementation of camel milk has reduced the level of blood glucose of diabetic albino rats (Baragob, 2015) and alloxan-induced diabetic dogs (Sboui *et al.*, 2010) and the effect was depending on the amount of camel milk. The hypo-glycemic activity of camel milk is attributed to the presence of various components including the existence of high concentration of insulin like substances such as half-cystine, in addition to the regulatory and small size immunoglobulins functions of camel milk on β-cell (Breitling, 2002). Moreover, camel milk does not react to acid and form coagulation in human stomach; this could be another reason for hypoglycemic effect in camel milk (Agrawal *et al.*, 2003).

Antimicrobial Activity

Camel milk was reported to contain a various antimicrobial agents including immunoglobulins, lactoperoxidase, lactoferrin, hydrogen peroxide and lysozyme (Al-Juboori *et al.*, 2013). The amount of these agents in camel milk is greater than that reported for other mammalian antibacterial proteins (Kappeler *et al.* 1999). Xanthine oxidoreductase (XOR) protein is another antimicrobial compound in camel milk which could play an important antimicrobial defensive role in the neonatal gut (Harrison, 2006). Other antimicrobial compound was also isolated from camel milk but not detected in cow milk such as peptidoglycan recognition protein (PGRP) (Kappeler *et al.*, 1999). Aforementioned components exist naturally in camel milk and have an antimicrobial effect against pathogenic strains including *Staphylococcus aureus*, *Listeria monocytogenes*, *Salmonella typhimurium*and *Escherichia coli* (Benkerroum *et al.*, 2004; El-Agamy *et al.*, 1992). Immunoglobulins are another natural protector in camel milk which functions against infections in the gut of newborns. These antimicrobial substances work with different inhibitory mechanisms, for instance, PGRP inactivate pathogenic strains by binding to peptidoglycan structures in the cell wall (Abd El-Salam & El-Shibiny, 2013).While, the inhibitory action of lactoferrin in camel milk against *S. typhimurium* is through binding iron and making it unavailable for its growth (Ochoa & Cleary, 2009). In contrast, the presence of lysozyme in camel milk was reported to prolong the gelation process of yoghurt due to the delay of yoghurt culture growth in camel milk (Jumah *et al.*, 2001). It is evident that antimicrobial substances in camel milk lose their complete activity after heat treatment at 100 °C for 30 min (El-Agamy, 2000).

Camel milk encrypts antimicrobial peptides in their primary structure and could be released using digestive or microbial proteolytic enzymes. The activity of these antimicrobial peptides depends on strain, incubation time and peptides molecular weight. Additional factors were also found to enhance the antimicrobial effect including structural activity (Gobbetti *et al.*, 2004). Whereas, the alteration of Asp (D) with Arg (R) and the addition of Lys (K) residues to the *C*-terminus of antimicrobial peptide were found to increase the bactericidal activity to Gram-negative bacteria (Pellegrini *et al.*, 2001). Camel milk inoculated with two added combined culture (*Lactobacillus acidophilus* and *Streptococcus thermophilus* or *Lactobacillus helveticus* and *Streptococcus thermophilus*) was found to exhibit varying degree of inhibition against *B. cereus*, *S. typhimurium* and *S. aureus* (Alhaj *et al.*, 2016). This effect was mainly found to depend on culture, incubation time and antimicrobial peptide molecular weight. However, the antimicrobial inhibition activity of camel milk containing *L. helveticus* and *S. thermophilus* was higher than that noticed in camel milk containing *L. acidophilus* and *S. thermophilus*. This is attributed to the nature of proteolytic system of *L. helveticus* which result in more antimicrobial peptides formation.

Antioxidant Activity

There is strong evidence between diabetic, cardiovascular diseases, aging, cancer and the imbalance of free radical levels in the body (Sah *et al.*, 2014; Shori, 2013). The formation of free radicals (superoxide anion radical and hydroxyl radical) is a normal result of aerobic organisms during respiration (Virtanen *et al.*, 2007). An excess of free radicals formation could led to cause cellular or tissue injury by oxidizing cellular proteins, enzymes, membrane lipids and DNA (Sah *et al.*, 2014). Under normal conditions, defense system shall prevent body from this damage using antioxidant enzymes and low molecular massnon-enzymatic antioxidant compounds (Virtanen *et al.*, 2007). Antioxidants peptides could be derived from various food proteins including milk and dairy products; these peptides contain 5-16 amino acid residues and considered to be safe, low cost, healthy and easily absorbed in small intestine (Sarmadia & Ismail, 2010). According to the recent information by IFIC about 34% of consumers get enough food contain potential antioxidant effect (IFIC, 2013). The antioxidant activity of camel milk has been approved through a number of *in vitro* studies (Al-Saleh *et al.*, 2014; Jrad *et al.*, 2014; Shori, 2013; Salami *et al.*, 2011) and *in vivo* studies (AL-Ayadhi & Elamin, 2013). Various methods based on radical scavenging inhibition (hydroxyl radical and DPPH) were adopted to determine the antioxidant activity of camel milk. The DPPH radical scavenging activity, total phenol compounds and reducing power of camel casein hydrolysate were reported to be greater than those of bovine casein hydrolysate and un-hydrolysed camel casein (Al-Saleh *et al.*, 2014). These findings were supported by a recent study, which showed that free radical scavenging of camel casein and camel casein hydrolysate were higher than those found for camel milk whole protein and its hydrolysate (Jrad *et al.*, 2014). This is attributed to the presence of camel β-casein (main casein in camel milk protein) which showed high antioxidant activity after hydrolysis with chymotrypsin (Salami *et al.*, 2011). Moreover, the exposure of free radical scavenging amino acid residues such as phenylalanine, tryptophan, methionine, tyrosine and cysteine were found to increase the oxidative stability of casein hydrolysate (Moure *et al.*, 2006).

Anti-Cancer Activity

According to the latest statistics of International Agency of Research on Cancer (IARC) in 2012 worldwide, the number of new cancer cases was 14.1 million, whereas the number of cancer deaths was 8.2 million. Moreover, people living with cancer (within 5 years of diagnosis) were 32.6 million (WHO, 2012). Colorectal cancer (CRC) is highly affected by the dietary and lifestyle factors thus could be substantially reduced by controlling the different risk factors, including the dietary ones. In general, the relation between dairy products and CRC are controversial (Gill & Rowland, 2003). There are some studies exhibited no significant effect associated between dairy products consumption and CRC. While, several studies suggested that increased consumption of dairy products including camel milk may elevate the risk of CRC (Amr *et al.*, 2015, Korashy *et al.,* 2012, Quita & Kurdi, 2010). Camel milk was reported to have superior chemo-preventive properties over cow milk, thus extensively consumed by cancer patients in the Middle East (Quita & Kurdi, 2010). The chemo-preventive effect of unfermented and fermented camel milk against different kind of cancers was studied using different cancer biomarkers. This effect is attributed to the bioactive components presence in milk and dairy products including conjugated linoleic acid, sphingolipids, calcium, lactoferrin, casein or addition of probiotic and prebiotic (Gill & Rowland, 2003). Camel milk has shown to inhibit the hepatic and breast cancers and to alleviate the hepatotoxicity induced by natural toxicants. Camel milk intubated to albino mice has significantly inhibited the micronucleated polychromatic erythrocytes (MnPCEs) in the bone marrow and increased the mitotic index induced by cisplatin chemotherapy (Quita & Kurdi, 2010). In another animal study, camel milk showed therapeutic effects to rats after aflatoxin B1 intoxication using amelioration of cancer blood biomarkers (Abdel Magjeed, 2005). In another research, camel milk has significantly inhibited cancer cells proliferation through the activation of caspase-3 mRNA and the induction of extrinsic and intrinsic apoptotic signaling pathways (Korashy *et al.,* 2012). Recently, Amr *et al.* (2015) has studied the chemopreventive potential of camel milk compared to bovine milk, however both milks exhibited chemopreventive potential on Fischer rates against preneoplastic lesions as expressed by ACF in the early stages of colon carcinogenesis.

Hypoallergenicity Activity

Some infants are born allergic to various food components including milk and even soy milk. Approximately 70% of sensation to food allergens is being disappeared at the age of six (Kulig *et al.*, 1999). On the other hand, up to 23% of children are sensitized without showing symptoms (Kirjanvainen, 2003). There is no doubt; mothers' milk is the ideal nutrition for newborn infants during the early months of life. Although, infants in many cases need to complete their necessary nutrition with some alternative formulae such as soy milk, goat milk or extensively hydrolyzed milk protein formulae (El-Agamy, 2007). Approximately 10-20% of children showed allergenicity to bovine milk are also expressed sensation to soy derivatives (El-Agamay *et al.*, 2009, Maldonado *et al.*, 1998, Businco *et al.*, 1992). Researchers have recently proposed camel milk proteins as alternative to children allergic to bovine milk. It is evident that high incidence of allergenicity in bovine milk is related to the high percentage of αs- casein (Taylor, 1986) and β-lactoglobulin (El-Agmay, 2007). In contrast, camel milk is hypo-allergic similar to mothers' milk due to the high percentage of β-casein, low percentage of αs- casein (El-Agamay *et al.,* 2009), similarity of immunoglobulins (Shabo *et al.,* 2005) and deficiency of β-lactoglobulin (Kappeler, 1998). Accordingly, camel milk is expected to cause a little hypersensitivity reactions (El-Agamay *et al.*, 2009). Nevertheless, no immunological similarity was found between camel and cow milk using ELISA technique (El-Agamay *et al.*, 2009). Therefore, camel milk could be proposed as a new protein source for children allergic to bovine milk.

BIOACTIVITY OF CAMEL MILK OLIGOSACCHARIDE

Like other milk sources, lactose is the dominant saccharide in camel milk and consist 4.4% of total milk composition (Al haj & Al Kanhal, 2010). Other substantial quantities of saccharides including neutral and acidic oligosaccharides, glucose, fructose, and glucosamine were also found in camel milk (Fox & McSweeney, 1998). Oligosaccharides are carbohydrates with a degree of polymerization contain a small number of saccharide units (between 3 and 14), most of these have lactose residue and some N-acetyl groups (Walstra *et al.*, 2008). The potential health claims of milk oligosaccharides and their proposed mechanisms are discussed by Boehm & Stahl (2007) and Kunz and Rudloff (2006). These claims are summarized as follows: modulate the intestinal flora, affect different gastrointestinal activities, effect on mineral absorption, anti-adhesion effect against pathogens, enhance the immune system, and enhance the growth of *Bifidobacterium bifidum*. In particular attention, 3'-GL oligosaccharide which is considered as a prebiotic component was detected in camel milk (Alhaj *et al.*, 2013). This oligosaccharide could be used as a food additive in infant formula (Urashima *et al.*, 2009).

The number and concentration of identified oligosaccharides in human milk is much higher than that reported for domestic mammalian animals including camel milk (Alhaj *et al.*, 2013; Fukuda *et al.*, 2010; Urashima *et al.*, 1997). Researchers (Boehm & Stahl, 2003) recorded eighty-seven oligosaccharides in human milk compared to thirteen and seven characterized oligosaccharides in Bactrian camel milk /colostrum (Fukuda *et al.*, 2010), and in Dromedary camel milk (Alhaj *et al.*, 2013), respectively. Furthermore, the concentration of oligosaccharides in camel and bovine milk compared to human milk was found to decrease during lactation (Finke, 2000; Martin *et al.*, 2001; Fukuda, *et al.*, 2010). On the other hand, significant homology and heterogeneity differences were reported in the oligosaccharides structure between human and camel milk (Alhaj *et al.*, 2013; Fukuda *et al.*, 2010; Mehra & Kelly, 2006). Two oligosaccharides; Sialyl -3'-galactosyllactose and sialyllacto-N-novopentaose-a were not detected in human milk/colostrum but detected in camel milk. In contrast, 3'-GL, LNnH, 3'-SL, 6'-SL and MSLNnH oligosaccharides are both detected in dromedary camel and human milk (Alhaj *et al.*, 2013). The following oligosaccharides, Sialyllacto-N-novopentaose-a, LNnH and MFLNnH, which contain Gal(β1–4)GlcNAc(N-acetyllactosamine), are categorized as Type II oligosaccharides and only found in Dromedary and Bactrian camel milk (Alhaj *et al.*, 2013). Accordingly, the presence or absence of Type I oligosaccharide that contain Gal(β1–3)GlcNAc (lacto-N-biose I) is expected to be the main significant contrast between human and camel or bovine milk oligosaccharide (Fukuda *et al.*, 2010).

BIOACTIVITY OF CAMEL CONJUGATED LINOLEIC ACID (CLA)

For many years the concept of eating dairy products was likely associated for being harmful to health due to the presence of saturated fat and cholesterol. This concept was misleading and often inaccurate because not all fatty acids or saturated fatty acids have the same biological effects. Researchers concluded that fatty acid within a whole diet context has to be considered individually to clarify the link between health and diet (Parodi, 2009; Lock *et al.*, 2008). Bauman *et al.* (2006) highlighted a number of bioactive components in milk fat (e.g. essential fatty acids including conjugated linoleic acid, vaccenic acid, butyric acid, sphingolipids, 13-methyltetradecanoic acid, stearic acid, ether lipids,omega-3 fatty acids and vitamins A, D). Conjugated linoleic acid (CLA) is the most important bioactive component in milk fat due to its inhibitory effect on cancer, immune function, inflammation, diabetes and atherosclerosis (Gnädig *et al.*, 2003). The concentration of CLA in camel milk fat is 4.56 mg/g which is greater than that reported for cow milk (Al-khdier *et al.*, 2014; Cardak *et al.*, 2003). This concentration was found to increase in camel milk through addition of some starter cultures including *Bifidobacterium angulatum*,

Bifidobacterium longum subsp. *Infantis* and *Lactobacillus delbrueckii* subsp. *bulgaricus* (Al-khdier *et al.*, 2014). More extensive research is needed to investigate the functional properties of CLA in camel milk fat. The current information is highly important but not enough to warrant a strong conclusion.

BIOACTIVITY OF D AND L AMINO ACID IN CAMEL MILK

Among the proteinaceous foodstuffs, milk is of major importance not only for infants but also for children and adults. This is attributed to its high nutritional value in terms of essential AAs and contents of calcium. Although L-amino acids are the major structure blocks of peptides and proteins of all living organisms; however, the corresponding stereoisomers (enantiomers) of L-amino acids is called D-amino acids which occur in low amounts in milk as well as most tissues of all mammals. In recent years, positive health effects of some D-amino acids established and some were used as pharmaceutical drugs including D-Asp stimulates testosterone synthesis, increases human sperm count and mobility, and is implicated in human pre-ovulatory follicular fluid (D'Aniello *et al.*, 2007, Topo *et al.*, 2009). The Mg-salt of DL-Asp is also used as magnesium supplement and protection against heart diseases, D-Ser is used to treat the schizophrenia and D-Phe for treatment of Parkinson's disease (Stenberg *et al.*, 2002).

In the last decades, many studies have analyzed the presence of D-amino acids in many processed foods. These studies assumed that D-amino acids are released in dairy products, fermented beverages and other products matured by the presence of some active bacteria (Brueckner & Hausch, 1990). However, raw milk is usually contaminated with microorganisms, such as anaerobic bacteria of the genera *Bacterioides, Ruminococcus* and *Butyrivibrio*. The low amount of free D-amino acids found in milk is significant and expected to be due to the result of the bacterial digestion and autolysis (Brückner & Fujii, 2010). The addition of cultures to camel milk of various dairy products has significantly enhanced the D-amino acid content. For example, the addition of three starter cultures (*Lactobacillus acidophilus* and *Streptococcus thermophilus; Lactobacillus helveticus* and *Streptococcus thermophilus; and Lactobacillus bulgaricus* and *Streptococcus thermophilus*) have relatively increased the concentration of D- Ala, D-Val, D-Orn, D-Lys and D-Arg in fermented camel milk (Alhaj, 2015). The amino acid content was varied depending on starter culture and fermentation process. The current available information on D-amino acid content in camel milk is scarce in the literature; further work is needed to highlight the importance of D-amino acid in camel milk.

CONCLUSION AND FUTURE RESEARCH

Camel milk is a good source of bioactive components for the people living in the arid and urban areas. The current available information is highly important but extensive research is required to support the present potential health claims and their proposed mechanisms. Functional products based on camel milk source are required in the commercial market due to increasing demand in recent years. These products have to be clinically proven, scientifically evident supported and exhibit no side effect after consumption. Consumers have to be given more awareness about the healthfulness and importance of camel milk.

REFERENCES

Abd El-Salam, M. H., & El-Shibiny, S. (2013). Bioactive Peptides of Buffalo, Camel, Goat, Sheep, Mare, and Yak Milks and Milk Products. *Food Reviews International*, *29*(1), 1–23. doi:10.1080/87559129.2012.692137

Abdel Magjeed, N. (2005). Corrective effect of milk camel on some cancer biomarkers in blood of rats intoxicated with aflatoxin B1. *Journal of Saudi Chemical Society*, *9*, 253–264.

Abdelgadir, W. S., Ahmed, T. K., & Dirar, H. A. (1998). The traditional fermented milk products of the Sudan. *International Journal of Food Microbiology*, *44*(1-2), 1–13. doi:10.1016/S0168-1605(98)00090-7 PMID:9849779

Abou-Soliman, N. H. (2005). *Studies on goat milk proteins: molecular and immunologicalcharacterization with respect to human health and nutrition*. (Ph.D. Thesis). Alexandria University, Egypt.

Agrawal, R. P., Budania, S., Sharma, P., Gupta, R., Kochar, D. K., Panwar, R. B., & Sahani, M. S. (2007). Zero prevalence of diabetes in camel milk consuming Raica community of northwest Rajasthan, India. *Diabetes Research and Clinical Practice*, *76*(2), 290–296. doi:10.1016/j.diabres.2006.09.036 PMID:17098321

Agrawal, R. P., Jain, S., Shah, S., Chopra, A., & Agarwal, V. (2011). Effect of camel milk on glycemic control and insulin requirement in patients with type 1 diabetes: 2-years randomized controlled trial. *European Journal of Clinical Nutrition*, *65*(9), 1048–1052. doi:10.1038/ejcn.2011.98 PMID:21629270

Al-Ayadhi, L. Y., & Elamin, N. E. (2013). Camel milk as a potential therapy as an antioxidant in autism spectrum disorder (ASD). *Evidence-Based Complementary and Alternative Medicine*, 1–8.

Al Haj, O. A., & Al Kanhal, H. A. (2010). Compositional, technological and nutritional aspects of dromedary camel milk. *International Dairy Journal*, *20*, 811-821.

Al-Juboori, A. J., Mohammed, M., Rashid, J., Kurian, J., & El Refaey S. (2013). Nutritional and medicinal value of camel (Camelus Dromedarius) milk. *Food & Environment II*, *170*, 221-232.

Al-Khdier, A. M., Al-Saleh, A. A., Abu-Tarboush, H. M., Ismail, E. A., & Metwalli, A. A. (2014). The ability of some starter cultures to increase the conjugated linoleic acid level in cow and camel milks. *Journal of Pure and Applied Microbiology*, *8*, 363–370.

Al-Saleh, A. A., Metwalli, A. A. M., Ismail, E. A., & Alhaj, O. A. (2014). Antioxidative activity of camel milk casein hydrolysates. *Journal of Camel Practice & Research*, *21*(2), 229–237. doi:10.5958/2277-8934.2014.00041.1

Alhaj, O. A. (2015). *Chromatographic determination of L- and D-amino acids in fermented camel milk*. Unpublished work, King Saud University, Kingdom of Saudi Arabia.

Alhaj, O. A., Brückner, H., & Al-Khalifa, A. S. (2012). Sequences of ACE-inhibitory precursor peptides from bacterial fermented milk of *Camelus dromedarius*. *Journal of Peptide Science*, *18*, S146–S147.

Alhaj, O. A., Kanekanian, A., & Peters, A. (2007). Investigation on whey proteins profile of commercially aviabale milk-based probiotics health drinks using fast protein liquid chromatography (FPLC). *British Food Journal*, *109*(6), 469–480. doi:10.1108/00070700710753526

Alhaj, O. A., Kanekanian, A., Peters, A., & Tatham, A. (2010). Hypocholesterolemic effect of *Bifidobacterium animalis* subsp. *Lactis* (Bb12) and trypsin casein hydrolysate. *Food Chemistry*, *123*(2), 430–435. doi:10.1016/j.foodchem.2010.04.061

Alhaj, O. A., Metwalli, A. A., Ismail, E. A., Ali, H. S., Al-Khalifa, A. S., & Kanekanian, A. D. (2016). *Angiotensin Converting Enzyme - inhibitory activity and antimicrobial effect of fermented camel milk (Camelusdromedarius).* Unpublished work, King Saud University, Kingdom of Saudi Arabia.

Alhaj, O. A., Metwalli, A. A. M., & Ismail, E. A. (2011). Heat stability of camel milk proteins after sterilization process. *Journal of Camel Practice & Research*, *18*, 277–282.

Alhaj, O. A., Taufik, E., Handa, Y., Fukuda, K., Saito, T., & Urashima, T. (2013). Chemical characterization of oligosaccharides in commercially pasteurized dromedary camel (*camelusdromedarius*) milk. *International Dairy Journal*, *28*(2), 70–75. doi:10.1016/j.idairyj.2012.08.008

Amr, A. M., Takruri, H. R., Shomaf, M. S., Alhaj, O. A., & Faris, M. E. (2015). *Chemopreventive potential of probiotic fermented camel (Camelusdromedarius) and bovine (Bostaurus) milks against Azoxymethane-Induced aberrant crypt foci in Fischer 344 Rats, unpublished work.* Amman, Jordan: University of Jordan.

Baragob, A. E. A. (2015). Composition and hypoglycemic effect of camel milk in streptozotocin–induced diabetic rats. *Biochemistry and Biotechnology Research*, *3*, 38–42.

Bauman, D. E., Mather, I. H., Wall, R. J., & Lock, A. L. (2006). Major advances associated with the biosynthesis of milk. *Journal of Dairy Science*, *89*(4), 1235–1243. doi:10.3168/jds.S0022-0302(06)72192-0 PMID:16537956

Benkerroum, N., Mekkaoui, M., Bennani, N., & Kamal, H. (2004). Antimicrobial activity of camel's milk against pathogenic strains of Escherichia coli and Listeria monocytogene. *International Journal of Dairy Technology*, *57*(1), 39–43. doi:10.1111/j.1471-0307.2004.00127.x

Boehm, G., & Stahl, B. (2003). Oligosaccharides. In Functional Dairy Products (pp. 203-243). Cambridge, UK: Woodhead Publishers.

Boehm, G., & Stahl, B. (2007). Oligosaccharides from Milk. *The Journal of Nutrition*, *137*, 847S–849S. PMID:17311985

Breitling, L. (2002). Insulin and anti diabetic activity of camel milk. *Journal of Camel Practice and Research*, *9*, 43–45.

Brückner, H., & Fujii, N. (2010). *D-Amino Acids in Chemistry, Life Sciences and Biotechnology*. Weinheim, Germany: Verlag Helvetica ChimicaActa, Zürich, Switzerland and Wiley-VCH.

Brueckner, H., & Hausch, M. (1990). D-amino acids in dairy products: Detection, origin and nutritional aspects. I. Milk, fermented milk, fresh cheese and acid crude cheese. *Milchwissenschaft. Milk Science International*, *45*, 357–360.

Businco, L., Bruno, G., Giampietro, P. G., & Cantoni, A. (1992). Allergenicity and nutritional adequacy of soy protein formulas. *The Journal of Pediatrics*, *121*(5), S21–S28. doi:10.1016/S0022-3476(05)81402-7 PMID:1447630

Cardak, A. D., Yetismeyen, A., & Bruckner, H. (2003). Quantitative comparison of free fatty acids in camel, goat and cow milk. *Milchwissenschaft. Milk Science International*, *58*, 127–130.

Claeys, W. L., Verraes, C., Cardoen, S., De Block, J., Huyghebaert, A., Raes, K., & Herman, L. et al. (2014). Consumption of raw or heated milk from different species: An evaluation of the nutritional and potential health benefits. *Food Control*, *42*, 188–201. doi:10.1016/j.foodcont.2014.01.045

D'Aniello, G., Grieco, N., Filippo, M. A., Capiello, F., Topo, E., D'Aniello, E., & Ronsini, S. (2007). Reproductive implicatin of D-aspartic acid in human pre-ovulatory follicular fluid. *Human Reproduction (Oxford, England)*, *22*(12), 3178–3183. doi:10.1093/humrep/dem328 PMID:17951582

Donkor, O. N., Henriksson, A., Singh, T. K., Vasiljevic, T., & Shah, N. P. (2007). ACE-inhibitory activity of probiotic yoghurt. *International Dairy Journal*, *17*(11), 1321–1331. doi:10.1016/j.idairyj.2007.02.009

El-Agamy, E. I. (2000). Effect of heat treatment on camel milk proteins with respectto antimicrobial factors: A comparison with cows' and buffalo milk proteins. *Food Chemistry*, *68*(2), 227–232. doi:10.1016/S0308-8146(99)00199-5

El-Agamy, E. I. (2007). The challenge of cow milk protein allergy. *Small Ruminant Research*, *68*(1-2), 64–72. doi:10.1016/j.smallrumres.2006.09.016

El-Agamy, E. I., Nawar, M., Shamsia, S. M., Awad, S., & Haenlein, G. F. W. (2009). Are camel milk proteins convenient to the nutrition of cow milk allergic children? *Small Ruminant Research*, *82*(1), 1–6. doi:10.1016/j.smallrumres.2008.12.016

El-Agamy, E. I., Ruppanner, R., Ismail, A., Champagne, C. P., & Assaf, R. (1992). Antibacterial and antiviral activity of camel milk protective proteins. *The Journal of Dairy Research*, *59*(02), 169–175. doi:10.1017/S0022029900030417 PMID:1319434

Euromonitor, I. (2010). *Cardiovascular health: A key area of functional food and drinks development.* London: Euromonitor International. Retrieved July 10, 2015, from http://www.euromonitor.com/cardiovascular-health-a-key-area-of-functional-food-and-drinks-development/report

FAO. (2008). *Camels and camel milk.* Retrieved June 5, 2015, from http://www.fao.org/docrep/003/x6528e/X6528E04.htm

FAOSTAT. (2013). *Camel milk.* Retrieved May 15, 2015 from http://faostat3.fao.org/home/E

Farah, Z. (1996). *Camel milk properties and products.* St. Gallen, Switzerland: SKAT, Swiss Centre for Developments Cooperation in Technology and Management.

Finke, B. (2000). *Isolierung und charakterisierung von oligosaccharide naushumanen und tierischen-milchen.* (Ph.D. thesis). University of Giessen, Shaker Verlag, Aachen, Germany.

Fox, P. F., & McSweeney, P. L. H. (1998). Lactose chapter. In *Dairy Chemistry and Biochemistry* (pp. 21–66). Thomson Science.

Fukuda, K., Yamamoto, A., Ganzorig, K., Khuukhenbaatar, J., Senda, A., Saito, T., & Urashima, T. (2010). Chemical characterization of the oligosaccharides in Bactrian camel (*Camelusbactrianus*) milk and colostrums. *Journal of Dairy Science*, *93*(12), 5572–5587. doi:10.3168/jds.2010-3151 PMID:21094729

Ghosh, D. (2009). Future perspectives of nutrigeonomics foods: Benefits vs risks. *Indian Journal of Biochemistry & Biophysics*, *46*, 31–36. PMID:19374251

Gill, C., & Rowland, I. (2003). Cancer. In Functional Dairy Products (pp. 19-53). Cambridge, UK: Woodhead Publishers.

Gnädig, S., Xue, Y., Berdeaux, O., Chardigny, J. M., & Sebedio, J. L. (2003). Conjugated linoleic acid (CLA) as a functional ingredient. In Functional Dairy Products (pp. 263-298). CRC Press.

Gobbetti, M., Minervini, F., & Rizzello, C. G. (2004). Angiotensin I-converting enzyme-inhibitory and antimicrobial bioactive peptides. *International Journal of Dairy Society*, *57*(2-3), 173–188. doi:10.1111/j.1471-0307.2004.00139.x

Harrison, R. (2006). Milk xanthine oxidase: Properties and physiological roles. *International Dairy Journal*, *16*(6), 546–554. doi:10.1016/j.idairyj.2005.08.016

Hilliam, M. (2003). Future for dairy products ingredients in the functional foods market. *Australian Journal of Dairy Technology*, *58*, 98–103.

IFIC. (2011). *Functional foods*. International Food Information Council Foundation. Retrieved July 12, 2015, from http://www.foodinsight.org

IFIC. (2013). *Functional Foods, consumer survey*. International Food Information Council Foundation. Retrieved July 17, 2015 from http://www.foodinsight.org

IFIC. (2015). *Food & health survey*. International Food Information Council Foundation. Retrieved July 20, 2015 from http://www.foodinsight.org

ILSI. (1999). Scientific concepts of functional foods in Europe: Consensus document. *The British Journal of Nutrition*, *81*(04), s1–s27. doi:10.1017/S0007114599000471 PMID:10999022

Jang, A., & Lee, M. (2005). Purification and identification of angiotensin converting enzyme inhibitory peptides from beef hydrolysates. *Meat Science*, *69*(4), 653–661. doi:10.1016/j.meatsci.2004.10.014 PMID:22063143

Jrad, Z., Girardet, J.-M., Adt, I., Oulahal, N., Degraeve, P., Khorchani, T., & El Hatmi, H. (2014). Antioxidant activity of camel milk casein. *Mljekarstvo*, *64*, 287–294. doi:10.15567/mljekarstvo.2014.0408

Jumah, R. Y., Shaker, R. R., & Abu-Jadayil, B. (2001). Effect of milk source on therheological properties of yoghurt during the gelation process. *International Journal of Dairy Technology*, *54*(3), 89–93. doi:10.1046/j.1364-727x.2001.00012.x

Kappeler, S. (1998). *Compositional and structural analysis of camel milk proteins with emphasis on protective proteins*. (Ph.D. Thesis). Swiss Federal Institute of Technology, Zürich, Switzerland.

Kappeler, S., Farah, Z., & Puhan, Z. (1999). Alternative splitting of lactophorin mRNA from lactating mammary gland of the camel (*Camelus dromedarius*). *Journal of Dairy Science*, *82*(10), 2084–2093. doi:10.3168/jds.S0022-0302(99)75450-0 PMID:10531593

Kappeler, S., Farah, Z., & Puhan, Z. (2003). 5'-Flanking regions of camel milk genesare highly similar to homologue regions of other species and can be divided into two distinct groups. *Journal of Dairy Science*, *86*(2), 498–508. doi:10.3168/jds.S0022-0302(03)73628-5 PMID:12647956

Khan, A. A., Alzohiary, M. A., & Mohieldein, A. H. (2012). Antidiabetic effects of camel milk in streptozotocin (STZ)-induced diabetic rats. *American Journal of Biochemistry and Molecular Biology*. DOI:10.3923/ajbmb.2012

Khaskheli, M., Arain, M. A., Chaudhry, S., Soomro, A. H., & Qureshi, T. A. (2005). Physico-chemical quality of camel milk. *Journal of Agriculture and Social Sciences*, *2*, 164–166.

Kirjanvainen, P. V. (2003). Probiotic and the management of food allergy. In Functional Dairy Products (pp. 108-131). Cambridge, UK: Woodhead Publishers.

Kitts, D., & Weiler, K. (2003). Bioactive proteins and peptides from food sources. Applications of bioprocesses used in isolation and recovery. *Current Pharmaceutical Design*, *9*(16), 1309–1323. doi:10.2174/1381612033454883 PMID:12769739

Konuspayeva, G., Faye, B., & Loiseau, G. (2009). The composition of camel milk: A meta-analysis of the literature data. *Journal of Food Composition and Analysis*, *22*(2), 95–101. doi:10.1016/j.jfca.2008.09.008

Korashy, H. M., Maayah, Z. H., Abd-Allah, A. R., El-Kadi, A. O. S., & Alhaider, A. A. (2012). Camel Milk Triggers Apoptotic Signaling Pathways in Human Hepatoma HepG2 and Breast CancerMCF7 Cell Lines through Transcriptional Mechanism. *Journal of Biomedicine & Biotechnology*, 1–9. doi:10.1155/2012/593195

Korhonen, H., & Pihlanto, A. (2003). Food-derived bioactive peptides - opportunities for designing future foods. *Current Pharmaceutical Design*, *9*(16), 1297–1308. doi:10.2174/1381612033454892 PMID:12769738

Kulig, M., Bergmann, R., Klettke, U., Wahn, V., Tacke, U., & Wahn, U. (1999). Natural course of sensitization to food and inhalant allergens during the first 6 years of life. *The Journal of Allergy and Clinical Immunology*, *103*(6), 1173–1179. doi:10.1016/S0091-6749(99)70195-8 PMID:10359902

Kunz, C., & Rudloff, S. (2006). Health promoting aspects of milk oligosaccharides. *International Dairy Journal*, *16*(11), 1341–1346. doi:10.1016/j.idairyj.2006.06.020

Kuwabara, Y., Nagai, S., Yoshimitsu, N., Nakagawa, I., Watanabe, Y., & Tamai, Y. (1995). Antihypertensive effect of the milk fermented by culturing with various lactic acid bacteria and yeast. *Journal of Fermentation and Bioengineering*, *80*(3), 294–295. doi:10.1016/0922-338X(95)90834-M

Léonil, J., Gagnaire, V., Mollé, D., Pezennec, S., & Bouhallab, S. (2000). Application of chromatography and mass spectrometry to the characterization of food proteins and derived peptides. *Journal of Chromatography. A*, *881*(1-2), 1–21. doi:10.1016/S0021-9673(00)00071-6 PMID:10905689

Li, G. H., Le, G. W., Shi, Y. H., & Shrestha, S. (2004). Angiotensin I-converting enzyme inhibitory peptides derived from food proteins and their physiological and pharmacological effects. *Nutrition Research (New York, N.Y.)*, *24*(7), 469–486. doi:10.1016/S0271-5317(04)00058-2

Lock, A. L., Destaillats, F., Kraft, J., & German, J. B. (2008). Introduction to the proceedings of the symposium 'Scientific update on dairy fats and cardiovascular disease'. *Journal of the American College of Nutrition*, *27*(6), 720S–722S. doi:10.1080/07315724.2008.10719749 PMID:19155431

López-Fandiño, R., Otte, J., & Van Camp, J. (2006). Review: Physiological, chemicaland technological aspects of milk-protein-derived peptides with antihypertensiveand ACE-inhibitory activity. *International Dairy Journal*, *16*(11), 1277–1293. doi:10.1016/j.idairyj.2006.06.004

Maldonado, J., Gil, A., Narbona, E., & Molina, J. A. (1998). Special formulas in infant nutrition: A review. *Early Human Development*, *53*, S23–S32. doi:10.1016/S0378-3782(98)00062-0 PMID:10102652

Martin, M. J., Martin-Sosa, S., Garcia-Pardo, L. A., & Hueso, P. (2001). Distribution of bovine sialoglycoconjugates during lactation. *Journal of Dairy Science*, *84*(5), 995–1000. doi:10.3168/jds.S0022-0302(01)74558-4 PMID:11384055

Mehra, R., & Kelly, P. (2006). Milk oligosaccharides: Structural and technological aspects[Review]. *International Dairy Journal*, *16*(11), 1334–1340. doi:10.1016/j.idairyj.2006.06.008

Meisel, H. (2004). Multifunctional peptides encrypted in milk proteins. *BioFactors (Oxford, England)*, *21*(1-4), 55–61. doi:10.1002/biof.552210111 PMID:15630170

Meisel, H., & Bockelmann, W. (1999). Bioactive peptides encrypted in milk proteins: Proteolytic activation and thropho-functional properties. *Antonie van Leeuwenhoek*, *76*(1/4), 207–215. doi:10.1023/A:1002063805780 PMID:10532380

Meisel, H., Walsh, D. J., Murray, B., & FitzGerald, R. J. (2006). ACE inhibitory peptides. In Y. Mine & F. Shahidi (Eds.), *Nutraceutical Proteins and Peptides in Health and Disease* (Vol. 4, pp. 269–315). Taylor & Francis Group Publisher.

Moslehishad, M., Ehsani, M. R., Salami, M., Mirdamadi, S., Ezzatpanah, H., Niasari, A. N., & Moosavi-Movahedi, A. A. (2013). The comparative assessment of ACE-inhibitory and antioxidant activities of peptide fractions obtained from fermented camel and bovine milk by *Lactobacillus rhamnosus* PTCC 1637. *International Dairy Journal*, *29*(2), 82–87. doi:10.1016/j.idairyj.2012.10.015

Moure, A., Domínguez, H., & Parajó, J. C. (2006). Antioxidant properties of ultrafiltration-recovered soy protein fractions from industrial effluents and their hydrolysates. *Process Biochemistry*, *41*(2), 447–456. doi:10.1016/j.procbio.2005.07.014

Ochoa, T. J., & Cleary, T. G. (2009). Effect of lactoferrin on enteric pathogens. *Biochimie*, *91*(1), 30–34. doi:10.1016/j.biochi.2008.04.006 PMID:18472012

Otte, J., Shalaby, S. M. A., Zakora, M., & Neilsen, M. S. (2007). Fractionation and identification of ACE-inhibitory peptides from α-lactalbumin and β-casein produced by thermolysin-catalysed hydrolysis. *International Dairy Journal*, *17*(12), 1460–1472. doi:10.1016/j.idairyj.2007.04.008

Pan, D., Luo, Y., & Tanokura, M. (2005). Antihypertensive peptides from skimmed milk hydrolysate digested by cell-free extract of Lactobacillus helveticus JCM1004. *Food Chemistry*, *91*(1), 123–129. doi:10.1016/j.foodchem.2004.05.055

Park, Y. W. (2009). Overview of bioactive components in milk and dairy products. In Y. W. Park (Ed.), *Bioactive Componentsin Milk and Dairy Products* (pp. 3–13). Blackwell Publishing. doi:10.1002/9780813821504.ch1

Parodi, P. W. (2009). Has the association between saturated fatty acids, serum cholesterol and coronary heart disease been over emphasized? *International Dairy Journal*, *19*(6-7), 345–361. doi:10.1016/j.idairyj.2009.01.001

Pellegrini, A., Dettling, C., Thomas, U., & Hunziker, P. (2001). Isolation and characterization of four bactericidal domains in the bovine β-lactoglobulin. *Biochemicaet Biophysica Acta*, *1526*(2), 131–140. doi:10.1016/S0304-4165(01)00116-7 PMID:11325534

Quan, S., Tsuda, H., & Miyamoto, T. (2008). Angiotensin I-converting enzyme inhibitory peptides in skim milk fermented with Lactobacillus helveticus 130B4 from camel milk in Inner Mongolia, China. *Journal of the Science of Food and Agriculture*, *88*(15), 2688–2692. doi:10.1002/jsfa.3394

Quita, S. M., & Kurdi, A. F. L. (2010). Antigenotoxic and anticytotoxic effect of camel milk in mice treated with cisplatin. *Saudi Journal of Biological Sciences*, *17*(2), 159–166. doi:10.1016/j.sjbs.2010.02.010 PMID:23961073

Sah, B. N. P., Vasiljevic, T., McKechnie, S., & Donkor, O. N. (2014). Effect of probiotics on antioxidant and antimutagenic activities of crude peptide extract from yogurt. *Food Chemistry*, *156*, 264–270. doi:10.1016/j.foodchem.2014.01.105 PMID:24629967

Salami, M., Moosavi-Movahedi, A. A., Ehsani, M. R., Yousefi, R., Haertlé, T., Chobert, J. M., & Niasari-Naslaji, A. et al. (2010). Improvement of the antimicrobial and antioxidant activities of camel and bovine whey proteins by limited proteolysis. *Journal of Agricultural and Food Chemistry*, *58*(6), 3297–3302. doi:10.1021/jf9033283 PMID:20175528

Salami, M., Moosavi-Movahedi, A. A., Moosavi-Movahedi, F., Ehsani, M. R., Yousefi, R., Farhadi, M., & Haertlé, T. et al. (2011). Biological activity of camel milk casein following enzymatic digestion. *The Journal of Dairy Research*, *78*(04), 471–478. doi:10.1017/S0022029911000628 PMID:21910944

Sarmadi, B. H., & Ismail, A. (2010). Antioxidative peptides from food proteins: A review. *Peptides*, *31*(10), 1949–1956. doi:10.1016/j.peptides.2010.06.020 PMID:20600423

Sboui, A., Khorchani, T., Djegham, M., Agrebi, A., Elhatmi, H., & Belhadj, O. (2010). Anti-diabetic effect of camel milk in alloxan-induced diabetic dogs: A dose–response experiment. *Journal of Animal Physiology and Animal Nutrition*, *94*(4), 540–546. doi:10.1111/j.1439-0396.2009.00941.x PMID:19906135

Shabo, Y., Barzel, R., Margoulis, M., & Yagil, R. (2005). Camel milk for food allergies in children. *Immunology and Allergies*, *7*, 796–798. PMID:16382703

Shalash, M. R. (1984). The production and utilization of camel milk. In W. R. Cockrill (Ed.), *The Camelid: An all-purpose animal* (pp. 196–208). Uppsala, Sweden: Scandinavian Institute of African Studies.

Shamsia, S. M. (2009). Nutritional and therapeutic properties of camel andhuman milks. *International Journal of Genetics and Molecular Biology*, *1*, 52-58.

Shori, A. B. (2013). Antioxidant activity and viability of lactic acid bacteria in soybean-yogurt made from cow and camel milk. *Journal of Taibahuniversity for Science*, *7*, 202-208.

Singh, M. B., Fotedar, R., & Lakshminarayana, J. (2008). Camel milk consumption pattern and its association with diabetes among Raika community of Jodhpur district of Rajasthan. *Ethno-Med*, *2*, 104–105.

Skeggs, L. T., Kahn, J. E., & Shumway, N. P. (1956). The preparation and function of the angiotensin-converting enzyme. *The Journal of Experimental Medicine*, *103*(3), 295–299. doi:10.1084/jem.103.3.295 PMID:13295487

Stenberg, M., Marko-Varga, G., & Oste, R. (2002). Enantio separation of D- and L-amino acids by a coupled system consisting of an ion-exchange column and a chiral column and determination of D-aspartic acid and d-glutamic acid in soy products. *Food Chemistry*, *79*(4), 507–512. doi:10.1016/S0308-8146(02)00215-7

Taylor, S. L. (1986). Immunological and allergic properties of cows' milk proteins in humans. *Journal of Food Protection*, *49*, 239–250.

Topo, E., Soricelli, A., D'Aniello, A., Ronsini, S., & D'Aniello, G. (2009). The role and molecular mechanism of D-aspartic acid in the release and synthesis of LH and testosterone in humans and rats. *Reproductive Biology and Endocrinology*, *7*(1), 120–131. doi:10.1186/1477-7827-7-120 PMID:19860889

Urashima, T., Kitaoka, M., Asakuma, S., & Messer, M. (2009). Milk oligosaccharides. In Advanced Dairy Chemistry. Lactose, Water, Salts and Minor Constituents (pp. 295-349). New York, NY: Springer Science Business Media.

Urashima, T., Murata, S., & Nakamura, T. (1997). Structural determination of monosialyltrisaccharides obtained from caprine colostrum. *Comparative Biochemistry and Physiology*, *116B*(4), 431–435. doi:10.1016/S0305-0491(96)00269-6 PMID:9149396

Virtanen, T., Pihlanto, A., Akkanen, S., & Korhonen, H. (2007). Development of antioxidant activity in milk whey during fermentation with lactic acid bacteria. *Journal of Applied Microbiology*, *102*(1), 106–115. doi:10.1111/j.1365-2672.2006.03072.x PMID:17184325

Walstra, P., Wouters, J. T. M., & Geurts, T. J. (2008). Milk for liquid consumption. In Dairy Science and Technology (pp. 421-444). CRC, Taylor & Francis.

WHO. (2012). *Estimated incidence, mortality and prevalence worldwide in 2012*. Retrieved May 23, 2015, from http://globocan.iarc.fr/Pages/fact_sheets_cancer.aspx

Yagil, R. (1987). Camel milk - A review. *Farm Animals*, *2*, 81–99.

Chapter 8
Pomegranate Peel and Fruit Extracts:
A Novel Approach to Avert Degenerative Disorders - Pomegranate and Degenerative Diseases

Tariq Ismail
Bahauddin Zakariya University, Pakistan

Saeed Akhtar
Bahauddin Zakariya University, Pakistan

Muhammad Riaz
Bahauddin Zakariya University, Pakistan

ABSTRACT

Pomegranate (Punica granatum L.), the fruit and its peel have been shown to hold tremendous potential for the treatment of various ailments. Incorporation of pomegranate, peel and their extracts, as key functional ingredients in various ethnopharmacological formulations are widely accepted in almost all cultures of the World. In addition to their disease ameliorating features, pomegranate and the peel extracts have gained significant popularity in functional food market as ingredient of choice in foods designed to prevent onset of various non-communicable diseases. Health promoting features of the pomegranate peel and fruit extracts define the scope of this natural reserve in global nutraceutical and functional food industry. On account of their unique phytochemicals profile, plentiful pool of antioxidants, dietary fibers, minerals and natural colors, both the valuable reserves have been remained as highly explored plant material in last two decades. Building levels of interest in this fruit has created a deeper insight among researchers to understand actual potential and pathways of pomegranate biomolecules reactivity in human models. The chapter in hand meticulously deals with pomegranate and its extracts as source of innovative healthy components responsible for averting cardiovascular diseases, inflammatory and non-inflammatory disorders, type 2 diabetes, gastric ulcers, various types of cancers and neurodegenerative disorders.

DOI: 10.4018/978-1-5225-0591-4.ch008

INTRODUCTION

Pomegranate (*Punica granatum* L.) from the plant family *Punicaceae* is a wonderful source of natural biomolecules implicated as ethnic or folk medicine for the treatment of various health ailments since centuries. Some very earlier studies on pharmacological properties of pomegranate, the bark, fruit and its various anatomical parts endeavor the entire plant and the fruiting body as convincing tools to treat microbiological infections, inflammatory and non-inflammatory diseases and several other degenerative disorders (Milin & Stanimirovic, 1950; Polunin & Stainton, 1985; Morton, 1987; Novarro et al., 1996). The fruit and the inedible fractions (peel and seeds) of pomegranate are biochemically composed of more than 124 different phytochemicals comprised of phenolics, flavonoids, anthocyanins, and a broad range of essential minerals and vitamins. Extensive review of literature in this highly explored domain correlate extraordinary phytochemical and microelemental profile of pomegranate all fractions to their strong antioxidant, anti-mutagenic, apoptotic and antimicrobial properties (Lansky et al. 2005; Li et al., 2006; Heber, 2011). Therapeutic properties of pomegranate are of broad prospects and are proposed to mitigate cardiovascular diseases (Shema-Didi et al., 2014), prostate cancer (Malik et al., 2005), colon cancer (Kasimsetty et al., 2010), breast cancer (Kim et al., 2002), skin melanoma (Pacheco-Palencia et al., 2008), neurodegenerative disorders (Subash et al., 2014), arthritis (Shukla et al., 2008), infertility (Atilgan et al., 2014), Oral and dental diseases (DiSilvestro et al., 2009), gastric damages (Moghaddam et al., 2013) and microbiological pathogenesis (Tanveer et al. 2015). The consumption patterns of the fruit and its various accessions vary in different cultures. The fruit or berry is conventionally manually peeled off to separate the juicy arils which are consumed with seeds or crushed to extract pleasant flavored juice rich in high molecular weight phytochemicals i.e. ellagiatannins, flavonoids. Phytochemical composition that defines characteristic role of pomegranate as pharmacological preparation varies with the fruit fraction, cultivar, harvesting time, geographical and climatic condition of the fruit cultivation region (Fischer et al. 2011; Kumari et al., 2012; Zhao et al., 2013). Refer to the to-date explored phytochemistry of the pomegranate fruit and its peel fraction (Figures 1 and 2), a unique class of phenolics i.e. ellagitannins comprising of punicalagin, punicalin, pedunculagin, corilagin, ellagic acid, gallagic acid, tellimagrandin I, casuarinin, granatin A and granatin B. Among some other promising biomolecules, the fruit and its various fractions have also been reported to hold potential levels of caffeic acid, catechin, gallocatechin, luteolin, kaempferol, delphinidin, cyanidin, pelarogonidin, *p*-coumaric acid and gallic acid (Akhtar et al. 2015). Mechanistic role of pomegranate biomolecules and the reactive substances responsible for site-specific inhibitory reactions are still not evidently defined. Interpretations of research made on fate of pomegranate macro biomolecules i.e. ellagitannins in human body and their conversion to recoverable bioactive fractions reveal urolithins (A, B, C & D) as the major stakeholders in mediating various ailments (Gonzalez-Sarrias et al. 2010; Kasimsetty et al. 2010). Gross comparison of free radicals scavenging properties further enlighten urolithins as potential antioxidants than the parent compounds i.e. punicalagin and ellagic acid (Bialonska et al. 2009).

To its audience, this chapter comprehensively defines pomegranate - a traditional medicine of various cultures as tremendously explored potential therapeutic agent of the modern age. Highlighting evidence based ethnic uses of the fruit and its various fractions, the readers are provided with up to date information on pomegranate application trends in therapeutics specifically in mitigating degenerative disorders.

Figure 1. Principle phenolics of pomegranate peel and fruit extracts

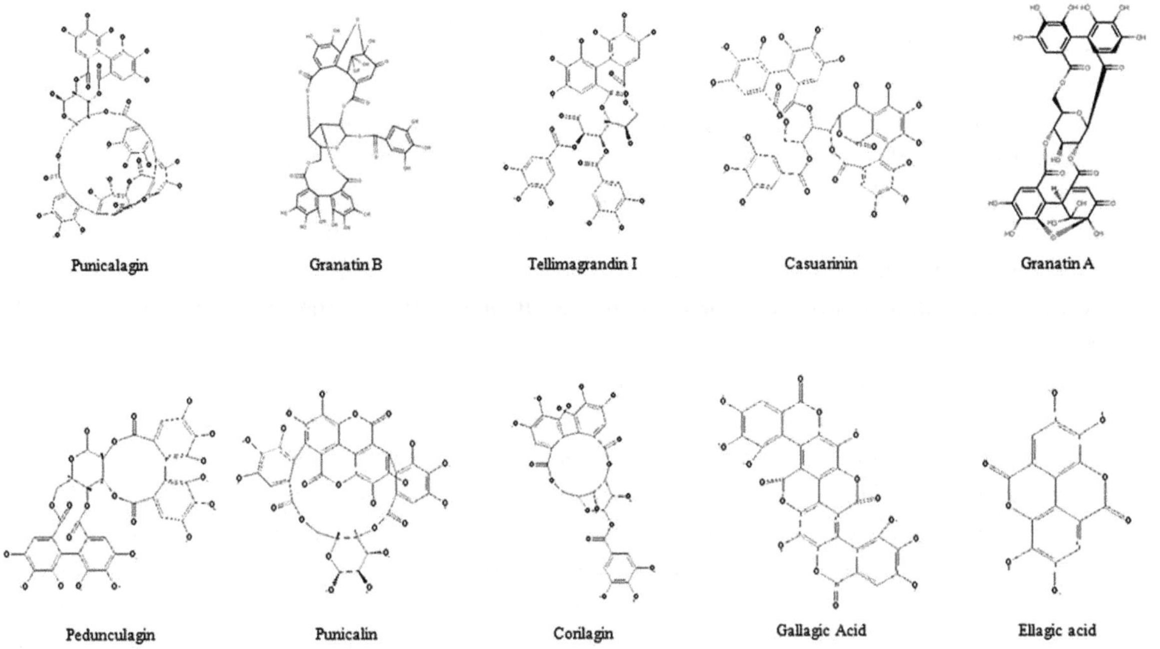

Source: Akhtar et al., 2015

Figure 2. Principle phenolics of pomegranate peel and fruit extracts

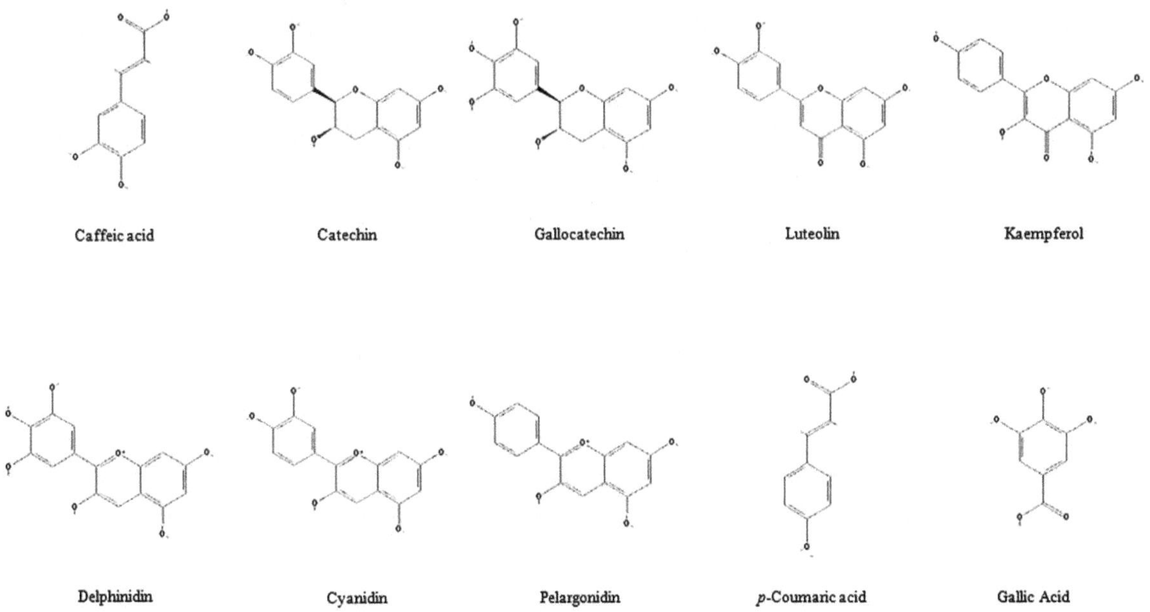

Source: Akhtar et al., 2015

BACKGROUND

Pomegranate: Ethnic Uses and Research Evidences

Pomegranate, the fruit and its various fractions bear some biologically active compounds that offer antidiarrheal properties. Phytochemical screening of extracts showing positive effect in diarrhea management reveals presence of a range of tannins, alkaloids and flavonoids. As witnessed from ethnic uses, antidiarrheal properties of pomegranate juice extracts have been evaluated *in vivo* in rats with castor oil induced diarrhea. The study consolidated protection of laboratory animal from diarrhea and reduced gastro intestinal transit time in dose dependent manner (Souli et al. 2015). Pomegranate peel water extracts offered at 100 – 400mg/kg b.w. have also been reported with reduction in acetylcholine concentration and ileum movement of rats having castor oil induced diarrhea (Qnais et al. 2007).

As has been reported by Lansky et al. (2004), aqueous decoctions of pomegranate rind, peel or hull have various ethnic uses in treatment of diarrhea, dysentery and stomatitis. Whereas, the extracts being treated as therapeutic rinsing agent have also been in application as mouthwash as well as douche and enema agent. Potent antibacterial features of pomegranate peel extracts make it very responsive remedy against gastro-intestinal infections associated with diarrhea, typhoid fever and foodborne illnesses (Pradeep et al. 2008). Widely practiced in ethnopharmacology, pomegranate peel and its various extracts are also in use as anthelmintic and anti-coccidiosis agent. In line with confirmation of pomegranate ethnic use as anti-coccidiosis agent, an *in vivo* study engaging a group of mice infected with 10^3 oocytes of *Eimeria papilla* was carried out by Dkhil (2013). The study endorsed pomegranate extracts as potent anti-coccidiosis and anthelmintic agent inhibiting 50% population of the infected agent after being treated with pomegranate extract @ 300mg/kg b.w.

Menopause associated with reduction or cessation of oestrogen and progesterone secretion is often characterized by low bone mass, bone tissue damages and bone fragility (Raisz 2005). Pomegranate bears estrogenic activity and hence is in application as folk medicine for preventing postmenopausal osteoporosis (Jurenka 2008). Traditional concept of pomegranate and its various extracts utilization as complementary and alternate medicine are believed to be the strong basis for the developments in modern medicine. Developmental exploration of pomegranate as pool of biomolecules bearing immense health significance could therefore be referred as a process of integrating traditional knowledge for the sake of stronger and efficacious therapeutic solutions.

POMEGRANATE: ANTI-DEGENERATIVE DISORDERS PROSPECTS

This section of the chapter comprehensively deals with the prospective use of pomegranate peel and fruit extracts as potential ethnopharmacological approach of the modern era to avert various degenerative disorders. A critical appraisal encompassing most recent updates on the subject has been made for the readers on following subsections:

1. Pomegranate: Wound Healing Properties,
2. Pomegranate: Anti-Inflammatory Properties,
3. Protective Role in Inflammatory and Non-Inflammatory Lungs Disorders,
4. Pomegranate and Gastric Health,

5. Pomegranate: Hypertension Mediating Features,
6. Pomegranate and Cardiovascular Diseases,
7. Pomegranate and Type 2 Diabetes,
8. Pomegranate: Preventive and Curative Approach in Various Types of Cancers,
9. Pomegranate and Neurodegenerative Disorders.

Pomegranate: Wound Healing Properties

Wound healing comprised of inflammatory, proliferative and remodeling phases is integration of biological and molecular process that involves a collaborative role of different kind of cells and tissues in cellular proliferation and extracellular matrix remodeling (Kirsner & Eaglstein, 1993; Falanga, 2005). As witnessed from several plant and animal based pharmacological models, plant based drugs formulation or Ayurvedics have been found very effective replacement of pharmacological drugs in external wound healing (Biswas & Mukherjee, 2003). A lot of research was placed in to find out wound healing potential of pomegranate, its various fraction and extracts based ointments after potential findings of Klein (2010) were being published as US patent. The findings proposed remarkable recovery of diabetic patients with chronic foot sores and lesions after being treated with pomegranate flower extracts, seed oil and rind powder based ointment for a period of 30 – 60 days. Microscopic and histological examination reveals pomegranate peel and peel extracts based gel formulations to increase hydroxyproline contents, collagen regeneration, increase fibroblast infiltration and epithelialization of the incised treated wounds (Murthy et al. 2004). Topical application of ointments carrying 5% pomegranate peel methanolic extracts on incised wounds in laboratory animals significantly improve healing score as compared to the negative control (Chidambara Murthy et al., 2004; Hayouni et al., 2011). Skin repairing properties add up cosmetical features to pomegranate and its various fractions. Pomegranate peel aqueous extracts perform skin repairing property in a polar manner and promote skin regeneration (Aslam et al. 2006). Quite similar to the standard drugs in skin epithelialization and regeneration, pomegranate and the peel extracts endeavor as potential ingredients in treating infected and relatively difficult to heal wounds.

Pomegranate: Anti-Inflammatory Properties

Inflammatory disorders are supposed to be the outcome of inflammatory cells hyperactivity, excessive levels of pro-inflammatory mediators and transcription factors including i.e. TNF-α, NF-kB, IL-1, IL-6, and IL-8 and hyper production of reactive oxygen as well as nitrogen species alike hydroxyl radicals, hydrogen peroxide, nitric oxide, singlet oxygen and peroxyl radicals (Conner et al. 1996; Babior, 2000; Nathan, 2006).

Ellagitannins, ellagic acid and metabolic product of the hydrolysable tannins are the major stakeholders among pomegranate phytochemicals pools bearing anti-inflammatory properties. Hydrolysable tannins rich pomegranate extracts exhibit significant potential in suppressing joint inflammation and is referred as a potent non-pharmacological therapy to avert arthritis associated health damages. Mechanistic role of pomegranate fruit or peel extracts in reducing joint inflammation is reduction in infiltration of joints by inflammatory cells and consequent alleviation of bone and cartilage destruction (Shukla et al. 2008). Reports on occurrence of acute colon inflammation cases are at hike whereas; microbiological infections, stress and simpler peptides associated allergic response are reportedly a few of the major inducible inflammatory factors (Rubio & Befrits, 2008).

Pomegranate has also been experienced in management of inflammatory bowl disease and the fruit extracts (250mg/kg/day) enriched with ellagic acid (10mg/kg/day) were found as a healthful remediation in managing cronh's disease induced in chronic rat models. The study consolidated reduction in overexpression of inducible nitric oxide synthase (iNOS) and cyclooxygenase-2 (COX-2) and prevented translocation of NF-kB (Rosillo et al. 2012). In an earlier study, Larrosa et al. (2010) identified Urolithins A as the vital compound to offer colon anti-inflammatory properties by maintaining their integrity in colon mucosa unlike pomegranate extracts. As discussed earlier, the extracts and urolihins inhibited oxidative stress in colon mucosa and suppressed expression of inflammatory markers including those of iNOS, COX-2, prostaglandin E2 (PGE-2) and prostaglandin E synthase.

Unlike anti-inflammatory pharmacological drugs, pomegranate phytochemicals e.g. ellagic acid have prolonged onset of anti-inflammatory response and duration of inhibitory action. Granatin B among some tested hydrolysable tannins has also been suggested as standard marker in identifying anti-inflammatory properties of pomegranate. The compound was reported to inhibit carrageenan induced mice paw edema by strongly inhibiting expression of iNOS, COX-2 and PGE-2 (Lee et al. 2010).

Protective Role in Inflammatory and Non-Inflammatory Lung Disorders

Certain epidemiological findings argue a correlation between respiratory disease and consumption of fruits. Anthocyanins and proanthocyanins are fruit derived phenolics that attenuate respiratory inflammation and other non-specific inflammations (Nyanhanda et al. 2014). Despite of unknown pharmacological targets and limited knowledge on mechanism of their action, pomegranate based phytochemical formulations have still a wide acceptability in management of critical malignancies like lungs inflammation. Acute lung injuries characterized by alveolar inflammation and accumulation of neutrophils in lungs has not find specific drug therapy yet. Pomegranate peel extracts attenuates lungs inflammation by inhibiting production of myeloperoxidase. One of pomegranate fractionated compound alike ellagic acid reduces recruitment of neutrophils in lung area and inhibits changes in vascular permeability (Cornelio Favarin et al. 2013). Bachoual et al. (2011) in his experiment on intratracheal endotoxin induced inflammation in mice and stated pomegranate peel aqueous extracts to reduce bronchoalveolar lavage fluid protein concentration, cellularity and neutrophil concentration. A similar kind of research also comment pomegranate extracts as alternate or supplementary therapeutic approach to manage pulmonary inflammation. The study evidently support poly lactic-co-glycolic acid microparticles encapsulated with pomegranate extracts to reduce leukocytes specifically eosinophils, as well as lungs protein and cytokines levels (de Oliveira et al. 2013). In addition to anti-inflammatory properties, hydroalcoholic seed extracts of pomegranate also exhibit ability to inhibit bleomycin induced lungs fibrosis (Hemmati et al. 2013) thus proclaiming the fruit extracts to inhibit pathological changes responsible for incompetent breathing.

Pomegranate and Gastric Health

Commercial standard drug formulations to cure gastric ulcers have generated un-predicted side effects in patients under treatments. Gastric ulcers being the painful condition have become a challenging health problem to be addressed as a priority. Development of natural plant based formulations have achieved significant popularity index as far as their antioxidant and anti-ulcer properties are concerned. Anti-ulcer index of pomegranate and extracts of its different fraction varies with phenolics and flavonoids concentration and type of cultivar (Gautam & Sharma, 2012: Moghaddam et al. 2014). Pomegranate peel extracts (500mg/kg B.W) on account of their potent free radicals scavenging properties have been witnessed to inhibit ~74% ethanol induced gastric ulceration. The study correlated reduction in degree of ulceration with increasing antioxidant pool of glutathione peroxidase, glutathione, superoxide dismutase and catalase (Ajaikumar et al. 2005). Generation of extra secretions from the adherent mucus of stomach walls has also been proposed as ulcer protective feature of tannin rich pomegranate extracts. Feeding gastric ulcer induced rat models with 50, 100 and 500mg/kg b.w. pomegranate tannins reduce alcohol induced malondialdehyde and nitric oxide levels and progressively (dose dependent manner) improves mucus secretions without impacting total acidity, acid output and gastric juice volume thus suggesting extra mucus secretions as ulcer protective features of fruit tannins (Lai et al. 2009).

Pomegranate: Hypertension Mediating Features

Seventh report by committee on prevention, detection, evaluation and treatment of high blood pressure; insights hypertension as most common disease among primary care patients (JNC-7 Guidelines, 2004). Hypertension being a risk factor in development of cardiovascular diseases and strokes were detected among more than 45 million people in USA (Ong et al. 2007). Life style modifications are better approach to prevent hypertension instead of exerting on pharmacological interventions to cure the disorder. Pomegranate, the fruit and highly valued extracts of inedible peel fraction on account of their potent antioxidant profile, are reportedly administrated for avoiding development of atherosclerotic lesions and delay in onset of aging and associated health disorders (Stow 2011). Pomegranate phytochemicals probably combat oxidative stress in patients diagnosed with hypertension. Administrating pomegranate juice extracts (100mg/kg B.W) for 4 weeks to wistar rats with angiotensin II induced hypertension diabetic rats reduced arterial blood pressure and other biochemical changes associated with diabetes. Moreover, histo-pathological examination of the treated diabetic rats identified preventive role of the juice extracts in averting tubular degenerative changes (Mohan et al. 2010). A 2 week study conducted in hypertensive patients (*n*-21) depicted consumption of 150ml of pomegranate juice between lunch and dinner significantly reduced systolic and diastolic blood pressure however; the treated individuals were not reported with any change in flow mediated dilation (Asgary et al. 2014). This endeavors that pomegranate may serve as an adjunct therapy instead of other pharmacological and non-pharmacological interventions for management of hypertension and to avoid consequent risks of cardiac stroke.

Pomegranate and Cardiovascular Diseases

Prolong consumption of pomegranate juice and administration of pomegranate extracts improves cardiac health. Available literature consolidates beneficial effects of pomegranate consumption on attenuating aging and stress mediated arterial hardening and reverting progression of atherosclerosis. Cardiovascular failure is amongst a few major causes of mortality in patients under renal replacement therapies (Kundhal & Lok, 2005). On account of various research reports, pomegranate juice has anti-atherogenic properties due to its ability to lower down production of angiotensin converting enzymes (ACE) that ultimately result in reduction of systolic blood pressure. Regular consumption of 100ml pomegranate juice for a period of one year has been reported to reduce systolic blood pressure and alter lipid profile (reduction in LDL levels) of haemodylasis patients thus favorably reducing risks of atherosclerosis and cardiac failure (Shema-Didi et al. 2014). Another *in vivo* study proclaiming antioxidant features of pomegranate juice to reduce ACE (~36%) and systolic blood pressure (~5%) on regular consumption of the fruit juice i.e. 50ml; and otherwise 1.5mmol of total phenols (Aviram & Dornfeld, 2001). Soluble fractions of pomegranate polyphenols including hydrolysable tannins and anthocyanins have been supposed to be linked with anti-atherosclerotic characteristics. A double blind study engaging patients with myocardial ischemia and coronary heart disease were conducted to review effect of consuming 240ml pomegranate juice daily for 3months, the report witness a significant reduction in stress induced ischemia in patients feed with pomegranate juices (Sumner et al. 2005).

Inverse relationship exists between consumption of plant polyphenols and cardiovascular disease. Pomegranate polyphenols either consumed in the form of fruit juice or decoctions of the inedible fractions somehow reduce oxidation of low density lipoprotein and subsequent inhibition of onward foam cell generation and atherosclerosis development. Treating patients diagnosed with increased intima – media thickness of the artery with pomegranate fruit, seed, and peel extracts, individually or in combination may reduce intima-media thickness in addition to reduction in size of atherosclerotic lesions. A randomized, double blind study on 146 human subject diagnosed with more than 1 major coronary heart disease risk factor, depicted pomegranate juice consumption might have slowed down progression of carotid intima-media thickness more specifically in subjects with higher rate of oxidative stress (Davidson et al. 2009; Aviram & Dornfeld, 2010). Accumulation of polyphenols inside the macrophages replacing lipid peroxides and interaction with LDL to scavenge reactive oxygen species are considered as possible mechanism of reducing atherosclerosis (Aviram et al. 2002). Arterial blockage may be a product of LDL oxidation and pomegranate juice, in dose dependent concentration has been reported to inhibit LDL oxidation by 43% whereas intake of fruit juice reduced macrophage uptake of oxidized LDL by 88% (Fuhrman & Aviram, 2005).

Pomegranate and Type 2 Diabetes

Traditionally pomegranate and its accessions like flowers are referred as traditional anti-diabetic therapy (Xu et al. 2009). Over the last decade, plentiful research on pomegranate established a link between the fruit and type 2 diabetes. Principle diabetes preventive role of pomegranate lies behind the fruit ability to scavenge reactive oxygen species responsible for pancreatic β-cells injury that ultimately leads toward development of type 2 diabetes (Hunt et al. 1990). Pomegranate extracts owing to their potent free radical scavenging properties (Tzulker et al. 2007), neutralize the effect of reactive oxygen species thereby preventing onset of type 2 diabetes. Human studies have identified diabetes preventive role of pomegranate juice and derived products to be associated with enhanced activity of certain antioxidant enzymes alike paraoxonase 1 (PON1) and inhibition of nuclear transcription factor (NF-κB) activation (Schubert et al. 2002; Rock et al. 2008). Rosenblat and the group (2006) in their study on diabetic patient revealed pomegranate juice to not alter serum glucose levels but significant reduction in serum TBARS and lipid peroxides levels. It further endorsed feeding pomegranate juice to diabetic patient improve serum thiol and PON1 activity.

Pomegranate: Preventive and Curative Approach in Various Types of Cancers

Highly prevalent in low and medium income countries, cancer is a leading cause of death in both the developed and developing nations. Incomplete or partially available health systems for the diagnosis and management of cancer in poor economies are the significant determinants for cancer related higher mortalities. Global estimates reflect 41% increase in cancer burden from 1975 to 2008 whereas 70% more cases are expected by 2030. Appropriate preventive strategies accompanied with earlier detection system have been warranted as viable strategies to cut down the cancer burden from world community (Kanavos, 2006; Sloan & Gelband, 2007; Ferlay et al., 2010).

Reactive oxygen species on account of their capability to generate various type of cancers are extensively linked with DNA damages and subsequent mutations and malignancies. Site specific generation of reactive oxygen species and inhibition by antioxidant mediated chelation of precursor metal ions (Chevion, 1988; Sies, 1997). Antioxidants thus either of synthetic or plant origin are viable approach to prevent onset of carcinogenesis. Pomegranate vide its high ranking biomolecules such as ellagic acid and punicalagin are supposed to arrest cancer cells growth by inducing multistep cell death program i.e. apoptosis. The fruit extracts possess a class of phenolics and other compounds of biomedical significance that can render anti-proliferative, anti-inflammatory and pro-apoptotic properties in prostate, breast, colon, lungs and several other types of cancers (Khan et al. 2009).

Prostate cancer has higher probability of occurrence among men in age greater than 50 hence; implementing natural products mediated chemoprevention strategy significantly improve patient quality of life by delaying rate of disease progression (Saleem et al. 2003). Pomegranate juice, pericarp extracts and compounds derived during fractionation of extracts affect human prostate cancer xenograft growth and cell proliferation probably vide apoptotic pathway. *In vitro* examination supports acute response of pomegranate juice and rind extracts in inhibiting proliferation of certain prostate cancer cell lines i.e. PC-3, LNCaP and DU 145 (Albrecht et al. 2004). Pure compounds isolated from aqueous and oil component of pomegranate individually exhibited *in vitro* inhibitory properties against PC-3 prostate cancer cell lines. Super additive role of punicic acid, luteolin, ellagic acid and caffeic acid was displayed by synergistic application of all fractions as compared to the individual ones in inhibiting invasion of PC-3 prostate cancer lines (Lansky et al. 2005).

Co-treatment of prostate cancer cells with pomegranate extracts inhibit cancer cell growth by offering an additive effect to lower down cancer cells proliferation. Pomegranate peel and arils extracts standardized with 37% punicalagin induced apoptosis and inhibited cells proliferation by 20% whereas IGFBP-3, a potent negative regulator exhibited 30% inhibition. The study further revealed a synergistic enhanced activity of pomegranate extracts (10μg/ml) and IGFBP-3 (1μg/ml) in inducing apoptosis and modulating tumor production (Koyama et al. 2010).

Despite of handful research, bioactive metabolites responsible for cancer treatment and prevention have not yet completely investigated. Discovered up till now are the urolithins - the only metabolic products of ellagitannins being produced by the activity of gut microbiota in colon. Studies on colorectal cancer patients fed with pomegranate extracts carrying varying ratios of punicalagin and ellagic acid vide detection from urine and plasma samples had demonstrated recovery of free and conjugate ellagic acid, 12 urolithins and gallic acid (Nuñez-Sánchez et al., 2014). Sizeable evidence of urolithins role in colorectal cancer treatment was also displayed in the same study where higher metabolites recovery was witnessed from patient with normal tissues as compared to the treated ones.

Antiestrogens including those of aromatase inhibitors are the available tools to treat breast cancer. Chemo treatment for blockade of estrogen synthesis and its action is the possible strategy to avert breast cancer development and inhibition of its proliferation (Brodie et al. 2006). Pomegranate juice and the fruit extracts have been witnessed *in vitro* and *in vivo* as viable chemopreventive strategy for breast cancer cells. Exposure of carcinogen to mammary glands treated with pomegranate juice polyphenols has been reported to initiate tumorigenesis to a lesser extent as compared to the control. The author (s) to this research consolidated 42% reduction in lesions being produced by the carcinogen in glands treated with pomegranate polyphenols (Mehta & Lansky, 2004). Six ellagitannins derivatives / metabolites were recorded by Adams et al. (2010) of whom urolithins B was the most efficacious in inhibiting aromatase activity in live cell assay. A similar study represented ellagic acid, luteolin and punicic acid as vital products of ellagitannins presenting increase in adhesion of cancer cells and reduction in their migration without putting any impact on normal cells (Rocha et al. 2012). Pomegranate extracts inhibits breast cancer cells (MCF-7) by inducing apoptosis. In a study by Jeune et al. (2005) a synergistically enhanced response of pomegranate extracts and genestein was produced while evaluating their efficacy against 48hrs cultured MCF-7 breast cancer cells. It further states co-treatment with extracts and genestein as more efficacious in inducing apoptosis as compared to the single treatment.

Over exposure of human skin to ultraviolet radiations have capability to generate certain disorders including those of sunburns, immunosuppression, hyperplasia, edema and skin cancers or melanoma. Natural products in line with their potential to act as cancer chemopreventive and carcinogenesis reversing approach, have been in application to prevent and treat melanoma as well (Pacheco-Palencia et al. 2008; Singh et al. 2014). Pomegranate extracts standardized to punicalagin inhibit UVA and UVB mediated damage to human skin fibroblast cells (SKU-1064). The study define 5 – 60mg/L concentration of extracts as effective in protecting skin fibroblast cells from death probably through reduction in activation of NF-kB and down regulation of caspase – 3 (a partial and /or major factor responsible for cleavage of key proteins). Pomegranate peel extracts have also been shown as good candidate in treating melanoma. Pomegranate peel extracts evaluated at concentration of 10 - 450µg/ml for their efficacy in melanoma cells (B16F10) revealed a positive anti-proliferative and angiogenesis inhibitory properties of extracts against melanoma cells in dose dependent manner (Dana & Rafiee, 2015). Better uptake of pomegranate biomolecules by the cancer cells, their hydrolysis and further sustainable release in cell cytoplasm are key properties for better chemo-preventive and curative role of the extracts in various types of cancers. In the light of the most recent updates on the subject, cancer chemopreventive and curative features of pomegranate extracts can be further improved by adopting advanced biomolecules extraction and processing techniques like nanoencapsulation.

Pomegranate and Neurodegenerative Disorders

Brain aging is generally characterized by a gradual loss in several physiological functions including cognitive properties, sensory and motor features. Alzheimer's disease in a row of neurodegenerative disorders is symptomized with progressive memory loss and cognitive impairment. Generation of neurofibrillary tangles, enhanced production and accumulation of amyloid β peptides are the two pathological hallmark of Alzheimer's disease (Subash et al. 2014; Asseburg et al. 2014). Several studies suggest neurotoxicity associated with amyloid β peptides is connected with oxidative stress. In this specific context fruits like pomegranate bearing significant antioxidant pool could serve as a better opportunity to enhance quality of life. A most recent work on pomegranate juice consumption on cognitive performance of transgenic and double Swedish amyloid precursor protein (APP) mutation mice model revealed daily allowance of 4% pomegranate juice in mice diet to reduce anxiety, improve memory, locomotor function and learning ability as compared to the mice models fed on standard feed (Subash et al. 2015). Another work on pomegranate ameliorative effects in Alzheimer's disease reveals the peel extracts of the fruit as gamma secretase modulator and favor diminution in Alzheimer's pathogenesis (Ahmed, 2013). Human studies further validate consumption of 8ounces of pomegranate juice daily for a period of four weeks improves functional brain memory in elder subjects for both the verbal and visual tasks (Bookheimer et al. 2013).

Consumption Trends and Lethality Levels

Pomegranate fruit, peel and the respective extracts have various consumption patterns alike as fresh and fermented juice, ripened and dry arils, peel powder tablets and capsules, powdered extracts and extracts based gels and ointments. Formation of tannin - salivary complex in mouth attribute astringency to peel and its extracts despite, a thoughtful consumption is necessitated to avoid undesirable effects. In Ayurveda's, pomegranate peel aqueous decoctions prepared by boiling peel in water for 10 – 40 min are deployed in treating diarrhea, dysentery, tapeworm infestation, oral apathae, hyperacidity and several other ailments. Pomegranate fruit and peel based formulations of the modern age include pure juice (100%), concentrates, extracts capsules (500 and 1000mg), freeze dried powdered extracts (500mg), spray dried encapsulated extracts, cosmeceutique skin care lotions and moisturizing gels (Aslam et al. 2006; Robert et al. 2010; Vlachojannis et al. 2015). A robust approach has also been observed in last couple of years among researchers for designing pomegranate peel and extracts based functional food formulations. Worldwide tremendous feedback has been given to pomegranate peel and their extracts in food based preparations as antioxidant, protein and lipid stabilizer, antimicrobial, color and texture enhancer, and above all, as nutraceutical and functional food component (Iqbal et al. 2008; Naveena et al. 2008; Altunkaya et al. 2013; Ismail et al. 2014; Singh & Immanuel, 2014).

Pomegranate and the peel extracts, alike other herbal extracts might have toxicological risks for its consumers that merit for systematic safety evaluation of the plant material. Intraperitoneal administration of pomegranate hydro-alcoholic extracts in laboratory animals reveals acute doses responsible for 50% mortality in tested animal as 731.1mg/kg b.w. (Vidal et al. 2003) and 1321mg/kg b.w (Qnais et al. 2007) whereas no observed adverse effect levels of extracts on oral administration were reported to be >2000mg/kg b.w. (Das & Sarma, 2014). The only available human study by Heber et al. (2007) on safety evaluation of pomegranate ellagitannins enriched supplements defines safer limit of dietary supplements consumption as 1420mg per day evidently highlighting protective role of pomegranate antioxidants in human body.

CONCLUSION

In vitro and *in vivo* investigations made on pomegranate and its extracts suggest the fruit and its extracts as heart-healthy diet and plentiful source of high molecular weight biomolecules responsible for protection against a range of mild infections to several life threatening degenerative disorders. To date, the fruit, peel and various extracts of pomegranate have been experienced as remarkable biomedical formulas and nutraceuticals and functional foods ingredient to deliver food enrichment, preservation, stabilization, and texture enhancement properties. Limitations exist in fruit and their extracts utilization owing to inadequate information on pomegranate biomolecules and drug interaction, organ and cell specific role of extracts and fractionated compounds in disease management. A fewer convincing research to utilize the plant material as ready to use therapeutic and functional food ingredient further urge for the need of safe and efficacious commercial preparations to improve quality of life.

REFERENCES

Adams, L. S., Zhang, Y., Seeram, N. P., Heber, D., & Chen, S. (2010). Pomegranate ellagitannin–derived compounds exhibit antiproliferative & antiaromatase activity in breast cancer cells in vitro. *Cancer Prevention Research (Philadelphia, Pa.)*, *3*(1), 108–113. doi:10.1158/1940-6207.CAPR-08-0225 PMID:20051378

Ahmed, A. H. (2013). The ability of pomegranate to ameliorate symptoms associated with Alzheimer's disease in aged transgenic mice. *Open Access Master's Theses*. Paper 146. Available at: http://digitalcommons.uri.edu/theses/146

Ajaikumar, K. B., Asheef, M., Babu, B. H., & Padikkala, J. (2005). The inhibition of gastric mucosal injury by *Punica granatum* L. (pomegranate) methanolic extract. *Journal of Ethnopharmacology*, *96*(1), 171–176. doi:10.1016/j.jep.2004.09.007 PMID:15588667

Akhtar, S., Ismail, T., Fraternale, D., & Sestili, P. (2015). Pomegranate peel and peel extracts: Chemistry and food features. *Food Chemistry*, *174*, 417–425. doi:10.1016/j.foodchem.2014.11.035 PMID:25529700

Albrecht, M., Jiang, W., Kumi-Diaka, J., Lansky, E. P., Gommersall, L. M., Patel, A., & Campbell, M. J. et al. (2004). Pomegranate extracts potently suppress proliferation, xenograft growth, & invasion of human prostate cancer cells. *Journal of Medicinal Food*, *7*(3), 274–283. doi:10.1089/jmf.2004.7.274 PMID:15383219

Altunkaya, A., Hedegaard, R. V., Brimer, L., Gökmen, V., & Skibsted, L. H. (2013). Antioxidant capacity versus chemical safety of wheat bread enriched with pomegranate peel powder. *Food & Function*, *4*(5), 722–727. doi:10.1039/c3fo30296b PMID:23429604

Asgary, S., Sahebkar, A., Afshani, M. R., Keshvari, M., Haghjooyjavanmard, S., & Rafieian-Kopaei, M. (2014). Clinical evaluation of blood pressure lowering, endothelial function improving, hypolipidemic & anti-inflammatory effects of pomegranate juice in hypertensive subjects. *Journal of Phytotherapy Research*, *28*(2), 193–199. doi:10.1002/ptr.4977 PMID:23519910

Aslam, M. N., Lansky, E. P., & Varani, J. (2006). Pomegranate as a cosmeceutical source: Pomegranate fractions promote proliferation & procollagen synthesis & inhibit matrix metalloproteinase-1 production in human skin cells. *Journal of Ethnopharmacology*, *103*(3), 311–318. doi:10.1016/j.jep.2005.07.027 PMID:16221534

Asseburg, H., Hagl, S., & Eckert, G. P. (2014). Nutritional approaches for healthy aging of the brain and the prevention of neurodegenerative diseases. In Pharma-Nutrition (pp. 457-479). Springer International Publishing. doi:10.1007/978-3-319-06151-1_23

Atilgan, D., Parlaktas, B., Uluocak, N., Gencten, Y., Erdemir, F., Ozyurt, H., & Aslan, H. et al. (2014). Pomegranate (*Punica granatum*) juice reduces oxidative injury & improves sperm concentration in a rat model of testicular torsion-detorsion. *Journal of Experimental & Therapeutic Medicine*, *8*(2), 478–482. PMID:25009604

Aviram, M., & Dornfeld, L. (2001). Pomegranate juice consumption inhibits serum angiotensin converting enzyme activity & reduces systolic blood pressure. *Atherosclerosis*, *158*(1), 195–198. doi:10.1016/S0021-9150(01)00412-9 PMID:11500191

Aviram, M., & Dornfeld, L. (2010). *U.S. Patent No. 7,645,469*. Washington, DC: U.S. Patent & Trademark Office.

Aviram, M., Dornfeld, L., Kaplan, M., Coleman, R., Gaitini, D., Nitecki, S., & Fuhrman, B. (2002). Pomegranate juice flavonoids inhibit low-density lipoprotein oxidation & cardiovascular diseases: Studies in atherosclerotic mice & in humans. *Drugs Under Experimental and Clinical Research*, *28*(2-3), 49–62. PMID:12224378

Aviram, M., Dornfeld, L., Rosenblat, M., Volkova, N., Kaplan, M., Coleman, R., & Fuhrman, B. et al. (2000). Pomegranate juice consumption reduces oxidative stress, atherogenic modifications to LDL, and platelet aggregation: Studies in humans and in atherosclerotic apolipoprotein E–deficient mice. *The American Journal of Clinical Nutrition*, *71*(5), 1062–1076. PMID:10799367

Babior, B. M. (2000). Phagocytes & oxidative stress. *The American Journal of Medicine*, *109*(1), 33–44. doi:10.1016/S0002-9343(00)00481-2 PMID:10936476

Bachoual, R., Talmoudi, W., Boussetta, T., Braut, F., & El-Benna, J. (2011). An aqueous pomegranate peel extract inhibits neutrophil myeloperoxiSarmae in vitro & attenuates lung inflammation in mice. *Journal of Food & Chemical Toxicology*, *49*(6), 1224–1228. doi:10.1016/j.fct.2011.02.024 PMID:21376769

Bialonska, D., Kasimsetty, S. G., Khan, S. I., & Ferreira, D. (2009). Urolithins, intestinal microbial metabolites of pomegranate ellagitannins, exhibit potent antioxidant activity in a cell-based assay. *Journal of Agricultural and Food Chemistry*, *57*(21), 10181–10186. doi:10.1021/jf9025794 PMID:19824638

Biswas, T. K., & Mukherjee, B. (2003). Plant medicines of Indian origin for wound healing activity: A review. *The International Journal of Lower Extremity Wounds*, *2*(1), 25–39. doi:10.1177/1534734603002001006 PMID:15866825

Bookheimer, S. Y., Renner, B. A., Ekstrom, A., Li, Z., Henning, S. M., Brown, J. A., & Small, G. W. et al. (2013). Pomegranate juice augments memory & FMRI activity in middle-aged & older adults with mild memory complaints. *Evidence-Based Complementary & Alternative Medicine. Article ID*, *946298*. doi:10.1155/2013/946298

Brodie, A., Sabnis, G., & Jelovac, D. (2006). Aromatase & breast cancer. *The Journal of Steroid Biochemistry and Molecular Biology*, *102*(1), 97–102. doi:10.1016/j.jsbmb.2006.09.002 PMID:17113978

Chevion, M. (1988). A site-specific mechanism for free radical induced biological damage: The essential role of redox-active transition metals. *Free Radical Biology & Medicine*, *5*(1), 27–37. doi:10.1016/0891-5849(88)90059-7 PMID:3075945

Chidambara Murthy, K. N., Reddy, V. K., Veigas, J. M., & Murthy, U. D. (2004). Study on wound healing activity of Punica granatum peel. *Journal of Medicinal Food*, *7*(2), 256–259. doi:10.1089/1096620041224111 PMID:15298776

Conner, E. M., & Grisham, M. B. (1996). Inflammation, free radicals, & antioxidants. *The Journal of Nutrition*, *12*(4), 274–277. doi:10.1016/S0899-9007(96)00000-8 PMID:8862535

Cornelio Favarin, D., Martins Teixeira, M., Lemos de Andrade, E., de Freitas Alves, C., Lazo Chica, J. E., Artério Sorgi, C., & Paula Rogerio, A. et al. (2013). Anti-inflammatory effects of ellagic acid on acute lung injury induced by acid in mice. *Mediators of Inflammation. Article ID, 164202*. doi:10.1155/2013/164202

Dana, N., & Rafiee, L. (2015). Antiangiogenic & antiproliferative effects of black pomegranate peel extract on melanoma cell line. *Research in Pharmaceutical Sciences*, *10*(2), 117–124. PMID:26487888

Das, S., & Sarma, P. H. U. L. E. N. (2014). A study on the anticonvulsant and antianxiety activity of ethanolic extract of punica granatum linn. *International Journal of Pharmacy and Pharmaceutical Sciences*, *6*(2), 389–392.

Davidson, M. H., Maki, K. C., Dicklin, M. R., Feinstein, S. B., Witchger, M. S., Bell, M., & Aviram, M. et al. (2009). Effects of consumption of pomegranate juice on carotid intima–media thickness in men & women at moderate risk for coronary heart disease. *The American Journal of Cardiology*, *104*(7), 936–942. doi:10.1016/j.amjcard.2009.05.037 PMID:19766760

de Oliveira, J. F., Garreto, D. V., da Silva, M. C., Fortes, T. S., de Oliveira, R. B., Nascimento, F. R., & Nicolete, R. et al. (2013). Therapeutic potential of biodegradable microparticles containing Punica granatum L.(pomegranate) in murine model of asthma. *Inflammation Research*, *62*(11), 971–980. doi:10.1007/s00011-013-0659-3 PMID:23979691

DiSilvestro, R. A., DiSilvestro, D. J., & DiSilvestro, D. J. (2009). Pomegranate extract mouth rinsing effects on saliva measures relevant to gingivitis risk. *Journal of Phytotherapy Research*, *23*(8), 1123–1127. doi:10.1002/ptr.2759 PMID:19170139

Dkhil, M. A. (2013). Anti-coccidial, anthelmintic & antioxidant activities of pomegranate (Punica granatum) peel extract. *Journal of Parasitology Research*, *112*(7), 2639–2646. doi:10.1007/s00436-013-3430-3 PMID:23609599

Falanga, V. (2005). Wound healing & its impairment in the diabetic foot. *Lancet*, *366*(9498), 1736–1743. doi:10.1016/S0140-6736(05)67700-8 PMID:16291068

Ferlay, J., Shin, H. R., Bray, F., Forman, D., Mathers, C., & Parkin, D. M. (2010). Estimates of worldwide burden of cancer in 2008: GLOBOCAN 2008. *International Journal of Cancer*, *127*(12), 2893–2917. doi:10.1002/ijc.25516 PMID:21351269

Fischer, U. A., Carle, R., & Kammerer, D. R. (2011). Identification and quantification of phenolic compounds from pomegranate (*Punica granatum* L.) peel, mesocarp, aril and differently produced juices by HPLC-DAD–ESI/MS^n. *Food Chemistry*, *127*(2), 807–821. doi:10.1016/j.foodchem.2010.12.156 PMID:23140740

Fuhrman, B., & Aviram, M. (2005).Pomegranate & cardiovascular diseases: pomegranate juice polyphenolic antioxidants protect against oxidative stress & atherosclerosis development.*International Symposium on Human Health Effects of Fruits & Vegetables*, *744*, 205-216.

Gautam, R. U. P. E. S. H., & Sharma, S. (2012). Antiulcer activity of *Punica granatum* Linn. in diabetic rats. *International Journal of Pharmacy & Pharmaceutical Sciences*, *4*, 459–461.

González-Sarrías, A., Giménez-Bastida, J. A., García-Conesa, M. T., Gómez-Sánchez, M. B., García-Talavera, N. V., Gil-Izquierdo, A., & Espín, J. C. et al. (2010). Occurrence of urolithins, gut microbiota ellagic acid metabolites & proliferation markers expression response in the human prostate gland upon consumption of walnuts & pomegranate juice. *Journal of Molecular Nutrition & Food Research*, *54*(3), 311–322. doi:10.1002/mnfr.200900152 PMID:19885850

Hayouni, E. A., Miled, K., Boubaker, S., Bellasfar, Z., Abedrabba, M., Iwaski, H., & Hamdi, M. et al. (2011). Hydroalcoholic extract based-ointment from *Punica granatum* L. peels with enhanced in vivo healing potential on dermal wounds. *Phytomedicine*, *18*(11), 976–984. doi:10.1016/j.phymed.2011.02.011 PMID:21466954

Heber, D., Seeram, N. P., Wyatt, H., Henning, S. M., Zhang, Y., Ogden, L. G., & Hill, J. O. et al. (2007). Safety and antioxidant activity of a pomegranate ellagitannin-enriched polyphenol dietary supplement in overweight individuals with increased waist size. *Journal of Agricultural and Food Chemistry*, *55*(24), 10050–10054. doi:10.1021/jf071689v PMID:17966977

Hemmati, A. A., Rezaie, A., & Darabpour, P. (2013). Preventive effects of pomegranate seed extract on bleomycin-induced pulmonary fibrosis in rat. *Jundishapur Journal of Natural Pharmaceutical Products*, *8*(2), 76–80. doi:10.17795/jjnpp-8821 PMID:24624192

Hunt, J. V., Smith, C. C., & Wolff, S. P. (1990). Autoxidative glycosylation & possible involvement of peroxides & free radicals in LDL modification by glucose. *Journal of Diabetes*, *39*(11), 1420–1424. doi:10.2337/diab.39.11.1420 PMID:2227114

Iqbal, S., Haleem, S., Akhtar, M., Zia-Ul-Haq, M., & Akbar, J. (2008). Efficiency of pomegranate peel extracts in stabilization of sunflower oil under accelerated conditions. *Food Research International*, *41*(2), 194–200. doi:10.1016/j.foodres.2007.11.005

Ismail, T., Akhtar, S., Riaz, M., & Ismail, A. (2014). Effect of pomegranate peel supplementation on nutritional, organoleptic & stability properties of cookies. *International Journal of Food Sciences and Nutrition*, *65*(6), 661–666. doi:10.3109/09637486.2014.908170 PMID:24725173

Jeune, M. L., Kumi-Diaka, J., & Brown, J. (2005). Anticancer activities of pomegranate extracts & genistein in human breast cancer cells. *Journal of Medicinal Food*, *8*(4), 469–475. doi:10.1089/jmf.2005.8.469 PMID:16379557

JNC-7 Guidelines. (2004). The seventh report of the joint national committee on prevention, detection, evaluation, & treatment of high blood pressure. National Heart, Lung, and Blood Institute (US). Report. No. 04-5230.

Jolly, C. I., Narayanan, S., & Prabhu, S. K. (2000). Antihypertensive activity of flowers of *Punica granatum* Linn. (Variety-Gulnar). *Indian Journal of Natural Products*, *16*(1), 3–7.

Jurenka, J. (2008). Therapeutic application of pomegranate (*Punica granatum*): *A Review. Alternative Medicine Review*, *13*, 128–144. PMID:18590349

Kanavos, P. (2006). The rising burden of cancer in the developing world. *Annals of Oncology, 17*(suppl 8), 15-23.

Kasimsetty, S. G., Bialonska, D., Reddy, M. K., Ma, G., Khan, S. I., & Ferreira, D. (2010). Colon cancer chemopreventive activities of pomegranate ellagitannins and urolithins. *Journal of Agricultural and Food Chemistry, 58*(4), 2180–2187. doi:10.1021/jf903762h PMID:20112993

Khan, G. N., Gorin, M. A., Rosenthal, D., Pan, Q., Bao, L. W., Wu, Z. F., & Merajver, S. D. et al. (2009). Pomegranate fruit extract impairs invasion & motility in human breast cancer. *Integrative Cancer Therapies, 8*(3), 242–253. doi:10.1177/1534735409341405 PMID:19815594

Kim, N. D., Mehta, R., Yu, W., Neeman, I., Livney, T., Amichay, A., & Lansky, E. et al. (2002). Chemopreventive & adjuvant therapeutic potential of pomegranate (*Punica granatum*) for human breast cancer. *Breast Cancer Research and Treatment, 71*(3), 203–217. doi:10.1023/A:1014405730585 PMID:12002340

Kim, N. D., Mehta, R., Yu, W., Neeman, I., Livney, T., Amichay, A., & Mansel, R. et al. (2002). Chemopreventive and adjuvant therapeutic potential of pomegranate (*Punica granatum*) for human breast cancer. *Breast Cancer Research and Treatment, 71*(3), 203–217. doi:10.1023/A:1014405730585 PMID:12002340

Kirsner, R. S., & Eaglstein, W. H. (1993). The wound healing process. *Journal of Dermatologic Clinics, 11*(4), 629–640. PMID:8222347

Klein & Mordechai. (n.d.). *Pomegranate-derived Products for the Treatment of Skin Sores & Lesions.* U.S. Patent Application, 12, 676-957.

Koyama, S., Cobb, L. J., Mehta, H. H., Seeram, N. P., Heber, D., Pantuck, A. J., & Cohen, P. (2010). Pomegranate extract induces apoptosis in human prostate cancer cells by modulation of the IGF–IGFBP axis. *Growth Hormone & IGF Research, 20*(1), 55–62. doi:10.1016/j.ghir.2009.09.003 PMID:19853487

Kumari, A., Dora, J., Kumar, A., & Kumar, A. (2012). Pomegranate (*Punica granatum*)-Overview. *International Journal of Pharmaceutical and Chemical Sciences, 1*(4), 1218–1222.

Kundhal, K., & Lok, C. (2005). Clinical epidemiology of cardiovascular disease in chronic kidney disease. *Nephron. Clinical Practice, 101*(2), 47–c52. doi:10.1159/000086221 PMID:15942250

Lai, S., Zhou, Q., Zhang, Y., & Shang, J. Yu. T. (2009). Effects of pomegranate tannins onexperimental gastric damages. *Zhongguo Zhong Yao Za Zhi, 34*(10), 1290–1294. PMID:19673398

Lansky, E., Shubert, S., & Neeman, I. (2004). Pharmacological and therapeutic properties of pomegranate. *Israel. CIHEAM-Options Mediterraneennes, 42*, 231–235.

Lansky, E. P., Harrison, G., Froom, P., & Jiang, W. G. (2005). Pomegranate (Punica granatum) pure chemicals show possible synergistic inhibition of human PC-3 prostate cancer cell invasion across Matrigel™. *Investigational New Drugs, 23*(2), 121–122. doi:10.1007/s10637-005-5856-7 PMID:15744587

Larrosa, M., González-Sarrías, A., Yáñez-Gascón, M. J., Selma, M. V., Azorín-Ortuño, M., Toti, S., & Espín, J. C. (2010). Anti-inflammatory properties of a pomegranate extract & its metabolite urolithin-A in a colitis rat model & the effect of colon inflammation on phenolic metabolism. *The Journal of Nutritional Biochemistry, 21*(8), 717–725. doi:10.1016/j.jnutbio.2009.04.012 PMID:19616930

Lee, C. J., Chen, L. G., Liang, W. L., & Wang, C. C. (2010). Anti-inflammatory effects of Punica granatum Linne invitro & in vivo. *Journal of Food Chemistry, 118*(2), 315–322. doi:10.1016/j.foodchem.2009.04.123

Li, Y., Guo, C., Yang, J., Wei, J., Xu, J., & Cheng, S. (2006). Evaluation of antioxidant properties of pomegranate peel extract in comparison with pomegranate pulp extract. *Food Chemistry*, *96*(2), 254–260. doi:10.1016/j.foodchem.2005.02.033

Mahmood, A. A., Sidik, K., Salmah, I., Suzainur, K. A. R., & Yusoff, K. M. (2004). Cytoprotective effects of honey and methanol extracts from *P. granatum* L. fruit peel and *N. sativa* L seeds on ethanol-induced gastric damage in rats. *Journal of Food Technology*, *2*(3), 136–141.

Malik, A., Afaq, F., Sarfaraz, S., Adhami, V. M., Syed, D. N., & Mukhtar, H. (2005). Pomegranate fruit juice for chemoprevention & chemotherapy of prostate cancer. *Proceedings of the National Academy of Sciences of the United States of America*, *102*(41), 14813–14818. doi:10.1073/pnas.0505870102 PMID:16192356

Mehta, R., & Lansky, E. P. (2004). Breast cancer chemopreventive properties of pomegranate (Punica granatum) fruit extracts in a mouse mammary organ culture. *European Journal of Cancer Prevention*, *13*(4), 345–348. doi:10.1097/01.cej.0000136571.70998.5a PMID:15554563

Milin, L., & Stanimarovic, S. (1950). Vitamins & pharmacology of pomegranate juice. *Medicinski Glasnik*, *4*(11-12), 259. PMID:14805886

Moghaddam, G., Sharifzadeh, M., Hassanzadeh, G., Khanavi, M., Dolatshahi, F., Sadeghi, N., & Hajimahmoodi, M. et al. (2014). Anti-Ulcerative Potential of Punica granatum L. hydroalcoholic peel extract. *Tropical Journal of Pharmaceutical Research*, *13*(7), 1093–1097. doi:10.4314/tjpr.v13i7.12

Mohan, M., Waghulde, H., & Kasture, S. (2010). Effect of pomegranate juice on Angiotensin II-induced hypertension in diabetic wistar rats. *Journal of Phytotherapy Research*, *24*(S2), 196–203. doi:10.1002/ptr.3090 PMID:20020514

Morton, J. (1987). Pomegranate. In J. F. Morton (Ed.), Fruits of Warm Climates (pp. 352–355). Wallingford, UK: CabDirect Publishing.

Murad, H. (2003). *U.S. Patent No. 6,630,163*. Washington, DC: U.S. Patent and Trademark Office.

Nathan, C. (2006). Neutrophils and immunity: Challenges and opportunities. *Nature Reviews. Immunology*, *6*(3), 173–182. doi:10.1038/nri1785 PMID:16498448

Navarro, V., Villarreal, M. L., Rojas, G., & Lozoya, X. (1996). Antimicrobial evaluation of some plants used in Mexican traditional medicine for the treatment of infectious diseases. *Journal of Ethnopharmacology*, *53*(3), 143–147. doi:10.1016/0378-8741(96)01429-8 PMID:8887021

Naveena, B. M., Sen, A. R., Kingsly, R. P., Singh, D. B., & Kondaiah, N. (2008). Antioxidant activity of pomegranate rind powder extract in cooked chicken patties. *International Journal of Food Science & Technology*, *43*(10), 1807–1812. doi:10.1111/j.1365-2621.2007.01708.x

Negi, P. S., Jayaprakasha, G. K., & Jena, B. S. (2003). Antioxidant and antimutagenic activities of pomegranate peel extracts. *Food Chemistry*, *80*(3), 393–397. doi:10.1016/S0308-8146(02)00279-0

Nuñez-Sánchez, M. A., García-Villalba, R., Monedero-Saiz, T., García-Talavera, N. V., Gómez-Sánchez, M. B., Sánchez-Álvarez, C., & Espín, J. C. et al. (2014). Targeted metabolic profiling of pomegranate polyphenols and urolithins in plasma, urine and colon tissues from colorectal cancer patients. *Molecular Nutrition & Food Research*, *58*(6), 1199–1211. PMID:24532260

Nyanhanda, T., Elaine, M. G., & Roger, D. H. (2014). Plant-derived foods for the attenuation of allergic airway inflammation. *Current Pharmaceutical Design*, *20*(6), 869–878. doi:10.2174/13816128113199990056 PMID:23701570

Ong, K. L., Cheung, B. M. Y., Man, Y. B., Lau, C. P., & Lam, K. S. L. (2007). Prevalence, awareness, treatment & control of hypertension among United States adults 1999–2004. *Hypertension*, *49*(1), 69–75. doi:10.1161/01.HYP.0000252676.46043.18 PMID:17159087

Pacheco-Palencia, L. A., Noratto, G., Hingorani, L., Talcott, S. T., & Mertens-Talcott, S. U. (2008). Protective effects of standardized pomegranate (*Punica granatum* L.) polyphenolic extract in ultraviolet-irradiated human skin fibroblasts. *Journal of Agricultural and Food Chemistry*, *56*(18), 8434–8441. doi:10.1021/jf8005307 PMID:18717570

Polunin, O., & Stainton, A. (1985). Pomegranate. In O. Polunin & A. Stainton (Eds.), Flowers of the Himalaya (pp. 532-534). New York: Oxford University Press.

Pradeep, B. V., Manojbabu, M. K., & Palaniswamy, M. (2008). Antibacterial activity of *Punica granatum* L. against gastro intestinal tract infection causing organisms. *Journal of Ethnobotanical Leaflets, 2008*(1), 143.

Qnais, E. Y., Elokda, A. S., Abu Ghalyun, Y. Y., & Abdulla, F. A. (2007). Antidiarrheal activity of the aqueous extract of *Punica granatum* (Pomegranate) peels. *Journal of Pharmaceutical Biology*, *45*(9), 715–720. doi:10.1080/13880200701575304

Raisz, L. G. (2005). Pathogenesis of osteoporosis: Concepts, conflicts, & prospects. *The Journal of Clinical Investigation*, *115*(12), 3318–3325. doi:10.1172/JCI27071 PMID:16322775

Robert, P., Gorena, T., Romero, N., Sepulveda, E., Chavez, J., & Saenz, C. (2010). Encapsulation of polyphenols and anthocyanins from pomegranate (Punica granatum) by spray drying. *International Journal of Food Science & Technology*, *45*(7), 1386–1394. doi:10.1111/j.1365-2621.2010.02270.x

Rocha, A., Wang, L., Penichet, M., & Martins-Green, M. (2012). Pomegranate juice & specific components inhibit cell & molecular processes critical for metastasis of breast cancer. *Breast Cancer Research and Treatment*, *136*(3), 647–658. doi:10.1007/s10549-012-2264-5 PMID:23065001

Rock, W., Rosenblat, M., Miller-Lotan, R., Levy, A. P., Elias, M., & Aviram, M. (2008). Consumption of wonderful variety pomegranate juice and extract by diabetic patients increases paraoxonase 1 association with high-density lipoprotein and stimulates its catalytic activities. *Journal of Agricultural and Food Chemistry*, *56*(18), 8704–8713. doi:10.1021/jf801756x PMID:18759451

Rosenblat, M., Hayek, T., & Aviram, M. (2006). Anti-oxidative effects of pomegranate juice (PJ) consumption by diabetic patients on serum and on macrophages. *Atherosclerosis*, *187*(2), 363–371. doi:10.1016/j.atherosclerosis.2005.09.006 PMID:16226266

Rosillo, M. A., Sánchez-Hidalgo, M., Cárdeno, A., Aparicio-Soto, M., Sánchez-Fidalgo, S., Villegas, I., & de la Lastra, C. A. (2012). Dietary supplementation of an ellagic acid-enriched pomegranate extract attenuates chronic colonic inflammation in rats. *Journal of Pharmacological Research*, *66*(3), 235–242. doi:10.1016/j.phrs.2012.05.006 PMID:22677088

Rubio, C. A., & Befrits, R. (2008). Colorectal cancer in Crohn's disease — review of a 56-year experience in Karolinska Institute University Hospital. *Journal of Environmental Pathology, Toxicology and Oncology*, *27*(4), 257–266. doi:10.1615/JEnvironPatholToxicolOncol.v27.i4.20 PMID:19105531

Saleem, M., Adhami, V. M., Siddiqui, I. A., & Mukhtar, H. (2003, September). Tea Beverage in Chemoprevention of Prostate Cancer: A Mini-Review. *Nutrition and Cancer*, *47*(1), 13–23. doi:10.1207/s15327914nc4701_2

Saleem, M., Adhami, V. M., Siddiqui, I. A., & Mukhtar, H. (2003). Tea beverage in chemoprevention of prostate cancer: A mini-review. *Journal of Nutrition & Cancer*, *47*(1), 13–23. doi:10.1207/s15327914nc4701_2 PMID:14769533

SaleemM.AdhamiV. M.SiddiquiI. A.MukhtarH. (2003) Tea

Schubert, S. Y., Neeman, I., & Resnick, N. (2002). A novel mechanism for the inhibition of NF-κB activation in vascular endothelial cells by natural antioxidants. *The FASEB Journal*, *16*(14), 1931–1933. PMID:12368228

Shema-Didi, L., Kristal, B., Sela, S., Geron, R., & Ore, L. (2014). Does pomegranate intake attenuate cardiovascular risk factors in hemodialysis patients. *The Journal of Nutrition*, *13*(1), 18. doi:10.1186/1475-2891-13-18 PMID:24593225

Shukla, M., Gupta, K., Rasheed, Z., Khan, K. A., & Haqqi, T. M. (2008). Consumption of hydrolyzable tannins-rich pomegranate extract suppresses inflammation & joint damage in rheumatoid arthritis. *The Journal of Nutrition*, *24*(7), 733–743. doi:10.1016/j.nut.2008.03.013 PMID:18490140

Sies, H. (1997). Oxidative stress: Oxidants and antioxidants. *Experimental Physiology*, *82*(2), 291–295. doi:10.1113/expphysiol.1997.sp004024 PMID:9129943

Singh, M., Suman, S., & Shukla, Y. (2014). *New enlightenment of skin cancer chemoprevention through phytochemicals: in vitro & in vivo studies & the underlying mechanisms.* BioMed Research International.

Singh, S., & Immanuel, G. (2014). Extraction of antioxidants from fruit peels & its utilization in paneer. *Journal of Food Processing Technology*, *5*, 1–5.

Sloan, F. A., & Gelband, H. (2007). *Cancer control opportunities in low-and middle-income countries.* National Academies Press.

Souli, A., Sebai, H., Rtibi, K., Chehimi, L., Sakly, M., Amri, M., & Marzouki, L. et al. (2015). Inhibitory effects of two varieties of tunisian pomegranate (*Punica granatum* L.) extracts on gastrointestinal transit in rat. *Journal of Medicinal Food*, *18*(9), 1007–1012. doi:10.1089/jmf.2014.0110 PMID:25775227

Stowe, C. B. (2011). The effects of pomegranate juice consumption on blood pressure & cardiovascular health. *Complementary Therapies in Clinical Practice*, *17*(2), 113–115. doi:10.1016/j.ctcp.2010.09.004 PMID:21457902

Subash, S., Braidy, N., Essa, M. M., Zayana, A. B., Ragini, V., Al-Adawi, S., & Guillemin, G. J. et al. (2015). Long-term (15 mo) dietary supplementation with pomegranates from Oman attenuates cognitive & behavioral deficits in a transgenic mice model of Alzheimer's disease. *The Journal of Nutrition*, *31*(1), 223–229. doi:10.1016/j.nut.2014.06.004 PMID:25441596

Subash, S., Essa, M. M., Al-Asmi, A., Al-Adawi, S., Vaishnav, R., Braidy, N., & Guillemin, G. J. (2014). Pomegranate from Oman alleviates the brain oxidative damage in transgenic mouse model of Alzheimer's disease. *Journal of Traditional & Complementary Medicine*, *4*(4), 232. doi:10.4103/2225-4110.139107 PMID:25379464

Sumner, M. D., Elliott-Eller, M., Weidner, G., Daubenmier, J. J., Chew, M. H., Marlin, R., & Ornish, D. et al. (2005). Effects of pomegranate juice consumption on myocardial perfusion in patients with coronary heart disease. *The American Journal of Cardiology*, *96*(6), 810–814. doi:10.1016/j.amjcard.2005.05.026 PMID:16169367

Tanveer, A., Farooq, U., Akram, K., Hayat, Z., Shafi, A., Nazar, H., & Ahmad, Z. (2015). Pomegranate extracts: A natural preventive measure against spoilage & pathogenic microorganisms. *Food Reviews International*, *31*(1), 29–51. doi:10.1080/87559129.2014.961074

Tzulker, R., Glazer, I., Bar-Ilan, I., Holl, D., Aviram, M., & Amir, R. (2007). Antioxidant activity, polyphenol content & related compounds in different fruit juices & homogenates prepared from 29 different pomegranate accessions. *Journal of Agricultural and Food Chemistry*, *55*(23), 9559–9570. doi:10.1021/jf071413n PMID:17914875

Vidal, A., Fallarero, A., Peña, B. R., Medina, M. E., Gra, B., Rivera, F., & Vuorela, P. M. et al. (2003). Studies on the toxicity of *Punica granatum* L.(Punicaceae) whole fruit extracts. *Journal of Ethnopharmacology*, *89*, 295–300. PMID:14611895

Vlachojannis, C., Zimmermann, B. F., & Chrubasik-Hausmann, S. (2015). Efficacy & safety of pomegranate medicinal products for cancer. *Journal of Evidence-Based Complementary & Alternative Medicine. Article ID*, *258598*. doi:10.1155/2015/258598

Xu, K. Z. Y., Zhu, C., Kim, M. S., Yamahara, J., & Li, Y. (2009). Pomegranate flower ameliorates fatty liver in an animal model of type 2 diabetes & obesity. *Journal of Ethnopharmacology*, *123*(2), 280–287. doi:10.1016/j.jep.2009.03.035 PMID:19429373

Zhao, X., Yuan, Z., Fang, Y., Yin, Y., & Feng, L. (2013). Characterization and evaluation of major anthocyanins in pomegranate (*Punica granatum* L.) peel of different cultivars and their development phases. *European Food Research and Technology*, *236*(1), 109–117. doi:10.1007/s00217-012-1869-6

Chapter 9
Yerba Mate:
Chemistry, Technology, and Biological Properties

Roberto Buffo
Universidad de San Pablo-T, Argentina

ABSTRACT

Yerba mate (Ilex paraguariensis) is a plant original from the subtropical regions of South America, present in Southern Brazil, Northeastern Argentina, Paraguay and Uruguay. It is primarily consumed as a beverage made by steeping the leaves of the plant in hot water. The growing interest in mate products has made it paramount that research on this herbal tea continues, as it has shown extraordinary possibilities not only as a consumer beverage but also in the nutraceutical industry. Yet, there is much to be done: human-based studies to support the properties verified in vitro and in vivo models with animas are scarce.

INTRODUCTION

Yerba mate (*Ilex paraguariensis*) is a plant original from the subtropical regions of South America, present in Southern Brazil, Northeastern Argentina, Paraguay and Uruguay. It was already being consumed by native South Americans at the time of arrival of Europeans. Nowadays the aqueous extract of yerba mate, product constituted exclusively from dried and crumbled leaves and branches of *Ilex paraguariensis* according to Brazilian and Argentinean legislations, is consumed widely in the region of origin at a rate of more than one liter per day by millions of people and constitutes a major alternative to coffee and tea (Mosimann et al, 2006). The product is prepared mainly as four different types of beverages: the *chimarrão* and *mate cocido* in the south of Brazil, Uruguay, Argentina and Paraguay; the *tereré*, popular in the central west of Brazil and Paraguay, and the *mate* tea, corresponding to Southeastern Brazil, Argentina and Uruguay. Both *chimarrão* and *tereré* are made with green dried and crumbled *mate* leaves, the first prepared with hot water, the second with cold water. Beverages are prepared by compacting a certain amount of leaves, previously moistened with water against the walls of a vessel made from a gourd called *cuia* or *mate* itself. The beverage is drunk by sucking through a metal pipe called *bombilla* which has a perforated, flattened disc at the end immersed in the infusion to act as a filter that prevents

DOI: 10.4018/978-1-5225-0591-4.ch009

the leaves from being consumed. *Mate* tea is prepared with roasted leaves and brewed as any other herbal tea, whereas *mate cocido* refers to green yerba mate leaves brewed as herbal tea commercialized in small bags (Mozzafera, 1997; Bastos et al, 2005).

Yerba mate can be cultivated and processed in a variety of ways. Plantations are the most popular growth environments because of ease of harvest and a more consistent production quality and quantity. Its processing occurs in six steps: harvesting, roasting, drying, milling, aging and blending/packaging. Leaves and small stems are harvested mechanically, divided into 100 kg sacks, and transported to a processing facility. Roasting, which inactivates enzymes and preserves sensory qualities, occurs by direct contact with fire at temperatures between 250 and 550ºC for 2 to 4 minutes. Drying takes place by exposure to hot air until moisture content of 3% is attained, typically during 12 to 14 hours. Dry product is then put into cement or cedar aging chambers for as long as 12 months: this helps to develop the typical flavor of *mate*. Aged product is ultimately milled to desired size before packaging (Isolabella et al, 2010).

PHYTOCHEMISTRY

Purine Alkaloids

Xantines are a class of purine alkaloids found in many different plants, including tea, coffee and cocoa. The ones found in yerba mate include theophylline (1,3-dimethylxantine), theobromine (3,7-dimethylxantine) and caffeine (1,3,7-trimethylxantine). Of the three, caffeine is found in the highest concentration, 1-2% of dry weight, followed by theobromine, 0.3-0.9% of dry weight. Some authors have questioned the presence of theophylline in yerba mate for considering that this compound is just an intermediate in the catabolism of caffeine in the plant (Ito et al, 1977; Athayde et al, 2000; Schubert et al., 2006).

The concentration of caffeine in relation to consumer consumption has been found to be approximately 78 mg of caffeine in one cup of *mate* infusion, around 150 ml, a value near that of coffee. However, the customary rate of *mate* consumption prepared through the traditional method presents intakes above 500 ml, thus resulting in 260 mg or more of total caffeine (Mozzafera, 1997). It has also been suggested that the drying process can significantly affect caffeine concentration as well as color and chlorophyll content of leaves: up to 30% and 70-80% of caffeine and chlorophyll, respectively. However, even though caffeine concentration was lower in dried leaves than in fresh product, there is evidence that when the former was use to make the infusion, significantly more caffeine and caffeoylquinic acids were being extracted in comparison with fresh leaves. This increased extraction of compounds is likely from the disruption of cells during drying. It may also be explained by a decrease in moisture and an increase in soluble solids during drying, thus leading to a greater amount of compounds dissolved into the infusion (Barros et al, 2000; Schubert et al, 2006).

Caffeoyl Derivatives

The compounds of this chemical family in yerba mate include caffeic acid, chlorogenic acid, 3,4-dicaffeoylquinic acid, 3,5-dicaffeoylquinic acid and 4,5-dicaffeoylquinic acid, primary constituents that account for the antioxidant capacity of *mate* tea, acting as hydrogen and electron donors and also as transition metal ion chelators (Carini et al, 1998; Filip et al, 2000).

Saponins

Saponins are bitter and highly water-soluble compounds found in many types of plants and are believed to be one of the main factors accounting for the distinct flavor of *mate* tea. Not only do they play a role in flavor but also are attributed to anti-inflamatory and hypocholesterolemic properties (Gnoatto et al, 2005). Several of these compounds, namely triterpenoid saponins with ursolic and oleanolic moieties have been isolated from the leaves of yerba mate. The hypocholesterolemic properties may be attributed to the saponin inhibition of passive diffusion of colic acid and formation of micelles that cannot be absorbed and are this excreted (Gosmann et al, 1995; Ferreira, 1997)

Minerals

Mate contains high concentrations of inorganic compounds. Presence of aluminum, chromium, copper, iron, manganese, nickel, potassium and zinc is of particular interest due to their importance in human metabolism and development. It should be noted that an inverse correlation was found between the amount of these minerals leached into a *mate* infusion and the tannin concentration: best leaching rates correspond to lower concentration values (Heck and De Mejia, 2007). Mineral contents from leaves also change drastically depending on agricultural practices. Use of fertilizers and quality of soil have an important impact on mineral composition of *mate* leaves and should be taken into account for the production of higher nutritional products (Bastos et al, 2007).

Adulterants

Adulterants of other *ilex* species may be incorporated into the final *mate* product, either intentionally or unintentionally. They can be problematic for the quality of the infusion due to their differing concentration of saponins. *Mate* prepared with *Ilex paraguariensis* showed to be the least bitter of all extracts prepared with adulterating species; thus, it is possible that their addition can have a significant effect on the bitterness of *mate* beverages. Not only do the adulterating plants contain greater concentrations of bitter compounds but the fruits of *Ilex paraguariensis* plants themselves also contain bitter saponins. If these fruits were incorporated into *mate* products they could also lead to an increase in bitterness and a decrease in overall quality (Reginatto et al, 1999; Taketa, 2004).

TECHNOLOGICAL CONSIDERATIONS

Flavor and Aroma

Driving forces behind sales and brand selection and consumer preference for *mate* brands is largely driven by smell and taste attributes. It has been shown that there is a direct correlation between consumer preference for taste and aroma of *mate* products to the appearance and organoleptic features of such products. Sensory panels require key terms to define these attributes. Some of the one that have been utilized include: bitter, astringent, acid, hay, green, humid, toasted and paper (Cruz et al, 2003).

Aroma compounds in yerba mate have also been characterized using gas chromatography/mass spectrometry. Among the 196 volatile chemical compounds found in *mate* teas only 144 are also present in green tea. Among the distinctive components we can mention 2-butoxy ethanol in high concentrations and 3,3,5-trimethyl cyclohexanone and related compounds (Kawakami and Kobayashi, 1991).

Roasting process of dried *mate* leaves have been shown to have a dramatic effect on their flavor and aroma. Roasted *mate* shows higher concentrations of furans, pyrazines and pyrroles compared to green *mate* likely due to Maillard reaction (Kawakami and Kobayashi, 1991). Bastos et al (2003) examined essential oil extracts from both green and roasted *mate* and found that the latter contains significantly less of the compounds responsible for the green-floral aroma, that is, limonene, characteristic of green *mate*. They also found an increase in compounds such as methyl furfural and furfural, likely responsible for the smoky characteristic of roasted *mate*. One of the defining characteristics of *mate* teas is the perception of bitterness, which can be attributed to caffeine (Ley et al, 2006), tannins (Drinkine et al, 2007) and saponins (Ma et al, 1989). It should in addition be noted that the presence of stems, often found in most varieties, could significantly reduce the bitter feature compared with those without stems (Calvino, 2005).

Compound Extraction

While yerba mate is primarily consumed in a beverage form made by steeping the leaves of the plant in hot water, its high concentration of beneficial compounds make it an interesting subject for extraction and purification of compounds for use in the nutraceutical industry. Sonication has proven to be highly effective to eliminate caffeine and theobromine from *mate* leaves. However, this method is affected by solvent polarity as well as extraction time and solvent-to-sample mass ratio. In addition, it requires the use of organic solvents such as methanol and hexane which can be rather troublesome when extracts are to be used for human consumption. The alternatives is the utilization of supercritical carbon dioxide extraction, which not only is a much safer and more inexpensive procedure, lowering solvent and energy requirements, but also yields higher rates of extracted caffeine (Saldana et al, 2002; Jacques et al, 2007).

FUNCTIONAL PROPERTIES

Antioxidant Capacity

It has been found that the consumption of *mate* tea significantly contributes to the overall antioxidant intake and provides high amounts of caffeoylquinic acid derivatives, with biological effects potentially beneficial for human health (Bravo et al, 2007). Yerba mate's ability to quench reactive oxygen species has been correlated to polyphenol concentration in the infusion. The compound that may be primarily responsible for this activity is chlorogenic acid (Anesini et al, 2006).

Ilex paraguariensis extracts are very potent inhibitors of low-density lipoproteins oxidation and have anti-mutagenic effects. This ability demonstrates their potential as chain-breaking antioxidants. It was suggested that the antioxidant activity may be related to the presence of polyphenolic compounds that might inhibit free-radical reactions through the chelation of transition-metal ions (Vinson et al, 1995; van Acker et al, 1996).

Mate extract has shown to be a potent inhibitor of oxidative stress caused by reacting oxygen species, considerably so for the liver and heart. The heart is susceptible to oxidative stress during post-ischemic reperfusion. Administering *mate* extract may decrease lipid oxidation in the heart by protecting myocardial tissue (Schinella et al, 2005).

It has also been reported that hyperglycemia is a cause for diabetic complications due to dicarbonyls involved in advanced glycation end-product formation. Oxidation has been linked to glycation and *mate* extracts show a dose-dependent inhibition of dicarbonyl action and products derived from Maillard reaction by modulating the activity of glucose-6-phosphatase involved in glucose metabolism (Lunceford and Gugliucci, 2005).

Weight Management and Obesity

Obesity is a growing concern in many countries and current research in many areas is directed at finding a way to curb the epidemic. *Mate* tea has been shown to have possible effects in the area of weight loss by decreasing the respiratory quotient, this increasing fat oxidation rates (Martinet et al, 1999). A herbal infusion made from *mate*, *guarana* and *damiana* showed drastic slowing of gastric emptying as well as a decrease in the perceived time for gastric fullness, thus increasing satiety. This was also followed by a substantial decrease in weight, after 45 days, in overweight patients (Andersen and Fogh, 2001). The potential for weight loss has led to the consideration of *mate* tea as a dietary supplement (Pittler and Ernst, 2004).

It has also been cited that the effect of yerba mate on weight loss could be related to caffeine concentration, contributing to lipolytic activity, or saponin concentration, interfering with cholesterol metabolism and delaying intestinal absorption of dietary fat (Dickel et al, 2007).

Antimicrobial and Oral Health

Compounds present in yerba mate possessing antimicrobial activity include caffeoyl derivatives, methylxantines and N-hexane extracts (alcohols and terpenes), against a broad spectrum of Gram-positive and Gram-negative bacteria (Kubo et al, 1993; Sari et al, 2007; Filip et al, 2010). However, contradictory information is available in the literature on which compounds might contribute to activity against specific microorganisms and whether may have additive or synergistic effects. It is likely that combinations of chemicals found in yerba mate extracts contribute together on antimicrobial activity against bacteria and/or fungi (e.g., rutin in the latter case) as evidenced by the ineffectiveness of activity of some individual compounds (Burris et al, 2012).

Cancer Prevention

In vitro and animal experiments have shown a protective effect of yerba mate against cancer, mostly related to inhibition of enzymes responsible for high rates of mitosis on tumor cells (Heck & De Mejia, 2007). Proteasome inhibitors identified in yerba mate include mainly caffeoylquinic acids; other compounds present in yerba mate showing cytotoxic properties against tumor cells are rutin and quercetin. Although the latter are found with small concentrations, they show the diversity of flavonoids of yerba mate that contribute to its overall anticancer potential (Alta et al, 2006).

Digestion Improvement

Research conducted in Argentina found that yerba mate does induce an increase in bile flow and enhance intestinal transit. According to the results obtained with four species of *Ilex* studied, choleretic activity of

Ilex paraguariensis was slow, gradual and sustained, whereas that of *Ilex brevicuspis* was rapid, reached a maximum and then decreased rapidly (Gorzalczany et al, 2001).

Anti-Fatigue and Stimulant Actions

Yerba mate is a central nervous system stimulant. Metabolic effects of *mate* appear to include the ability to maintain aerobic breakdown of carbohydrates during exercise for long periods of time. As a result, more calories are burned, thereby increasing cardiac efficiency and delaying the build-up of lactic acid. Indeed, a US Patent of 2002 cites yerba mate as inhibitor of monoamine oxidase (MAO) activity by 40-50% *in vitro*. The underlying study suggests that *mate* might be useful for treating a variety of disorders such as "depression, disorders of attention and focus, disorders of mood and emotional behavior, Parkinson's disease, extrapyramidal disorders, hypertension, substance abuse, eating disorders, withdrawal syndromes and cessation of smoking" (Bastos et al, 2007).

Circulatory Systems and Hypocholesterolemic Effect

Stein et al (2005) have suggested that the antioxidant activity of *mate* infusions might be responsible, in part, for the decrease in plasma level of cholesterol and triglycerides and that the induced vasodilatation observed for both aqueous and acidified butanol fraction from yerba mate are mediated by the release of endothelium-derived substances.

Gorgen et al (2005) have reported that *Ilex paraguariensis* is able to interfere in the circulatory system, acting as a diuretic and hypotensive agent. The chronic ingestion of their aqueous extracts promoted a decrease of ATP, ADP and AMP hydrolysis in rat blood serum. Thus, it seems that this treatment can alter the nucleotidase pathway, modulating the balance in the purine levels which can induce relevant effects, for example in the cardiovascular system.

Chimarrão Ingestion and Cancer Incidence

The high esophagus cancer incidence in some South American locations where population traditionally consumes *chimarrão* was an epidemiological concern during the 1980s-1990s. However, no studies could find a positive correlation between *chimarrão* drinking and cancer. The main issue may be the temperature in which *chimarrão* is drunk, that leads to lesions in tissues. Confusion factors such as smoking, alcohol drinking and meat barbecue consumption were factors blurring results in epidemiological studies (Bastos et al, 2007).

One important problem in yerba mate production chain is the contamination of *mate* products with polycyclic aromatic hydrocarbons (PAH) that are potential carcinogenic compounds. They originate from the burning of wood traditionally used in the drying process. These compounds are hydrophobic and their contents in *mate* infusions are usually very low, but become important due to the large amount drunk per day per person (Bastos et al, 2007).

Fagundes et al (2006) evaluated the degree and sources of PAH exposure of the inhabitants of Southern Brazil. These authors measured 1-hydroxypyrene glucuronide, a metabolite derived from PAH in the urine of two hundred healthy adults (half male, half female; half smokers, half non-smokers). They suggested that both tobacco smoke and *mate* drinking contribute to high levels of benzo-α-pyrene exposure, a potential factor associated with esophageal cancer. They also stated that the increased metabolite presence in urine might be related not just with thermal injury but also with contaminants. This fact helps in explaining the increased risk of cancer previously reported in the region.

In a case-control study conducted in Argentina to investigate bladder cancer and *mate* consumption involving 114 pairs concluded that *mate* with *bombilla* consumed for the last 20 years by the subjects was associated with bladder cancer in ever-smokers but not in never-smokers. *Mate cocido* had no relationship with bladder cancer (Bates et al, 2007).

CONCLUSION

Yerba mate has been consumed for centuries but it has only been scientifically studied in the last two decades. The growing interest in *mate* products has made it paramount that research on this herbal tea continues, as it has shown extraordinary possibilities not only as a consumer beverage but also in the nutraceutical industry. Yet, there is much to be done: human-based studies to support the properties verified *in vitro* and *in vivo* models with animas are scarce. Besides, a necessary effort towards the improvement of the production chain is required to certificate quality with consistency. Nowadays most of the *mate* products lack quality in one way or another: huge differences in chemical composition from one harvest to another, the possible contamination with aromatic polycyclic hydrocarbons and the lack of microbiological control. Increasing number of *mate* products, growing interest by countries whose population and the nowadays more active research on the chemistry and functional properties of yerba mate may impulse a new era for this traditional South American product on the perspective of "environmentally correct, socially fair and economically feasible" from both producers and consumers (Bastos et al, 2007, Heck and De Mejia, 2007, Burris et al, 2012).

REFERENCES

Alta, M., Ramos, S., Mateos, B., Granado-Serrano, A. B., Bravo, L., & Goya, L. (2006). Quercetin Protects Human Hepatoma Hepg2 Against Oxidative Stress Induced By Tert-Butyl Hydroperoxide. *Toxicology and Applied Pharmacology*, *212*(2), 110–118. doi:10.1016/j.taap.2005.07.014 PMID:16126241

Andersen, T., & Fogh, W. J. (2001). Weight Loss and Delayed Gastric Emptying Following a South American Herbal Preparation in Overweight Patients. *Journal of Human Nutrition and Dietetics*, *14*(3), 243–250. doi:10.1046/j.1365-277X.2001.00290.x PMID:11424516

Anesini, C., Ferraro, G., & Filip, R. (2006). Peroxidase-Like Activity of *Ilex Paraguariensis. Food Chemistry*, *97*(3), 459–464. doi:10.1016/j.foodchem.2005.05.025

Athayde, M. I., Coelho, G. C., & Schenkel, E. P. (2000). Caffeine and Theobromine in Epicuticular Wax of *Ilex Paraguariensis* St.Hil. *Phytochemistry*, *55*(7), 853–857. doi:10.1016/S0031-9422(00)00324-1 PMID:11190409

Barros, S. G. S., Ghisolfi, E. S., Luz, L. P., Barlem, G. G., Vidal, R. M., Wolff, F. H., & Prolla, J. C. et al. (2000). Mate (Chimarrão) É Consumido Em Alta Temperature Por População Sob Risco Para O Carcinoma Epidermóide De Esófago. *Arquivos de Gastroenterologia*, *37*(1), 25–30. doi:10.1590/S0004-28032000000100006 PMID:10962624

Bastos, D. H. M., Moura de Oliveira, D., Texeira Matsumoto, R. L., Oliveira Carvalho, D., & Lima Ribeiro, M. (2007). *Yerba mate*: Pharmacological Properties, Research and Biotechnology. *Med. Arom. Plant Sci. Biotech.*, *1*(1), 37–46.

Bastos, D. M. H., Fornari, A. C., Queiroz, Y. S., Soares, R. A. M., & Torres, E. A. F. S. (2005). The Chlorogenic Acid and Caffeine Content of Yerba Mate (*Ilex Paraguariensis*) Beverages. *Acta Farm. Bonaer.*, *24*, 91–95.

Bastos, D. M. H., & Torres, E. A. F. S. (2003). Bebidas à Base de Erva-Mate (*Ilex Paraguariensis*) e Saúde Pública. *Nutrire: Rev. Soc. Bras. Aliment. Nutri.*, *26*, 77–89.

Bates, M. N., Hopenhayn, C., Rey, O. A., & Moore, L. E. (2007). Bladder Cancer and Mate Consumption in Argentina: A Case-Control Study. *Cancer Letters*, *246*(1-2), 268–273. doi:10.1016/j.canlet.2006.03.005 PMID:16616809

Bravo, I., Goya, L., & Lecumberri, E. (2007). LC/MS Characterization of Phenolic Constituents of Mate (*Ilex paraguariensis* St Hil.) and Its Antioxidant Activity Compared to Commonly Consumed Beverages. *Food Research International*, *11*, 401–407.

Burris, K. P., Harte, F. M., Michael Davidson, P., Neal Stewart, C. Jr, & Zivanovic, S. (2012). Composition and Bioactive Properties of Yerba Mate (*Ilex paraguariensis* A. St.-Hil.): A review. *Chilean J. Agric. Res.*, *72*(2), 268–274. doi:10.4067/S0718-58392012000200016

Calvino, A. (2005). Note: Caffeine Content and Dynamical Bitterness of Yerba Mate *Ilex paraguariensis* Infusions. *Food Science & Technology International*, *11*(6), 401–407. doi:10.1177/1082013205060624

Carini, M., Facino, R. M., Aldini, G., Calloni, M., & Colombo, L. (1998). Characterization of Phenolic Antioxidants from Mate (*Ilex paraguariensis*) by Liquid Chromatography Mass Spectrometry and Liquid Chromatography Tandem Mass Spectrometry. *Rapid Communications in Mass Spectrometry*, *12*(22), 1813–1819. doi:10.1002/(SICI)1097-0231(19981130)12:22<1813::AID-RCM379>3.0.CO;2-#

Cruz, M. J. S., Garitta, L. V., & Hough, G. (2003). Note: Relationships of consumer acceptability and sensory attributes of Yerba Mate (*Ilex paraguariensis* St. Hil.) using preference mapping. *Food Science & Technology International*, *9*(5), 347–362. doi:10.1177/1082013203038376

Dickel, M. I., Rates, S. M., & Ritter, M. R. (2007). Plants Popularly Used for Losing Weight Purposes in Porto Alegre, South Brazil. *Journal of Ethnopharmacology*, *109*(1), 60–71. doi:10.1016/j.jep.2006.07.003 PMID:16963210

Drinkine, J., Lopes, P., Kennedy, J. A., Teissedre, P. L., & Saucier, C. (2007). Ethylidene-Bridged Flavan-3-ols in Red Wine and Correlation With Wine Age. *Journal of Agricultural and Food Chemistry*, *55*(15), 6292–6299. doi:10.1021/jf070038w PMID:17602645

Fagundes, R. B., Abnet, C. C., Strickland, P. T., Kamangar, F., Roth, M. J., Taylor, P. R., & Dawsey, S. M. (2006). Higher Urine 1-Hydroxy Pyrene Glucuronide (1-OHPG) is Associated with Tobacco Smoke Exposure and Drinking Mate in Healthy Subjects from Rio Grande do Sul, Brazil. *BMC Cancer*, *6*(1), 139–145. doi:10.1186/1471-2407-6-139 PMID:16729889

Ferreira, F., Vázquez, A., Güntner, C., & Moyna, P. (1997). Inhibition of the Passive Diffusion of Chol. Acid by the *Ilex Paraguariensis* St. Hil. saponins. *Phytotherapy Research*, *11*(1), 79–81. doi:10.1002/(SICI)1099-1573(199702)11:1<79::AID-PTR34>3.0.CO;2-R

Filip, R., Lotito, S. B., Ferraro, G., & Praga, C. G. (2000). Antioxidant Activity of *Ilex paraguariensis* and Related Species. *Nutrition Research (New York, N.Y.)*, *20*(10), 1437–1446. doi:10.1016/S0271-5317(00)80024-X

Gorgen, M., Turatti, K., Medeiros, A. R., Buffon, A., Bonan, C. D., Sarkis, J. J., & Pereira, G. S. (2005). Aqueous Extract of *Ilex paraguariensis* Decreases Nucleotide Hydrolysis in Rat Blood Serum. *Journal of Ethnopharmacology*, *97*(1), 73–77. doi:10.1016/j.jep.2004.10.015 PMID:15652278

Gorzalczany, S., Filip, R., Alonso, M. R., Mino, J., Ferraro, G. E., & Acevedo, C. (2001). Choleretic Effect and Intestinal Propulsion of 'Mate' (*Ilex paraguariensis*) and its Substitutes or Adulterants. *Journal of Ethnopharmacology*, *75*(2-3), 291–294. doi:10.1016/S0378-8741(01)00179-9 PMID:11297866

Gosmann, G., Guillaume, D., Taketa, A. T., & Schenkel, E. P. (1995). Triterpenoid Saponins from *Ilex paraguariensis*. *Journal of Natural Products*, *58*(3), 438–441. doi:10.1021/np50117a015 PMID:7775986

Heck, C. I., & De Mejia, E. G. (2007). Yerba Mate Tea (*Ilex paraguariensis*): A Comprehensive Review on Chemistry, Health Implications and Technological Considerations. *Journal of Food Science*, *72*(9), 138–151. doi:10.1111/j.1750-3841.2007.00535.x PMID:18034743

Isolabella, S., Cogoi, L., Lopes, P., Anesini, C., Ferraro, G., & Filip, R. (2010). Study of the Bioactive Compounds Variation During Yerba Mate (*Ilex paraguariensis*) Processing. *Food Chemistry*, *122*(3), 695–699. doi:10.1016/j.foodchem.2010.03.039

Ito, E., Crozier, A., & Ashihara, H. (1997). Theophylline Metabolism in Higher Plants. *Biochimica et Biophysica Acta*, *1336*(2), 323–330. doi:10.1016/S0304-4165(97)00045-7 PMID:9305805

Jacques, R. A., dos Santos Freitas, I., Perez, V. F., Dariva, C., de Oliveira, A. P., de Oliveira, J. V., & Caramao, E. B. (2007). The Use of Ultrasound in the Extraction of *Ilex paraguariensis* Leaves: A Comparison with Maceration. *Ultrasonics Sonochemistry*, *14*(1), 6–12. doi:10.1016/j.ultsonch.2005.11.007 PMID:16439181

Kawakami, M., & Kobayashi, A. (1991). Volatile Constituents of Green Mate and Roasted Mate. *Journal of Agricultural and Food Chemistry*, *39*(7), 1275–1279. doi:10.1021/jf00007a016

Kubo, K., Saito, M., Tadokoro, T., & Mackawa, A. (1997). Changes in Susceptibility of Tissues to Lipid Peroxidation after Ingestion of Various Levels of Docosahexanoic Acid and Vitamin E. *The British Journal of Nutrition*, *78*(04), 655–669. doi:10.1079/BJN19970181 PMID:9389890

Ley, J. P., Blings, M., Paetz, S., Krammer, G. B., & Bertram, H. J. (2006). New bitter-masking compounds: Hydroxylated benzoic acid amides of aromatic amines as structural analogues of homoeriodictyol. *Journal of Agricultural and Food Chemistry*, *54*(22), 8574–8579. doi:10.1021/jf0617061 PMID:17061836

Lunceford, N., & Gugliucci, A. (2005). *Ilex paraguariensis* extracts inhibit AGE formation more efficiently than green tea. *Fitoterapia*, *76*(5), 419–427. doi:10.1016/j.fitote.2005.03.021 PMID:15894431

Ma, W. W., Heinstein, P. P., & McLaughlin, J. L. (1989). Additional Toxic, Bitter Saponins from the Seeds of *Chenopodium quinoa. Journal of Natural Products*, *52*(5), 1132–1135. doi:10.1021/np50065a035 PMID:2607350

Mosimann, A. L., Wilhelm-Filho, D., & Da Silva, E. L. (2006). Aqueous extract of *Ilex paraguariensis* attenuates the progression of atherosclerosis in cholesterol-fed rabbits. *BioFactors (Oxford, England)*, *26*(1), 59–70. doi:10.1002/biof.5520260106 PMID:16614483

Mozzafera, P. (1997). Mate Drinking: Caffeine and Phenolic Acid Intake. *Food Chemistry*, *60*(1), 67–71. doi:10.1016/S0308-8146(96)00311-1

Pittler, M. H., & Ernst, E. (2004). Dietary supplements for body-weight reduction: A systematic review. *The American Journal of Clinical Nutrition*, *79*, 529–536. PMID:15051593

Reginatto, F. H., Athayde, M. L., Gosmann, G., & Schenkel, E. P. (1999). Methylxantines Accumulation in *Ilex* Species – Caffeine and Theobromine in Erva-Mate (*Ilex paraguariensis*) and Other *Ilex* Species. *Journal of the Brazilian Chemical Society*, *10*(6), 443–446. doi:10.1590/S0103-50531999000600004

Saldana, M. D., Zetzl, C., Mohamed, R. S., & Brunner, G. (2002). Extraction of Methylxantines from Guarana seeds, Mate leaves, and Cocoa Beans using Supercritical Carbon Dioxide and Ethanol. *Journal of Agricultural and Food Chemistry*, *50*(17), 4820–4826. doi:10.1021/jf020128v PMID:12166966

Sari, F., Turkmen, N., Polat, G., & Velioghi, Y. S. (2007). Total polyphenol, antioxidant and antibacterial activities of black mate tea. *Food Science and Technology Research*, *13*(3), 265–269. doi:10.3136/fstr.13.265

Schinella, G. R., Troiani, G., Davila, V., de Buschiazzo, P. M., & Tournier, H. A. (2000). Antioxidant Effects of an Aqueous Extract of *Ilex Paraguariensis. Biochemical and Biophysical Research Communications*, *269*(2), 357–360. doi:10.1006/bbrc.2000.2293 PMID:10708556

Schubert, A., Zanin, F. F., Pereira, D. F., & Athayde, M. L. (2006). Variação anual de metilxantinas totais em amostras de *Ilex paraguariensis* St. Hill. (erva-mate) en Ijuí e Santa Maria, Estado do Rio Grande do Sul. *Quimica Nova*, *29*(6), 1233–1236. doi:10.1590/S0100-40422006000600016

Stein, F. L. P., Schimidt, B., & Furlong, E. B. (2005). Vascular Responses to Extractable Fractions of *Ilex paraguariensis* in Rats Fed Standard and High Cholesterol Diets. *Biological Research for Nursing*, *7*(2), 146–156. doi:10.1177/1099800405280521 PMID:16267376

Takeda, A. T. (2004). Triterpenes and Triperpenoidal Glycosides from the Fruits of *Ilex Paraguariensis* (Mate). *Journal of the Brazilian Chemical Society*, *15*(2), 205–211. doi:10.1590/S0103-50532004000200008

Vinson, J. A., Jang, J., Dabbagh, Y. A., Serry, M. M., & Cai, S. (1995). Plant Polyphenols Exhibit Lipoprotein-Bound Antioxidant Activity using an *in vitro* Oxidation Model for Heart Disease. *Journal of Agricultural and Food Chemistry*, *43*(11), 2798–2799. doi:10.1021/jf00059a004

von Acker, S. A., de Groot, M. J., van der Berg, D. J., Tromp, M. N., Donne-Op den Keider, G., van der Vijgh, W. J., & Bast, A. (1996). A Quantum Chemical Explanation of the Antioxidant Activity of Flavonoids. *Chemical Research in Toxicology*, *9*(8), 1305–1312. doi:10.1021/tx9600964 PMID:8951233

Chapter 10
Health Benefits and Risks of Rice

Md Zakir Hossain Howlader
University of Dhaka, Bangladesh

Hossain Uddin Shekhar
University of Dhaka, Bangladesh

ABSTRACT

Rice is a fundamental food in many cultural cuisines around the world, and it is an important cereal crop that feeds more than half of the world's population. The two main categories are white rice and whole grain rice or bow ice. Whole grain rice is not processed very much, so it is high in nutritional value, whereas white rice is processed so that the bran or outer covering is removed, leaving it with less nutritional value. People choose different styles of rice for particular flavors, depending on their culinary needs, the availability, and the potential for healthy benefits as well.

INTRODUCTION

Rice is the seed of the grass species *Oryza sativa* (Asian rice) or *Oryza glaberrima* (African rice). As a cereal grain, it is the most widely consumed staple food for a large part of the world's human population, especially in Asia. It is the agricultural commodity with the third-highest worldwide production, after sugarcane and maize, according to 2012 FAOSTAT data (FAOSTAT, 2012). After corn, rice (Oryza sativa, L.) is the second most widely produced cereal crop in the world, with global paddy production reaching 720 million metric tons in 2012; yet it leads all cereals in supplying caloric energy to humans, accounting for 20% of the global dietary energy intake (FAO, 2004). Rice is grown in over 100 countries and on every continent except Antarctica, extending from 50° north latitude to 40° south latitude, and from sea level to an altitude of 3000 m (Juliano, 1993; Khush, 1997; Maclean, 2002). It is also grown under an extremely wide range of air temperatures (17–33°C) (Maclean, 2002; De Datta, 1981).

Rice is a semi-aquatic annual grass plant that includes approximately 22 species of the genus *Oryza,*of which 20 are wild. Two species of rice are important for human consumption: *O. sativa* and *O. glaberrima*. *O. sativa* was first grown in Southeast Asia, somewhere in India, Myanmar, Thailand,

DOI: 10.4018/978-1-5225-0591-4.ch010

North Vietnam, or China, between 8000 and 15,000 years ago. *O. glaberrima* is thought to have been domesticated from its wild ancestor *Oryza barthii* by people living in the floodplains of the Niger River in Africa about 3000 years ago. Today, rice is cultivated on every continent except Antarctica. Of the two cultivated species, *O. sativa* is more widely grown, including in Asia, North and South America, the European Union, the Middle East, and Africa. Cultivation of *O. glaberrima* is confined to Africa, where it is fast being replaced by *O. sativa*.

Thousands of *O. sativa* cultivars are grown in more than 100 countries. They can be classified into three widely cultivated ecological varieties: the long-grained indica variety grown in tropical and sub-tropical Asia; the short/medium-grained japonica rice cultivated in temperate regions such as Japan and northern China; and the medium grained javonica rice grown in the Philippines and the mountainous areas of Madagascar and Indonesia (IRRI, 2013). Rice is cultivated in a variety of water regimes and soil types, such as saline, alkaline, and acid–Sulphur soils. Irrigated lowland systems where rice is grown in bunded fields can produce two to three crops per year, and nearly three-quarters of the world rice production. Rain-fed lowland rice is grown in bunded fields that are flooded with rainwater. The areas of greatest poverty in South Asia, parts of Southeast Asia, and essentially all of Africa use rain-fed lowland farming to produce 20% of the world's rice. Upland rice farming done in dry land conditions produces 4% of the world's total rice production (IRRI, 2013).

RICE PRODUCTION

The world dedicated 162.3 million hectares in 2012 for rice cultivation and the total production was about 738.1 million tonnes. The average world farm yield for rice was 4.5 tonnes per hectare, in 2012(FAO, 2014). Rice is a major food staple and a mainstay for the rural population and their food security. It is mainly cultivated by small farmers in holdings of less than 1 hectare. Rice is also a wage commodity for workers in the cash crop or non-agricultural sectors. Rice is vital for the nutrition of much of the population in Asia, as well as in Latin America and the Caribbean and in Africa; it is central to the food security of over half the world population. Developing countries account for 95% of the total production, with China and India alone responsible for nearly half of the world output. (FAO, 2003).

Figure 1. Left: O. sativa with small wind-pollinated flowers; right: O. sativa, in different growing stages

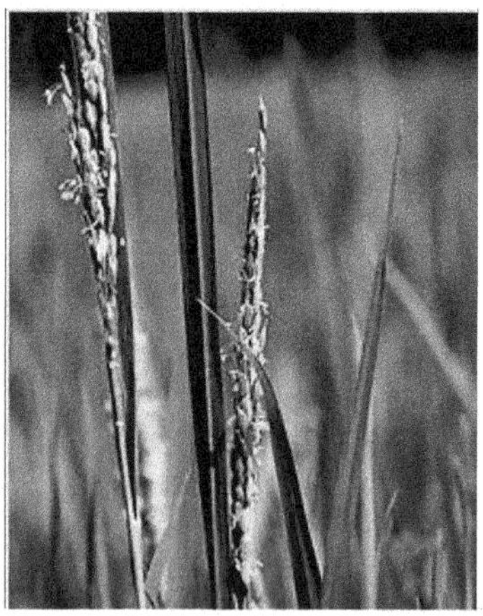

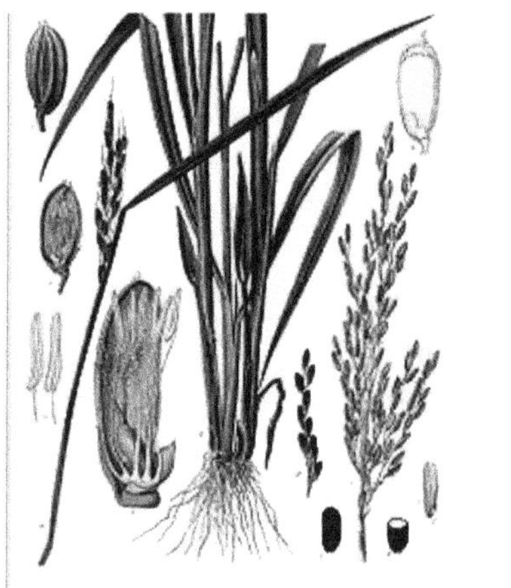

Figure 2. Rice can come in many shapes, colours, and sizes.
Photo by the IRRI.

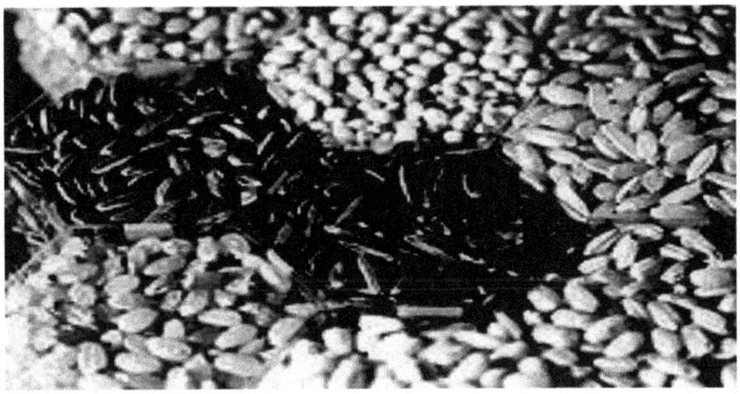

Record increases in rice production occurred during the last three decades of the twentieth century. The Green Revolution between the 1940s and the late 1960s resulted in an increase in agriculture production among the developing countries, mainly achieved through the transfer of a series of research and technology initiatives (FAO, 2006). While populations of low-income countries increased by 90% between 1966 and 2000, paddy rice production during the same period increased by 130%. World production of rice has risen steadily from about 200 million tonnes of paddy rice in 1960 to over 678 million tonnes in 2009. The three largest producers of rice in 2009 were China (197 million tonnes), India (131 Mt), and Indonesia (64 Mt) (Table 1).

About 84% of the rice-production growth has been attributed to modern farming technologies that have produced semi-dwarf, early-maturing rice varieties that can be planted up to three times per year and are responsive to nitrogen fertilizers (Khush, 2004; Maclean, 2002). These new rice varieties grown in irrigated land in half of the world's harvested area contribute to nearly three-quarters of the world's total rice production. Yield levels have doubled or tripled from the pre-Green Revolution average in many Asian countries. In Asia, the demand for rice is expected to increase by 70% over the next 30 years, driven

Table 1. Top 10 rice producers by country, 2012 (million metric ton)

China	204.3
India	152.6
Indonesia	69.0
Vietnam	43.7
Thailand	37.8
Bangladesh	33.9
Mayanmar	33.0
Philippines	18.0
Brazil	11.5
Japan	10.7

FAOSTAT, 2014.

primarily by population growth. (Hossain, 1997). Rice is currently grown in over a hundred countries that produce more than 715 million tons of paddy rice annually (480 million tons of milled rice;) (FAO, 2013). Fifteen countries account for 90% of the world's rice harvest. China and India alone account for around 50% of the rice grown. Together with Indonesia, Bangladesh, Vietnam, Myanmar, Thailand, the Philippines, Japan, Pakistan, Cambodia, the Republic of Korea, Nepal, and Sri Lanka, Asian countries account for 90% of the world's total rice production (Muthayya, S, 2012). Other major non-Asian rice producing countries include Brazil, the United States, Egypt, Madagascar, and Nigeria, which together account for 5% of the rice produced globally (FAO, 2013). In Africa, rice is the fastest growing food staple. Total cereal production in Africa has risen steadily from 9.3% in 1961 to 15.2% in 2007 (IRRI, 2013). However, only 54% of the rice consumption is supplied locally.

As of 2009 world food consumption of rice was 531.6 million metric tons of paddy equivalent (354,603 of milled equivalent), while the far largest consumers were China consuming 156.3 million metric tons of paddy equivalent (29.4% of the world consumption) and India consuming 123.5 million metric tons of paddy equivalent (23.3% of the world consumption) (Table 2) (FAO, FAOSTAT, 2012).

PROCESSING OF RICE

Rice (*Oryza sativa*) is one of the most important cereal crops in the world. It is a dietary staple that provides the bulk of daily calories for many companion animals and humans. The bran fraction of rice is a nutrient-rich by-product that has been primarily used as a low-cost feed for livestock and a fiber source in pet food. By-products from processing of rice can include rice hulls, rice bran, rice polishings, and broken rice grains. Rice is harvested from fields in the form of paddy rice in which each kernel is fully enveloped by a tough, fibrous hull. After the rice is dried, the first stage of the milling process is removal of the hull, which yields brown rice. Next, the outer layer is removed from the brown rice kernels to yield white rice. The separated outer (brown) layer is designated as rice bran (Elizabeth, 2011).

Table 2. food consumption of rice by country, 2009 (million metric ton of paddy equivalent)

World Total	531.6
China	156.3
India	123.5
Bangladesh	50.4
Indonesia	45.3
Vietnam	18.4
Philippines	17.0
Thailand	13.7
Japan	10.2
Myanmar	10.0
Brazil	10.0

FAO, FAOSTAT, 2012.

Rice Milling

Paddy rice is the end product of the harvesting and threshing of rice grains. It is usually harvested with about 20% moisture and dried down to about 14% so that it can be safely stored. The paddy rice is made up of an outer husk layer, germ and bran layers, and the endosperm. Various levels of milling can remove the outermost husk layer to yield brown rice kernels or further remove the bran and germ layers to yield white rice kernels. Milling can be undertaken using a single-pass, single-stage village mill in a one-step process or through amultistage process that involves the rice grain passing through a number of different operations and machines from paddy to brown or white rice (IRRI, 2013). On average, paddy rice produces 25% husk, 10% bran and germ, and 65% white rice (Chen et al., 1998).

Rice milling, however, results in the loss of a significant proportion of a number of B vitamins and minerals that are found predominately in the outer germ and bran layers (Figure 3) (Baurenfiend et al., 1991). Rice is a poor source of vitamins and minerals, and the milling process further depletes the grains of these micronutrients. Populations that subsist on rice are at high risk of vitamin and mineral deficiency (VMD). There are, however, opportunities to fortify rice with vitamins and minerals using various techniques to reduce losses during milling and/or add these micronutrients to milled rice. Nutrient losses during milling can be minimized by a process called partially steamed before drying and milling, resulting in some of the B vitamins migrating further into the grain (Manful, 2007).

Figure 3. Percent milling losses of vitamins and minerals from paddy rice to white rice
Baurenfiend et al., 1991.

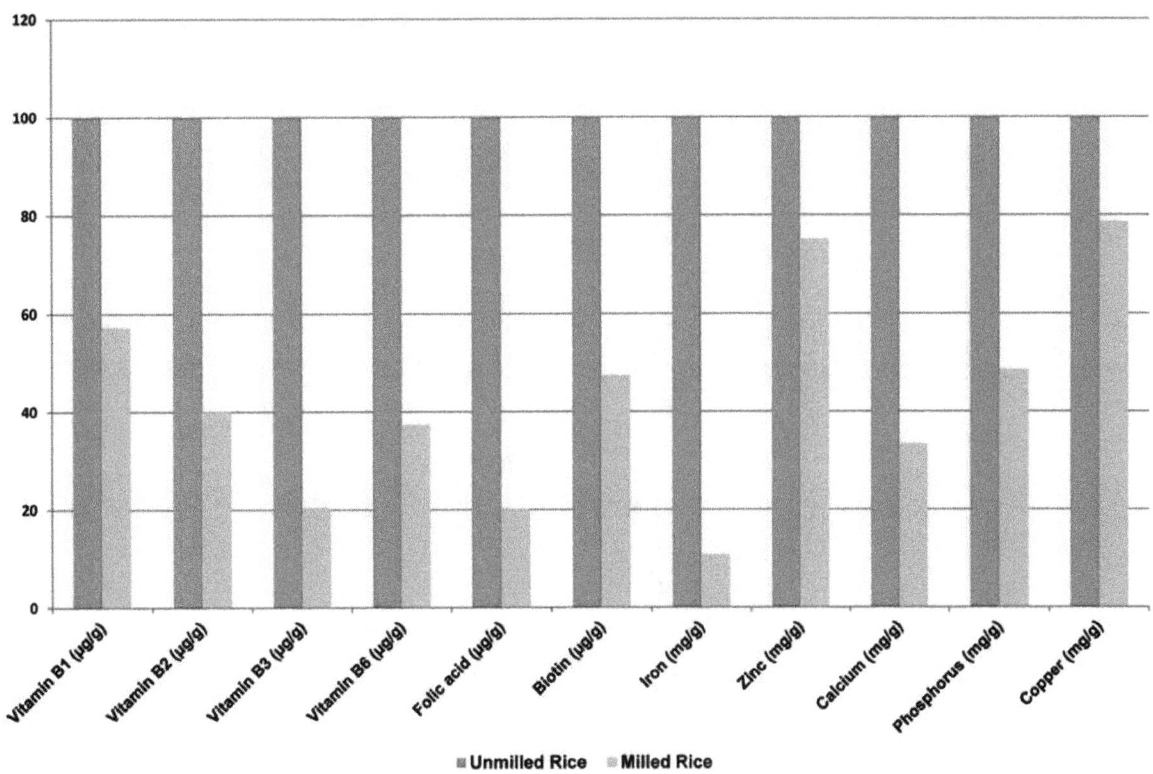

GRAIN STRUCTURE AND COMPOSITION

The rice grain (rough rice or paddy) consists of an outer protective covering, the hull, and the rice caryopsis or fruit (brown, cargo, dehulled or dehusked rice), (Figure 5). Brown rice consists of the outer layers of pericarp, seed-coat and nucellus; the germ or embryo; and the endosperm. The endosperm consists of the aleurone layer and the endosperm proper, consisting of the subaleurone layer and the starchy or inner endosperm. The aleurone layer encloses the embryo. Pigment is confined to the pericarp (Juliano & Bechtel, 1985).

The hull (husk) constitutes about 20 percent of the rough rice weight, but values range from 16 to 28 percent. The distribution of brown rice weight is pericarp 1 to 2 percent, aleurone plus nucellus and seed-coat 4 to 6 percent, germ 1 percent, scutellum 2 percent and endosperm 90 to 91 percent (Juliano, 1972). The aleurone layer varies from one to five cell layers; it is thicker at the dorsal than at the ventral side and thicker in short-grain than in long-grain rices (del Rosario et al., 1968). The aleurone and embryo cells are rich in protein bodies, containing globoids or phytate bodies, and in lipid bodies (Tanaka et al., 1973; Tanaka, Ogawa & Kasai, 1977).

The endosperm cells are thin-walled and packed with amyloplasts containing compound starch granules. The two outermost cell layers (the subaleurone layer) are rich in protein and lipid and have smaller amyloplasts and compound starch granules than the inner endosperm. The starch granules are polyhedral and mainly 3 to 9, µm in size, with unimodal distribution. Protein occurs mainly in the form of spherical protein bodies 0.5 to 4 µm in size throughout the endosperm (del Rosario et al., 1968; Bechtel & Pomeranz, 1978), but crystalline protein bodies and small spherical protein bodies are localized in the subaleurone

Figure 4. Longitudinal section of rice grain
Juliano, 1985b.

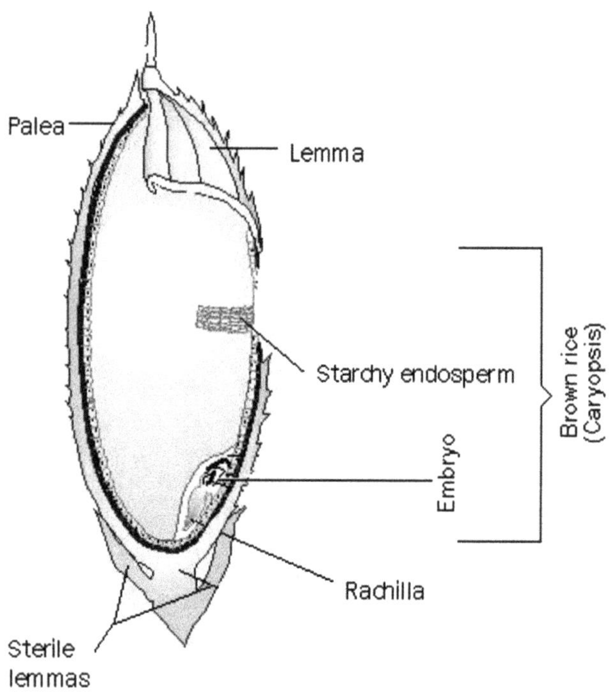

Figure 5. Schematic diagram of various protein bodies and compound starch granule in the endosperm subaleurone layer
Coffman & Juliano, 1987.

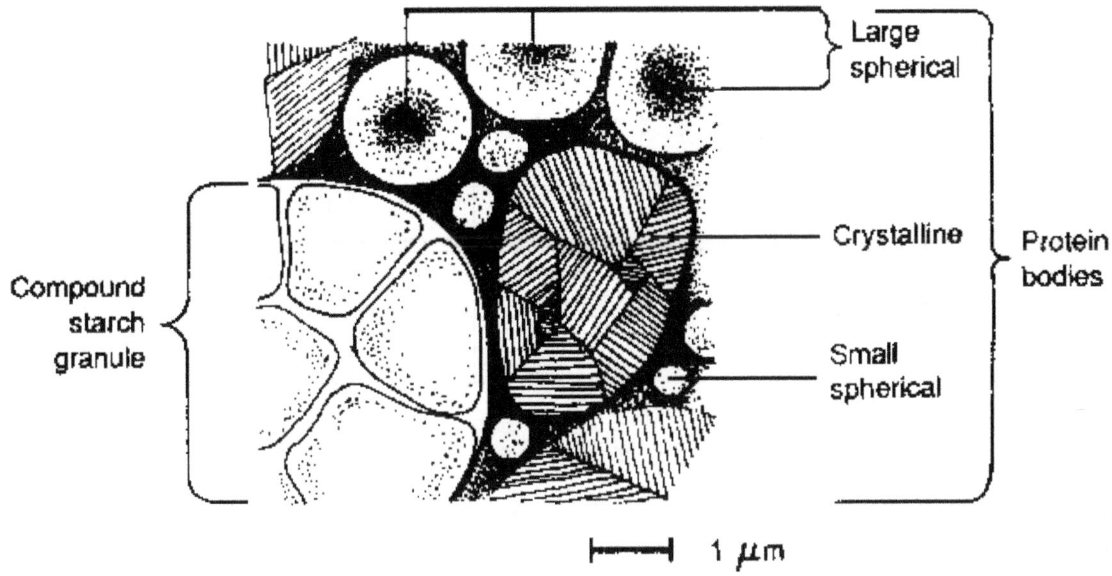

layer. The large spherical protein body corresponds to PB -I of Tanaka et al. (1980) and the crystalline protein body is identical to PB-II. Both PB-I and PB-II are distributed throughout the rice endosperm.

Non-waxy rice (containing amylose in addition to amylopectin) has a translucent endosperm, whereas waxy (0 to 2 percent amylose) rice has an opaque endosperm because of the presence of pores between and within the starch granules. Thus, waxy grain has about 95 to 98 percent the grain weight of non-waxy grain.

Gross Nutrient Composition

Among the milling fractions of rice, the bran has the highest energy and protein content and the hull has the lowest. Only the brown rice fraction is edible. Abrasive or friction milling to remove the pericarp, seed-coat, testa, aleurone layer and embryo to yield milled rice results in loss of fat, protein, crude and neutral detergent fibre, ash, thiamine, riboflavin, niacin and α-tocopherol. Available carbohydrates, mainly starch, are higher in milled rice than in brown rice. The gradients for the various nutrients are not identical as evidenced from analysis of successive milling fractions of brown rice and milled rice (Barber, 1972). Dietary fibre is highest in the bran layer (and the hull) and lowest in milled rice (Table 3). Density and bulk density are lowest in the hull, followed by the bran, and highest in milled rice because of the low oil content.

The B vitamins are concentrated in the bran layers, as is a-tocopherol (vitamin E), (Table 4). The rice grain has no vitamin A, vitamin D or vitamin C (FAO, 1954). The locational gradient in the whole rice grain is steeper for thiamine than for riboflavin and niacin, resulting in a lower percent retention of thiamine (vitamin B1) in milled rice (Table 4). About 50 percent of the total thiamine is in the scutellum and 80 to 85 percent of the niacin is in the pericarp plus aleurone layer (Hinton & Shaw, 1954).

Table 3. Proximate composition of rough rice and its milling fractions at 14 percent moisture

Rice Fraction	Crude Protein (g N x 5. 95)	Crude Fat (g)	Crude Fibre (g)	Crude Ash (g)	Available Carbohydrates (g)	Neutral Detergent Fibre (g)	Energy Content		Density (g/ml)	Bulk Density (g/ml)
							(kJ)	(kcal)		
Rough rice	5.8-7.7	1.5-2.3	7.2-10.4	2.9-5.2	64-73	16.4-19.2	1580	378	1.17-1.23	0.56-0.64
Brown rice	7.1-8.3	1.6-2.8	0.6-1.0	1.0-1.5	73-87	2.9-3.9	1520-1 610	363-385	1.31	0.68
Milled rice	6.3-7.1	0.3-0.5	0.2-0.5	0.3-0.8	77-89	0.7-2.3	1460-1 560	349-373	1.44-1.46	0.78-0.85
Rice bran	11.3-14.9	15.0-19.7	7.0-11.4	6.6-9.9	34-62	24-29	670-1 990	399-476	1.16-1.29	0.20-0.40
Rice hull	2.0-2.8	0.3-0.8	34.5-45.9	13.2-21.0	22-34	66-74	1110-1 390	265-332	0.67-0.74	0.10-0.16

Juliano, 1985b.

The embryo accounts for more than 95 percent of total tocopherols (of which α-tocopherols account for one-third) and nearly one-third of the oil content of the rice grain (Gopala Krishna, Prabhakar & Sen, 1984). By calculation, 65 percent of the thiamine of brown rice is in the bran, 13 percent in the polish and 22 percent in the milled rice fraction (Juliano & Bechtel, 1985). Corresponding values for riboflavin are 39 percent in the bran, 8 percent in the polish and 53 percent in the milled rice fraction. Niacin distribution is 54 percent in the bran, 13 percent in the polish and 33 percent in the milled rice fraction.

The minerals (ash) are also concentrated in the outer layers of brown rice or in the bran fraction (Table 4). A major proportion (90 percent) of the phosphorus in bran is phytin phosphorus. Potassium and magnesium are the principal salts of phytin. The ash distribution in brown rice is 51 percent in the bran, 10 percent in the germ, 10 percent in the polish and 28 percent in the milled rice fraction; iron, phosphorus and potassium show a similar distribution (Resurrecciόn, Juliano & Tanaka, 1979). However,

Table 4. Vitamin and mineral content of rough rice and its milling fractions at 14 percent moisture

Rice Fraction	Thiamine (mg)	Riboflavin (mg)	Niacin (mg)	α - Tocopherol (mg)	Calcium (mg)	Phosphorus (g)	Phytin P (g)	Iron (mg)	Zinc (mg)
Rough rice	0.26-0.33	0.06-0.11	2.9-5.6	0.90-2.00	10-80	0.17-0.39	0.18-0.21	1.4-6.0	1.7-3.1
Brown rice	0.29-0.61	0.04-0.14	3.5-5.3	0.90-2.50	10-50	0.17-0.43	0.13-0.27	0.2-5.2	0.6-2.8
Milled rice	0.02-0.11	0.02-0.06	1.3-2.4	75-0.30	10-30	0.08-0.15	0.02-0.07	0.2-2.8	0.6-2.3
Rice bran	1.20-2.40	0.18-0.43	26.7-49.9	2.60-13.3	30-120	1.1-2.5	0.9-2.2	8.6-43.0	4.3-25.8
Rice hull	0.09-0.21	0.05-0.07	1.6-4.2	0	60-130	0.03-0.07	0	3.9-9.5	0.9-4.0

Juliano, 1985.

some minerals show a relatively more even distribution in the grain: milled rice retained 63 percent of the sodium, 74 percent of the calcium and 83 percent of the Kjeldahl N content of brown rice (Juliano, 1985b).

Starch

Starch is the major constituent of milled rice at about 90 percent of the dry matter. Starch is a polymer of D-glucose linked α -(1-4) and usually consists of an essentially linear fraction, amylose, and a branched fraction, amylopectin. Branch points are α -(1-6) linkages. Innovative techniques have now shown rice amylose to have two to four chains with a number-average degree of polymerization (DP_n) of 900 to glucose units and a ß-amylolysis limit of 73 to 87 percent (Hizukuri et al., 1989). It is a mixture of benched and linear molecules with DP_n of 1100 to 1700 and 700 to 900, respectively. The branched fraction constitutes 25 to 50 percent by number and 30 to 60 percent by weight of amylose. The iodine affinity of rice amyloses is 20 to 21 percent by weight.

Based on colorimetric starch-iodine colour absorption standards at 590 to 620 nm, milled rice is classified as waxy (1 to 2 percent), very low amylose (2 to 12 percent), low amylose (12 to 20 percent), intermediate (20 to 25 percent) and high (25 to 33 percent) amylose rice, (Juliano, 1979, 1985b). Recent studies showed that the maximum true amylose content is 20 percent and that additional iodine binding is due to the long linear chains in amylopectin (Takeda, Hizukuri & Juliano, 1987). Hence colorimetric amylose values are now termed "apparent amylose content". The waxy endosperm is opaque and shows air spaces between the starch granules, which have a lower density than non-waxy granules. The structure of the starch granule is still not well understood, but crystallinity and staling are attributed to the amylopectin fraction.

Protein

Endosperm (milled rice) protein consists of several fractions comprising 15 percent albumin (water soluble) plus globulin (salt soluble), 5 to 8 percent prolamin (alcohol soluble) and the rest glutelin (alkali soluble), (Juliano, 1985b). Using sequential protein extraction, the mean ratio for 33 samples was found to be 9 percent prolamin, 7 percent albumin plus globulin and 84 percent glutelin (Huebner et al.,

Table 5. Amino acid content of rough rice and its milling fractions at 14 percent moisture (g per 16 g N)

Rice Fraction	Histidine	Isoleucine	Leucine	Lysine + Cysteine	Methionine + Tyrosine	Phenylalanine	Threonine	Tryptophan	Valine	Amino Acid Score[a]
Rough rice	1.5-2.8	3.0-4.8	6.9-8.8	3.2-4.7	4.5-6.2	9.3-10.8	3.0-4.5	1.2-2.0	4.6-7.0	55-81
Brown rice	2.3-2.5	3.4-4.4	7.9-8.5	3.7-4.1	4.4-4.6	8.6-9.3	3.7-3.8	1.2-1.4	4.8-6.3	64-71
Milled rice	2.2-2.6	3.5-4.6	8.0-8.2	3.2-4.0	4.3-5.0	9.3-10.4	3.5-3.7	1.2-1.7	4.7-6.5	55-69
Rice bran	2.7-3.3	2.7-4.1	6.9-7.6	4.8-5.4	4.2-4.8	7.7-8.0	3.8-4.2	0.6-1.2	4.9-6.0	83-93
Rice hull	1.6-2.0	3.2-4.0	8.0-8.2	3.8-5.4	3.5-3.7	6.6-7.3	4.2-5.0	0.6	5.5-7.5	66-93

Juliano, 1985b.

1990). The mean prolamin content of seven IRRI milled rices was 6.5 percent of their total protein (IRRI, 1991b). The lysine content of rice protein is 3.5 to 4.0 percent, one of the highest among cereal proteins.

Rice bran proteins are richer in albumin than endosperm proteins and are found as distinct protein bodies containing globoids in the aleurone layer and the germ. These structures are different from endosperm protein bodies. Tanaka et al. (1973) reported the presence of 66 percent albumin, 7 percent globulin and 27 percent prolamin plus glutelin in aleurone protein bodies. Ogawa, Tanaka and Kasai (1977) reported the presence of 98 percent albumin in embryo protein bodies.

The endosperm protein is localized mainly in protein bodies (Figure 6). The crystalline (PB-II) protein bodies are rich in glutelin, and the large spherical protein bodies (PB-I) are rich in prolamin. Ogawa et al. (1987) estimated that endosperm storage proteins were composed of 60 to 65 percent PB-II proteins, 20 to 25 percent PB-I proteins and 10 to 15 percent albumin and globulin in the cytoplasm. Rice starch granule amylose binds up to 0.7 percent protein that is mainly the waxy gene protein or granule-bound starchy synthase, with a molecular mass of about 60 kilodaltons (kd), (Villareal & Juliano, 1989b).

Rice glutelin consists of three acidic or α- subunits of 30 to 39 kd and two basic or β-subunits of 19 to 25 kd (Kagawa, Hirano & Kikuchi, 1988). The two kinds of subunits are formed by cleavage of a 57-kd polypeptide precursor (Sugimoto, Tanaka & Kasai, 1986). Prolamin consists mainly (90 percent) of the 13- kd subunit plus two minor subunits of 10 and 16 kd (Hibino et al., 1989). The essential amino acid contents of the glutelin and prolamin subunits (Table 6) showed lysine as limiting in these polypeptides except in the 13-kd prolamin subunit, which has 5.5 percent lysine and is limiting in methionine plus cysteine. Thus, glutelin has a better amino acid score than prolamin except for the 16-kd prolamin subunit. The 10-kd prolamin subunit has a high (6.8 percent) cysteine content.

Lipid

The lipid or fat content of rice is mainly in the bran fraction (20 percent, dry basis), specifically as lipid bodies or spherosomes in the aleurone layer and bran; however, about 1.5 to 1.7 percent is present in milled rice, mainly as non-starch lipids extracted by ether, chloroform-methanol and cold water-saturated

Table 6. Aminogram (g/16 g N) of the acidic and basic subunits of rice glutelin and the major and minor subunits of prolamin

Amino Acid	Glutelin Subunits[a]		Prolamin Subunits		
	30-39 kd (Acidic)	19-25 kd (Basic)	13 kd	10 kd	16 kd
Histidine	2.2-2.5	2.6-2.7	2.0-2.4	1.7	4.2
Isoleucine	3.2-3.3	4.1-4.9	3.8-5.4	1.6	3.6
Leucine	6.4-7.5	7.0-8.5	17.9-26.4	4.7	8.1
Lysine	2.2-3.0	3.0-4.1	0.4-5.5	1.0	3.3
Methionine + cystine[b]	0.2-1.9	0.1-2.4	0.7-1.2	22.5	5.3
Phenylalanine + tyrosine	10.0-10.5	10.1-10.8	12.7-21.6	4.3	7.6
Threonine	2.8-3.7	2.5-3.7	1.8-2.8	6.8	2.7
Valine	5.1-5.7	5.7-7.0	2.7-3.9	4.4	3.9
Amino acid score[c] (%)	38-52	52-71	7-8[d]	18	57

butanol (Juliano & Goddard, 1986; Tanaka et al., 1978). Protein bodies, particularly the core, are rich in lipids (Choudhury & Juliano, 1980; Tanaka et al., 1978). The major fatty acids of these lipids are linoleic, oleic and palmitic acids (Hemavathy & Prabhaker, 1987; Taira, Nakagahra & Nagamine, 1988). Essential fatty acids in rice oil are about 29 to 42 percent linoleic acid and 0.8 to 1.0 percent linolenic acid (Jaiswal, 1983). The content of essential fatty acids may be increased with temperature during grain development, but at the expense of reduction in total oil content (Taira, Taira & Fujii, 1979).

Non-Starch Polysaccharides

Non-starch polysaccharides consist of water soluble polysaccharides and insoluble dietary fibre (Juliano, 1985b). They can complex with starch and may have a hypocholesterolaemic effect (Normand, Ory & Mod, 1981; Normand et al., 1984). The endosperm has a lower content of dietary fibre than the rest of brown rice (Shibuya, 1989). Reported values for neutral detergent fibre are 0.7 to 2.3 percent (Juliano, 1985b). In addition, the endosperm or milled rice cell wall has a low lignin content but a high content of pectic substances or pectin. Endosperm pectin has a higher uronic acid content but a lower arabinose-to-xylose ratio than the other grain tissues. The hemicellulose of endosperm also has a lower arabinose-toxylose ratio than the three other grain tissues.

HEALTH BENEFITS OF RICE

Rice has been part of the human diet for thousands of years. Historical evidence suggests that rice may have been produced and consumed up to 10,000 years ago. This, alongside its current global status as the world's most important human food, makes rice production responsible for feeding more people over a longer period than any other crop.

The health benefits of rice include its ability to provide fast and instant energy, regulate and improve bowel movements, stabilize blood sugar levels, and slow down the aging process, while also providing an essential source of vitamin B1 to the human body. Other benefits include its ability to boost skin health, increase the metabolism, aid in digestion, reduce high blood pressure, help weight loss efforts, improve the immune system and provide protection against dysentery, cancer, and heart disease. Rice is a fundamental food in many cultural cuisines around the world, and it is an important cereal crop that feeds more than half of the world's population.

Brown rice has a greater food value than white, since the outer brown coatings contain the proteins and minerals; the white endosperm is chiefly carbohydrate. As a food rice is low in fat and (compared with other cereal grains) in protein. The miracle rices have grains richer in protein than the old varieties.

Rice, being one of the most produced and consumed cereals in the world, has an important role in the relation between the diet and health. Several compounds with antioxidant activity have been identified in rice, including phenolic compounds, tocopherols, tocotrienols and γ-oryzanol (Iqbal et al., 2005). The phenolic compounds are mainly associated with the pericarp in rice, hence, the milling process reduces the concentration of these compounds in the grain. Besides, grains with darker pericarp colour, such as red and black rice, contain higher amounts of polyphenols (Tian et al., 2004; Zhou et al., 2004). The concentration of total phenolics in the grain has been positively associated with the antioxidant activity (Itani et al., 2002; Goffman & Bergman, 2004; Zhang et al., 2006), with potential beneficial effects on health, such as reduction of oxidative stress (Ling et al., 2001; Hu et al., 2003), aid in the prevention of cancer (Hudson et al., 2000; Hu et al., 2003; Hyun & Chung, 2004; Chen et al., 2006), in the control of blood lipids and related diseases, which may help in the prevention of cardiovascular problems (Ling et al., 2001), and in the prevention of the complications of diabetes (Morimitsu et al., 2002; Yawadio et al., 2007).

The antioxidant compounds in rice were classified into six groups:

1. Phenolic acids,
2. Flavonoids,
3. Anthocyanins and proanthocyanidins,
4. Tocopherols and tocotrienols (vitamin E),
5. γ-oryzanol, and
6. Phytic acid.

The first three groups are referred to collectively as phenolic compounds. Phenolic compounds may exert their antioxidant activity in different ways. They may directly scavenge some reactive species, including hydroxyl, peroxyl and superoxide radicals, acting as chain breaking antioxidants. They may suppress lipid peroxidation recycling other antioxidants, such as α-tocopherol. Some phenolic compounds may bind pro-oxidant metals, such as iron and copper, preventing the formation of free radicals from these pro-oxidants while simultaneously maintaining their capacity to scavenge free radicals (Moran et al., 1997; Kris-Etherton et al.,2003; Halliwell, 2007). Besides, the effects of some phenolics are related to the increase in the activity of antioxidant enzymes (Chiang et al., 2006) and induction of the synthesis of antioxidant proteins (Chung et al., 2006).

ANTIOXIDANT ACTIVITY AND BIOLOGICAL EFFECT

The concentration of total phenolics in the rice grains has been positively correlated with the antioxidant activity (Itani et al., 2002; Goffman & Bergman, 2004; Zhang et al., 2006). In red pericarp grains, a high correlation was observed between this activity and the content of proanthocyanidins, but in the case of black pericarp grains the correlation depended on the content of anthocyanins (Oki et al., 2002). These results suggested that the phenolic compounds were among the main responsible ones for the antioxidant activity of rice grains (Goffman & Bergman, 2004). Usually, grains with red and black pericarp presented higher antioxidant activity than those with light brown pericarp colour (Nam et al., 2005). Goffman and Bergman (2004), evaluating the genotypes with different pericarp colour, observed the values of antioxidant activity between 10.0 and 13.1μM TE (Trolox equivalent) g-1 bran for the grains with light brown pericarp, between 119.9 and 312.3μM TE g-1 bran for red pericarp grains and between 56.3 e 345.3μM TE g-1 bran for black pericarp grains. These results also demonstrated that, besides the variation in the antioxidant activity among grains with different pericarp colour, variation in a group of grains with the same pericarp colour was also observed. Besides the difference in the total antioxidant activity, differences have also been observed among the genotypes in the ability to scavenge the reactive oxygen species. Nam et al. (2005) reported reduction in the concentration of superoxide anions by competitively inhibiting xanthine oxidase (enzyme that induces the formation of reactive oxygen species in the cells), and scavenged hydroxyl radicals through direct mechanism. On the other hand, another genotype scavenged superoxide anions without affecting the activity of xanthine oxidase, and reduced hydroxyl radicals through binding ferrous ion. This showed that the antioxidant compounds present in these grains might act in different ways to reduce the oxidative stress in the organism and, with that, help in the prevention of several diseases.

The reduction of the oxidative stress by polyphenols in rice grains was observed in in vitro and ex vivo studies, indicated by the reduction in the production of nitric oxide (Hu et al., 2003) and in the concentration of reactive oxygen species (Hu et al., 2003; Chiang et al., 2006). Simultaneously to the reduction in the indicators of oxidation, an increase in the antioxidant capacity was observed, including higher total antioxidant capacity and increased activity of antioxidant enzymes, such as superoxide dismutase and catalase (Chiang et al., 2006). Studies with cell cultures have shown that phenolic compounds in the rice may also be associated with antimutagenic, anticarcinogenic and antimetastasis activities, due to their ability to directly protect the DNA against the damage and affect cell proliferation (Hu et al., 2003; Chen et al., 2006). Using the extracts obtained from the rice grains with light brown pericarp colour, a reduction in the number of viable cells and colony formation of breast and colon cancer cells was observed (Hudson et al., 2000).

Although in vitro studies can give some information about the antioxidant activity and possible biological effects of rice phenolics, the relevance of this information to antioxidant effectiveness in the organism is very limited without data on their bioavailability and metabolism (Collins, 2005). The bioavailability differs greatly from one polyphenol to another due to several factors, such as food matrix, concentration of the polyphenol in the food, background diet and interindividual variations, affecting the concentration of active metabolites in the organism (Manach et al., 2005; Zhao & Moghadasian, 2008). However, few studies have been developed to evaluate the antioxidant properties of rice phenolics in vivo, and most of them used animal models instead of humans. Studies with animals have shown beneficial effects of the consumption of the colored fraction (pericarp) of rice grains on the control of blood lipids and related diseases, helping in the prevention of cardiovascular problems. In these studies, with apolipoprotein (apo)E-deficient mice (Xia et al., 2003) and hypercholesterolemic rabbits (Ling et al., 2001), the supplementation of the diet with the pericarp of the rice reduced the occurrence of atherosclerotic plaques. This effect was related to different mechanisms, including the increase in the antioxidant capacity of the organism (Ling et al., 2001), reduction in the total cholesterol concentration in the blood (Xia et al.,2003), reduction in the ratio between LDL and HDL cholesterol (Ling et al., 2001; Xia et al., 2003), reduction in the accumulation of cholesterol in the aorta tissue and reduction in the oxidation of LDL cholesterol (Xia et al., 2003).

Rice possesses different compounds with antioxidant activity, including polyphenols, but variations are observed in the concentration of these compounds in the grains, mainly due to genotype, pericarp colour and processing. Although rice is not among the foods with higher concentrations of phenolic compounds, it may be an important source of these compounds due to its wide utilization in feeding.

Flavonoid Composition of Rice

Similar to phenolic acid, flavonoids are synthesized by the phenylpropanoid metabolic pathway. Most flavonoids have absorption maxima at 370 nm. Flavonoids consist of a 15-carbon skeleton that is organized in two aromatic rings (A- and B-rings) interlinked by a three-carbon chain (structure C6-C3-C6). Flavonoids are recognized for both their ability to donate electrons and to stop chain reactions. These activities are attributed to the phenolic hydroxyls, particularly in the 3′OH and 4′OH of the three-carbon chain (Ramarathnam et al. 1989a; Hudson et al. 2000; Kim et al. 2010; Cho et al. 2013). Of the seven flavonoids that are usually reported in rice, tricin appears to be the major flavonoid in the bran, accounting for 77% of all seven flavonoids (131.5 mg/100 g). The other flavonoids are present in the following order: luteolin (14%) > apigenin (6%) > quercetin (3%) > isorhamnetin (1%) > kaempferol (<1%) > myricetin (<1%).

Anthocyanin and Proanthocyanidin Composition of Rice

Anthocyanins, another class of flavonoids, which exhibit maximum absorbance in the green/blue spectrum at 510 nm, are water-soluble glycosides of polyhydroxyl and polymethoxyl derivatives of 2-phenylbenzopyrylium or flavylium (2-phenylchromenylium) salts. About 18 anthocyanins have been identified in rice, of which only four have been quantified (cyanidin-3-O-glucoside, peonidin-3-O-glucoside, cyanidin-3-O-rutinoside, and cyanidin-3-O-galactoside). The mean value of the sum of the four anthocyanins in pigmented rice varieties is 1252.7 mg/100 g and 345.8 mg/100 g for the bran and the whole grain, respectively. The anthocyanin content of rice varies more widely than does the phenolic acid content. (Hirawan et al. 2011; Goufo et al. 2014a; Sriseadka et al. 2013).

Tocopherol and Tocotrienol Composition of Rice

Tocotrienols and tocopherols are known collectively as vitamin E or tocols as they share a common basic structural unit based on an amphiphilic 6-chromanol ring and a terpenoid side chain located at position 2 of the ring. The chromanol head group can be joined to a saturated phytyl side chain to form tocopherols, or to an unsaturated geranylgeranyl side chain to form tocotrienols. The head group can then be methylated in different configurations, resulting in four alternative forms (a, b, c, and d). The free hydroxyl group on the chromanol ring is responsible for the antioxidant properties, and the hydrogen atom from this group can be donated to free radicals, resulting in a resonance-stabilized vitamin E radical (Qureshi et al. 2000; Xu et al. 2001; Kim 2005). In nonpigmented rice varieties, the mean vitamin E content is 14.5, 247.2, 60.2, and 3.0 mg/kg for the endosperm, bran, whole grain, and husk, respectively. A positive correlation between c-tocotrienol and vitamin E content was observed, but only a loose correlation between the total tocopherol and total tocotrienol content was found (Sookwong et al. 2007). Overall, tocotrienols account for 47–80% of the total vitamin E content, and tocopherols for 20–53%. In heated rice bran, two novel tocotrienols were isolated and characterized as desmethyl and didesmethyl tocotrienols (Qureshi et al. 2000). The unsaturated tocotrienols were found to have greater antioxidant properties, which are probably related to the fact that their structures have fewer methyl groups and hence lower steric hindrance impeding their penetration into membranes.

Steryl Ferulate (γ-Oryzanol) Composition of Rice

Gamma-oryzanol is a mixture of steryl ferulates, which are formed by esterification of the hydroxyl group of sterols (campesterol, stigmasterol, b-sitosterol) or triterpene alcohols (cycloartanol, cycloartenol, 24-methylenecycloartanol, cyclobranol) with the carboxylic acid group of ferulic acid (Jeng et al. 2012). Sterols with a saturated steroid skeleton are known

as stanols, whereas compounds containing a double bond between C5 and C6 or between C7 and C8 are referred to as sterols. Methyl groups at C4 affect the antioxidant properties of steryl ferulates (Mandak & Nystrom 2012). On the basis of their absorbance maxima at 330 nm, at least 25 components of γ

-oryzanol have been identified so far, with five of them comprising about 95% of the total γ -oryzanol content (Miller & Engel 2006). In nonpigmented rice varieties, the mean value of these five components is 58.9, 3067.1, and 288.6 mg/kg for the endosperm, bran, and whole grain, respectively.

Several studies have reported health benefits of γ -oryzanol, such as its antioxidant activity, improvement of plasma lipid pattern, reduction of total plasma cholesterol and increase of HDL cholesterol levels, and inhibition of the platelet aggregation (Cicero and Gaddi, 2001). Gamma aminobutyric acid (GABA) is a non-protein amino acid compound that is synthesized from glutamic acid by glutamate decarboxylase (GAD). GABA is a neurotransmitter in the brain and spinal cord of mammals (Banchuen et al., 2009). It can regulate blood pressure, heart rate, sensations of pain and anxiety, lipid levels in serum and assist in insulin secretion to prevent diabetes. In addition to rice grain, several studies on bioactive compounds of germinated rice have also been reported (Varanyanond et al. 2005; Lin & Lai, 2011).

RISKS OF RICE CONSUMPTION

Eating white rice on a regular basis may increase the risk for type 2 diabetes, according to new Harvard School of Public Health (HSPH) research. HSPH researchers from the Department of Nutrition—led by Emily Hu,—reviewed four earlier studies involving more than 352,000 people from China, Japan, the United States, and Australia who were tracked between four and 22 years. The researchers found that people who ate the most rice—three to four servings a day—were 1.5 times more likely to have diabetes than people who ate the least amount of rice. In addition, for every additional large bowl of white rice a person ate each day, the risk rose 10 percent. The link was stronger for people in Asian countries, who eat an average of three to four servings of white rice per day. People in Western countries eat, on average, one to two servings a week (Hu et al. 2012).

Rice has been a staple food in Asian countries for centuries. By the twentieth century, the advance of grain-processing technology made it possible for large scale production of refined grains (Miller, 2002) . Through refining processes, the outer bran and germ portions of intact rice grains (i.e., brown rice) is removed to produce white rice that primarily consists of starchy endosperm. Although not entirely consistent, consumption of white rice, in general, generates a stronger postprandial blood glucose response as measured by the glycemic index (GI) than the same amount of brown rice. A systematic review found that the mean GI was 64 $\pm$ 7 for white rice and 55 $\pm$ 5 for brown rice (Foster-Powell, 2002). Higher dietary GI has been consistently associated with elevated risk of type 2 diabetes (T2D) in prospective cohort studies (Schulze, 2004; Villegas, 2007). The prevalence of type 2 diabetes is increasing rapidly worldwide (Wild et al. 2004). Control of body weight by balancing energy intake and energy expenditure is of major importance for the prevention of type 2 diabetes, but the role of specific dietary factors in the etiology of type 2 diabetes is less well established (Steyn et al. 2004).

Rice and Heavy Metal Contamination

Rice consumption has been identified as an important route of arsenic exposure among populations not living in arsenic-endemic regions (Gilbert-Diamond, 2011; Davis, 2012; Oguri, 2014), as well as populations in arsenic-endemic regions, such as Bangladesh, Taiwan, and India, where groundwater is heavily contaminated by arsenic (Ohno, 2007; Signes-Pastor, 2008).

Chronic exposure to arsenic, especially inorganic arsenic, may be atherogenic through multifaceted detrimental effects on blood pressure, systemic inflammation, oxidative stress, and endothelial dysfunction (Jomova et al. 2011). In arsenic-endemic regions, high arsenic concentration in drinking water was associated with increased risk of CVD (Moon et al. 2012; Liao et al. 2012; Chen, 2011). However, findings from non–arsenic-endemic areas were mixed. In 3 ecological studies, regional arsenic concentration in groundwater was associated with an increased CVD risk in Spain and the United States (Meliker et al. 2007, Medrano et al. 2010, Lisabeth et al. 2010), although in other 2 ecological studies in the United States, such a positive association was not found (Engel et al. 1994; Lewis et al. 1999). In the only prospective study, higher urinary concentration of inorganic plus methylated organic arsenic species was associated with elevated risks of CVD, CAD, and stroke among U.S. adults living in Arizona, Oklahoma, and the Dakotas, independently of age, sex, educational levels, smoking status, BMI, and plasma concentration of LDL cholesterol (Moon et al. 2013).

The 2012 Consumer Reports claimed that "samples of white rice, brown rice and rice breakfast cereals that many U.S. adults and children eat may contain worrisome levels of arsenic." (Consumer Reports Magazine, 2012). A positive association between rice consumption and arsenic level in human body has been observed in previous studies in US (Davis et al. 2012; Glilbert-Diamond et al, 2011). While arsenic is a naturally occurring element found in air, soil, water, and foods, inorganic arsenic has been associated with various types of cancers, including those of the lung, liver, bladder, kidney and skin (Chen et al. 2010).

During 18 to 26 years follow-up for over 280,000 US men and women, results from three prospective cohorts suggested the intakes of total rice, white rice or brown rice were not significantly associated with the risk of overall cancers. While arsenic and inorganic arsenic are carcinogenic to humans, it remains unknown whether arsenic associated with rice consumption increases risks of developing cancers. They did not find statistically significant associations between rice consumption and overall cancer risk in adult men or women (Ran Zhang et al. 2016).

Rice and Cardiovascular Disease

Data regarding associations between rice consumption and risk of cardiovascular disease (CVD) are sparse and mixed. In a Japanese population who consumed white rice as a staple food, greater rice consumption was associated with lower mortality from CVD, especially coronary artery disease (CAD), in men, whereas in women, the association was not evident (Eshak et al. 2011). In another Japanese study, there was a null association of risk of CVD, CAD, and stroke with rice consumption, although rice was the major source of arsenic intake in this Japanese population (Eshak et al. 2014; Sawada et al. 2013). In contrast, among Chinese adults, greater carbohydrate intake mostly from white rice was associated with higher CAD incidence (Yu et al. 2013). In these well-characterized large cohorts of U.S. male and female health professionals, there was no significant associations between rice consumption and risk of developing CVD or CAD independently of demographic, lifestyle, and dietary risk factors of CVD. These null associations were largely similar between whites and Asians. Higher white rice consumption has not been shown to increase the risk of cardiovascular diseases but may be associated with increased risk of metabolic syndrome.

CONCLUSION

Rice is a good source of various biologically active compounds including phenolic antioxidants. Antioxidants are the essential nutrients that help protect human body against the free radicals. Stabilized rice bran has over 100 antioxidants and co-factors which means it contains a wide range of nutrients required for natural health maintenance. Antioxidants also play a role in the body's cell protection system and help to boost immune system and cardiovascular function. Phytonutrients in rice bran possessing antioxidant and other reported beneficial physiological properties include: ferulic acid, its esterified derivative (γ-oryzanol), and unsaponifiable components such as tocopherol (vitamin E) and tocotrienol (as a form of vitamin E) . The nutrients in rice have known potential for reducing the risk of coronary heart disease, reducing tumor incidence, cancer risk, lowering blood pressure, reduces the rate of cholesterol and fat absorption, delaying gastrointestinal emptying and providing gastrointestinal health. Thus diet with the regular inclusion of cereals can contribute much to health promotion and disease prevention. Studies have shown that nutraceutical combination (red yeast rice, berberine and policosanols) improves aortic stiffness in low-moderate risk hypercholesterolemic patients. Evidence is accumulating that consumption of whole grains may reduce risk of chronic diseases including various types of cancer (Jacobs et al. 1988), cardiovascular diseases (Jacobs et al. 2004), and type 2 diabetes (Fung et al. 2002; Montonen et al. 2003; van Dam et al. 2006). Foods are considered to be whole grains if all components of the kernel, i.e., the bran, germ, and endosperm, are present in their natural proportions. Both the fiber-rich bran outer coating and the inner germ are rich in micronutrients and phytochemicals, whereas the endosperm middle layer mainly consists of starch. In the refining process, components of the grain that are part of the bran and germ are lost, including fiber, minerals, vitamins, lignans, and other phytochemicals. These components may offer important health benefits, including beneficial effects on glucose metabolism.

Into the future, rice will remain an important food staple for billions of people. To help ensure that rice can contribute to the healthy diets of rice consumers worldwide, IRRI has studied the glycemic index of rice and is developing healthier rice. IRRI also responds to concerns about contamination in rice.

REFERENCES

A 2 Z Project. (2008). *Rice fortification in developing countries: a critical review of the technical and economic feasibility*. Washington, DC: Academy for Educational Development. Retrieved from http://www.oecd.org/env/ehs/biotrack/46815658.pdf

Anderson, A. J., & Wynn, J. P. (2001). Microbial polyhydroxyalkanoates, polysaccharides and lipids. Cambridge University Press.

Anton, J., Meseguer, I., & Rodriguez-Valera, F. (1988). Production of an extracellular polysaccharide by Haloferax mediterranei. *Applied and Environmental Microbiology*, *54*, 23812386. PMID:16347749

Arsenic in your food. (2012). *Consumer Reports Magazine*.

Association of OfficialAnalytical Chemists (AOAC). (1995). *Official methods of analysis*. AOAC International.

Barber, S. (1972). Milled rice and changes during aging. In D. F. Houston (Ed.), *Rice chemistry and technology* (pp. 215–263). St Paul, MN: Am. Assoc. Cereal Chem.

Barber, S., Camacho, J., Cerni, R., Tortosa, E., & Primo, E. (1974). Process for the stabilization of rice bran I Basic research studies. In *Proceedings of Rice byproducts utilization.*

Baurenfiend, J. C., & DeRitter, E. (1991). Foods considered for nutrient addition: cereal grain products. In *Nutrient Additions to Food*. Academic Press.

Bechtel, D. B., & Pomeranz, Y. (1978). Ultrastructure of the mature ungerminated rice (Oryza sativa) caryopsis. The starchy endosperm. *American Journal of Botany*, *65*, 684–691.

Bhathena, S. J., & Velasquez, M. T. (2002). Beneficial role of dietary phytoestrogens in obesity and diabetes. *The American Journal of Clinical Nutrition*, *76*, 1191–1201. PMID:12450882

Bingham, S. A., Day, N. E., Luben, R., Ferrari, P., Slimani, N., Norat, T., & Riboli, E. et al. (2003). Dietary fiber in food & protection against colorectal cancer in the European Prospective Investigation into Cancer & Nutrition (EPIC): An observational study. *Lancet*, *361*, 1496–1501. doi:10.1016/S0140-6736(03)13174-1 PMID:12737858

Buffa, C. W. (1976). Rice bran wax, a new wax for cosmetics, drugs & toiletries. *Cosmet Toiletries*, *91*, 14–16.

Cassidy, A., Mukamal, K. J., Liu, L., Franz, M., Eliassen, A. H., & Rimm, E. B. (2013). High anthocyanin intake is associated with a reduced risk of myocardial infarction in young and middle-aged women. *Circulation*, *127*(2), 188–196. doi:10.1161/CIRCULATIONAHA.112.122408 PMID:23319811

Chandrashekar, P., Kumar, P. K. P., Ramesh, H. P., Lokesh, B. R., & Krishna, A. G. G. (2014). Hypolipidemic effect of oryzanol concentrate and low temperature extracted crude rice bran oil in experimental male wistar rats. *Journal of Food Science and Technology*, *51*(7), 1278–1285. doi:10.1007/s13197-012-0628-9 PMID:24966420

Chen, C. L., Chiou, H. Y., Hsu, L. I., Hsueh, Y. M., Wu, M. M., Wang, Y. H., & Chen, C. J. (2010). Arsenic in drinking water and risk of urinary tract cancer: A follow-up study from northeastern Taiwan. *Cancer Epidemiology, Biomarkers & Prevention*, *19*(1), 101–110. doi:10.1158/1055-9965.EPI-09-0333 PMID:20056628

Chen, H., Siebenmorgen, T., & Griffin, K. (1998). Quality characteristics of long-grain rice milled in two commercial systems. *Cereal Chemistry.*, *75*(4), 560–565. doi:10.1094/CCHEM.1998.75.4.560

Chen, P., Kuo, W., Chiang, C., Chiou, H., Hsieh, Y., & Chu, S. (2006). Black rice anthocyanins inhibit cancer cells invasion via repressions of MMPs and uPA expression. *Chemico-Biological Interactions*, *163*(3), 218–229. doi:10.1016/j.cbi.2006.08.003 PMID:16970933

Chen, Y., Graziano, J. H., Parvez, F., Liu, M., Slavkovich, V., Kalra, T., & Ahsan, H. et al. (2011). Arsenic exposure from drinking water and mortality from cardiovascular disease in Bangladesh: Prospective cohort study. *BMJ (Clinical Research Ed.)*, *342*(may05 2), d2431. doi:10.1136/bmj.d2431 PMID:21546419

Chiang, A., Wu, H., Yeh, H., Chu, C., Lin, H., & Lee, W. (2006). Antioxidant effects of black rice extract through the induction of superoxide dismutase and catalase activities. *Lipids*, *41*(8), 797–803. doi:10.1007/s11745-006-5033-6 PMID:17120934

Choi, H. J., Kim, J., & Jhon, M. S. (1999). Viscoelastic characterization of biodegradable poly (3-hydroxy butyrate-co-3-hydroxy valerate). *Polymer*, *40*, 4135–4138. doi:10.1016/S0032-3861(98)00627-2

Choi, Y., Jeong, H. S., & Lee, J. (2007). Antioxidant activity of methanolic extracts from some grains consumed in Korea. *Food Chemistry*, *103*(1), 130–138. doi:10.1016/j.foodchem.2006.08.004

Choudhury, N. H., & Juliano, B. O. (1980). Effect of' amylose content on the lipids of mature rice grain. *Phytochemistry*, *19*(7), 1385–1389. doi:10.1016/0031-9422(80)80179-8

Chung, M. J., Walker, P. A., & Hogstrand, C. (2006). Dietary phenolic antioxidants, caffeic acid and Trolox, protect rainbow trout gill cells from nitric oxide-induced apoptosis. *Aquatic Toxicology (Amsterdam, Netherlands)*, *80*(4), 321–328. doi:10.1016/j.aquatox.2006.09.009 PMID:17113165

Davis, M. A., Mackenzie, T. A., Cottingham, K. L., Gilbert-Diamond, D., Punshon, T., & Karagas, M. R. (2012). Rice consumption and urinary arsenic concentrations in U.S. children. *Environmental Health Perspectives*, *120*(10), 1418–1424. doi:10.1289/ehp.1205014 PMID:23008276

De, B. K., & Bhattacharyya, D. K. (1998). Physical refiningof rice bran oil in relation to degumming & dewaxing. *Journal of the American Oil Chemists' Society*, *75*(11), 1683–1686. doi:10.1007/s11746-998-0112-x

De Datta, S. K. (1981). *Principles and Practices of Rice Production*. New York, NY: John Wiley and Sons, Inc.

De Deckere, E. A. M., & Korver, O. (1996). Minor constituents of rice brain oil as functional foods. *Nutrition Reviews*, *54*(11), S120–S126. doi:10.1111/j.1753-4887.1996.tb03831.x PMID:9110588

del Rosario, A. R., Briones, V. P., Vidal, A. J., & Juliano, B. O. (1968). Composition and endosperm structure of developing and mature rice kernel. *Cereal Chemistry*, *45*, 225–235.

Dexter, P. B. (1998). *Rice fortification for developing countries*. Fayetteville, AR: OMNI/USAID. Retrieved from http://www.mostproject.org/PDF/rice4.pdf

Engel, R. R., & Smith, A. H. (1994). Arsenic in drinking water and mortality from vascular disease: An ecologic analysis in 30 counties in the United States. *Archives of Environmental & Occupational Health*, *49*(5), 418–427. doi:10.1080/00039896.1994.9954996 PMID:7944575

Eshak, E. S., Iso, H., Date, C., Yamagishi, K., Kikuchi, S., Watanabe, Y., & Tamakoshi, A. et al. (2011). JACC Study Group. Rice intake is associated with reduced risk of mortality from cardiovascular disease in Japanese men but not women. *The Journal of Nutrition*, *141*(4), 595–602. doi:10.3945/jn.110.132167 PMID:21346103

Eshak, E. S., Iso, H., Yamagishi, K., Kokubo, Y., Saito, I., Yatsuya, H., & Tsugane, S. et al. (2014). Rice consumption is not associated with risk of cardiovascular disease morbidity or mortality in Japanese men and women: A large population-based, prospective cohort study. *The American Journal of Clinical Nutrition*, *141*(1), 199–207. doi:10.3945/ajcn.113.079038 PMID:24740204

FAO. (1954). *Rice and rice diets – a nutritional survey* (rev. ed.). Rome: FAO.

FAO (Food and Agriculture Organization of the United Nations). (2004). Rice is life.*Proceedings of the FAO Rice Conference*. Food and Agriculture Organization of the United Nations.

FAOSTAT (The Statistics Division of the Food and Agriculture Organization of the United Nations). (2012). *Database of Food and Agricultural Organization*. Available from: http://faostat3.fao.org/

Firestone, D. (1997) Officialmethods & recommended practices of the AOCS (5th ed.). AOCS Press.

Food and Agricultural Organisation. (2013). *FAOSTAT Database*. Rome: Food and Agricultural Organization.

Food and Agriculture Organization. (2006). *Rice International commodity profile*. Rome: Food and Agricultural Organization. Retrieved from http://www.fao.org/fileadmin/templates/est/COMM_MARKETS_MONITORI G/Rice/Documents/Rice_Profile_Dec-06.pdf

Food and Nutrition Press. (2013). *FAORiceMarket Monitor*. Accessed June 29, (2013). http://www.fao.org/economic/est/publications/rice-ublications/rice%20marketmonitor-FoodandAgricultureOrganization

Foster-Powell, K., Holt, S. H., & Brand-Miller, J. C. (2002). International table of glycemic index and glycemic load values. *The American Journal of Clinical Nutrition*, *76*(1), 5–56. PMID:12081815

Fry, A. C., Bonner, E., Lewis, D. L., Johnson, R. L., Stone, M. H., & Kraemer, W. J. (1997). The effects of gamma-oryzanol supplementation during resistance exercise training. *International Journal of Sport Nutrition*, *7*, 318–329. PMID:9407258

Fukushi, J. (1966). Antioxidant effects of oryzanol. In Edible rice bran oil part – III. Hokkaido-Ritsu Eisei Kenkyushoho.

Fung, T. T., Hu, F. B., Pereira, M. A., Liu, S., Stampfer, M. J., Coldtz, G. A., & Willet, W. C. (2002). Whole-grain intake and the risk of type 2 diabetes: A prospective study in men. *The American Journal of Clinical Nutrition*, *76*, 535–540. PMID:12197996

Gilbert-Diamond, D., Cottingham, K. L., Gruber, J. F., Punshon, T., Sayarath, V., Gandolfi, A. J., & Karagas, M. (2011). Rice consumption contributes to arsenic exposure in US women. *Proceedings of the National Academy of Sciences of the United States of America*, *108*(51), 20656–20660. doi:10.1073/pnas.1109127108 PMID:22143778

Goffman, F. D., & Bergman, C. J. (2004). Rice kernel phenolic content and its relationship with antiradical efficiency. *Journal of the Science of Food and Agriculture*, *84*(10), 1235–1240. doi:10.1002/jsfa.1780

Gopala Krishna, A. G., Khatoon, S., Sheila, P. M., Sarmandal, C. V., & Indira, T. N. (2001). Effect of refining crude rice bran oil on the retention of oryzanol in the refined oil. *Journal of the American Oil Chemists' Society*, *78*(2), 127–131. doi:10.1007/s11746-001-0232-0

Gopala Krishna, A. G., Prabhakar, J. V., & Sen, D. P. (1984). Effect of degree of milling on tocopherol content of rice bran. *Journal of Food Science and Technology*, *21*, 222–224.

Hammond N (1994). Functional & nutritional characteristics of rice bran extracts. *Cereal Foods World*, *39*, 752-754.

Hanmoungjai, P., Pyle, D. L., & Niranjan, K. (2001). Enzymatic process for extracting oil & protein from rice bran. *Journal of the American Oil Chemists' Society*, *78*(8), 817–821. doi:10.1007/s11746-001-0348-2

Hegsted, M., & Windhauser, M. M. (1993). Reducing human heart disease risk with rice bran. *Louisiana Agriculture*, *36*, 22–23.

Heim, K. E., Tagliaferro, A. R., & Bobilya, D. J. (2002). Flavonoid antioxidants: Chemistry, metabolism and structure-activity relationships. *The Journal of Nutritional Biochemistry*, *13*(10), 527–584. doi:10.1016/S0955-2863(02)00208-5 PMID:12550068

Hemavathy, J., & Prabhakar, J. V. (1987). Lipid composition of rice (*Oryza sativa* L.) bran. J. *Journal of the American Oil Chemists' Society*, *64*(7), 1016–1019. doi:10.1007/BF02542441

Henon, G., Recseg, K., & Kovari, K. (2001). Wax analysis of vegetable oils using liquid chromatography on a double adsorbent layer of silica gel & silver nitrate impregnated silica gel. *Journal of the American Oil Chemists' Society*, *78*(4), 401–410. doi:10.1007/s11746-001-0275-2

Hibino, K., Kidzu, T., Masumura, T., Ohtsuki, K., Tanaka, K., Kawabata, K., & Fujii, S. (1989). Amino acid composition of rice prolamin polypeptides. *Agricultural and Biological Chemistry*, *53*, 513–518.

Hinton, J. J. C., & Shaw, B. (1954). The distribution of nicotinic acid in the rice grain. *The British Journal of Nutrition*, *8*(01), 65–71. doi:10.1079/BJN19540010 PMID:13140830

Holden, J. M., Bhagwat, S. A., Haytowitz, D. B., Gebhardt, S. E., Dwyen, J. T., Peterson, J., & Balentine, D. et al. (2005). Development of a database of critically evaluated flavonoids data: Application of USDA's data quality evaluation system. *Journal of Food Composition and Analysis*, *18*(8), 829–844. doi:10.1016/j.jfca.2004.07.002

Hossain, M. (1997). Rice supply and demand in Asia: a socioeconomic and biophysical analysis. In *Proceedings of the Second International Symposium on Systems Approaches for Agricultural Development*. doi:10.1007/978-94-011-5416-1_20

Houston, M. C. (2005). Nutraceuticals, vitamins, antioxidants, and minerals in the prevention and treatment of hypertension. *Progress in Cardiovascular Diseases*, *47*(6), 396–449. doi:10.1016/j.pcad.2005.01.004 PMID:16115519

Hu, C., Zawistowski, J., Ling, W., & Kitts, D. D. (2003). Black rice (*Oryza sativa* L. *indica*) pigmented fraction suppresses both reactive oxygen species and nitric oxide in chemical and biological model systems. *Journal of Agricultural and Food Chemistry*, *51*(18), 5271–5277. doi:10.1021/jf034466n PMID:12926869

Hu, E., Pan, A., Malik, V., & Sun, Q. (2012). White rice consumption and risk of type 2 diabetes: Meta-analysis and systematic review. *BMJ (Clinical Research Ed.)*, *344*(mar15 3), e1454. doi:10.1136/bmj.e1454 PMID:22422870

Huang, T., Duan, K., Huang, S., & Chen, C. W. (2006). Production of polyhydroxyalkanoates from inexpensive extruded rice bran & starch by Haloferax mediterranei. *Journal of Industrial Microbiology & Biotechnology*, *33*(8), 701–706. doi:10.1007/s10295-006-0098-z PMID:16491353

Hudson, E. A., Dinh, P. A., Kokubun, T., Simmonds, M. S. J., & Gescher, A. (2000). Characterization of potentially chemopreventive phenols in extracts of brown rice that inhibit the growth of human breast and colon cancer cells. *Cancer Epidemiology, Biomarkers & Prevention*, *9*, 1163–1170. PMID:11097223

Huebner, F. R., Bietz, J. A., Webb, B. D., & Juliano, B. O. (1990). Rice cultivar identification by high-performance liquid chromatography of endosperm proteins. *Cereal Chemistry*, *67*, 129–135.

Hyun, J. W., & Chung, H. S. (2004). Cyanidin and malvidin from *Oryza sativa* cv. Heugjinjubyeo mediate cytotoxicity against human monocytic leukemia cells by arrest of G2/M phase and induction of apoptosis. *Journal of Agricultural and Food Chemistry*, *52*(8), 2213–2217. doi:10.1021/jf030370h PMID:15080622

International Fund for Agricultural Development, World Food Programme, Food and Agricultural Organization. (2012). *The State of Food Insecurity in the World (2012). Economic growth is necessary but not sufficient to accelerate reduction of hunger and malnutrition*. Rome: Food and Agricultural Organization. Accessed June 29, 2013. http://www.fao.org/publications/sofi/(2012)/en/

International Organization for Standardization. Geneva, Switzerland (ISO) 13299 Sensory Analysis Methodology. (1998). General guidance for establishing a sensory profile. ISO.

International Rice Research Institute. (2013). *Rice knowledge bank*. Los Ba˜nos, the Philippines: Author. Retrieved from http://www.knowledgebank.irri.org/rkb/rice-milling.html

International Rice Research Institute. (2013). *World Rice Statistics (2013)*. Los Ba˜nos, the Philippines: IRRI. Retrieved from http://irri.org/index.php?option=com_k2&view=item&id=9081&Itemid=100481&lang=en

Iqbal, S., Bhanger, M. I., & Anwar, F. (2005). Antioxidant properties and components of some commercially available varieties of rice bran in Pakistan. *Food Chemistry*, *93*(2), 265–272. doi:10.1016/j.foodchem.2004.09.024

IRRI. (1990). *(199lb). Program report for*. Manila: IRRI.

Itani, T., Tatemoto, H., Okamoto, M., Fujii, K., & Muto, N. (2002). A comparative study on antioxidative activity and polyphenol content of colored kernel rice. *Journal of Japanese Society of Nutrition and Food Science*, *49*(8), 540–543. doi:10.3136/nskkk.49.540

Ito, M. (2003). Characterization of natural waxes & their application to cosmetic foundations. *Fragrance Journal*, *31*, 38–46.

Iwama, F., & Maruta, S. (1969). Composition of hard portion of crude rice bran wax. *Kogyo Kagaku Zassh*, *722*, 605–2608.

Jacobs, D. R. Jr, & Gallaher, D. D. (2004). Whole grain intake and cardiovascular disease: A review. *Current Atherosclerosis Reports*, *6*(6), 415–423. doi:10.1007/s11883-004-0081-y PMID:15485586

Jacobs, D. R. Jr, Marquart, L., Slavin, J., & Kushi, L. H. (1998). Whole-grain intake andcancer: An expanded review and meta-analysis. *Nutrition and Cancer*, *30*(2), 85–96. doi:10.1080/01635589809514647 PMID:9589426

Jaiswal, P. K. (1983). Specification of rice bran oil and extractions. In *Rice bran oil: status and prospects. Proceedings of a seminar*. Oil Technologists' Association of India.

Johnson, L. A., & Lusas, E. W. (1983). Comparison of alternative solvents for oil extraction. *Journal of the American Oil Chemists' Society*, *60*(2), 229–242. doi:10.1007/BF02543490

Jomova, K., Jenisova, Z., Feszterova, M., Baros, S., Liska, J., Hudecova, D., & Valko, M. et al. (2011). Arsenic: Toxicity, oxidative stress and human disease. *Journal of Applied Toxicology*, *31*, 95–107. PMID:21321970

Juliano, B. O. (1972). The rice caryopsis and its composition. In D. F. Houston (Ed.), *Rice chemistry and technology* (pp. 16–74). St Paul, MN: American Association of Cereal Chemistry.

Juliano, B. O. (1979). The chemical basis of rice grain quality. In *Proceedings, Workshop on Chemical Aspects of Rice Grain Quality*. Los Baños, Laguna, the Philippines: IRRI.

Juliano, B. O. (Ed.). (1985b). *Rice: chemistry and technology* (2nd ed.). St Paul, MN: American Association of Cereal Chemistry.

Juliano, B. O. (1993). *Rice in Human Nutrition*. Rome: Food and Agriculture Organization of the United Nations.

Juliano, B. O., & Bechtel, D. B. (1985). The rice grain and its gross compo sition. In B. O. Juliano (Ed.), *Rice chemistry and technology* (2nd ed.; pp. 17–57). St Paul, MN: American Association of Cereal Chemistry.

Juliano, B. O., & Goddard, M. S. (1986). Cause of varietal difference in insulin and glucose responses to ingested rice. *Qualitas Plantarum Plant Foods for Human Nutrition*, *36*(1), 35–41. doi:10.1007/BF01091751

Kagawa, H., Hirano, H., & Kikuchi, E. (1988). Variation in glutelin seed storage protein in rice (*Oryza sativa* L.). *Japanese Journal of Breeding*, *38*, 327-332.

Khush, G. (1997). Origin, dispersal, cultivation and variation of rice. *Plant Molecular Biology*, *35*(1/2), 25–34. doi:10.1023/A:1005810616885 PMID:9291957

Khush, G. (2004). *Harnessing science and technology for sustainable rice based production systems.* Presented at the FAO Rice Conference, Rome, Italy.

Kochhar, S. P. (2000). Stable and healthful frying oil for the 21st century. *Inform (Silver Spring, Md.)*, *11*, 642–647.

Koji, I. (2009). Present condition and problems of rice industry under socio-economic transformation in Cambodia. PhD dissertation. Japan: Graduate School of International Development,Nagoya University. Retrieved from http://www2.gsid.nagoya-u.ac.jp/blog/anda/files/2009/06/21_ishikawa.pdf

Lebesi, D. M., & Tzia, C. (2009). Effect of the addition of dietary fiber& edible cereal bran sources on the baking & sensory characteristics of cupcakes. *Food and Bioprocess Technology*, *4*(5), 710–722. doi:10.1007/s11947-009-0181-3

Lewis, D. R., Southwick, J. W., Ouellet-Hellstrom, R., Rench, J., & Calderon, R. L. (1999). Drinking water arsenic in Utah: A cohort mortality study. *Environmental Health Perspectives*, *107*(5), 359–365. doi:10.1289/ehp.99107359 PMID:10210691

Liao, Y. T., Chen, C. J., Li, W. F., Hsu, L. I., Tsai, L. Y., Huang, Y. L., & Wang, S. L. et al. (2012). Elevated lactate dehydrogenase activity and increased cardiovascular mortality in the arsenic-endemic areas of southwestern Taiwan. *Toxicology and Applied Pharmacology*, *262*(3), 232–237. doi:10.1016/j.taap.2012.04.028 PMID:22569360

Lichtenstein, A. H., Ausman, L. M., Carrasco, W., Gualtieri, L. J., Jenner, J. L., Ordovas, J. M., & Schaefer, E. J. et al. (1994). Rice br.an oil consumption & plasma lipid levels in moderately hypercholesterolemic humans Ar*terio.sclerosis*. *Thrombosis, and Vascular Biology*, *14*, 549–556. doi:10.1161/01.ATV.14.4.549

Lisabeth, L. D., Ahn, H. J., Chen, J. J., Sealy-Jefferson, S., Burke, J. F., & Meliker, J. R. (2010). Arsenic in drinking water and stroke hospitalizations in Michigan. *Stroke*, *41*(11), 2499–2504. doi:10.1161/STROKEAHA.110.585281 PMID:20947858

Maclean, J. L., Dawe, D. C., Hardy, B., & Hettel, G. P. (Eds.). (2002). Rice Almanac. CABI Publishing.

Manful, J. T., Swetman, A. A., Coker, R. D., & Drunis, A. (2007). Changes in the thiamine and riboflavin contents of rice during artisanal parboiling in Ghana. *Tropical Science*, *47*(4), 211–217. doi:10.1002/ts.215

Medrano, M. A., Boix, R., Pastor-Barriuso, R., Palau, M., Damián, J., Ramis, R., & Navas-Acien, A. et al. (2010). Arsenic in public water supplies and cardiovascular mortality in Spain. *Environmental Research*, *110*(5), 448–454. doi:10.1016/j.envres.2009.10.002 PMID:19880104

Meliker, J. R., Wahl, R. L., Cameron, L. L., & Nriagu, J. O. (2007). Arsenic in drinking water and cerebrovascular disease, diabetes mellitus, and kidney disease in Michigan: A standardized mortality ratio analysis. *Environmental Health*, *6*(1), 4. doi:10.1186/1476-069X-6-4 PMID:17274811

Miller, G., Prakash, A., & Decker, E. (2002). *Whole-grain foods in health and disease*. St. Paul, MN: American Association of Cereal Chemists.

Mishra, A., Gopalakrishna, A. G., & Prabhakar, J. V. (1988). Factors affecting refining losses in rice (Oryza sativa L.) bran oil. *Journal of the American Oil Chemists' Society*, *65*(10), 1605–1609. doi:10.1007/BF02912563

Moghadasian, M. H., & Frohlich, J. J. (1999). Effects of dietary phytosterols on cholesterol metabolism & atherosclerosis: Clinical & experimental evidence. *The American Journal of Medicine*, *107*(6), 588–594. doi:10.1016/S0002-9343(99)00285-5 PMID:10625028

Montonen, J., Knekt, P., Jarvinen, R., Aromaa, A., & Reunanen, A. (2003). Whole grain and fiber intake and the incidence of type 2 diabetes. *The American Journal of Clinical Nutrition*, *77*(3), 622–629. PMID:12600852

Moon, K., Guallar, E., & Navas-Acien, A. (2012). Arsenic exposure and cardiovascular disease: An updated systematic review. *Current Atherosclerosis Reports*, *14*(6), 542–555. doi:10.1007/s11883-012-0280-x PMID:22968315

Moon, K. A., Guallar, E., Umans, J. G., Devereux, R. B., Best, L. G., Francesconi, K. A., & Navas-Acien, A. et al. (2013). Association between exposure to low to moderate arsenic levels and incident cardiovascular disease: A prospective cohort study. *Annals of Internal Medicine*, *159*, 649–659. PMID:24061511

Morimitsu, Y., Kubota, K., Tashiro, T., Hashizume, E., Kamiya, T., & Osawa, T. (2002). Inhibitory effect of anthocyanins and colored rice on diabetic cataract formation in the rat lenses. *International Congress Series*, *1245*, 503–508. doi:10.1016/S0531-5131(02)00919-6

Muthayya, S., Hall, J., Bagriansky, J., Sugimoto, J., Gundry, D., Matthias, D., & Maberly, G. et al. (2012). Rice Fortification—an emerging opportunity to contribute to the elimination of vitamin and mineral deficiency worldwide. *Food and Nutrition Bulletin*, *33*(4), 296–307. doi:10.1177/156482651203300410 PMID:23424896

Nam, S. H., Choi, S. P., Kang, M. Y., Kozukue, N., & Friedman, M. (2005). Antioxidative, antimutagenic, and anticarcinogenic activities of rice bran extracts in chemical and cell assays. *Journal of Agricultural and Food Chemistry*, *53*(3), 816–822. doi:10.1021/jf0490293 PMID:15686439

Normand, E. L., Ory, R. L., & Mod, R. R. (1981). Interactions of several bile acids with hemicelluloses from several varieties of rice. *Journal of Food Science*, *46*(4), 1159–1161. doi:10.1111/j.1365-2621.1981.tb03014.x

Normand, F. L., Ory, R. L., Mod, R. R., Saunders, R. M., & Gumbmann, M. R. (1984). Influence of rice hemicelluloses and α-cellulose on lipid and water content of rice faeces and on blood lipids. *Journal of Cereal Science*, *2*(1), 37–42. doi:10.1016/S0733-5210(84)80006-5

Normile, D. (2004). Yangtze seen as earliest rice site. *Science*, *275*(5298), 309. doi:10.1126/science.275.5298.309

Ogawa, M., Kumamaru, T., Satoh, H., Iwata, N., Omura, T., Kasai, Z., & Tanaka, K. (1987). Purification of protein body-I of rice seed and its polypeptide composition. *Plant & Cell Physiology*, *28*, 1517–1527.

Oki, T., Masuda, M., Kobayashi, M., Nishiba, Y., Furuta, S., Suda, I., & Sato, T. (2002). Polymeric procyanidins as radical-scavenging components in red-hulled rice. *Journal of Agricultural and Food Chemistry*, *50*(26), 7524–7529. doi:10.1021/jf025841z PMID:12475265

Organisation for Economic Co-operation and Development. (1999). *Consensus document on the biology of Oryza sativa (rice). Report No. ENV/JM/MONO(99)26.* OCED Environmental health and Safety Publications. Paris: Organisation for Economic Co-operation and Development.

Port'eres, R. (1962). Berceauxagricolesprimairessur le continent africain. *Journal of African History*, *3*(02), 195–210. doi:10.1017/S0021853700003030

Port'eres, R. (1976). African cereals: Eleusine, fonio, black fonio, teff, Brachiaria, Paspalum, Pennisetum, and African rice. In Origins of African Plant Domestication. Academic Press.

Pulido, R., Bravo, L., & Saura-Calixto, F. (2000). Antioxidant activity of dietary polyphenols as determined by a modified ferric reducing/antioxidant power assay. *Journal of Agricultural and Food Chemistry*, *48*(8), 3396–3402. doi:10.1021/jf9913458 PMID:10956123

Raghuram, T. C., Rao, U. B., & Rukmini, C. (1989). Studies on hypolipidemic effects of dietary rice bran oil in human subjects. *Nutrition Reports International*, *39*, 889–895.

Resurreccion, A. P., Juliano, B. O., & Tanaka, Y. (1979). Nutrient content and distribution in milling fractions of rice grain. *Journal of the Science of Food and Agriculture*, *30*(5), 475–481. doi:10.1002/jsfa.2740300506 PMID:470348

Ryan, E. P. (2011). Bioactive food components and health properties of rice bran. *Journal of the American Veterinary Medical Association*, *238*(5), 593–600. doi:10.2460/javma.238.5.593 PMID:21355801

Sawada, N., Iwasaki, M., Inoue, M., Takachi, R., Sasazuki, S., Yamaji, T., & Tsugane, S. et al. (2013). Dietary arsenic intake and subsequent risk of cancer: The Japan Public Health Center–based (JPHC) Prospective Study. *Cancer Causes & Control*, *24*(7), 1403–1415. doi:10.1007/s10552-013-0220-2 PMID:23666560

Schulze, M. B., Liu, S., Rimm, E. B., Manson, J. E., Willett, W. C., & Hu, F. B. (2004). Glycemic index, glycemic load,and dietary fiber intake and incidence of type 2 diabetes in younger and middle-aged women. *The American Journal of Clinical Nutrition*, *80*(2), 348–356. PMID:15277155

Sengupta, R., & Bhattacharyya, D. K. (1996). Enzymatic extraction of mustard seed & rice bran. *Journal of the American Oil Chemists' Society*, *73*(6), 687–692. doi:10.1007/BF02517941

Sharp CQ, Kitchens KJ (1990). Using rice bran in yeast bread in a home baker. *Cereal Foods World*, *35*, 1021-1024.

Shibuya, N. (1989). Comparative studies on the cell wall polymers obtained from different parts of rice grains. In N. G. Lewis & M. G. Paice (Eds.), *Plant cell wall polymers: biogenesis and biodegradation, Symp. No. 399* (pp. 333–344). Washington, DC: American Chemical Society. doi:10.1021/bk-1989-0399.ch024

Sierra, S., Lara-Villoslada, F., Olivares, M., Jiménez, J., Boza, J., & Xaus, J. (2005). Increased immune response in mice consuming rice bran oil. *European Journal of Nutrition*, *44*(8), 509–516. doi:10.1007/s00394-005-0554-y PMID:15719157

Song, Y., He, K., Levitan, E. B., Manson, J. E., & Liu, S. (2006). Effects of oral magnesium supplementation on glycaemic control in Type 2 diabetes: Ameta-analysis of randomized double-blind controlled trials. *Diabetic Medicine*, *23*(10), 1050–1056. doi:10.1111/j.1464-5491.2006.01852.x PMID:16978367

Steyn, N. P., Mann, J., Bennett, P. H., Temple, N., Zimmet, P., Tuomilehto, J., & Louheranta, A. et al. (2004). Diet, nutrition and the prevention of type 2 diabetes. *Public Health Nutrition*, *7*(1a), 147–165. doi:10.1079/PHN2003586 PMID:14972058

Sugimoto, T., Tanaka, K., & Kasai, Z. (1986). Molecular species in the protein body II (PB-II) of developing rice endosperm. *Agricultural and Biological Chemistry*, *50*, 3031–3035.

Taira, H., Nakagahra, M., & Nagamine, T. (1988). Fatty acid composition of indica, sinica, japonica, and japonica groups of nonglutinous brown rice. *Journal of Agricultural and Food Chemistry*, *36*(1), 45–47. doi:10.1021/jf00079a011

Taira, H., Taira, H., & Fujii, K. (1979). Influence of cropping season on lipid content and fatty acid composition of lowland nonglutinous brown rice. *Nihon Sakumotsu Gakkai Kiji*, *48*(3), 371–377. doi:10.1626/jcs.48.371

Takeda, Y., Hizukuri, S., & Juliano, B. O. (1987). Structures of rice amylopectin with low and high affinities for iodine. *Carbohydrate Research*, *168*(1), 79–88. doi:10.1016/0008-6215(87)80008-3

Tanaka, K., Ogawa, M., & Kasai, Z. (1977). The rice scutellum. II. A comparison of scutellar and aleurone electron-dense particles by transmission electron microscopy including energy-dispersive X-ray analysis. *Cereal Chemistry*, *54*, 684–689.

Tanaka, K., Sugimoto, T., Ogawa, M., & Kasai, Z. (1980). Isolation and characterization of two types of protein bodies in the rice endosperm. *Agricultural and Biological Chemistry*, *44*, 1633–1639.

Tanaka, K., Yoshida, T., Asada, K., & Kasai, Z. (1973). Subcellular particles isolated from aleurone layer of rice seeds. *Archives of Biochemistry and Biophysics*, *155*(1), 136–143. doi:10.1016/S0003-9861(73)80016-5 PMID:4712443

Tanaka, Y., Resurrecci6n, A. P., Juliano, B. O., & Bechtel, D. B. (1978). Properties of whole and undigested fraction of protein bodies of milled rice. *Agricultural and Biological Chemistry*, *42*, 2015–2023.

Teng, P. S., Kropff, M. J., Ten Berge, H. F. M., Dent, J. B., Lansigan, F. P., & Van Laar, H. H. (1997). Approaches at the Farm and Regional Levels. Los Ba˜nos: International Rice Research Institute.

Vali, S. R., Ju, Y., Kaimal, T. N. B., & Chern, Y. (2005). A process for the preparation of food grade rice bran wax & determination of its composition. *Journal of the American Oil Chemists' Society*, *82*(1), 57–64. doi:10.1007/s11746-005-1043-z

van Dam, R. M., Hu, F. B., Rosenberg, L., Krishnan, S., & Palmer, J. R. (2006). Dietary calcium and magnesium, major food sources, and risk of type 2 diabetes in U.S. black women. *Diabetes Care*, *29*(10), 2238–2243. doi:10.2337/dc06-1014 PMID:17003299

Varraso, R., Kabrhel, C., Goldhaber, S. Z., Rimm, E. B., & Camargo, C. A. Jr. (2012). Prospective study of diet and venous thromboembolism in US women and men. *American Journal of Epidemiology*, *175*(2), 114–126. doi:10.1093/aje/kwr377 PMID:22180874

Villareal, C. P., & Juliano, B. O. (1989). b. Comparative level of waxy gene product of endosperm starch granules of different rice ecotypes. *Starch*, *41*(10), 369–371. doi:10.1002/star.19890411002

Villegas, R., Liu, S., Gao, Y. T., Yang, G., Li, H., Zheng, W., & Shu, X. O. (2007). Prospective study of dietary carbohydrates, glycemic index, glycemic load, and incidence of type 2 diabetes mellitus in middleaged Chinese women. *Archives of Internal Medicine*, *167*(21), 2310–2316. doi:10.1001/archinte.167.21.2310 PMID:18039989

Wang, T., Hicks, K. B., & Moreau, R. (2002). Antioxidant activity of phytosterols, oryzanol & other phytosterol conjugates. *Journal of the American Oil Chemists' Society*, *79*(12), 1201–1206. doi:10.1007/s11746-002-0628-x

Weickert, M. O., Mohlig, M., Schofl, C., Arafat, A. M., Otto, B., Viehoff, H., & Pfeiffer, A. F. (2006). Cereal. fiber improves whole-body insulin sensitivity in overweight and obese women. *Diabetes Care*, *29*(4), 775–780. doi:10.2337/diacare.29.04.06.dc05-2374 PMID:16567814

Wells, J. H. (1993). Utilization of rice bran & oil in human diets. *Louisiana Agriculture*, *36*, 4–8.

Wild, S., Roglic, G., Green, A., Sicree, R., & King, H. (2004). Global prevalence of diabetes: Estimates for the year 2000 and projections for 2030. *Diabetes Care*, *27*(5), 1047–1053. doi:10.2337/diacare.27.5.1047 PMID:15111519

Yasuhiko, T., & Fumio, I. (1988). Recent technical advances in rice bran oil processing (II About refining process).Transactions of the Kokushikan Univ. *Faculty of Engineering*, *21*, 118–124.

Yawadio, R., Tanimori, S., & Morita, N. (2007). Identification of phenolic compounds isolated from pigmented rices and their aldose reductase inhibitory activities. *Food Chemistry*, *101*(4), 1616–1625. doi:10.1016/j.foodchem.2006.04.016

Yoon, S. H., & Rhee, J. S. (1982). Composition of waxes from crude rice bran oil. *Journal of the American Oil Chemists' Society*, *59*(12), 561–563. doi:10.1007/BF02636324

Yu, D., Shu, X. O., Li, H., Xiang, Y. B., Yang, G., Gao, Y. T., & Zhang, X. (2013). Dietary carbohydrates, refined grains, glycemic load, and risk of coronary heart disease in Chinese adults. *American Journal of Epidemiology*, *178*(10), 1542–1549. doi:10.1093/aje/kwt178 PMID:24008907

Zhang, M., Guo, B., Zhang, R., Chi, J., We, Z., Xu, Z., & Tang, X. (2006). Separation, purification and identification of antioxidant compositions in black rice. *Agricultural Sciences in China*, *5*(6), 431440. doi:10.1016/S1671-2927(06)60073-4

Zhang, R., Zhang, X., Wu, K., Wu, H., Sun, Q., Hu, F. B., & Giovannucci, E. L. (2016). Rice consumption and cancer incidence in US men and women. *International Journal of Cancer*, *138*(3), 555–564. doi:10.1002/ijc.29704 PMID:26219234

Zhao, Z., & Moghadasian, M. H. (2008). Chemistry, natural sources, dietary intake and pharmacokinetic properties of ferulic acid: A review. *Food Chemistry*, *109*(4), 691–702. doi:10.1016/j.foodchem.2008.02.039 PMID:26049981

Zhou, Z., Robards, K., Helliwell, S., & Blanchard, C. (2004). The distribution of phenolic acids in rice. *Food Chemistry*, *87*(3), 401–406. doi:10.1016/j.foodchem.2003.12.015

Chapter 11
Soy and Soy Products, Isoflavones, Equol, and Health

Baltasar Mayo
IPLA-CSIC, Spain

Lucía Guadamuro
IPLA-CSIC, Spain

Ana Belén Flórez
IPLA-CSIC, Spain

Susana Delgado
IPLA-CSIC, Spain

ABSTRACT

In Asian countries, soybeans have been used as food and food ingredients for centuries and their consumption have been associated with beneficial health effects. In addition to their nutritive value, soybeans have many active chemical compounds, among which isoflavones are the most important. Isoflavones are plant-derived phytoestrogens, chemically comparable in their structure and properties to human estrogens. For isoflavones to become bioavailable, their activation and/or conversion into more active metabolites, such equol from daidzein, must occur. Equol is the isoflavone metabolite with the greatest estrogenic activity and antioxidant capacity. Epidemiological studies have suggested that high intakes of isoflavones reduce the symptoms of menopause as well as the incidence of hormone-dependent and aging-associated diseases such as osteoporosis, cardiovascular disease and cancer. This chapter reviews soy consumption, isoflavone metabolism, and briefly summarizes the results of recent clinical trials on, and meta-analyses of, the effects of isoflavone consumption on human health.

GENERAL INTRODUCTION

Soy ("Shu" in ancient Chinese) -*Glycine max* (Linnaeus-Merril)- is an annual herbaceous legume of the family *Fabaceae*. It is native to China, where it has been cultivated for some 5000 years (Qiu & Chang, 2010). Originally, soy was a subtropical crop, but numerous varieties have now been adapted to very different climates. The United States, Brazil, Argentina and China are the current leaders in soybean production. Like some other long-domesticated crops, the relationship between modern cultivated soy and wild-growing species can no longer be traced back with any degree of certainty.

From a nutritional point of view, dry, mature, raw soybeans typically contain 8.5% moisture, 36.5% protein, 30 carbohydrates, 20% lipids and about 5% ash (National Nutrient Reference Database of the

DOI: 10.4018/978-1-5225-0591-4.ch011

United States Department of Agriculture [USDA]; http://ndb.nal.usda.gov/). Soybean oil contains large amounts of monounsaturated (22.8%) and polyunsaturated (57.7%) fatty acids. Soy protein ranks the highest among vegetable proteins; its nutritional value equals that of milk and egg proteins (Food and Agriculture Organization/World Health Organization, 2013). In addition, soybeans contain large amounts of many bioactive polyphenols (Kang et al., 2010), among which the phytoestrogenic isoflavones are the most important; their consumption has been associated with positive health effects (del Rio et al., 2013; Crozier et al., 2009).

The consumption of soy and soy-derived products varies widely between human communities (Mulligan et al., 2013; Zamora-Ros et al., 2012; Boker et al., 2002). Those of Asian countries (especially China, Japan and Korea), where soy and soy products have been used for centuries as food and food ingredients (Qiu & Chang, 2010; Guan et al., 2008), remain the largest consumers. A soy protein intake of approximately 6-11 g/day, along with a soy isoflavone intake of 25-50 mg/day, has been reported for elderly Japanese people (Messina et al., 2006). Large surveys undertaken in the USA and Europe have reported intakes ten times lower than in Asian nations (Bai et al., 2013; Peeters et al., 2007; Boker et al., 2002). Nonetheless, the growing evidence of the multiple health benefits of soy has raised interest in its consumption (Jing & Wei-Jie, 2015; He & Chen, 2013; Wei et al., 2012; de Cremoux et al., 2010; Harland & Haffner, 2008).

Soy Products

Soybeans can be eaten freshly boiled or steamed or after processing in different ways. Traditional Asian soy products are typically divided into two categories, unfermented (e.g., soymilk, tofu and okara) and fermented (e.g., soy sauce, natto, miso, and tempeh) (He & Chen, 2013). Soymilk is produced by soaking dried soybeans in water and then grinding them. It contains amounts of protein and fat similar to those seen in cow's milk, but it is free of lactose and cholesterol. Tofu is a curd made by coagulating soy protein using mineral salts (calcium, magnesium) or an acid (glucono-δ-lactone). The precipitation of soy protein produces a jelly-like curd similar to a fresh cottage cheese. This curd can then be converted into different types of product. Okara is the residual solid that results from soymilk extraction. It typically contains 80% moisture, 3.2% protein and 1.7% fat. It is used as a food ingredient in Asia, although it is most commonly employed as a livestock feed. Soy sauce is the most common seasoning in China and was in use at least as early as 160 AD (He & Chen, 2013). Traditional soy sauce is manufactured by fermenting a mix of wheat and soybean. This involves several microorganisms, including *Aspergillus*, lactic acid bacteria and yeasts. The resulting sauce has a very complex flavor and aroma, the products of chemical and biochemical reactions that occur during manufacturing and ripening. Natto is a traditional Japanese soy food made by fermenting boiled soybeans with *Bacillus subtillis* Natto strains. The smell, flavor and slimy texture of natto resemble those of some very strong cheeses. Tempeh is a fermented soybean product from Indonesia. It is made by fermenting dehulled and partially cooked soybeans with a *Rhizopus* mold. The extensive network formed by its mycelium binds the soybean together to form a block, producing a fermented soybean loaf. Miso is a popular Japanese food made by fermenting rice and soybeans with a mixture of molds, yeast and bacteria. Traditional miso manufacture starts by fermenting cooked rice with koji spores (i.e., spores from *Aspergillus oryzae*). This is followed by a second fermentation of the fermented rice with cooked soybeans, involving a mix of molds, yeasts and bacteria, to yield a paste with a complex flavor.

Phenolic Compounds, Phytoestrogens, and Isoflavones

Phenolic compounds are chemical substances characterized by having at least one aromatic ring containing one or more hydroxyl groups. Over 8000 phenolic structures have been reported in the plant kingdom, many of which end up in our food (Crozier et al., 2009). They can be classified into two broad groups: flavonoids and non-flavonoids. Non-flavonoids are a heterogeneous group of phenolic compounds ranging from simple molecules, such as benzoic acid and hydroxycinnamates, to more complex compounds such as stilbenes, lignans, hydrolysable tannins, gallotannins and ellagitannins, among others (del Rio et al., 2013; Crozier et al., 2009). Flavonoids are polyphenolic compounds comprising 15 carbons and involving two aromatic rings connected by a three carbon bridge (Figure 1). The main subclasses of

Figure 1. Structure of the flavonoid skeleton and the main flavonoid classes; major soy isoflavones are also depicted.

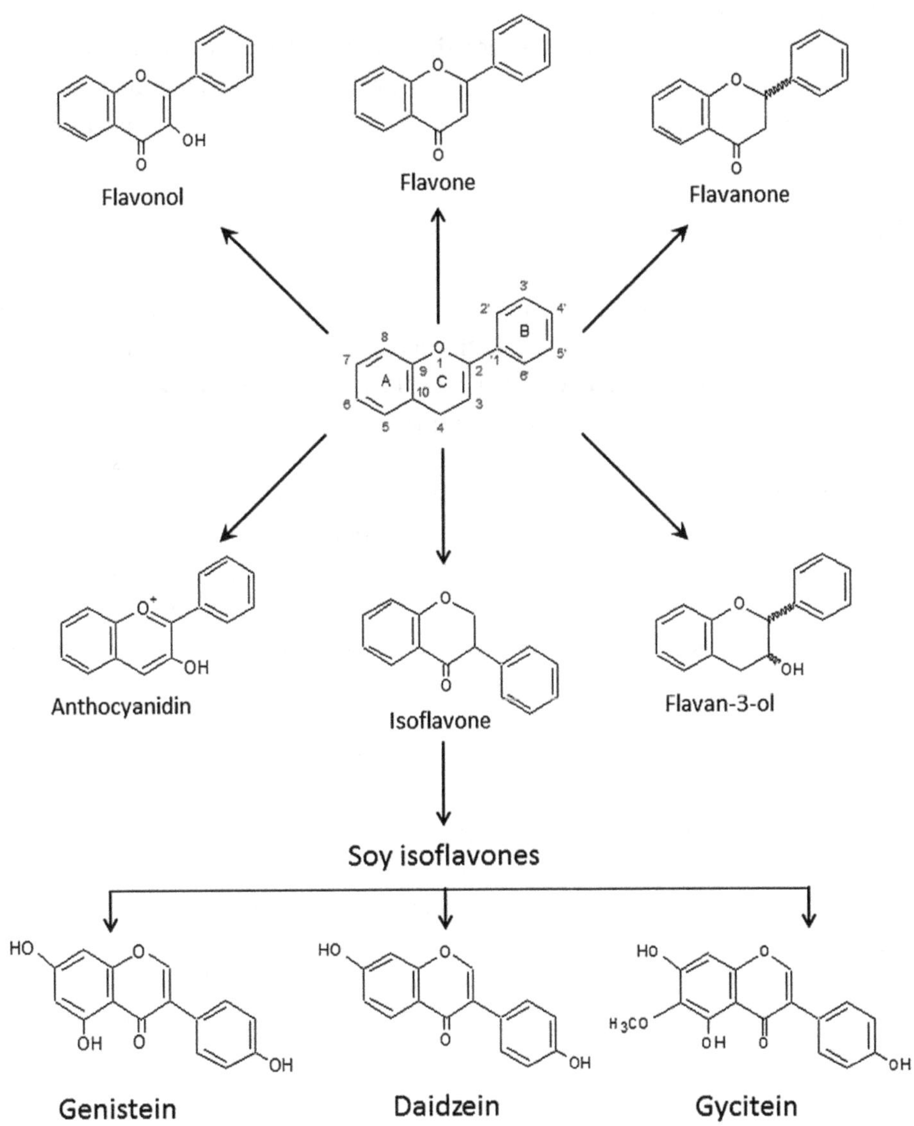

dietary flavonoids are flavanols, flavones, flavan-3-ols, anthocyanidins, flavanones, and isoflavones (del Rio et al., 2013). Databases such as the Phenol-Explorer Database (www.phenol-explorer.eu) and the USDA Flavonoid Database (http://www.ars.usda.gov/News/docs.htm?docid=6231), have substantially contributed to the understanding of human exposure to phenolic compounds.

Phytoestrogens -also called estrogen-like molecules and non-steroidal estrogens- are a heterogeneous group of phenolic compounds whose structures resemble that of 17-β-estradiol (Pilšáková et al., 2010). Over 100 phytoestrogens are known. They are divided, according to their chemical structure, into flavonoids (apigenin, quercitin, narigenin), isoflavones (genistein, daidzein, formontein, biochanin A), lignans (enterodiol, enterolactone), coumestans (coumestanol), and stilbenes (resveratrol) (Crozier et al., 2009). Of these, the isoflavones and the stilbene resveratrol have been the most intensively investigated (Bilal et al., 2014). In foods, phytoestrogens are present as mixtures, usually as poorly-absorbable or biologically-inactive glycoside conjugates with carbohydrate moieties (del Rio et al., 2013). Their bioavailability depends strongly on their transformation by enzymes produced by the gastrointestinal microbiota (with some help from tissue-produced enzymes) (Landete et al., 2015; Selma et al., 2009; Aura, 2008; Nielsen & Williamson, 2007).

There is considerable epidemiological evidence to indicate that diets rich in phytoestrogen-containing foods reduce the risk of a number of chronic diseases, notably cardiovascular and neurodegenerative diseases and cancer (Bilal et al., 2014; Wada et al., 2013; Pilšáková et al., 2010; Peeters et al., 2007).

ISOFLAVONES

Isoflavones are phenolic compounds with two aromatic planar rings (A and B) connected by a three-carbon bridge (usually called ring C). Unlike that seen in flavonoids, ring B is attached to carbon 3 rather than carbon 2 (Figure 1). Isoflavones are found in over 300 plants (Aguiar et al., 2007), mostly in the roots and seeds, but soybeans are the richest sources (Kaufman et al., 1997); dried soybeans contain 1.2-4.2 mg/g (Zhang et al., 2014; Thompson et al., 2006). The exact concentration depends on the soil in which the plants are grown, the climate, stage of ripening, and the level of processing to which the beans are subjected (Caldwell et al., 2005). Like other phenolic compounds, soy isoflavones are found mostly as glycoconjugates (>80%). The majority of soy isoflavone-glycosides, i.e., genistin, daidzin and glycitin, are found in dried beans at concentrations of 4.4, 3.9 and 0.7 μmol g^{-1} respectively (Zhang et al., 2014). These β-glycosides are not readily absorbed in the intestine and have low estrogenic activity, and must be hydrolyzed to become bioavailable (bioavailability refers to the proportion of the absorbed dose of a molecule, or the metabolites produced from it, reaching the appropriate molecular targets [Nielsen & Williamson, 2007]) and thus attain their full biological activity (Crozier et al., 2009; de Cremoux et al., 2010). Enzyme action on the isoflavone-glycosides mentioned above converts them into the isoflavone aglycones genistein, daidzein and glycitein respectively (Figure 1).

In cells, aglycones undergo metabolic transformation into sulfated, glucuronided and methylated metabolites which pass into the bloodstream. They may then be further metabolized in the liver or secreted in the bile to return to the small intestine (Franke et al., 2014; Gardana et al., 2014; Schwen et al., 2012). Isoflavones that remain unabsorbed, and those returned to the small intestine via the bile, reach the colon where they are deconjugated by bacterial enzymes and then either absorbed or further metabolized by microbial action (Franke et al., 2014; Gardana et al., 2014; Schwen et al., 2012; Atkinson et al., 2005; Simons et al., 2005; Steer et al., 2003).

Though the European Food Safety Authority (EFSA) has recently refuted claims regarding the effects of isoflavones on body function (European Food Safety Authority, 2012), high soy and isoflavone intakes have repeatedly been associated with many beneficial health effects (see below). However, no studies on the long-term effects of isoflavone treatment have ever been performed, and little is also known about the changes in metabolic markers of health during isoflavone interventions (Charles et al., 2009; Decroos et al., 2006).

Soy, Isoflavones, Isoflavone Extracts and Functional Foods

Functional foods are those that provide health benefits beyond basic nutrition, thus contributing to the maintenance and prolongation of a healthy state (Katan & de Roos, 2004). The presence of biologically active proteins and isoflavones has led to soy-derived foods being regarded as functional foods. For example, soy-based foods have been used to treat menopause symptoms (Brouns, 2002). In the USA, the Food and Drug Administration has allowed manufacturers of soy foods to make a heart health claim since 1999 if their products contain a mandatory 6.26 g of soy protein per serving (Food and Drug Administration, 1999). Combining soy with a probiotic food usually results in the enhanced bioavailability of isoflavone aglycones (Champagne et al., 2010; Wei et al., 2007); the use of isoflavone-activating microorganisms might therefore further improve the health benefits of soy. However, current probiotics were neither selected for their glycosidic properties nor for any other isoflavone-activating ability (Gareau et al., 2010).

Beyond consumption of soy, isoflavones are broadly ingested as concentrated extracts. Many commercial brands are currently on the market shelves (12st Century®, Fisiogen®, SoyLife™, AllNatural®, LifeExtension®, etc.). They are prepared by different extraction methods, contain variable amounts of soy isoflavones and different proportions of isoflavone-glycosides and aglycones.

Metabolism of Isoflavones

The predominance of endogenous phenolic-deglycosylating bacteria in the intestine, such as *Bacteroides* and *Clostridium* spp., suggests that deglycosylation is not the limiting step in the *in vivo* activation of isoflavones (Landete et al., 2015; Aura, 2008). In fact, intestinal lactic acid bacteria (LAB) and bifidobacteria are also involved in the conversion of isoflavone glycosides into aglycones (Champagne et al., 2010; Rekha & Vijayalakshmi, 2010; Otieno and Shah, 2007; Tsangalis et al., 2002). Indeed, genome sequencing of LAB and bifidobacteria has revealed an impressive array of genes coding for glycosidases, including β-glucosidases, which are thought to be involved in aglycone production (Klaenhammer et al., 2002; Schell et al., 2002).

Isoflavone aglycones may be further transformed in the intestine by dehydroxylation, reduction, C-ring cleavage or demethylation (Setchell et al., 2002) (Figure 2). For example, genistein can be converted into dihydrogenistein, 6'-hydroxy-*O*-desmethylangolensin, *p*-ethyl phenol (Hosoda et al., 2011; Steer et al., 2003) or 5'-hydroxy equol (Heinonen et al., 2003), while glycitein can be converted into dihydroglycitein, dihydro-6,7,4'-trihydroxyisoflavone, 5'-*O*-methyl-*O*-desmethylangolensin or 6-*O*-methyl-equol (Simons et al., 2005). The major microbial metabolites of daidzein are hydroxydaidzein (DHD) and equol (Rüfer et al., 2008; Atkinson et al., 2005). However, the evolution of isoflavone-metabolizing populations in the gut during soy/isoflavone intake is not yet known. Neither is it known how isoflavones interact with the majority of microbial populations in the gastrointestinal tract.

Figure 2. Metabolism of isoflavone-glucosides, genistin and daidzin, by the human microbiota

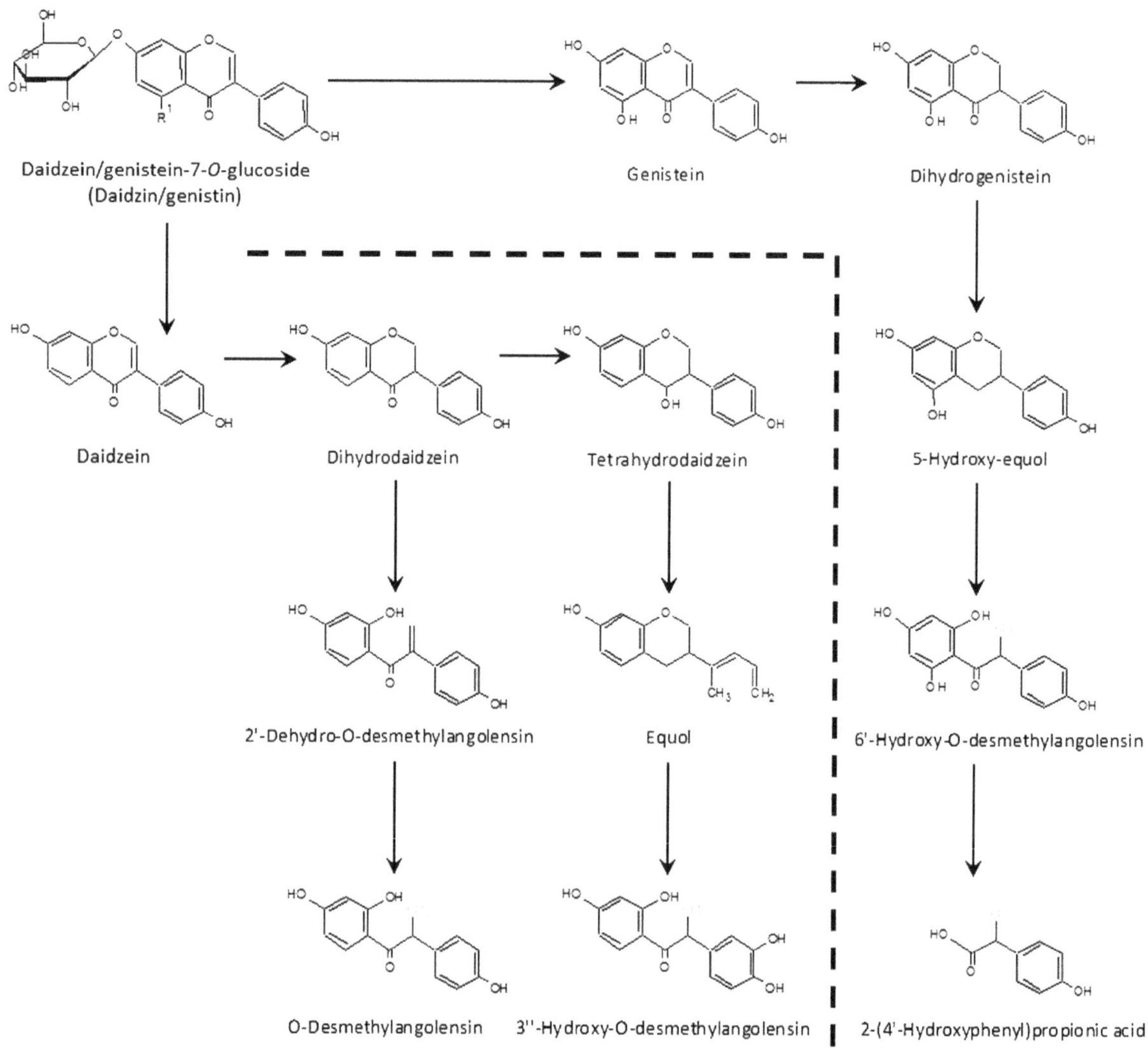

The intestinal degradation of isoflavones into biologically inactive compounds, such as the conversion of daidzein into *O*-desmethylangolensin (*O*-DMA), can also occur (Gardana et al., 2014). *O*-DMA and equol are likely produced by different bacteria, and those involved might even differ between individuals. Identifying the microbial species/strains involved in the conversion of isoflavones into more active compounds would help in the design of strategies aimed at increasing the size of desirable populations, enhancing desirable isoflavone transformation, and minimizing isoflavone degradation. These strategies might include the modulation of intestinal populations via the use of prebiotics (Steer et al., 2003) and probiotics (Ding & Shah, 2010), or even extreme interventions such as microbiota transplantation (Decroos et al., 2006). Recent high-throughput, culture-independent microbial techniques, such as metagenomics, metaproteomics and metatranscriptomics, should help unravel isoflavone metabolism (Kemperman et al., 2010).

Isoflavones and Human Intestinal Microbiota

There is strong evidence that diet greatly influences the composition of the intestinal microbiota (Graf et al., 2015). Indeed, fat and fiber have striking effects on microbial diversity (Martinez et al., 2010; Jumpertz et al., 2011). The impact of many microcomponents of the diet, however, including phenolic compounds, is much less well known. Substantiating results obtained using traditional microbial methods, recent molecular studies have revealed extensive diversity among the microbial gut communities of different individuals (Morgan et al., 2013; Qin et al., 2010). Not surprisingly, this diversity influences the isoflavone catabolic pathways that can be followed (Decross et al., 2006).

Research into the response of gut populations to isoflavone consumption *in vivo* is still needed. Isoflavones have some antimicrobial activity (Hummelova et al., 2015), though not as much as that of other polyphenols (caffeic acid, epicatechin, catechin, gallic acid, anthocyanins, etc.) (Landete, 2012), and this can modulate the diversity and composition of the gut microbiota (Figure 3). For example, isoflavone consumption may inhibit the growth of pathogens or increase the size of beneficial populations, contributing towards health benefits (Clavel & Mapesa, 2013; de Cremoux et al., 2010). However, studies on how isoflavones influence the composition and activity of the gut microbial community, and its effect on human health, are scarce (Clavel et al., 2005; Bolca et al., 2007; Nakatsu et al., 2014). Further, the results currently available are difficult to compare, the consequence of differences in treatment regimens, target groups and the analytical techniques employed. Understanding how microorganisms and metabolites interact and elicit a physiological response (or lack thereof) is, however, crucial if the results of observational and interventional studies are to be properly interpreted.

A bifidogenic effect of isoflavones has been reported in some studies (Clavel et al., 2005; Nakatsu et al., 2014). In equol producers, increases in the population size of *Clostridium* clusters have been observed (Clavel et al., 2005; Possemiers et al., 2007), and in general enterobacteria populations have been shown to decline during isoflavone treatment (Guadamuro et al., 2015; Figure 3). However, such effects may depend on the baseline sizes of particular populations, which vary widely between subjects (Morgan et al., 2013). The use of NGS will be crucial in the identification of core responses to the intake of soy isoflavones at the entire gut microbiome level (Nakatsu et al., 2014).

EQUOL

Extracted from the urine of pregnant mares back in 1932, equol [$C_{15}H_{12}O(OH)_2$] was the first isoflavonoid to be identified (Marrian & Haslewood, 1932). Later, in 1982 it was the first to be detected in human urine and blood (reviewed by Setchell et al., 2001). Equol is a metabolite of daidzein (Figure 2) and has a stronger estrogenic activity than any other isoflavone aglycone or other isoflavone metabolite (Sánchez-Calvo et al., 2013; Setchell et al., 2002), as well as the strongest antioxidant action and antiandrogenic effects. Chemically, equol is more stable than its precursor molecule daidzein, and more easily absorbed by the colon (Yuan et al., 2007; Setchell et al., 2002). The antiandrogenic properties of equol are unique. It binds specifically to 5α-dihydrotestosterone receptors, but not to testosterone, dehydropiandrosterone or androgen receptors (Lund et al., 2004). The non-planar chemical structure of equol might, at least in part, be responsible for its strong estrogenic activity (Crozier et al., 2009). All the animal species tested so far (mouse, rat, sheep, chicken and other fowl, goat, cow) produce equol in response to soy consumption (Setchell et al., 2002). However, equol is produced by only 30-50% of the

Figure 3. Microbial counts of three microbial populations (total colonic bacteria, bifidobacteria, and enterobacteria) in 16 women during isoflavone treatment. Results are expressed as the difference in counts between different times of treatment and basal counts. Thus increments and decrements are presented as up and down bars, respectively. Samples at month 1, 3 and 6 of isoflavone supplementation are color coded.

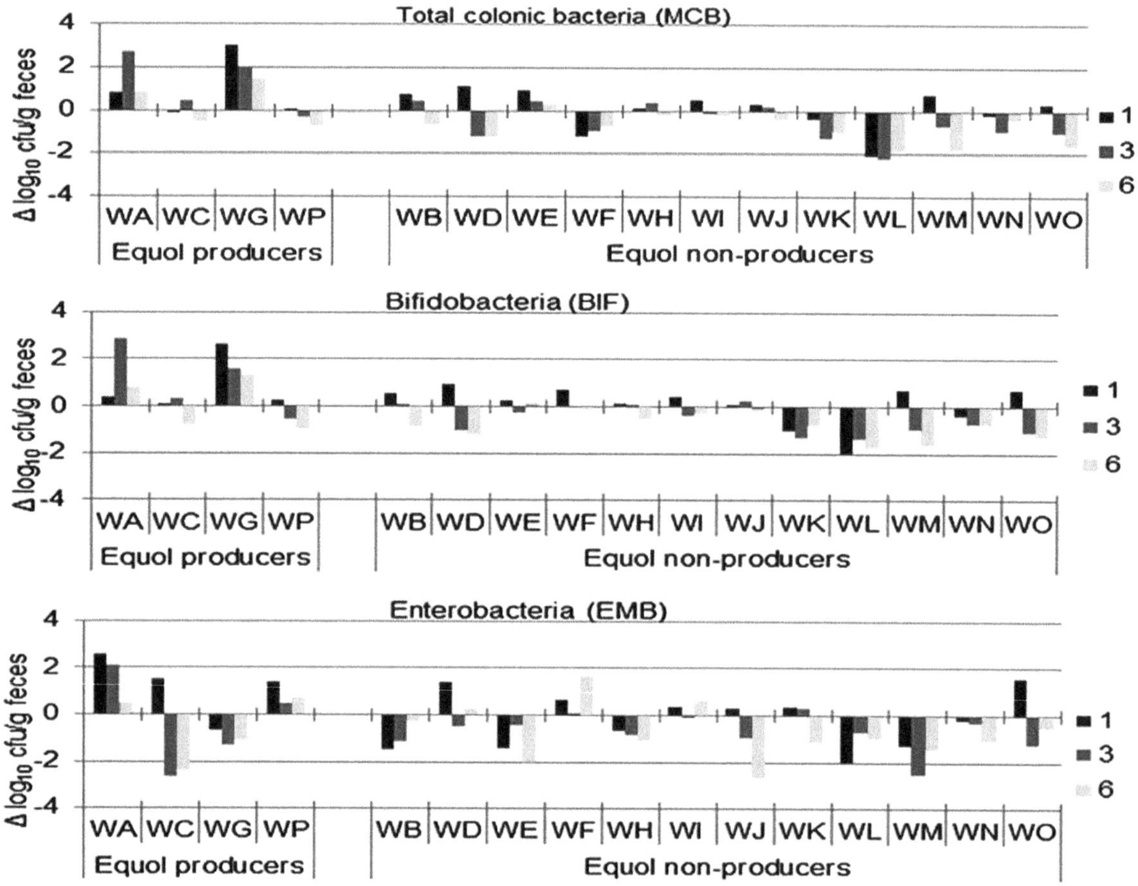

members in Western populations (Bolca et al., 2007; Peeters et al., 2007; Hall et al., 2007; Setchell and Cole, 2006) –these may be the only people in these populations who can fully benefit from isoflavone consumption. In contrast, 80 to 90% of subjects produce *O*-DMA from daidzein (Atkinson et al., 2005).

Equol Production Phenotype

Observational and interventional studies have reported inconsistent results on the stability of the equol production phenotype. Some authors propose that equol production status is a rather stable, i.e., that once an individual is an equol producer, he or she remains an equol producer (Wiseman et al., 2004; Setchell et al., 2003). Indeed, the possibility that equol production might be under some degree of genetic control has been suggested (Atkinson et al., 2005). However, several studies have reported that long-term soy ingestion can convert equol non-producers into equol producers (Franke et al., 2012; Lu et al.,

1996), and that the phenotype might be lost if soy consumption is ended. Thus, equol production may be stable in many but not all individuals (Akaza et al., 2004). Another topic of debate is whether other dietary components influence the capacity to produce equol (Frankenfeld, 2011; Franke et al., 2012). For instance, the frequency of equol producers among vegetarians has been reported significantly higher than among non-vegetarians (59% vs. 25%), suggesting that dietary components other than soy itself influence equol synthesis (Setchell & Cole, 2006). In this sense, Decroos et al. (2005) suggested that equol production was stimulated to a large extent by the hydrogen produced in the gut by endogenous intestinal populations. These authors also showed that equol production was enhanced in the presence of propionate and butyrate, and that a diet rich in carbohydrates might therefore stimulate equol production (Decross et al., 2005). Further, the consumption of milk and dairy products with daidzein has been significantly correlated with equol excretion (Frankefeld, 2011), as has the consumption of resistant starch and daidzein in ovariectomized mice (Tousen et al., 2011). Similarly, combining daidzein and lactulose consumption has been reported to promote equol production in sows via the modulation of the intestinal microbiota (Zheng et al., 2014). These findings suggest that equol formation can be increased via the modification of dietary habits.

Antibiotics have also been shown to both increase and decrease equol production (Atkinson et al., 2004; Franke et al., 2012), strongly suggesting that equol-producing microorganisms differ from one person to another.

Equol-Producing Microorganisms

Equol is an optically active molecule with asymmetric carbon atoms giving rise to different enantiomers. However, only S-equol has been detected as the result of bacterial daidzein conversion (Schwen et al., 2012; Jackson et al., 2011; Setchell et al., 2005). Bacterial equol biosynthesis seems to involve the intermediates dihydrodaidzein and tetrahydrodaidzein via a process involving three reductase enzymes (Figure 2).

Though limited, our knowledge of the microorganisms that produce equol from daidzein is growing (Setchell & Clerici, 2010; Yuan et al., 2007; Atkinson et al., 2005; Setchell et al., 2002). Initially, bacterial mixtures capable of producing this compound were described (Decross et al., 2005; Wang et al., 2007). However, in the last decade, a number of individual strains capable of forming equol from daidzein have been identified from either human or animal sources (Tsuji et al., 2010; Maruo et al., 2008; Yokoyama & Suzuki, 2008;Yu et al., 2008; Uchiyama et al., 2007; Wang et al., 2005). A few equol-producing bacteria also act on genistein, generating 5-hydroxy equol (Abiru et al., 2013; Matthies et al., 2012; Jin et al., 2010; Matthies et al., 2009).

Equol is not detected in the urine or plasma samples of most infants under 12 months of age fed breast or cow's milk (Brown et al., 2014; Cao et al., 2009), suggesting that equol-producing bacteria are late arrivers to the gastrointestinal ecosystem. It is not known whether equol production is a family-, species-, or strain-specific character (Clavel & Mapesa, 2013). Nearly all of the equol-producing microbes isolated so far have fallen into the family Coriobacteriaceae (Clavel et al., 2014), hinting at the functional specialization of these bacteria in the gut. Besides metabolizing isoflavones, the members of this family also metabolize steroid hormones and bile acids (Ridlon et al., 2006), increasing the likelihood of their having a physiological role in the gut environment. The family Coriobacteriaceae includes genera such as *Adlercreutzia, Assacharobacter, Eggerthella, Enterorhabdus, Paraeggerthela* and *Slackia* (Clavel et al., 2014). *Adlercreutzia equolifaciens* (Maruo et al., 2008), *Assacharobacter celatus* (Minamida et al., 2008), *Enterorhabdus mucosicola* (Clavel et al., 2009), *Slackia isoflavoniconvertens* (Matthies et al., 2009) and *Slackia equolifaciens* (Jin et al., 2010) are reported to be equol- and 5-hydroxy equol-producing bacteria (Table 1). Some isolates have been identified only at the genus level and are named after their strain code, e.g., *Eggerthela* sp. YY7918 (Yokoyama et al., 2011), *Paraeggerthela* sp. SNR40-432 (Abiru et al., 2013) or *Slackia* sp. NATTS (Sugiyama et al., 2014).

Only one non-Coriobacteriaceae, equol-producing strain of intestinal origin has been identified: *Lactococcus garvieae* (Uchiyama et al., 2007). Interestingly, this is the only equol-producing bacterium that possesses hydrolases able to act on isoflavone glycosides (the members of Coriobacteriaceae do not generally utilize carbohydrates) (Clavel et al., 2014). The *L. garvieae* genes involved in the production of equol have been cloned and characterized (Shimada et al., 2012; Shimada et al., 2011; Shimada et al., 2010), and found similar to sequences encoding equol-related reductases in *S. isoflavoniconvertens* (Schröder et al., 2013), *Eggerthella* spp. (Yokoyama et al., 2011), *Slackia* spp. NATTS (Tsuji et al., 2012; Shimada et al., 2012; Shimada et al., 2011; Shimada et al., 2010). This argues strongly for the recent horizontal transfer of equol-generating capacity from a member of the Coriobacteriaceae to *L. garvieae*. This is further supported by the specific codon usage and high GC content of the equol-associated genes (68%) (Shimada et al., 2011; Shimada et al., 2010), which greatly exceeds the genomic GC content of *L. garvieae* (39%).

Isolated strains with well characterized isoflavone-converting phenotypes could be used in the colonization of experimental animals (Matthies et al., 2012). This might prove the involvement of these microorganisms in the conversion of isoflavones, and help reveal the dynamics of the reaction. Well-characterized producer strains might then be used in large-scale biotechnological production of equol. In fact, the scant number of studies on the *in vivo* effects of equol has frequently been attributed to the high cost of the compound's production (Selvaraj et al., 2004).

Table 1. Well-characterized cultivable bacteria strains capable of converting the isoflavone daidzein to equol

Species	Strain	End Metabolite	Origin	Reference
Adlercreutzia equolifaciens	FJC-B9^{T}	Equol	Human faeces	Maruo et al. 2008
Asaccharobacter celatus	do03^{T}	Equol	Rat cecum	Minamida et al. 2008
Enterorhabdus mucosicola	Mt1-B8^{T}	Equol	Mouse ileal mucosa	Clavel et al. 2009
Lactococcus garvieae	20-92	Equol	Human faeces	Shimada et al. 2010
Slackia equolifaciens	DZE^{Ta}	Equol	Human faeces	Jin et al. 2010
Slackia isoflavoniconvertens	HE8^{Ta}	Equol	Human faeces	Matthies et al. 2012
Catenibacterium sp.	D1	Equol	Human faeces	Yu et al. 2008
Eggerthella sp.	YY7918	Equol	Human faeces	Yokoyama et al. 2011
Eggerthella sp.	D2	Equol	Human faeces	Yu et al. 2008
Eggerthella sp.	Julong 732[b]	Equol	Human faeces	Kim et al. 2009
Slackia sp.	NATTS	Equol	Human faeces	Tsuji et al. 2010

[a]These strains are also able to produce 5-hydroxy equol from the isoflavone genistein.

[b]From dihydrodaidzein only; this strain does not act over daidzein.

Molecular Aspects of Equol Formation

Next generation sequencing (NGS) techniques have facilitated the characterization of the genomes of some equol-producing isolates (Yokoyama et al., 2011; Tho et al., 2013) and helped to reveal the biochemical pathways involved in the synthesis of equol and 5-hydroxy equol from their precursor molecules (Schröder et al., 2013; Tsuji et al., 2012; Shimada et al., 2010). At least three enzymes -a daidzein-dependent NADP reductase, a dehydrodaidzein reductase and a tetrahydrodaidzein reductase– are reported to be used by *S. isoflavoniconvertens* (Schröder et al., 2013). The first enzyme of the pathway has been shown to participate in the formation of dihydrogenistein (Figure 2), a key step in the production of 5-hydroxy equol. Interestingly, 5-hydroxy equol has greater antioxidant activity than its precursor genistein (Arora et al., 1998). In both *S. isoflavoniconvertens* and *E. mucosicola*, the enzymes involved in both equol and 5-hydroxy equol production are induced by the presence of isoflavones (Schröder et al., 2013; Matthies et al., 2008). In *S. isoflavoniconvertens* the genes coding for isoflavone-converting enzymes are present in a cluster of about 10.5 kbp, in which eight open reading frames have been identified (Schröder et al., 2013).

EFFECTS OF ISOFLAVONES ON HEALTH

It is beyond the scope of this work to provide an exhaustive appraisal of all the possible health effects of isoflavones. Systematic reviews of human trials, prospective human trials, observational human studies, animal models, *in vitro* studies, and laboratory analyses suggest that soy foods and isoflavones may prevent or provide relief from menopausal symptoms and many other disease conditions (Figure 4). The interested reader is directed towards excellent reviews by Jin and Wei-Jie (2015), He and Chen (2013), Wei et al. (2012), Harland and Haffner (2008), Perabo et al. (2008), among others.

Both *in vitro* and *in vivo* studies have examined the effects of isoflavones on human health and their mode of action (Llaneza et al., 2010; Charles et al., 2009; Hermenegildo et al., 2005; Atkinson et al., 2004) (Figure 4). Although only *in vivo* human trials can provide definitive proof of any such effects, batch fecal fermentations (static models) (Atkinson et al., 2004), human gastrointestinal models (continuous models) (Islam et al., 2014), cell cultures (Lehmann et al., 2005), animal models (Allred et al., 2005) and human interventions (Liu et al., 2014; Llaneza et al., 2010; Charles et al., 2009) provide approximations. Static and continuous fermentors simulating the human gut provide easy-to-operate, cost-effective systems for assessing the metabolic conversion of isoflavones in the presence of human-derived microbiota, and for evaluating the effect of environmental conditions (temperature, pH, etc.) on the production of certain metabolites, including equol (Decroos et al., 2006; Atkinson et al., 2004). Cell cultures and animal models are commonly used to assess the availability (Steensma et al., 2004) and toxicity (Guan et al., 2008; Lehmann et al., 2005) of isoflavones, their *in vivo* metabolism (Matthies et al., 2012), and their efficacy in the treatment of diseases (Yanagihara et al., 2013; Handem et al., 2011; Gilani et al., 2009). Investigations involving the use of volunteers, however, provide the best conditions for studying the interactions of isoflavones with the human genetic background and personal gastrointestinal microbiota. Only such experimentation allows the impact of soy and isoflavone consumption on health to be properly examined (Yuan et al., 2007; Atkinson et al., 2005). Unfortunately, most human intervention studies so far have suffered from small sample sizes, short trial durations, and the use of

Figure 4. Potential beneficial health effects reported for soy isoflavones and principal study models for the different health benefits

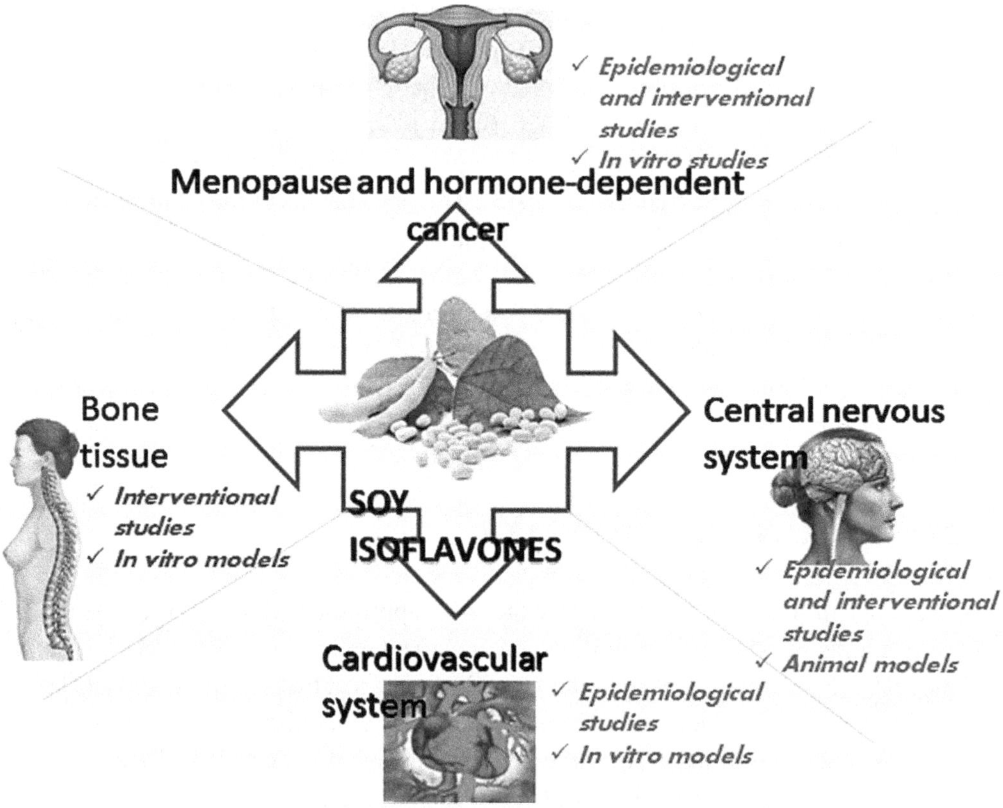

isoflavones from various sources, with different aglycone content, etc. Recently, several studies compared the efficacy of pure S-equol with that of isoflavones for the relief of several diseases (Aso et al., 2012; Jenks et al., 2012; Oyama et al., 2012).

Isoflavones and Menopause Symptoms

Asian women suffer fewer hot flashes (or flushes), night sweats and other discomforts of menopause (insomnia, fatigue, vaginal dryness) than Caucasian women, something that has been associated with high soy food intakes (Messina, 2000). Isoflavones received further attention as a possible treatment of menopause symptoms after the publication of the Women's Health Initiative results (2010), which showed a higher incidence of breast and uterus cancer and cardiovascular diseases among women whose menopause symptoms had been treated by hormone replacement therapy (Borrelli & Ernst, 2010; Molla et al., 2011). However, the most recent reviews and meta-analyses report the results of isoflavone treatment studies to be far from conclusive (Bolaños et al., 2010; Messina, 2010; Taku et al., 2010; Jacobs et al., 2009). Interpersonal differences in the intestinal microbiota may well account (at least in part) for the discrepancies seen (Qin et al., 2010). Such differences could give rise to different microbial isoflavone-derived metabolites being produced (Franke et al., 2014; Peeters et al., 2007), explaining the apparent lack of effectiveness seen in some studies. Recent clinical trials examining the efficacy of S-equol (10 mg/day for 8-12 weeks) as a treatment for hot flashes have reported symptoms to be significantly reduced compared to placebo treatment (Newton et al., 2015; Crawford et al., 2013; Aso et al., 2012; Jenks et al., 2012). Moreover, in one of the latest systematic reviews, the authors concluded that "extracts containing high levels of genistein appeared to reduce the number of daily hot flushes and need to be investigated further" (Lethavy et al., 2013).

Isoflavones and the Cardiovascular System

In Asian countries, the incidence of cardiovascular diseases is about eight times lower than in Western countries (Yamori, 2006; Appleby et al., 2004). Besides genetic factors, this large difference is assumed to have a nutritional basis. Soy is an important component of the diet of Asian populations, but since the introduction of the health claims made for soy protein many Europeans have bought soy foods as healthy choices, and they are now regarded as mainstream foods (Rosell et al., 2004). Systematic reviews and meta-analyses have suggested soy protein (circa 25 g/day) should be added to the diet of subjects with normal cholesterol levels or mild hypercholesterolemia; small but significant reductions in total and LDL (bad) cholesterol (ca. 6%) have been reported when this is done (Harland & Haffner, 2008; Reynols et al., 2006). Soy protein contains variable amounts of isoflavones (Mantovani et al., 2009), limiting the interpretation of experiments based on soy intake. Isoflavones taken alone, however, have been shown to exert a protective effect on the cardiovascular system (Taku et al., 2008). Growing evidence suggests that they may help regulate vasoactivity (Hermenegildo et al., 2005), lipid metabolism, and cholesterol transport (González-Granillo et al., 2012; Pilšáková et al., 2010).

Isoflavones and Bone

Low serum 17-β-estradiol levels are associated with reduced calcium availability and the activation of bone resorption-accelerating cytokines, leading to the dominance of bone resorption over bone synthesis, and eventually to osteoporosis (Wei et al., 2012). Osteoporosis can be a considerable problem for menopausal women, but a growing body of evidence suggests that isoflavones can help prevent it (Wei et al., 2012; Cassidy et al., 2006). A recent meta-analysis of the results of randomized control trials concluded that isoflavone intervention significantly attenuated spinal bone loss in menopausal women, inhibited bone resorption and stimulated bone formation (Wei et al., 2102; Taku et al., 2011; Taku et al., 2010). However, other authors report no evidence of any prevention of the decline of lumbar spine or proximal femur bone mineral density in postmenopausal women receiving 300 mg/day isoflavones (Tai et al., 2012). Endogenous (genetic background, intestinal microbiota) and exogenous (type of isoflavone, content, life style, etc.) factors influencing patient responsiveness might explain these conflicting results (Ho et al., 2008).

Isoflavones and Hormone-Dependent Cancers

The incidence of prostate, colon and some breast cancers is much lower in Asian countries than in the West (Mahmoud et al., 2014; Fritz et al., 2013; He & Cheng, 2013; Sugiyama et al., 2013; Perabo et al.,

2008). Environmental factors appear to contribute strongly to the development of these tumors. Indeed, Asian immigrants to Western countries who change their dietary habits suffer from these forms of cancer more frequently and at similar rates to Westerners (He and Chen, 2013). It is thought that soy consumption might, via isoflavone, be related to this reduction in risk. Following the ingestion of isoflavones by human volunteers, daidzein, genistein and their metabolites have been detected in prostate (Hong et al., 2002) and breast (Maubach et al., 2003) tissues. Soy isoflavones and their metabolites are similar to endogenous estrogens and may affect the growth of tumors via both hormonally mediated (agonism and antagonism of estradiol receptors, interference with estrogen metabolism, estrogenic activity) and non-hormonally mediated (epigenetic processes, activation of peroxisome proliferator-activated receptors, induction of apoptosis, stimulation of autophagy, etc.) mechanisms (He & Chen, 2013; Pilšáková et al., 2010).

Isoflavones and the Central Nervous System

Little is known about the influence of phytoestrogens on the brain (although like estradiol, isoflavones pass through the blood-brain barrier) or human behavior, but studies conducted in animals have shown isoflavones to have potentially beneficial effects on age-related problems such as reduced learning ability, memory and anxiety (Sarkasi et al., 2008; Lephart et al., 2002). Epidemiological studies again reveal lower rates of dementia in Asian populations (Liu et al., 2003). Human studies have focused mostly on the effects of isoflavones on cognitive functions (Fournier et al., 2007), and in general beneficial effects have been reported. The long-term administration of soy or isolated isoflavones has been associated with improved learning, logical thinking and planning ability in menopausal women (Karvaj et al., 2007; Kreijkamp-Kaspers et al., 2007; Duffy et al., 2003).

Isoflavones and Other Health Benefits

Isoflavones and equol have also been suggested to have an anti-aging effect on the skin, to provide protection against UV damage, to modulate obesity and diabetes type-2, and to ameliorate chronic kidney disease (Jing & Wei-Jie, 2015; Jackson et al., 2011; Charles et al., 2009; Yuan et al., 2007).

MODE OF ACTION OF ISOFLAVONES

If isoflavones are to be used as therapeutic agents or ingredients in functional foods for the prevention and cure of disease, unraveling their molecular mode of action is crucial. Human-derived cell lines afford a model for examining aspects of the cross-talk between isoflavones and host cells, and could provide clues on the molecular mechanisms at work. Isoflavones bind to the alpha (ERα) and beta (ERβ) estrogen receptors (Oseni et al., 2008), classifying them as selective estrogen receptor modulators (SERMs) rather than real estrogens. The affinity of genistein for ERβs is comparable to that shown by 17-β-estradiol (Morito et al., 2001), while the affinity of other isoflavones is some 100-500 times lower. Isoflavones exhibit estrogenic or anti-estrogenic effects depending on the concentration of endogenous estrogen present, as well as the amount and type of estrogen receptors (Yuan et al., 2007). They can activate both genomic and non-genomic estrogen signaling pathways, which may interact with the metabolism of steroid hormones and affect different tissues depending on the distribution of estrogen receptors around the body (Pilšáková et al., 2010). It has been reported that both genistein and daidzein partially regulate compound-specific target genes affecting both ERα-dependent and ERα-independent transcription expression (Satih et al., 2010). Further, isoflavones have the potential to reduce estradiol bioavailability by increasing levels of the circulating sex hormone-binding globulin (Low et al., 2006). They have also been shown to inhibit tyrosine kinases and DNA topoisomerase, which may account for their purported anti-cancer activity (Crozier et al., 2009). Antioxidant and metal ion-chelating properties of isoflavones have also been reported (Wang et al., 2008; Mitchell et al., 1998).

Isoflavones have been reported to accumulate in the tissues, which could well help modulate the biological functions of target cells (Maubach et al., 2003; Hong et al., 2002). In prostatic fluid, for example, daidzein is concentrated 2.2-fold and equol 45-fold (Hedlund et al., 2003) compared to plasma levels.

Isoflavones may also interact with the host biochemistry through epigenetic effects. Genistein exhibits epigenetic effects via genomic DNA methylation, which may reduce the growth of breast cancer cells (Li et al., 2009).

Of all isoflavone metabolites, equol has been the most investigated. Equol has been shown highly antioxidant in a number of cellular models (Choi and Kim, 2014; Wei et al., 2011). It is also reported to induce acute endothelium- and nitric oxide (NO)-dependent relaxation of the aortic rings (Joy et al., 2006), and is a potent activator of the human and mouse pregnane X receptor (PXR). Equol can prevent oxidized LDL-stimulated apoptosis in human umbilical vein endothelial cells at physiological concentrations (Kamiyama et al., 2009) and the oxidative stress induced by lipopolysaccharides in chicken macrophages (Gou et al., 2015). Further, equol has been proposed to modulate endothelial redox signaling and NO release, involving transactivation of epidermal growth factor receptor kinase and the reorganization of the F-actin cytoskeleton (Rowlands et al., 2011). These actions of equol may provide the bases of therapeutic strategies for restoring endothelial function in, for example, cardiovascular disease.

CONCLUSION

Soy has been used as a source of high-quality protein and other nutrients in Asian countries for hundreds of years. Soy isoflavones are soy-derived compounds structurally similar to estrogens, and have some of the same effects. The current interest in dietary isoflavones has primarily been driven by epidemiological studies suggesting that diets rich in these phytoestrogens are beneficial to human health. However the correlations observed cannot establish relationships of cause and effect. Further, much of the current evidence for isoflavone-related disease prevention derives from *in vitro* or animal experiments, and the direct extrapolation of their results to humans is controversial. There is therefore an urgent need to assess the real health benefits of isoflavones in humans. Certainly, the most recent reviews and meta-analyses show the results of most clinical trials to be far from conclusive. Research on the molecular mechanisms underlying the purported beneficial effects of isoflavones is also needed if these compounds are to receive support as functional ingredients.

ACKNOWLEDGMENT

Studies at the authors' laboratory on isoflavones have been supported by projects from the Spanish Ministry of Economy and Competitiveness (MINECO) (AGL2011-24300 and AGL-2014-57820-R) and Plan for Science, Technology and Innovation 2013-2017 of the Asturias Principality, co-funded by FEDER (GRUPIN14-137). L. Guadamuro and A.B. Flórez were supported by research contracts of FPI Program from MINECO (BES-2012-062502) and JAE-Doc Program from CSIC, respectively.

REFERENCES

Abiru, Y., Ueno, T., & Uchiyama, S. (2013). Isolation and characterization of novel S-equol-producing bacteria from brines of stinky tofu, a traditional fermented soy food in Taiwan. *International Journal of Food Sciences and Nutrition*, *64*(8), 936–943. doi:10.3109/09637486.2013.816936 PMID:23869769

Aguiar, C. L., Baptista, A. S., Alencar, S. M., Haddad, R., & Eberlin, M. N. (2007). Analysis of isoflavonoids from leguminous plant extracts by RPHPLC/DAD and electrospray ionization mass spectrometry. *International Journal of Food Sciences and Nutrition*, *58*(2), 116–124. doi:10.1080/09637480601149350 PMID:17469767

Akaza, H., Miyanaga, N., Takashima, N., Naito, S., Hirao, Y., Tsukamoto, T., & Pantuck, A. J. et al. (2004). Comparisons of percent equol producers between prostate cancer patients and controls: Case-controlled studies of isoflavones in Japanese, Korean and American residents. *Japanese Journal of Clinical Oncology*, *34*(2), 86–89. doi:10.1093/jjco/hyh015 PMID:15067102

Allred, C. D., Twaddle, N. C., Allred, K. F., Goeppinger, T. S., Churchwell, M. I., Ju, Y. H., & Doerge, D. R. et al. (2005). Soy processing affects metabolism and disposition of dietary isoflavones in ovariectomized BALB/c mice. *Journal of Agricultural and Food Chemistry*, *53*(22), 8542–8550. doi:10.1021/jf051246w PMID:16248551

Appleby, P. N., Spencer, E. A., & Key, T. J. (2004). Soy intake and blood cholesterol concentrations: A cross-sectional study of 1033 pre- and postmenopausal women in the Oxford arm of the European Prospective Investigation into Cancer and Nutrition. *The American Journal of Clinical Nutrition*, *80*, 1391–1396. PMID:15531691

Arora, A., Nair, M. G., & Strasburg, G. M. (1998). Antioxidant activities of isoflavones and their biological metabolites in a liposomal system. *Archives of Biochemistry and Biophysics*, *356*(2), 133–141. doi:10.1006/abbi.1998.0783 PMID:9705203

Aso, T., Uchiyama, S., Matsumura, Y., Taguchi, M., Nozaki, M., Takamatsu, K., Ishizuka, B., Kubota, T., Mizunuma, H., & Ohta, H. (2012). A natural S-equol supplement alleviates hot flushes and other menopausal symptoms in equol nonproducing postmenopausal Japanese women. *Journal of Womens Health (Larchmt)*, *21*, 92-100

Atkinson, C., Berman, S., Humbert, O., & Lampe, J. W. (2004). In vitro incubation of human feces with daidzein and antibiotics suggests interindividual differences in the bacteria responsible for equol production. *The Journal of Nutrition*, *134*, 596–599. PMID:14988453

Atkinson, C., Frankenfeld, C. L., & Lampe, J. W. (2005). Gut bacterial metabolism of the soy isoflavone daidzein: Exploring the relevance to human nutrition. *Experimental Biology and Medicine*, *230*, 155–170. PMID:15734719

Aura, A.-M. (2008). Microbial metabolism of dietary phenolic compounds in the colon. *Phytochemistry Reviews*, *7*(3), 407–429. doi:10.1007/s11101-008-9095-3

Bai, W., Wang, C., & Ren, C. (2013). Intakes of total and individual flavonoids by U.S. adults. *International Journal of Food Sciences and Nutrition*, *65*(1), 9–20. doi:10.3109/09637486.2013.832170 PMID:24020353

Bilal, I., Chowdhury, A., Davidson, J., & Whitehead, S. (2014). Phytoestrogens and prevention of breast cancer: The contentious debate. *World Journal of Clinical Oncology*, *5*(4), 705–712. doi:10.5306/wjco.v5.i4.705 PMID:25302172

Boker, L. K., Van der Schouw, Y. T., De Kleijn, M. J., Jacques, P. F., Grobbee, D. E., & Peeters, P. H. (2002). Intake of dietary phytoestrogens by Dutch women. *The Journal of Nutrition*, *132*, 1319–1328. PMID:12042453

Bolaños, R., Del Castillo, A., & Francia, J. (2010). Soy isoflavones versus placebo in the treatment of climacteric vasomotor symptoms: Systematic review and meta-analysis. *Menopause (New York, N.Y.)*, *17*, 660–666. PMID:20464785

Bolca, S., Possemiers, S., Herregat, A., Huybrechts, I., Heyerick, A., De Vriese, S., & Van de Wiele, T. et al. (2007). Microbial and dietary factors are associated with the equol producer phenotype in healthy postmenopausal women. *The Journal of Nutrition*, *137*, 2242–2246. PMID:17885005

Borrelli, F., & Ernst, E. (2010). Alternative and complementary therapies for the menopause. *Maturitas*, *66*(4), 333–343. doi:10.1016/j.maturitas.2010.05.010 PMID:20580501

Brouns, E. (2002). Soya isoflavones: A new and promising ingredient for the health foods sector. *Food Research International*, *35*(2-3), 187–193. doi:10.1016/S0963-9969(01)00182-X

Brown, N. M., Galandi, S. L., Summer, S. S., Zhao, X., Heubi, J. E., King, E. C., & Setchell, K. D. (2014). S-(-)equol production is developmentally regulated and related to early diet composition. *Nutrition Research (New York, N.Y.)*, *34*(5), 401–409. doi:10.1016/j.nutres.2014.03.005 PMID:24916553

Caldwell, C. R., Britz, S. J., & Mirecki, R. M. (2005). Effect of temperature, elevated carbon dioxide, and drought during seed development on the isoflavone content of dwarf soybean [*Glycine max* (L.) Merrill] grown in controlled environments. *Journal of Agricultural and Food Chemistry*, *53*(4), 1125–1129. doi:10.1021/jf0355351 PMID:15713029

Cao, Y., Calafat, A. M., Doerge, D. R., Umbach, D. M., Bernbaum, J. C., Twaddle, N. C., & Rogan, W. J. et al. (2009). Isoflavones in urine, saliva, and blood of infants: Data from a pilot study on the estrogenic activity of soy formula. *Journal of Exposure Science & Environmental Epidemiology*, *19*(2), 223–234. doi:10.1038/jes.2008.44 PMID:18665197

Cassidy, A., Albertazzi, P., Lise Nielsen, I., Hall, W., Williamson, G., Tetens, I., & Branca, F. et al. (2006). Critical review of health effects of soyabean phyto-oestrogens in post-menopausal women. *The Proceedings of the Nutrition Society*, *65*(01), 76–92. doi:10.1079/PNS2005476 PMID:16441947

Champagne, C. P., Tompkins, T. A., Buckley, N. D., & Green-Johnson, J. M. (2010). Effect of fermentation by pure and mixed cultures of *Streptococcus thermophilus* and *Lactobacillus helveticus* on isoflavone and B-vitamin content of a fermented soy beverage. *Food Microbiology*, *27*(7), 968–972. doi:10.1016/j.fm.2010.06.003 PMID:20688240

Charles, C., Yuskavage, J., Carlson, O., John, M., Tagalicud, A. S., Maggio, M., & Basaria, S. et al. (2009). Effects of high-dose isoflavones on metabolic and inflammatory markers in healthy postmenopausal women. *Menopause (New York, N.Y.)*, *16*(2), 395–400. doi:10.1097/gme.0b013e3181857979 PMID:18981951

Choi, E. J., & Kim, G. H. (2014). The antioxidant activity of daidzein metabolites, *O*-desmethylangolensin and equol, in HepG2 cells. *Molecular Medicine Reports*, *9*, 328–332. PMID:24154619

Clavel, T., Charrier, C., Braune, A., Wenning, M., Blaut, M., & Haller, D. (2009). Isolation of bacteria from the ileal mucosa of TNFdeltaARE mice and description of *Enterorhabdus mucosicola* gen. nov., sp. nov. *International Journal of Systematic and Evolutionary Microbiology*, *59*(7), 1805–1812. doi:10.1099/ijs.0.003087-0 PMID:19542111

Clavel, T., Fallani, M., Lepage, P., Levenez, F., Mathey, J., Rochet, V., & Coxam, V. et al. (2005). Isoflavones and functional foods alter the dominant intestinal microbiota in postmenopausal women. *The Journal of Nutrition*, *135*, 2786–2792. PMID:16317121

Clavel, T., Lepage, P., & Charrier, C. (2014). The family *Coriobacteriaceae*. In E. Rosenberg, E. F. DeLong, S. Lory, E. Stackebrandt, & F. Thompson (Eds.), *The Prokaryotes-Actinobacteria* (pp. 201–238). Berlin: Springer-Verlag.

Clavel, T., & Mapesa, J. O. (2013). Phenolics in human nutrition: importance of the intestinal microbiome for isoflavone and lignin bioavailability. In K. G. Ramawat & J. M. Merillon (Eds.), *Handbook of Natural Products*. Berlin: Springer-Verlag. doi:10.1007/978-3-642-22144-6_94

Crawford, S. L., Jackson, E. A., Churchill, L., Lampe, J. W., Leung, K., & Ockene, J. K. (2013). Impact of dose, frequency of administration, and equol production on efficacy of isoflavones for menopausal hot flashes: A pilot randomized trial. *Menopause (New York, N.Y.)*, *20*(9), 936–945. doi:10.1097/GME.0b013e3182829413 PMID:23511704

Crozier, A., Jaganath, I. B., & Clifford, M. N. (2009). Dietary phenolics: Chemistry, bioavailability and effects on health. *Natural Product Reports*, *26*(8), 1001–1043. doi:10.1039/b802662a PMID:19636448

de Cremoux, P., This, P., Leclercq, G., & Jacquot, Y. (2010). Controversies concerning the use of phytoestrogens in menopause management: Bioavailability and metabolism. *Maturitas*, *65*(4), 334–339. doi:10.1016/j.maturitas.2009.12.019 PMID:20080366

Decroos, K., Eeckhaut, E., Possemiers, S., & Verstraete, W. (2006). Administration of equol-producing bacteria alters the equol production status in the Simulator of the Gastrointestinal Microbial Ecosystem (SHIME). *The Journal of Nutrition*, *136*, 946–952. PMID:16549455

Decroos, K., Vanhemmens, S., Cattoir, S., Boon, N., & Verstraete, W. (2005). Isolation and characterisation of an equol-producing mixed microbial culture from a human faecal sample and its activity under gastrointestinal conditions. *Archives of Microbiology*, *183*(1), 45–55. doi:10.1007/s00203-004-0747-4 PMID:15578160

del Rio, D., Rodriguez-Mateos, A., Spencer, J. P., Tognolini, M., Borges, G., & Crozier, A. (2013). Dietary (poly)phenolics in human health: Structures, bioavailability, and evidence of protective effects against chronic diseases. *Antioxidants & Redox Signalling*, *18*(14), 1818–1892. doi:10.1089/ars.2012.4581 PMID:22794138

Ding, W. K., & Shah, N. P. (2010). Enhancing the biotransformation of isoflavones in soymilk supplemented with lactose using probiotic bacteria during extended fermentation. *Journal of Food Science*, *75*(3), M140–M149. doi:10.1111/j.1750-3841.2010.01526.x PMID:20492303

Duffy, R., Wiseman, H., & File, S. E. (2003). Improved cognitive function in postmenopausal women after 12 weeks of consumption of a soya extract containing isoflavones. *Pharmacology, Biochemistry, and Behavior*, *75*(3), 721–729. doi:10.1016/S0091-3057(03)00116-3 PMID:12895690

European Food Science Authority. (2012). Scientific Opinion on the substantiation of health claims related to soy isoflavones and maintenance of bone mineral density (ID 1655) and reduction of vasomotor symptoms associated with menopause (ID 1654, 1704, 2140, 3093, 3154, 3590) (further assessment) pursuant to Article 13(1) of Regulation (EC) No 1924/2006. *EFSA Journal*, *10*, 2847.

Food and Agriculture Organization/World Health Organization. (2013). Dietary protein quality evaluation in human nutrition. Report of an FAO expert consultation. Food and Agriculture Organization. *Food and Nutrition Paper, 92*.

Food and Drug Administration. (1999). Food labeling, health claims, soy protein, and coronary heart disease. *Federal Register*, *57*, 699–733.

Fournier, L. R., Ryan Borchers, T. A., Robison, L. M., Wiediger, M., Park, J. S., Chew, B. P., & Beerman, K. A. et al. (2007). The effects of soy milk and isoflavone supplements on cognitive performance in healthy, postmenopausal women. *The Journal of Nutrition, Health & Aging*, *11*, 155–164. PMID:17435957

Franke, A. A., Lai, J. F., & Halm, B. M. (2014). Absortion, distribution, metabolism, and excretion of isoflavonoids after soy intake. *Archives of Biochemistry and Biophysics*, *59*, 24–28. doi:10.1016/j.abb.2014.06.007 PMID:24946051

Franke, A. A., Lai, J. F., Halm, B. M., Pagano, I., Kono, N., Mack, W. J., & Hodis, H. N. (2012). Equol production changes over time in postmenopausal women. *The Journal of Nutritional Biochemistry*, *23*(6), 573–579. doi:10.1016/j.jnutbio.2011.03.002 PMID:21775122

Frankenfeld, C. L. (2011). *O*-desmethylangolensin: The importance of equol's lesser known cousin to human health. *Advances in Nutrition*, *2*(4), 317–324. doi:10.3945/an.111.000539 PMID:22332073

Fritz, H., Seely, D., Flower, G., Skidmore, B., Fernandes, R., Vadeboncoeur, S., & Fergusson, D. et al. (2013). Soy, red clover, and isoflavones and breast cancer: A systematic review. *PLoS ONE*, *8*(11), e81968. doi:10.1371/journal.pone.0081968 PMID:24312387

Gardana, C., Canzi, E., & Simonetti, P. (2014). R(-)-*O*-desmethylangolensin is the main enantiomeric form of daidzein metabolite produced by human in vitro and in vivo. *Journal of Chromatography. B, Analytical Technologies in the Biomedical and Life Sciences*, *953-954*, 30–37. doi:10.1016/j.jchromb.2014.01.048 PMID:24561352

Gareau, M. G., Sherman, P. M., & Walker, W. A. (2010). Probiotics and the gut microbiota in intestinal health and disease. *Nature Reviews in Gastroenterology and Hepatology*, *7*(9), 503–514. doi:10.1038/nrgastro.2010.117 PMID:20664519

Gilani, G. S., Nimal Ratnayke, W. M., Mueller, R., & Mazza, G. (2009). Effects of source of protein and supplementary extracted isoflavones and anthocyanins on longevity of Stroke-prone Spontaneously Hypertensive (SHRSP) rats. *The Journal of Toxicological Sciences*, *34*(3), 335–341. doi:10.2131/jts.34.335 PMID:19483387

González-Granillo, M., Steffensen, K. R., Granados, O., Torres, N., Korach-André, M., Ortiz, V., & Tovar, A. R. et al. (2012). Soy protein isoflavones differentially regulate liver X receptor isoforms to modulate lipid metabolism and cholesterol transport in the liver and intestine in mice. *Diabetologia*, *55*, 2469–2478. PMID:22739758

Gou, Z., Jiang, S., Zheng, C., Tian, Z., & Lin, X. (2015). Equol inhibits LPS-induced oxidative stress and enhances the immune response in chicken HD11 macrophages. *Cellular Physiology and Biochemistry*, *36*(2), 611–621. doi:10.1159/000430124 PMID:25997976

Graf, D., Di Cagno, R., Fåk, F., Flint, H. J., Nyman, M., Saarela, M., & Watzl, B. (2015). Contribution of diet to the composition of the human gut microbiota. *Microbial Ecology in Health and Disease*, *26*, 26164. PMID:25656825

Guadamuro, L., Delgado, S., Redruello, B., Flórez, A. B., Suárez, A., Martínez-Camblor, P., & Mayo, B. (2015). Equol status and changes in faecal microbiota in menopausal women receiving long-term treatment for menopause symptoms with a soy-isoflavone concentrate. *Frontiers in Microbiology*, *6*, 777. doi:10.3389/fmicb.2015.00777 PMID:26300856

Guan, L., Huang, Y., & Chen, Z. Y. (2008). Developmental and reproductive toxicity of soybean isoflavones to immature SD rats. *Biomedical and Environmental Sciences*, *21*(3), 197–204. doi:10.1016/S0895-3988(08)60029-X PMID:18714816

Hall, M. C., O'Brien, B., & McCormack, T. (2007). Equol producer status, salivary estradiol profile and urinary excretion of isoflavones in Irish Caucasian women, following ingestion of soymilk. *Steroids*, *72*(1), 64–70. doi:10.1016/j.steroids.2006.10.010 PMID:17157887

Hamden, K., Jaouadi, B., Carreau, S., Aouidet, A., & Elfeki, A. (2011). Therapeutic effects of soy isoflavones on α-amylase activity, insulin deficiency, liver-kidney function and metabolic disorders in diabetic rats. *Natural Product Research*, *25*(3), 244–255. doi:10.1080/14786411003683117 PMID:21108110

Harland, J. I., & Haffner, T. A. (2008). Systematic review, meta-analysis and regression of randomised controlled trials reporting an association between an intake of circa 25 g soya protein per day and blood cholesterol. *Atherosclerosis*, *200*(1), 13–27. doi:10.1016/j.atherosclerosis.2008.04.006 PMID:18534601

He, F. J., & Chen, J. Q. (2013). Consumption of soybean, soy foods, soy isoflavones and breast cancer incidence: Differences between Chinese women and women in Western countries and possible mechanisms. *Food Science and Human Wellness*, *2*(3-4), 146–161. doi:10.1016/j.fshw.2013.08.002

Hedlund, T. E., Johannes, W. U., & Miller, G. J. (2003). Soy isoflavonoid equol modulates the growth of benign and malignant prostatic epithelial cells *in vitro*. *The Prostate*, *54*(1), 68–78. doi:10.1002/pros.10137 PMID:12481257

Heinonen, S., Hoikkala, A., Wähälä, K., & Adlerreutz, H. (2003). Metabolism of the soy isoflavones daidzein, genistein and glycitein in human subjects. Identification of new metabolites having an intact isoflavonoid skeleton. *The Journal of Steroid Biochemistry and Molecular Biology*, *87*(4-5), 285–299. doi:10.1016/j.jsbmb.2003.09.003 PMID:14698210

Hermenegildo, C., Oviedo, P. J., García-Pérez, M. A., Tarín, J. J., & Cano, A. (2005). Effects of phytoestrogens genistein and daidzein on prostacyclin production by human endothelial cells. *The Journal of Pharmacology and Experimental Therapeutics*, *315*(2), 722–728. doi:10.1124/jpet.105.090456 PMID:16046614

Ho, S. C., Chan, S. G., Yip, Y. B., Chan, C. S., Woo, J. L., & Sham, A. (2008). Change in bone mineral density and its determinants in pre- and perimenopausal Chinese women: The Hong Kong Perimenopausal Women Osteoporosis Study. *Osteoporosis International*, *19*(12), 1785–1796. doi:10.1007/s00198-008-0614-2 PMID:18437272

Hong, S. J., Kim, S. I., Kwon, S. M., Lee, J. R., & Chung, B. C. (2002). Comparative study of concentration of isoflavones and lignans in plasma and prostatic tissues of normal control and benign prostatic hyperplasia. *Yonsei Medical Journal*, *43*(2), 236–241. doi:10.3349/ymj.2002.43.2.236 PMID:11971218

Hosoda, K., Furuta, T., & Ishii, K. (2011). Metabolism and disposition of isoflavone conjugated metabolites in humans after ingestion of kinako. *Drug Metabolism and Disposition: the Biological Fate of Chemicals*, *39*(9), 1762–1767. doi:10.1124/dmd.111.038281 PMID:21622628

Hummelova, J., Rondevaldova, J., Balastikova, A., Lapcik, O., & Kokoska, L. (2015). The relationship between structure and *in vitro* antibacterial activity of selected isoflavones and their metabolites with special focus on anti-staphylococcal effect of demethyltexasin. *Letters in Applied Microbiology*, *60*(3), 242–247. doi:10.1111/lam.12361 PMID:25421722

Islam, M. A., Punt, A., Spenkelink, B., Murk, A. J., Rolaf van Leeuwen, F. X., & Rietjens, I. M. (2014). Conversion of major soy isoflavone glucosides and aglycones *in vitro* intestinal models. *Molecular Nutrition & Food Research*, *58*(3), 503–515. doi:10.1002/mnfr.201300390 PMID:24668774

Jackson, R. L., Greiwe, J. S., & Schwen, R. J. (2011). Emerging evidence of the health benefits of S-equol, an estrogen receptor β agonist. *Nutrition Reviews*, *69*(8), 432–448. doi:10.1111/j.1753-4887.2011.00400.x PMID:21790611

Jacobs, A., Wegewitz, U., Sommerfeld, C., Grossklaus, R., & Lampen, A. (2009). Efficacy of isoflavones in relieving vasomotor menopausal symptoms. A systematic review. *Molecular Nutrition & Food Research*, *53*(9), 1084–1097. doi:10.1002/mnfr.200800552 PMID:19653225

Jenks, B. H., Iwashita, S., Nakagawa, Y., Ragland, K., Lee, J., Carson, W. H., & Uchiyama, S. et al. (2012). A pilot study on the effects of S-equol compared to soy isoflavones on menopausal hot flash frequency. *Journal of Women's Health*, *21*(6), 674–782. doi:10.1089/jwh.2011.3153 PMID:22409590

Jin, J. S., Kitahara, M., Sakamoto, M., Hattori, M., & Benno, Y. (2010). *Slackia equolifaciens* sp. nov., a human intestinal bacterium capable of producing equol. *International Journal of Systematic and Evolutionary Microbiology*, *60*(8), 1721–1724. doi:10.1099/ijs.0.016774-0 PMID:19734283

Jing, Z., & Wei-Jie, Y. (2015). Effects of soy protein containing isoflavones in patients with chronic kidney disease: A systematic review and meta-analysis. *Clinical Nutrition (Edinburgh, Lothian)*. doi:10.1016/j.clnu.2015.03.012 PMID:25882339

Joy, S., Siow, R. C., Rowlands, D. J., Becker, M., Wyatt, A. W., Aaronson, P. I., & Mann, G. E. et al. (2006). The isoflavone equol mediates rapid vascular relaxation: Ca2+-independent activation of endothelial nitric-oxide synthase/Hsp90 involving ERK1/2 and Akt phosphorylation in human endothelial cells. *The Journal of Biological Chemistry*, *281*(37), 27335–27345. doi:10.1074/jbc.M602803200 PMID:16840783

Jumpertz, R., Le, D. S., Turnbaugh, P. J., Trinidad, C., Bogardus, C., Gordon, J. I., & Krakoff, J. (2011). Energy-balance studies reveal associations between gut microbes, caloric load, and nutrient absorption in humans. *The American Journal of Clinical Nutrition*, *94*(1), 58–65. doi:10.3945/ajcn.110.010132 PMID:21543530

Kamiyama, M., Kishimoto, Y., Tani, M., Utsunomiya, K., & Kondo, K. (2009). Effects of equol on oxidized low-density lipoprotein-induced apoptosis in endothelial cells. *Journal of Atherosclerosis and Thrombosis*, *16*(3), 239–249. doi:10.5551/jat.1057 PMID:19638716

Kang, J., Badger, T. M., Ronis, M. J., & Wu, X. (2010). Non-isoflavone phytochemicals in soy and their health effects. *Journal of Agricultural and Food Chemistry*, *58*(14), 8119–8133. doi:10.1021/jf100901b PMID:20578706

Karvaj, M., Beno, P., & Fedor-Freybergh, P. G. (2007). Positive effect of flavonoids to cardiovascular and central nervous system. *Neuroendocrinology Letters*, *28*, 1–3. PMID:18030258

Katan, M. B., & de Roos, N. M. (2004). Promises and problems of functional foods. *Critical Reviews in Food Science and Nutrition*, *44*(5), 369–377. doi:10.1080/10408690490509609 PMID:15540650

Kaufman, P. B., Duke, J. A., Brielmann, H., Boik, J., & Hoyt, J. E. (1997). A comparative survey of leguminous plants as sources of the isoflavones, genistein and daidzein: Implications for human nutrition and health. *Journal of Alternative and Complementary Medicine (New York, N.Y.)*, *3*(1), 7–12. doi:10.1089/acm.1997.3.7 PMID:9395689

Kemperman, R. A., Bolca, S., Loger, L. C., & Vaughan, E. E. (2010). Novel approaches for analyzing gut microbes and dietary polyphenols: Challenges and opportunities. *Microbiology*, *156*(11), 3224–3231. doi:10.1099/mic.0.042127-0 PMID:20724384

Kim, M., Kim, S. I., Han, J., Wang, X. L., Song, D. G., & Kim, S. U. (2009). Stereospecific biotransformation of dihydrodaidzein into (3S)-equol by the human intestinal bacterium *Eggerthella* strain Julong 732. *Applied and Environmental Microbiology*, *75*(10), 3062–3068. doi:10.1128/AEM.02058-08 PMID:19304836

Klaenhammer, T., Altermann, E., Arigoni, F., Bolotin, A., Breidt, F., Broadbent, J., & Siezen, R. J. et al. (2002). Discovering lactic acid bacteria by genomics. *Antonie van Leeuwenhoek*, *82*(1/4), 29–58. doi:10.1023/A:1020638309912 PMID:12369195

Kreijkamp-Kaspers, S., Kok, L., Grobbee, D. E., de Haan, E. H., Aleman, A., & van der Schouw, Y. T. (2007). Dietary phytoestrogen intake and cognitive function in older women. *The Journals of Gerontology. Series A, Biological Sciences and Medical Sciences*, *62*(5), 556–562. doi:10.1093/gerona/62.5.556 PMID:17522362

Landete, J. M. (2012). Updated knowledge about polyphenols: Functions, bioavailability, metabolism, and health. *Critical Reviews in Food Science and Nutrition*, *52*(10), 936–948. doi:10.1080/10408398.2010.513779 PMID:22747081

Landete, J. M., Arqués, J., Medina, M., Gaya, P., De La Rivas, B., & Muñoz, R. (2015). Bioactivation of Phytoestrogens: Intestinal Bacteria and Health. *Critical Reviews in Food Science and Nutrition*, 00. doi:10.1080/10408398.2013.789823 PMID:25848676

Lehmann, L., Esch, H. L., Wagner, J., Rohnstock, L., & Metzler, M. (2005). Estrogenic and genotoxic potential of equol and two hydroxylated metabolites of Daidzein in cultured human Ishikawa cells. *Toxicology Letters*, *158*(1), 72–86. doi:10.1016/j.toxlet.2005.02.011 PMID:15993745

Lephart, E. D., West, T. W., Weber, K. S., Rhees, R. W., Setchell, K. D., Adlercreutz, H., & Lund, T. D. (2002). Neurobehavioral effects of dietary soy phytoestrogens. *Neurotoxicology and Teratology*, *24*(1), 5–16. doi:10.1016/S0892-0362(01)00197-0 PMID:11836067

Lethavy, A., Marjoribanks, J., Kronenberg, F., Roberts, H., Eden, J., & Brown, J. (2013). Phytoestrogens for menopausal vasomotor symptoms[Review]. *Cochrane Database of Systematic Reviews*, *12*(no. CD001395). doi:10.1002/14651858.CD001395.pub4 PMID:24323914

Li, Y., Liu, L., Andrews, L. G., & Tollefsbol, T. O. (2009). Genistein depletes telomerase activity through cross-talk between genetic and epigenetic mechanisms. *International Journal of Cancer*, *125*(2), 286–296. doi:10.1002/ijc.24398 PMID:19358274

Liu, L., Guo, X. E., Zhou, Y. Q., & Xia, J. L. (2003). Prevalence of dementia in China. *Dementia and Geriatric Cognitive Disorders*, *15*(4), 226–230. doi:10.1159/000068784 PMID:12626856

Liu, Z. M., Ho, S. C., Woo, J., Chen, Y. M., & Wong, C. (2014). Randomized controlled trial of whole soy and isoflavone daidzein on menopausal symptoms in equol-producing Chinese postmenopausal women. *Menopause (New York, N.Y.)*, *21*(6), 653–660. doi:10.1097/GME.0000000000000102 PMID:24149925

Llaneza, P., González, C., Fernández-Iñarrea, J., Alonso, A., Díaz, F., Arnott, I., & Ferrer-Barriendos, J. (2010). Soy isoflavones, diet and physical exercise modify serum cytokines in healthy obese postmenopausal women. *Phytomedicine*, *18*(4), 245–250. doi:10.1016/j.phymed.2010.07.011 PMID:20732799

Low, Y. L., Dunning, A. M., Dowsett, M., Luben, R. N., Khaw, K. T., Wareham, N. J., & Bingham, S. A. (2006). Implications of gene-environment interaction in studies of gene variants in breast cancer: An example of dietary isoflavones and the D356N polymorphism in the sex hormone-binding globulin gene. *Cancer Research*, *66*(18), 8980–8983. doi:10.1158/0008-5472.CAN-06-2432 PMID:16982738

Lu, L. J. W., Anderson, K. E., Graddy, J. J., & Nagamani, M. (1996). Effects of soya consumption for one month on steroid hormones in premenopausal women: Implications for breast cancer risk reduction. *Cancer Epidemiology, Biomarkers & Prevention*, *5*, 63–70. PMID:8770469

Lund, T. D., Munson, D. J., Haldy, M. E., Setchell, K. D., Lephart, E. D., & Handa, R. J. (2004). Equol is a novel anti-androgen that inhibits prostate growth and hormone feedback. *Biology of Reproduction*, *70*(4), 1188–1195. doi:10.1095/biolreprod.103.023713 PMID:14681200

Mahmoud, A. M., Yang, W., & Bosland, M. C. (2014). Soy isoflavones and prostate cancer: A review of molecular mechanisms. *The Journal of Steroid Biochemistry and Molecular Biology*, *140*, 116–132. doi:10.1016/j.jsbmb.2013.12.010 PMID:24373791

Mantovani, D., Cardozo Filho, L., Santos, L. C., de Souza, V. L., & Watanabe, C. S. (2009). Chromatographic quantification of isoflavone content from soy derivates using HPLC technique. *Journal of Chromatographic Science*, *47*(9), 766–769. doi:10.1093/chromsci/47.9.766 PMID:19835685

Marrian, G. F., & Haslewood, G. A. (1932). Equol, a new inactive phenol isolated from the keto-hydroxyoestrin fraction of mares' urine. *The Biochemical Journal*, *26*(4), 1227–1232. doi:10.1042/bj0261227 PMID:16744928

Martinez, I., Kim, J., Duffy, P. R., Schlegel, V. L., & Walter, J. (2010). Resistant starches types 2 and 4 have differential effects on the composition of the fecal microbiota in human subjects. *PLoS ONE*, *5*(11), e15046. doi:10.1371/journal.pone.0015046 PMID:21151493

Maruo, T., Sakamoto, M., Ito, C., Toda, T., & Benno, Y. (2008). *Adlercreutzia equolifaciens* gen. nov., sp. nov., an equol-producing bacterium isolated from human faeces, and emended description of the genus *Eggerthella. International Journal of Systematic and Evolutionary Microbiology*, *58*(5), 1221–1227. doi:10.1099/ijs.0.65404-0 PMID:18450717

Matthies, A., Blaut, M., & Braune, A. (2009). Isolation of a human intestinal bacterium capable of daidzein and genistein conversion. *Applied and Environmental Microbiology*, *75*(6), 1740–1744. doi:10.1128/AEM.01795-08 PMID:19139227

Matthies, A., Clavel, T., Gütschow, M., Engst, W., Haller, D., Blaut, M., & Braune, A. (2008). Conversion of daidzein and genistein by an anaerobic bacterium newly isolated from the mouse intestine. *Applied and Environmental Microbiology*, *74*(15), 4847–4852. doi:10.1128/AEM.00555-08 PMID:18539813

Matthies, A., Loh, G., Blaut, M., & Braune, A. (2012). Daidzein and genistein are converted to equol and 5-hydroxy-equol by human intestinal *Slackia isoflavoniconvertens* in gnotobiotic rats. *The Journal of Nutrition*, *142*(1), 40–66. doi:10.3945/jn.111.148247 PMID:22113864

Maubach, J., Bracke, M. E., Heyerick, A., Depypere, H. T., Serreyn, R. F., Mareel, M. M., & De Keukeleire, D. (2003). Quantitation of soy-derived phytoestrogens in human breast tissue and biological fluids by high-performance liquid chromatography. *Journal of Chromatography. B, Analytical Technologies in the Biomedical and Life Sciences*, *784*(1), 137–144. doi:10.1016/S1570-0232(02)00789-4 PMID:12504192

Messina, M. (2000). Soyfoods and shoybean phyto-oestrogens (isoflavones) as possible alternatives to hormone replacement therapy. *European Journal of Cancer*, *36*, S71–S77. doi:10.1016/S0959-8049(00)00233-1 PMID:11056326

Messina, M. (2010). A brief historical overview of the past two decades of soy and isoflavone research. *The Journal of Nutrition*, *140*(7), 1350S–1354S. doi:10.3945/jn.109.118315 PMID:20484551

Messina, M., Nagata, C., & Wu, A. H. (2006). Estimated Asian adult soy protein and isoflavone intakes. *Nutrition and Cancer*, *55*(1), 1–12. doi:10.1207/s15327914nc5501_1 PMID:16965235

Minamida, K., Ota, K., Nishimukai, M., Tanaka, M., Abe, A., Sone, T., & Asano, K. et al. (2008). *Asaccharobacter celatus* gen. nov., sp. nov., isolated from rat caecum. *International Journal of Systematic and Evolutionary Microbiology*, *58*(5), 1238–1240. doi:10.1099/ijs.0.64894-0 PMID:18450720

Mitchell, J. H., Gardner, P. T., McPhail, D. B., Morrice, P. C., Collins, A. R., & Duthie, G. G. (1998). Antioxidant efficacy of phytoestrogens in chemical and biological model systems. *Archives of Biochemistry and Biophysics*, *360*(1), 142–148. doi:10.1006/abbi.1998.0951 PMID:9826439

Molla, M. D., Hidalgo-Mora, J. J., & Soteras, M. G. (2011). Phytotherapy as alternative to hormone replacement therapy. *Frontiers in Bioscience*, *3*(1), 191–204. doi:10.2741/s144 PMID:21196369

Morgan, X. C., Segata, N., & Huttenhower, C. (2013). Biodiversity and functional genomics in the human microbiome. *Trends in Genetics*, *29*(1), 51–58. doi:10.1016/j.tig.2012.09.005 PMID:23140990

Morito, K., Hirose, T., Kinjo, J., Hirakawa, T., Okawa, M., Nohara, T., & Masamune, Y. et al. (2001). Interactions of phytoestrogens with estrogen receptors alpha and beta. *Biological & Pharmaceutical Bulletin*, *24*(4), 351–356. doi:10.1248/bpb.24.351 PMID:11305594

Mulligan, A. A., Kuhnle, G. G., Lentjes, M. A., van Scheltinga, V., Powell, N. A., McTaggart, A., & Khaw, K. T. et al. (2013). Intakes and sources of isoflavones, lignans, enterolignans, coumestrol and soya-containing foods in the Norfolk arm of the European Prospective Investigation into Cancer and Nutrition (EPIC-Norfolk), from 7 d food diaries, using a newly updated database. *Public Health Nutrition*, *16*(08), 1454–1462. doi:10.1017/S1368980012003904 PMID:22939391

Nakatsu, C. H., Arsmstrong, A., Cavijo, A. P., Martin, B. R., Barnes, S., & Weaver, C. M. (2014). Fecal bacterial community changes associated with isoflavone metabolites in postmenopausal women after soy bar consumption. *PLoS ONE*, *9*, e108924. PMID:25271941

Newton, K. M., Reed, S. D., Uchiyama, S., Qu, C., Ueno, T., Iwashita, S., & Lampe, J. W. et al. (2015). A cross-sectional study of equol producer status and self-reported vasomotor symptoms. *Menopause (New York, N.Y.)*, *22*(5), 489–495. doi:10.1097/GME.0000000000000363 PMID:25380274

Nielsen, I. L., & Williamson, G. (2007). Review of the factors affecting bioavailability of soy isoflavones in humans. *Nutrition and Cancer*, *57*(1), 1–10. doi:10.1080/01635580701267677 PMID:17516857

Oseni, T., Patel, R., Pyle, J., & Jordan, V. C. (2008). Selective estrogen receptor modulators and phytoestrogens. *Planta Medica*, *74*(13), 1656–1665. doi:10.1055/s-0028-1088304 PMID:18843590

Otieno, D. O., & Shah, N. P. (2007). Endogenous β-glucosidases and β-galactosidases activities from selected probiotic microorganisms and their role in isoflavone biotransformation in soymilk. *Journal of Applied Microbiology*, *103*(4), 910–917. doi:10.1111/j.1365-2672.2007.03438.x PMID:17897193

Oyama, A., Ueno, T., Uchiyama, S., Aihara, T., Miyake, T., Kondo, S., & Matsunaga, K. (2012). The effects of natural S-equol supplementation on skin aging in postmenopausal women: A pilot randomized placebo-controlled trial. *Menopause (New York, N.Y.)*, *19*(2), 202–210. doi:10.1097/gme.0b013e318227427b PMID:21934634

Peeters, P. H. M., Slimani, N., van der Schouw, Y. T., Grace, P. B., Navarro, C., Tjonneland, A., & Bingham, S. A. et al. (2007). Variations in plasma phytoestrogen concentrations in European adults. *The Journal of Nutrition*, *137*, 1294–1300. PMID:17449595

Perabo, F. G., Von Löw, E. C., Ellinger, J., von Rücker, A., Müller, S. C., & Bastian, P. J. (2008). Soy isoflavone genistein in prevention and treatment of prostate cancer. *Prostate Cancer and Prostatic Diseases*, *11*(1), 6–12. doi:10.1038/sj.pcan.4501000 PMID:17923857

Pilšáková, L., Riečanský, I., & Jagla, F. (2010). The physiological actions of isoflavone phytoestrogens. *Physiological Research*, *59*, 651–664. PMID:20406033

Possemiers, S., Bolca, S., Eeckhaut, E., Depypere, H., & Verstraete, W. (2007). Metabolism of isoflavones, lignans and prenylflavonoids by intestinal bacteria: Producer phenotyping and relation with intestinal community. *FEMS Microbiology Ecology*, *61*(2), 372–383. doi:10.1111/j.1574-6941.2007.00330.x PMID:17506823

Qin, J., Li, R., Raes, J., Arumugam, M., Burgdorf, K. S., Manichanh, C., & Wang, J. et al. (2010). A human gut microbial gene catalogue established by metagenomic sequencing. *Nature*, *464*(7285), 59–65. doi:10.1038/nature08821 PMID:20203603

Qiu, L. J., & Chang, R. Z. (2010). The origin and history of soybean. In G. Singh (Ed.), *The Soybean: Botany, Production and Uses*. Oxford, UK: CABI Publishing. doi:10.1079/9781845936440.0001

Rekha, C. R., & Vijayalakshmi, G. (2010). Bioconversion of isoflavone glycoside to aglycones, mineral bioavailability and vitamin B complex in fermented soymilk by probiotic bacteria and yeast. *Journal of Applied Microbiology*, *109*(4), 1198–1208. doi:10.1111/j.1365-2672.2010.04745.x PMID:20477889

Reynolds, K., Chin, A., Lees, K. A., Nguyen, A., Bujnowski, D., He, J., & Rosell, M. S. (2006). A meta-analysis of the effect of soy protein supplementation on serum lipids. *The American Journal of Cardiology*, *98*(5), 633–640. doi:10.1016/j.amjcard.2006.03.042 PMID:16923451

Ridlon, J. M., Kang, D. J., & Hylemon, P. B. (2006). Bile salt biotransformations by human intestinal bacteria. *Journal of Lipid Research*, *47*(2), 241–259. doi:10.1194/jlr.R500013-JLR200 PMID:16299351

Rosell, M. S., Appleby, P. N., Spencer, E. A., & Key, T. J. (2004). Soy intake and blood cholesterol concentrations: A cross-sectional study of 1033 pre- and postmenopausal women in the Oxford arm of the European Prospective Investigation into Cancer and Nutrition. *The American Journal of Clinical Nutrition*, *80*, 1391–1396. PMID:15531691

Rowlands, D. J., Chapple, S., Siow, R. C., & Mann, G. E. (2011). Equol-stimulated mitochondrial reactive oxygen species activate endothelial nitric oxide synthase and redox signaling in endothelial cells: Roles for F-actin and GPR30. *Hypertension*, *57*(4), 833–840. doi:10.1161/HYPERTENSIONAHA.110.162198 PMID:21300668

Rüfer, C. E., Bub, A., Möseneder, J., Winterhalter, P., Stürtz, M., & Kulling, S. E. (2008). Pharmacokinetics of the soybean isoflavone daidzein in its aglycone and glucoside form: A randomized, double-blind, crossover study. *The American Journal of Clinical Nutrition*, *87*, 1314–1323. PMID:18469255

Sánchez-Calvo, J. M., Rodríguez-Iglesias, M. A., Molinillo, J. M. G., & Macías, F. A. (2013). Soy isoflavones and their relationship with microflora: Beneficial effects on human Health in equol producers. *Phytochemistry Reviews*, *12*(4), 979–1000. doi:10.1007/s11101-013-9329-x

Sarkaki, A., Amani, R., Badavi, M., Moghaddam, A. Z., Aligholi, H., Safahani, M., & Haghighizadeh, M. H. (2008). Pre-treatment effect of different doses of soy isoflavones on spatial learning and memory in an ovariectomized animal model of Alzheimer's disease. *Pakistan Journal of Biological Sciences*, *11*, 1114–1119. doi:10.3923/pjbs.2008.1114.1119 PMID:18819549

Satih, S., Chalabi, N., Rabiau, N., Bosviel, R., Fontana, L., Bignon, Y. J., & Bernard-Gallon, D. J. (2010). Gene expression profiling of breast cancer cell lines in response to soy isoflavones using a pangenomic microarray approach. *OMICS: A Journal of Integrative Biology*, *14*(3), 231–238. doi:10.1089/omi.2009.0124 PMID:20455703

Schell, M. A., Karmirantzou, M., Snel, B., Vilanova, D., Berger, B., Zwahlen, M. C., … Arigoni, F. (2002). The genome sequence of *Bifidobacterium longum* reflects its adaptation to the human gastrointestinal tract. *Proceedings of the Natural Academy of Science, USA 99*. doi:10.1073/pnas.212527599

Schröder, C., Matthies, A., Engst, W., Blaut, M., & Braune, A. (2013). Identification and expression of genes involved in the conversion of daidzein and genistein by the equol-forming bacterium *Slackia isoflavoniconvertens*. *Applied and Environmental Microbiology*, *79*(11), 3494–3502. doi:10.1128/AEM.03693-12 PMID:23542626

Schwen, R. J., Nguyen, L., & Jackson, R. L. (2012). Elucidation of the metabolic pathway of S-equol in rat, monkey and man. *Food and Chemical Toxicology*, *50*(6), 2074–2083. doi:10.1016/j.fct.2012.03.048 PMID:22449546

Selma, M. V., Espín, J. C., & Tomás-Barberán, F. A. (2009). Interaction between phenolics and gut microbiota: Role in human health. *Journal of Agricultural and Food Chemistry*, *57*(15), 6485–6501. doi:10.1021/jf902107d PMID:19580283

Selvaraj, V., Zakroczymski, M. A., Naaz, A., Mukai, M., Ju, Y. H., Doerge, D. R., & Cooke, P. S. et al. (2004). Estrogenicity of the isoflavone metabolite equol on reproductive and non-reproductive organs in mice. *Biology of Reproduction*, *71*(3), 966–972. doi:10.1095/biolreprod.104.029512 PMID:15151933

Setchell, K. D., Brown, N. M., Desai, P., Zimmer-Nechemias, L., Wolfe, B. E., Brashear, W. T., & Heubi, J. E. et al. (2001). Bioavailability of pure isoflavones in healthy humans and analysis of commercial soy isoflavone supplements. *The Journal of Nutrition*, *131*, 1362S–1375S. PMID:11285356

Setchell, K. D., & Clerici, C. (2010). Equol: History, chemistry, and formation. *The Journal of Nutrition*, *140*(7), 1355S–1362S. doi:10.3945/jn.109.119776 PMID:20519412

Setchell, K. D., Clerici, C., Lephart, E. D., Cole, S. J., Heenan, C., Castellani, D., & Heubi, J. E. et al. (2005). S-equol, a potent ligand for estrogen receptor beta, is the exclusive enantiomeric form of the soy isoflavone metabolite produced by human intestinal bacterial flora. *The American Journal of Clinical Nutrition*, *81*, 1072–1079. PMID:15883431

Setchell, K. D., & Cole, S. J. (2006). Method of defining equol-producer status and its frequency among vegetarians. *The Journal of Nutrition*, *136*, 2188–2193. PMID:16857839

Setchell, K. D., Faughnan, M. S., Avades, T., Zimmer-Nechemias, L., Brown, N. M., Wolfe, B. E., & Cassidy, A. et al. (2003). Comparing the pharmacokinetics of daidzein and genistein with the use of 13C-labeled tracers in premenopausal women. *The American Journal of Clinical Nutrition*, *77*, 411–419. PMID:12540402

Setchell, K. D. R., Brown, N. M., & Lydeking-Olsen, E. (2002). Clinical importance of the metabolite equol. A clue to the effectiviness of soy and its isoflavones. *The Journal of Nutrition*, *132*, 3577–3584. PMID:12468591

Shimada, Y., Takahashi, M., Miyazawa, N., Abiru, Y., Uchiyama, S., & Hishigaki, H. (2012). Identification of a novel dihydrodaidzein racemase essential for biosynthesis of equol from daidzein in *Lactococcus* sp. strain 20-92. *Applied and Environmental Microbiology*, *78*(14), 4902–4907. doi:10.1128/AEM.00410-12 PMID:22582059

Shimada, Y., Takahashi, M., Miyazawa, N., Ohtani, T., Abiru, Y., Uchiyama, S., & Hishigaki, H. (2011). Identification of two novel reductases involved in equol biosynthesis in *Lactococcus* strain 20-92. *Journal of Molecular Microbiology and Biotechnology*, *2*(3-4), 160–172. doi:10.1159/000335049 PMID:22286043

Shimada, Y., Yasuda, S., Takahashi, M., Hayashi, T., Miyazawa, N., Sato, I., & Hishigaki, H. et al. (2010). Cloning and expression of a novel NADP(H)-dependent daidzein reductase, an enzyme involved in the metabolism of daidzein, from equol-producing *Lactococcus* strain 20-92. *Applied and Environmental Microbiology*, *76*(17), 5892–5901. doi:10.1128/AEM.01101-10 PMID:20639368

Simons, A. L., Renouf, M., Hendrich, S., & Murphy, P. A. (2005). Metabolism of glycitein (7;4'-dihydroxy-6-methoxy-isoflavone) by human gut microflora. *Journal of Agricultural and Food Chemistry*, *53*(22), 8519–8525. doi:10.1021/jf051546d PMID:16248547

Steensma, A., Noteborn, H. P., & Kuiper, H. A. (2004). Comparison of Caco-2, IEC-18 and HCEC cell lines as a model for intestinal absorption of genistein, daidzein and their glycosides. *Environmental Toxicology and Pharmacology*, *16*(3), 131–139. doi:10.1016/j.etap.2003.11.008 PMID:21782699

Steer, T., Johnson, I. T., Gee, J. M., & Gibson, G. R. (2003). Metabolism of the soyabean isoflavone glycoside genistin in vitro by the human gut bacteria and the effect of prebiotics. *The British Journal of Nutrition*, *90*(03), 635–642. doi:10.1079/BJN2003949 PMID:13129470

Sugiyama, Y., Masumori, N., Fukuta, F., Yoneta, A., Hida, T., Yamashita, T., & Tsukamoto, T. et al. (2013). Influence of isoflavone intake and equol-producing intestinal flora on prostate cancer risk. *Asian Pacific Journal of Cancer Prevention*, *14*(1), 1–4. doi:10.7314/APJCP.2013.14.1.1 PMID:23534704

Sugiyama, Y., Nagata, Y., Fukuta, F., Takayanagi, A., Masumori, N., Tsukamoto, T., & Mori, M. et al. (2014). Counts of *Slackia* sp. strain NATTS in intestinal flora are correlated to serum concentrations of equol both in prostate cancer cases and controls in Japanese men. *Asian Pacific Journal of Cancer Prevention*, *15*(6), 2693–2697. doi:10.7314/APJCP.2014.15.6.2693 PMID:24761887

Tai, T. Y., Tsai, K. S., Tu, S. T., Wu, J. S., Chang, C. I., Chen, C. L., & Wu, C. H. et al. (2012). The effect of soy isoflavone on bone mineral density in postmenopausal Taiwanese women with bone loss: A 2-year randomized double-blind placebo-controlled study. *Osteoporosis International*, *23*(5), 1571–1580. doi:10.1007/s00198-011-1750-7 PMID:21901480

Taku, K., Melby, M. K., Kurzer, M. S., Mizuno, S., Watanabe, S., & Ishimi, Y. (2010). Effects of soy isoflavone supplements on bone turnover markers in menopausal women: Systematic review and meta-analysis of randomized controlled trials. *Bone*, *47*(2), 413–423. doi:10.1016/j.bone.2010.05.001 PMID:20452475

Taku, K., Melby, M. K., Nishi, N., Omori, T., & Kurzer, M. S. (2011). Soy isoflavones for osteoporosis: An evidence-based approach. *Maturitas*, *70*(4), 333–338. doi:10.1016/j.maturitas.2011.09.001 PMID:21958941

Taku, K., Umegaki, K., Ishimi, Y., & Watanabe, S. (2008). Effects of extracted soy isoflavones alone on blood total and LDL cholesterol: Meta-analysis of randomized controlled trials. *Journal of Therapeutics and Clinical Risk Management*, *4*, 1097–1103. PMID:19209289

Tho, H., Oshima, K., Suzuki, T., Hattori, M., & Morita, H. (2013). Complete genome sequence of the equol-producing bacterium *Adlerkreutzia equolifaciens* DSM 19450. *Genome Announcements*, *1*, e00742. PMID:24051320

Thompson, L. U., Boucher, B. A., Liu, Z., Cotterchio, M., & Kreiger, N. (2006). Phytoestrogen content of foods consumed in Canada, including isoflavones, lignans, and coumestan. *Nutrition and Cancer*, *54*(2), 184–201. doi:10.1207/s15327914nc5402_5 PMID:16898863

Tousen, Y., Abe, F., Ishida, T., Uehara, M., & Ishimi, Y. (2011). Resistant starch promotes equol production and inhibits tibial bone loss in ovariectomized mice treated with daidzein. *Metabolism: Clinical and Experimental*, *60*(10), 1425–1432. doi:10.1016/j.metabol.2011.02.009 PMID:21550090

Tsangalis, D., Ashton, J. F., McGill, A. E. J., & Shah, N. P. (2002). Enzymic transformation of isoflavone phytoestrogens in soy milk by β-glucosidase producing bifidobacteria. *Journal of Food Science*, *67*(8), 3104–3113. doi:10.1111/j.1365-2621.2002.tb08866.x

Tsuji, H., Moriyama, K., Nomoto, K., & Akaza, H. (2012). Identification of an enzyme system for daidzein-to-equol conversion in *Slackia* sp. strain NATTS. *Applied and Environmental Microbiology*, *78*(4), 1228–1236. doi:10.1128/AEM.06779-11 PMID:22179235

Tsuji, H., Moriyama, K., Nomoto, K., Miyanaga, N., & Akaza, H. (2010). Isolation and characterization of the equol-producing bacterium *Slackia* sp. strain NATTS. *Archives of Microbiology*, *192*(4), 279–287. doi:10.1007/s00203-010-0546-z PMID:20237913

Uchiyama, S., Ueno, T., & Suzuki, T. (2007). Identification of a newly isolated equol-producing lactic acid bacterium from the human feces. *Journal of Intestinal Microbiology*, *21*, 217–220. doi:10.11209/jim.21.217

Wada, K., Nakamura, K., Tamai, Y., Tsuji, M., Kawachi, T., Hori, A., & Nagata, C. et al. (2013). Soy isoflavone intake and breast cancer risk in Japan: From the Takayama study. *International Journal of Cancer*, *133*, 952–960. PMID:23389819

Wang, D., Wang, L., Zhu, F., Zhu, J., Chen, X. D., Zou, L., & Li, L. et al. (2008). *In vitro and in vivo* studies on the antioxidant activities of the aqueous extracts of Douchi (A traditional Chinese slat fermented soybean food). *Food Chemistry*, *17*(4), 1421–1428. doi:10.1016/j.foodchem.2007.09.072

Wang, X. L., Hur, H. G., Lee, J. H., Kim, K. T., & Kim, S. I. (2005). Enantioselective synthesis of S-equol from dihydrodaidzein by a newly isolated anaerobic human intestinal bacterium. *Applied and Environmental Microbiology*, *71*(1), 214–219. doi:10.1128/AEM.71.1.214-219.2005 PMID:15640190

Wang, X. L., Kim, H. J., Kang, S. I., Kim, S. I., & Hur, H. G. (2007). Production of phytoestrogen S-equol from daidzein in mixed culture of two anaerobic bacteria. *Archives of Microbiology*, *187*(2), 155–160. doi:10.1007/s00203-006-0183-8 PMID:17109177

Wei, P., Liu, M., Chen, Y., & Chen, D.-D. (2012). Systematic review of soy isoflavone supplements on osteoporosis in women. *Asian Pacific Journal of Tropical Medicine*, *5*(3), 243–248. doi:10.1016/S1995-7645(12)60033-9 PMID:22305793

Wei, Q.-K., Chen, T.-R., & Chen, J.-T. (2007). Using *Lactobacillus* and *Bifidobacterium* to produce the isoflavone aglycones in fermented soymilk. *International Journal of Food Microbiology*, *117*(1), 120–124. doi:10.1016/j.ijfoodmicro.2007.02.024 PMID:17477997

Wei, X. J., Wu, J., Ni, Y. D., Lu, L. Z., & Zhao, R. Q. (2011). Antioxidant effect of a phytoestrogen equol on cultured muscle cells of embryonic broilers. *In Vitro Cellular & Developmental Biology. Animal*, *47*(10), 735–741. doi:10.1007/s11626-011-9464-x PMID:22083625

Wiseman, H., Casey, K., Bowey, E. A., Duffy, R., Davies, M., Rowland, I. R., & Clarke, D. B. et al. (2004). Influence of 10 wk of soy consumption on plasma concentrations and excretion of isoflavonoids and on gut microflora metabolism in healthy adults. *The American Journal of Clinical Nutrition*, *80*, 692–699. PMID:15321810

Women's Health Initiative. (2010). *Findings from the WHI Postmenopausal Hormone Therapy Trials.* Retrieved from: http://www.nhlbi.nih.gov/whi/

Yamori, Y. (2006). Food factors for aterosclerosis prevention: Asian perspective derived from analyses of worldwide dietary biomarkers. *Experimental and Clinical Cardiology*, *11*, 94–98. PMID:18651042

Yanagihara, K., Takigahira, M., Mihara, K., Kubo, T., Morimoto, C., Morita, Y., & Seyama, T. et al. (2013). Inhibitory effects of isoflavones on tumor growth and cachexia in newly established cachectic mouse models carrying human stomach cancers. *Nutrition and Cancer*, *65*(4), 578–589. doi:10.1080/01635581.2013.776089 PMID:23659450

Yokoyama, S., Oshima, K., Nomura, I., Hattori, M., & Suzuki, T. (2011). Complete genomic sequence of the equol-producing bacterium *Eggerthella* sp. strain YY7918, isolated from adult human intestine. *Journal of Bacteriology, 193*(19), 5570–5571. doi:10.1128/JB.05626-11 PMID:21914883

Yokoyama, S., & Suzuki, T. (2008). Isolation and characterization of a novel equol-producing bacterium from human feces. *Bioscience, Biotechnology, and Biochemistry, 72*(10), 2660–2666. doi:10.1271/bbb.80329 PMID:18838805

Yu, Z. T., Yao, W., & Zhu, W. Y. (2008). Isolation and identification of equol-producing bacterial strains from cultures of pig faeces. *FEMS Microbiology Letters, 282*(1), 73–80. doi:10.1111/j.1574-6968.2008.01108.x PMID:18328079

Yuan, J.-P., Wang, J.-H., & Liu, X. (2007). Metabolism of dietary soy isoflavones to equol by human intestinal microbiota. Implications for health. *Molecular Nutrition & Food Research, 51*(7), 765–781. doi:10.1002/mnfr.200600262 PMID:17579894

Zamora-Ros, R., Knaze, V., Luján-Barroso, L., Kuhnle, G. G., Mulligan, A. A., Touillaud, M., & González, C. A. (2012, August). Dietary intakes and food sources of phytoestrogens in the European Prospective Investigation into Cancer and Nutrition (EPIC) 24-hour dietary recall cohort. *European Journal of Clinical Nutrition, 66*(8), 932–941. doi:10.1038/ejcn.2012.36 PMID:22510793

Zhang, J., Ge, Y., Han, F., Li, B., Yan, S., Sun, J., & Wang, L. (2014). Isoflavone content of soybean cultivars from maturity group 0 to VI grown in Northern and Southern China. *Journal of the American Oil Chemists' Society, 91*(6), 1019–1028. doi:10.1007/s11746-014-2440-3 PMID:24882872

Zheng, W., Hou, Y., Su, Y., & Yao, W. (2014). Lactulose promotes equol production and changes the microbial community *in vitro* of daidzein by fecal inocula of sows. *Anaerobe, 25*, 47–52. doi:10.1016/j.anaerobe.2013.11.011 PMID:24315807

Chapter 12
Application of the Dietary Processed Sulfur Supplementation for Enhancing Nutritional and Functional Properties of Meat Products

Chi-Ho Lee
Konkuk University, South Korea

ABSTRACT

In recent years, the consumer demands for healthier meat and meat products with reduced level of fat, cholesterol, decreased contents of sodium chloride and nitrite, improved composition of fatty acid profile and incorporated health enhancing ingredients are rapidly increasing worldwide and prevent the risk of diseases. This review focuses on strategies to investigate the changes in physical, physicochemical and microbial properties of meat and meat products in dietary processed sulfur fed animals. Overall, this review focuses on sulfur supplementation to pigs, growth performance of pigs and meat quality, enhancing the nutritional and functional values, shelf-life extension, improve sensory quality characteristics and health benefit etc. This review further discusses the current status, consumer acceptance, and market for functional foods from the global viewpoints. Future prospects for functional meat and meat products are also discussed.

INTRODUCTION

Meat and meat products are important sources for protein, fat, essential amino acids, minerals and vitamin and other nutrients (Biesalski, 2005). Pork meat is usually consumed than any other meat products in South Korea. In 2012, approximately, 50% of the total meat consumption was pork compared to 22% of beef meat and 28% of poultry meat. Meat consumption has increased from 17.8kg per person to 19.3 kg per person in 2010 (Ministry for Food, Agriculture, Forestry and Fisheries. 2011). Recently, there

DOI: 10.4018/978-1-5225-0591-4.ch012

has been a major shift in Korean consumer's preference for leaner and more functional meat. Especially, consumers become more concerned about nutrition and functional health that changed the consumption patterns of meat and meat products. The carcass and meat quality attributes could be affected by the differences in dietary components, such as fatty acids composition, genetic type, age, and other supplements including green tea, Korean ginseng, garlic etc. Limited scientific reports are available for the effects of the processed sulfur concentration of the diet on meat quality. Especially, garlic is an important spice which is inevitable in Korean food. Garlic contains plentiful di-allyl sulfide of pungent taste and is generally found in plant compounds that give certain distinguishable odors to onions, a green onion, leek, garlic (Stanley *et al.*, 1998). Garlic has been used by Koreans for major spices in ordinary diets. Sulfur has been used as a traditional healing material for infirm patients (Stanley *et al.*, The Miracle of MSM., a Berkley book/published by The Berkley Publishing Group, New York 10014). Recently, consumers prefer to the animal functional foods with low fat and high meat quality products rather than high saturated fatty acids containing meat products. The palatability of pork is positively associated with oleic acids of marbling fats (Kim *et al.*, 2015). Therefore, advanced technology needs to be considered for increasing the oleic acid, amino acids with umami, and water holding capacity with meat quality, and for decreasing the saturated fatty acids in pig performance and pork products.

Dry-cured ham was made of pork, solar salt, fresh air, and fermentation in Southern Europe 2000 years ago, and hind leg surface was rubbed with salt and other additives to remove moisture (Mikami *et al.*, . 2007). Drying typically took 6–12 months or more (Mikami *et al.*, 2007). Dry-cured ham reduces weight by about 18% during ripening periods (typically 20–35% for Spanish ham) and concentrates the unique taste and aroma (Mikami *et al.*, 2007). The unique aroma and flavor is produced by enzymatic action and chemical reactions that occur during the long ripening period (Mikami *et al.*, 2007).

Sulfur has four isotopes with atomic numbers of 16, 17, 18 and 20. Processed sulfur was made by heating and melting to material or light mineral, separated the upper liquid sulfur and cooled material. It usually contained selenium and tellurium (Lee *et al.*, 2010). In Chinese medicine, sulfur has effects on homeostasis, nerve paralysis, and cold hands and feet and promotes a stronger muscle skeletal system (Stanley *et al.*, 1998). Western medicine has used sulfur for local irritants, constipation, hemorrhoids and skin diseases. It was also used to treat for dysentery, cholera, and typhoid before the development of antibiotics as it inhibits the growth of pathogenic microorganisms (Stanley *et al.* 1998). However, sulfur is highly toxic, and it is necessary to process the sulfur to remove toxic property for use as a medicine. Sulfur can cause side effects if ingested by humans or animals (Lee *et al.*, 2010). Methyl sulfonyl methane is found *Allium hookeri*, garlic, and green onion. (Lee *et al.*, 2009). Sulfur is also a component of sulfuric amino acids, collagen, polysaccharides, glycoproteins, and glutathione.

This review was to investigate the changes in physical, physicochemical and microbial properties of carcass and meat products in dietary processed sulfur fed pigs.

EFFECTS OF THE PROCESSED SULFUR SUPPLEMENTATION ON THE GROWTH PERFORMANCE AND MEAT QUALITY IN PIGS

When weaning pigs and growing-finishing pigs take sulfur supplementation, two different level of 0.1% (T1), 0.3% (T2) processed sulfur was added to commercial feed (control) to study the effects on the productivity and meat quality of pigs (Ha Young Noh. 2014). The weight, daily gain, daily feed intake and feed efficiency of weaning pigs by taking processed sulfur supplementation showed no significant difference between the treatments. However, T1 and T2 in 1st week with reduced feed intake, tended to increase daily feed intake and improve feed efficiency compared to the control. In 2nd week, daily gain was lowered but did not show any significant difference compared to the treatments. In 4th week, T1 and T2 for weight and daily gain increased compared to the control and T1 for feed efficiency was highly improved. The addition of 0.1% processed sulfur supplementation could be used for weaning pigs as the appropriate level.

The results of weight, daily gain, daily feed intake and feed efficiency of growing-finishing pigs with processed sulfur supplementation showed no significant difference between the treatments. However, weight was increased in T1 and T2 during in the weaning and growing period. However, daily gain was lowered with processed sulfur supplementation. T1 was the highest as 33.4 kg/day/head in daily feed intake and T2 was the lowest. There was no significant difference in feed efficiency.

In hematological assay of growing-finishing pigs fed processed sulfur, most of the survey items did not show significant difference. However, total protein in T1(6.37 g/dl) was significantly higher than the control (5.73 g/dl) and T2(5.77 g/dl. T1 (2.67 g/dl) for globulin content had significantly higher than other treatments. T1 had higher HDL-Cholesterol concentration of 36.20 mg/dl which was higher than other treatments. T1 had the creatinine content of 2.03 mg/dl which was significantly lower than the control (2.30 mg/dl). T2contained the uric acid of 0.63 mg/dl and triglyceride of 32.20 mg/dl which were significantly lower than other treatments.

Analysis of blood fatty acids of growing-finishing pigs with processed sulfur supplementation represented that the control had higher total SFA (42.05%), while T2 had higher total MUFA (51.08%) and w6 (9.30%) than T1 and control. T2 was also the highest in total w3 fatty acid.

Carcass grade and characteristics for processed sulfur fed pigs indicated that the backfat thickness for T1 and T2 were 23.54 and 25.07 mm, respectively, which were higher than the control. The control did not have 1+A grade, whereas T1 and T2 had 9.8and 4.5%of 1+A grade in carcass, respectively. Thus, the addition of 0.1% processed sulfur supplementation might be suggested as an appropriate level in growing-finishing pigs for carcass grade.

There were no significant differences in moisture and crude protein contents among the treatments. T2 had relatively lower the crude fat content, heating loss, and expressible drip than the control and T1. The pH value of growing pigs was significantly lower in T2. Chromaticity of growing pigs showed no significant difference in brightness among the control and processed sulfur supplementation treatment, whereas growing pigs by taking processed sulfur supplementation had significantly higher red color intensity than the control. T2 had the lowest value of thiobarbituric acid reactive substances (TBARS) after 5 days storage compared to the control and T1. Amino acid composition of growing pigs showed no significant difference in total amino acid composition among the treatment, while the higher methionine and cysteine contents were found in growing pigs with processed sulfur supplementation. Fatty acid composition of growing pigs had no significant difference in saturated fatty acids among the treatment. However, T2 contained significantly lower saturated and higher total w3 fatty acids than the control and T1. Although T2 had lower marbling score than the control, T2 had higher aroma and juiciness scores than compared to the control and T1. It would suggest that the addition of 0.3% processed sulfur supplementation might be regarded as an appropriate level of the desirable nutritional and sensory propertiesfor growing pigs.

Sulfur Effects on the Carcass of Beef Cattle

The beef cattle NRC (2000) recommends 0.15% sulfur to support adequate growth of beef cattle. Sulfur is required for growth and metabolism of many ruminal bacteria, particularly cellulolytic bacteria (Spears et al., 1976). Additionally, S is needed as a component of the S amino acids methionine, cysteine, and cystine, as well as the B vitamins thiamine and biotin (NRC, 2000).

Processed Sulfur Effects on Broilers and Ducks

Processed sulfur-fed broilers gained weight with decreased saturated fatty acids (Park et al. 2010). Increased weight was also found in broiler when fed with dietary 0.2% sulfur supplementation (Shin et al. 2013). Sulfur feeding also decreased total fat content and undesirable odors, and increased texture property of meat (Park et al. 2003). The 0.15% Processed sulfur-fed broilers had more weight, increased gain weight and feed consumption compared to the control (Kim et al., 2013). Decreased crude fat, triglyceride, and abdominal fat contents were also found in sulfur fed broilers (Park et al., 2003; Wallis, 1999; Shin 2013). Processed sulfur fed ducks had higher polyunsaturated fatty acids than the control (Park et al., 1999)

Processed Sulfur Effects on Pork Meats

Few studies were available for the processed sulfur effects on carcass and meat quality in Korea. Lee et al (2009) informed that the physicochemical, meat color and texture properties of pork loin are not affected by Methyl Sulfonyl Methane (MSM) supplementation from comparison the quality characteristics of pork from finishing pigs fed different levels of MSM. Loughmiller et al., (1998) reported that dietary sulfur amino acids and methionine on growth performance and carcass characteristics of finishing gilts resulted in the reduction in body weight according to the increased dietary sulfur amino acids supplementation. Detoxified effect of processed sulfur has been proved by toxicity test with animal model (Kim et al 2006). Moreover, it was previously reported that feeding 0.1% processed sulfur fed pigs was efficient for growing performance (Jang et al. 2006). Recently, sulfur has been used to feed pigs in order to produce good quality of meat products (Cho et. al. 2015). Sulfur compounds are also known for high antioxidant activity to increase the shelf life of meat products (Cho et. al. 2015).

PROCESSED SULFUR EFFECTS ON FUNCTIONAL PROPERTIES OF DRY CURED HAM DURING STORAGE

Sulfur is the eighth most abundant element in all living organisms and is the major ingredientof essential amino acids, such as thiamine and biotin, being absorbed and utilized by the body (Kim et al., 2005). Processed Sulfur was made by heating and melting to material or light mineral to separate the upper liquid sulfur and obtained from the cooled material, which contain selenium and tellurium (Lee *et al.*, 2010). In Chinese medicine, sulfur has the effects on hemostasis, nerve paralysis, and cold hands and feet. It also promotes a stronger musculoskeletal system (Lee *et al.*, 2009). In western medicine, sulfur has been used for local irritants, constipation, hemorrhoids and skin diseases, and was also used to treat for dysentery, cholera, and typhoid before the development of antibiotics as it inhibits the growth of pathogenic microorganisms (Block, 1986, 1992; Kumar *et al.*, 1998). However, sulfur is known for highly toxic, and thus it is necessary for sulfur to remove toxic property being used as a proper medicine. Sulfur may cause side effects if ingested by humans or animals (Choi *et al.*, 2002; Park *et al.*, 2010; Barrenrine *et al.*, 1958; Bouchard *et al.*, 1973).Methyl sulfonyl methane is found in *Allium hookeri*, garlic, and green onion. (Son *et al.*, 2012). Sulfur is also the main component of sulfuric amino acids, collagen, polysaccharides, glycoproteins, and glutathione and is essential for the action of steroid hormones and various growth factors (Park *et al.*, 2010).

Proximate Analysis

Changes in physicochemical, microbiological and sensory properties of dry cured ham during storage in processed sulfur fed pigs were investigated by Kim *et al.* (2014). Dry cured ham products were manufactured from processed sulfur (PS)-fed pigs according to the level of dietary PS. Three groups were used:CON, commercial basal dietary fed pigs; T1, 0.1% PS dietary fed pigs and T2, 0.3% PS dietary fed pigs. During the drying and ripening process, moisture content of CON, T1 and T2 significantly decreased from 71–73% to 50–55%, and crude protein, crude fat and ash contents significantly increased after 10 months storage. Moisture content in T2 was significantlyhigher than CON and crude fat content of T1 and T2 was significantly lower than that of CON. Lee et al (2009) and Li et al (2013) reported that feeding sulfur to pigs showed improve of water holding capacity and lower fat content in meat. In addition, a decrease in weight loss increased moisture content of dry cured ham during the drying and ripening period (Holden *et al.* 1998; Yeh & Liu, 2001). Therefore, the higher moisture content and reduced lipid level of T1 and T2 at 10 month seemed to be influenced by dietary sulfur supplement.

pH, Water Activity, and TBARS

pH values of dry cured ham in all groups increasedsignificantly at 4 months and remained stable during the ripening period.Previous studies indicated that lactic acid bacteria do not play an important role in dry cured ham preparation with salt added during storage (Molina *et al.* 1989; Jose *et al.* 2010). Initial pH value was not significantly different among CON, T1 and T2 groups. However, the pH of T1 and T2 was significantly lower than CON at 8 months. Several researches were investigated for increased pH in meat products during storage. Liberation of free amino acids, accumulation of ammonia or electrolyte changes during the ripening process can result in an increased pH value (Wardow *et al.* 1973; Hamm, 1974; Deymer & Vandekerckhove, 1979; Park *et al.* 1997).

Water activity of all dry cured ham significantly decreased from 0.99 to 0.92% during the drying and ripening period. The a_w of T2 was significantly higher than CON at 10 months. Dry cured hams made from processed sulfur-fed pigs may have increased lipid oxidation stability due to the negative relationship between a_w and lipid oxidation during the manufacture of dry cured meat products (Fanco *et al.* 2002; Lee *et al.* 2009).

TBA values for T1, T2 and CON significantly increased from 0.29 to 0.40 mg MDA/kg during processing. TBA values during the ripening of dry cured hams beyond 10 months were 0.29–0.44 mg MDA/kg (Cilla *et al.* 2006). A significant difference was observed between CON and sulfur-fed pigs (T1 and T2). Dietary sulfur-fed pigs showed increased antioxidant ability in dry cured ham. Glutathione is known as asulfur-containing protein that scavenges free radicals, and is synthesized throughout the trans-sulfuration pathway (Gulizar, 2004; Song *et al.* 2013; Martha & Iori, 2011). Changes in crude fat content and TBA values of all groups showed a positive relationship during storage (r = 0.56). Comparable results on lipid content and the level of lipid oxidation in meat products were also reported by Ismail *et al* (2009) and Veronica *et al* (2014).

VBN (Volatile Basic Nitrogen)

The value of VBN in CON, T1 and T2 groups increased significantly during the drying and ripening period. Previous studies indicated that some microbes have the ability to decompose proteins that generate volatile nitrogen compounds in meat products (Cilla *et al.* 2006; Darmadji *et al.* 1990). Other studies also reported that the concentration of free amino acids and peptides could increase during the ripening period, and free amino acids convert to biogenic amines during the ripening process (Virgili *et al.* 2007; Martuscelli *et al.* 2009). T1 and T2 had a significantly higher VBN value than CON at 4 and 10 months. A significant positive correlation was found between VBN and the level of dietary sulfur fed to pigs. Other studies indicated that sulfur-containing amino acids might be involved in the formation of cross-links or disulfide bonds between proteins (Marinaane *et al.* 2011; Stadman & Levine, 2003; Kim *et al.* 2000).

Microbial Counts during Ripening

A total aerobic bacterium of T2 was significantly lower than CON during storage. This could be attributed to the antimicrobial effect of sulfur. Antimicrobial activity of sulfur compounds has been studied by adding garlic to meat products (Yin & Cheng, 2003; Sallam *et al.*, 2004). Total aerobic and lactic acid bacteria colonies of all groups increased significantly until 4 months, and then tended to decline during the drying and ripening period. A decrease in water activity of dry cured ham could inhibit the growth of microorganisms during ripening process. Furthermore, growth of lactic bacteria had progressed during the fermentation process, and adecrease in pH value of dry cured ham by lactic acids showed antioxidant ability (Egan, 1983; Lin & Yen, 1999). These tendencies were also observed by Jose *et al.* (2010) and Vilar *et al.* (2000).

Changes in Fatty Acids during the Storage

Fatty acid composition is important to the taste and flavor of dry cured ham (Pastorelli *et al*, 2003). Lipid degradation occurs during the drying and ripening period, and fat content and fatty acid composition affect the texture and appearance of dry cured ham (Ruiz-Carrascal *et al.* 2000; Seong *et al.* 2010). The most plentiful saturated fatty acids in dry cured ham were palmitic acid (23.18–24.24%), stearic acid (13.73–14.72%) and myristic acid (1.07–1.17%). T1 and T2 showed significantly lower concentrations of linoleic acid than CON. Many lipid oxidation products such as hexanal are formed from linoleic acid (Frankel 1984). Oleic acid concentrations in CON at the initial phase were significantly higher than T1 and T2. After fermentation, oleic acid of T1 and T2 was significantly higher than CON. Lunt and Smith (1991) reported that high oleic acid concentration improves the taste of meat and impacts positive sensory score. According to Ruiz *et al* (2000), high fat concentration in dry cured ham positively affects the ratio of oleic acid to unsaturated fatty acids. The saturated fatty acid of CON was significantly higher than T1 and T2, and PUFA of T1 and T2 was significantly higher than CON in raw meat. Cameron and Enser (1991) reported that an increase in the MUFA/PUFA ratio enhances the taste of meat. In this study, MUFA/PUFA of T1 and T2 was significantly higher than CON. The polyunsaturated fatty acid/saturated fatty acid (PUFA/SFA ratio) in sulfur groups (0.35- 0.39) were significantly lower than CON (0.43). One of the most important indicators for evaluating nutritional quality of meat products is the PUFA/SFA ratio. COMA (1984) recommended a PUFA/SFA ratio of 0.4–0.45.

Significant differences of Δ-9- desaturase (16) index among CON, T1 and T2 were not found in the state of raw meat. However, Δ-9- desaturase (18) index of T1 was significantly lower than that of the control and T2. Nevertheless, Δ-9- desaturase (16) index of T2 was significantly lower than that of the control group from dry cured loin, whereas Δ-9- desaturase (18) index of T1 and T2 was significantly higher than that of the control group. Pogge, Lonergan and Hansen (2014) exhibited that increasing the desaturase activity of beef was affected by dietary sulfur addition.

Change in Free Amino Acids during Storage

The concentration of free amino acids in T1, T2 and CON significantly increased during the drying and ripening period. Previous studies reported that free amino acid content is generated by proteolysis activity during storage (Toldra *et al.* 2000; Armenteros *et al.* 2012). Proteolysis activity is catalyzed by cathepsins and calpains, which affect the formation of flavor compounds and precursors (Seong *et al.* 2010; Careri *et al.* 1993). Total free amino acid content of T1 and T2 were significantly higher than CON. An increase in the amount of free amino acids was related to enhance sensory quality of meat products, such as attractive flavor and texture (Toldra *et al.* 1995). Due to the level of dietary processed sulfur, the methionine concentration of T1 and T2 was significantly higher than CON. Song *et al* (2013) found that high sulfur content in diet-fed pigs leads to higher methionine content than a normal diet-fed pig. In addition, methionine can be involved in the formation of glutathione, which is an antioxidant of sulfur-containing compounds (Gulizar 2004). Our results showed significant and negative correlations between methionine content and TBA value ($r = -0.924$) at 10 months. Glutamic acid (Glu) content of T2 was significantly higher than T1 and CON, and Glu and Asp content of T1 was significantly higher than CON.

Descriptive Sensory Test

Sensory attribute scores of dry cured ham after 10 months of processing showed that the redness of T1 was significantly higher than CON, while no difference was observed between T1 and T2. Brightness of T2 was significantly higher than CON. The color of meat products was affected by changes in pH value and the reaction of pigment enzyme activities with oxygen (Lawrie, 1985). Studies have indicated that sulfur-containing compounds such as furans and disulfides influence flavor characteristics (Donald *et al.* 1994; Yang *et al.* 2012). In this study, the off-odor score of CON was significantly higher than T1. Aroma score of T1 and T2 was higher than CON. However, there were no significant differences among groups. Meat flavor from sulfur-fed pigs could be improved by intramuscular fat content and oxidized products from lipids (Carrapiso *et al.* 2002; Ruiz *et al.* 2002; Lee *et al.* 2009). The juiciness score of T2 was significantly higher than CON. The bitterness of T1 was better than CON, and no significantdifference was observed between T2 and CON. Sweetness of T1 was significantly higher than CON, which suggests that the combination of Glu and Asp concentration in T1 could enhance umami taste of dry cured ham (Misako *et al.* 2002; Kenzo 2009).

CONCLUSION

Processed sulfur supplementation could improve economics for the livestock farms with increasing carcass weight, yield rate, and carcass grade, and enhancing the nutritional and functional values of meat. Long term supplementation with processed sulfur can be an effective means of an antioxidant in dry cured ham due to the reduction of lipid oxidation. Moreover, dietary processed sulfur could contribute to improve sensory quality characteristics with reducing the intensity of off odor and increasing palatability. Processed sulfur treatment might enhance proteolysis activity during storage by increasing free amino acids in dry cured ham made from processed sulfur fed pigs. Fatty acid composition of dry cured ham made from processed sulfur-fed pigs could be beneficial to health. Overall, this review demonstrates that sulfur supplementation to pigs can improve growth performance of pigs and meat quality of dry cured ham products with extended shelf-life during storage.

REFERENCES

Ahn, D. U., Olsonm, D. G., Chen, J. X., Wu, C., & Lee, J. I. (1998). Effect of muscle type packaging and irradiation on lipid oxidation volatile production, and color in raw pork patties. *Meat Science*, *47*(1), 27–39. doi:10.1016/S0309-1740(97)00101-0 PMID:22063182

Bart, D. & Rex, G. H. (2002). Redox control of the transsulfuration and glutathione biosynthesis pathways. *Protein and Amino Acid Metabolism*, *5*, 85-92.

Bartolmew, D. T., & Blumer, J. N. (1977). Microbial interactions in country-style hams. *Journal of Food Science*, *42*(2), 498–502. doi:10.1111/j.1365-2621.1977.tb01531.x

Biesalski, H. K. (2005). Meat as a component of a healthy diet—Are there any risks or benefits if meat is avoided in the diet? *Meat Science*, *70*(3), 509–524. doi:10.1016/j.meatsci.2004.07.017 PMID:22063749

Boles, J. A., Shand, P. J., Patience, J. F., McCurdy, A. R., & Schaefer, A. L. (1993). Acid base status of stress susceptible pigs affects sensory quality of loin roasts. *Journal of Food Science*, *58*(6), 1254–1257. doi:10.1111/j.1365-2621.1993.tb06159.x

Brewer, M. S., Ikins, W. G., & Harbers, C. A. Z. (1992). TBA values, sensory characteristics, and volatiles in ground pork during long term frozen storage: Effects of packaging. *Journal of Food Science*, *57*(3), 558–580. doi:10.1111/j.1365-2621.1992.tb08042.x

Cho, H. S., Park, W. J., Hong, G. E., Kim, J. H., Ju, M. G., & Lee, C. H. (2015). Antioxidant activity of Allium hookeri root extract and its effect on lipid stability of sulfur-fed pork patties. *Korean J. Food Sci. An.*, *35*(1), 32–40. PMID:26761799

Cho, J. H., Min, B. J., Kwon, O. S., Shon, K. S., Jin, Y. G., Kim, H. J., & Kim, I. H. (2005). Effect of MSM (Methyl Sulfonyl Methane) supplementation on growth performance and digestibility of CA and N in pigs. *Journal of Korean Soc. Food Sci. Nutr.*, *34*(3), 361–365. doi:10.3746/jkfn.2005.34.3.361

Cho, W. M., Yang, S. H., Lee, S. M., Jang, S. S., Kim, H. C., Hong, S. K., & Kim, H. S. (2012). Effects of different additives on the growth performance and carcass characteristics of Holstein steers. *Journal of Life Science*, *22*(22), 61–166.

Choi, J. H., & Han, I. K. (1974). Effects of substitution of sodium on sodium sulphate for methionine on performance and nutrient metabolism of broiler chickens. *Korean Journal of Animal Sciences*, *16*, 20–36.

Chung, T. K., & Baker, D. H. (1992). Efficiency of dietary methionine utilization by young pigs. *The Journal of Nutrition*, *122*, 1862–1869. PMID:1512636

Drewnoski, M. E., Pogge, D. J., & Hanse, S. L. (2014). *Journal of Animal Science*. American Society of Animal Science. Retrieved from http://www.journalofanimalscience.org/content/early/2014/06/30/jas.2013-7242

Emery, R. S., Smith, C. K., & Huffman, C. F. (1957). Utilization of inorganic sulfate by rumen microorganisms. I. incorporation of inorganic sulfate into amino acids. APP. *Microbiol*, *5*, 360–363. PMID:13488436

Folch, J., Lees, M., & Sloane-Stanley, G. H. (1957). A simple method for the isolation and purification of total lipids from animal tissue. *The Journal of Biological Chemistry*, *226*, 497. PMID:13428781

Jang, H. D., Yoo, J. S., Chae, S. J., Park, S. I., Jung, J. C., & Kim, H. J. Kim & Seok, H. B. (2006). Effect of dietary methyl sulfonyl methane on growth performance and meat quality characteristics in growing finishing pigs. *Korean Journal of International Agriculture*, *18*, 116–120.

Jung, D. H., & Jung, S. H. (2005). *Garlic Science, World science, Israel Goldberg, Functional Foods*. New York: Chapman & Hall.

Jung, K. H. (2004). *Effect of the processed sulfur on the growth performance, antivirus and meat quality in pigs*. Chonnam University.

Kerr, B. J., Weber, T. E., Ziemer, C. J., Spence, C., Cotta, M. A., & Whitehead, T. R. (2011). Effect of dietary inorganic sulfur level on growth performance, fecal composition, and measures of inflammation and sulfate-reducing bacteria in the intestine of growing pigs. *Journal of Animal Science*, *89*(2), 426–437. doi:10.2527/jas.2010-3228 PMID:20952529

Kim, G. S., Jung, Y. R., Lee, N. J., Hong, S. H., Yu, J. H., Jeong, J. H., & Kang, J. K. (2006). The composition of the toxicity of processed sulfur with non processed sulfur in Sprague-Dawley rats. *J. Vet. Med. Biotechnol.*, *7*, 183–190.

Kim, J. H., Lee, H. R., Pyun, C. W., Hong, G. H., Kim, S. K., & Lee, C. H. (2015). Changes in physiochemical, microbiological and sensory properties of dry-cured ham in processed sulfur-fed pigs. *Journal of Food Processing and Preservation*, *39*(6), 829–839. doi:10.1111/jfpp.12293

Kim, J. H., Pyun, C. W., Hong, G. H., Kim, S. K., Yang, C. Y., & Lee, C. H. (2014). Changes in physiochemical and microbiological properties of isoflavone-treated dry-cured sausage from sulfur-fed pork during storage. *Journal of Animal Sciences and Technology*, *56*(1), 21. doi:10.1186/2055-0391-56-21 PMID:26290710

Lee, J., Lee, H. J., Park, J. D., Lee, S. K., Lee, S. I., Lim, H. D., & Kim, E. C. et al. (2008). Anti-cancer activity of highly purified sulfur in immortalized and malignant human oral keratinocytes. *Toxicology In Vitro*, *22*(1), 87–95. doi:10.1016/j.tiv.2007.08.016 PMID:17920232

Lee, J. I., Min, H. K., Lee, J. W., Jeong, J. D., Ha, Y. J., Kwack, S. C., & Park, J. S. (2009). Changes in the quality of loin from pigs supplemented with dietary methyl sulfonyl methane during cold storage. *Korean J. Food Sci*, *2*(2), 229–237. doi:10.5851/kosfa.2009.29.2.229

Lee, J. S., Kwon, J. K., Han, S. H., An, I. J., Kim, S. J., Lee, S. H., & Jung, J. Y. et al. (2010). Toxicity study of detoxification sulfur at 3 months post-treatment in rats. *J F Hyg Safety*, *25*, 263–268.

Loughmiller, J. A., Nelssen, J. L., Goodband, R. D., Tokach, M. D., Titgemeyer, E. C., & Kim, I. H. (1998). Influence of dietary total sulfur amino acids and methionine on growth performance and carcass characteristics of finishing gilts. *Journal of Animal Science*, *76*(8), 2129–2137. PMID:9734863

Loughmiller, J. A., Tokach, M. D., Goodband, R. D., Nelssen, J. L., Titgemeyer, E. C., Kim, I. H., & Dritz, S. (1996). Dietary total sulfur amino acid requirement for optimal growth performance and carcass characteristics in finishing gilts. In *Kansas State University Swine Day. Report of Progress* (pp. 133–135). Kansas State University.

Mikami, M., Sekikawa, M., & Shimada, K. I. (2007). Non-heated meat products (Dry cured ham). *FFI Journal.*, *212*(7), 572–582.

Ministry for food, agriculture, forestry and fisheries. (2011). *Main statistic information for food, agriculture, forestry and fisheries*. Author.

Mortensen, J. Z., Schmidt, E. B., Nielsen, A. H., & Dyerberg, J. (1983). The effect of N-6 and N-3 polyunsaturated fatty acids on hemostasis, blood lipids and blood pressure. *Thrombosis and Haemostasis*, *50*, 543–546. PMID:6636033

Nimni, M. E., Han, B., & Cordoba, F. (2007). Are we getting enough sulfur in our diet. *Nutrition and Metabolism (Lond)*, *4*, 24.

Noh, H. Y. (2014). *Effects of the processed sulfur supplementation on the growth performance and meat quality in pigs*. Konkuk University.

Park, J. H., Ryu, M. S., Lee, Y. E., Song, G. S., & Ryu, K. S. (2003). A comparison of fattening performance, physic-chemical properties of breast meat, vaccine titers in cross bred meat type hybrid chicks fed sulfur. *Korean Journal of Poultry Science*, *30*, 211–217.

Pogge, D., & Hansen, S. L. (2012). Effect of vitamin C on performance and antioxidant capacity of cattle fed varying concentrations of dietary sulfur. *Animal Industry Report*, *658*, 21.

Rozenn, N. L., Irena, B. K., Dariush, M., Lewis, H. K., Russell, P. T., & David, S. S. (2003). N-3 Polyunsaturated fatty acids, fatal ischemic heart disease, and nonfatal myocardial infarction in older adults: The Cardiovascular health study. *The American Journal of Clinical Nutrition*, *77*, 319–325. PMID:12540389

SAS Institute. (2002). SAS User's Guide: Statistics. Cary, NC: SAS Institute Inc.

Shin, J. S., Kim, M. A., & Lee, S. H. (2013). Comparison of physiological changes in broiler chicken fed with dietary processed sulfur. *Korean Journal of Food Preservation.*, *20*(2), 278–283. doi:10.11002/kjfp.2013.20.2.278

Song, R., Chen, C., Wang, L., Johnston, J., Kerr, B. J., Weber, T. E., & Shurson, G. C. (2013). High sulfur content in corn dried distillers grains with soluble protects against oxidized lipids by increasing sulfur-containing antioxidants in nursery pigs. *Journal of Animal Science*, *91*(6), 2715–2728. doi:10.2527/jas.2012-5350 PMID:23482577

Stanley W., Jacob, M. D., Ronald M., Lawrence, M.D. & Zucker, M. (1998). *The Miracle of MSM*. The Berkley Publishing Group.

Van Weerdn, E. J., & Schutte, J. B. (1976). Relation between methionine and inorganic sulphate in broiler rations. *Poultry Science*, *55*(4), 1476–1748. doi:10.3382/ps.0551476 PMID:951375

Wallis, I. R. (1999). Dietary supplements of methionine increase breast meat yield and decrease abdominal fat in growing broiler chickens. *Australian Journal of Experimental Agriculture*, *39*(2), 131–141. doi:10.1071/EA98130

Witte, V. C., Krause, G. F., & Bailey, M. E. (1970). A new extraction method for determining 2-thiobarbituric acid values of pork and beef during storage. *Journal of Food Science*, *35*(5), 582–585. doi:10.1111/j.1365-2621.1970.tb04815.x

Chapter 13
Food in Health Preservation and Promotion:
A Special Focus on the Interplay between Oxidative Stress and Pro-Oxidant/Antioxidant

Saikat Sen
Assam Downtown University, India

Raja Chakraborty
Assam Downtown University, India

ABSTRACT

Association between food and health is complex. Healthy food can promote and maintain good human health. Healthy food and nutrition is a key regulating factor for boosting the immunity and therapeutic effectiveness of a treatment strategy. Oxidative stress is well involved in the pathogenesis of diverse diseases and aging. Food always considered as good source of nutrients, protein, fat, carbohydrates, vitamins, minerals and antioxidants. Consumed as part of a normal diet, phytochemicals present in food like vitamins (vitamin C & E), minerals (like, zinc, selenium), phytoconstituents (phenolic compounds, flavonoids, carotenoids) confer additional health benefits, by virtue of their antioxidant property. A diet rich that rich in antioxidant molecule reduces the risk of several oxidative stress related diseases. Numerous antioxidant molecules isolated from food showed the curative and health promotion effect. This chapter majorly deals with the role antioxidant/pro-oxidant substances present in different foods on human body.

INTRODUCTION

Good health is elemental to living a productive life, meeting basic needs and contributing to healthy society. The components of health are numerous and their interactions with food are complex. Healthy diet is essential for the success of physical and mental potential for all individuals. Good food, physical activity and healthy lifestyle are the basic requirement for preservation and promotion of health. A good

DOI: 10.4018/978-1-5225-0591-4.ch013

diet is about receiving the correct amount of nutrients, bioactive molecules to maintain good health. Foods not only contain protein, fat, carbohydrates, vitamins and minerals but also supply essential biomolecules like antioxidants which are boosting our health. A good food can support human health and improve health potential, and yet can also be an important factor influencing ill health.

In 1980s the name antioxidants came into spotlight when it identified as miracle substances for good health. Food contains numerous biomolecule (antioxidant), which prevent free radical induce diseases, increase immunity and also act as anti-aging molecule. Regular intake of fruits and vegetables has also been shown to protect human from number of diseases, and concurrent scientific investigations have confirmed that antioxidant substances present in those fruits and vegetables are playing a central role for their beneficial effect (Wahlqvist, 2013; Sen & Chakraborty, 2015). Fruits, vegetables and other food can boost the antioxidant capacity of body and thus helpful for human.

REDOX HOMEOSTASIS AND OXIDATIVE STRESS

ROS/RNS and Redox Homeostasis

Cellular redox homeostasis can be described as a normal physiological situation specifically the maintenance of normal level of free radical/reactive species in *in vivo* condition through the genetic control and array of enzymatic systems. In normal physiologic conditions, cells regulate the redox balance through production and elimination of reactive oxygen species (ROS) and reactive nitrogen species (RNS). Cells are well equipped with different enzymatic and non-enzymatic antioxidant systems to maintain the normal level of ROS/RNS in body by scavenging ROS/RNS, so that redox homeostasis sustains (Sen & Chakraborty, 2011; Trachootham, Lu, Ogasawara, Valle & Huang, 2008; Valko et al., 2007).

ROS and RNS consist of free radicals and different reactive species. Free radicals can be generated in both endogenous and exogenous environment. Production of free radicals in *in vivo* condition is continuous process as a part of normal physiology. Several process or system of our body like immune system, metabolic process (lipid peroxidation, metabolism of arachidonic acid, platelets, and macrophages), inflammation, and stress generates reactive species continuously. Drugs (adriamycin, bleomycin, mitomycin C, nitrofurantoin), chemicals (carbon tetrachloride, chloroform, paraquat, benzo pyrene, cleaning products, glue, paints, paint thinners, perfumes, and pesticides), smoking of tobacco products, radiation, pollution and some food are responsible for generation of free radicals (Sen, Chakraborty, Sridhar, Reddy, & De, 2010; Sen & Chakraborty, 2011). Generation of free radical also increased in pathological condition. ROS and RNS are essential for body in low/moderate concentration. It acts as intercellular signal molecules and also participate in immune mechanism. But at high concentration they induce molecular damage (Valko et al., 2007; Zorov et al., 2005). Table 1 describes different ROS and RNS along with their properties.

Oxidative Stress and Diseases

Normal physiological and biochemical function of cell maintain by the steady state concentration of reactive species, which determined by the balance between the generation and removal of reactive species by various antioxidants. Redox state cannot explain only as the state of redox pair, but it also demonstrates the redox environment of a cell. Usually in normal conditions, redox state of a biological system

Table 1. Properties of different reactive oxygen and nitrogen species

Reactive Oxygen Species (ROS)		
Oxygen-centered radicals	Superoxide anion ($O_2^{\bullet -}$)	• It is a reduced form of molecular oxygen that formed in mitochondria as initial free radical. • $O_2^{\bullet -}$ contribute majorly in generation of other reactive species like H_2O_2, $^{\bullet}OH$, $^1O_2$, $OONO^-$. • $O_2^{\bullet -}$ can reduce the activity of catalase and glutathione peroxidase • One superoxide dismutase (SOD) converts two $O_2^{\bullet -}$ into one H_2O_2 and one oxygen molecule.
	Hydroxyl radical ($^{\bullet}OH$)	• $^{\bullet}OH$ is the neutral form of the hydroxide ion, which is highly reactive (half-life of approximately 10^{-9} s) and responsible for damage of lipid, polypeptides, proteins, DNA base. • $^{\bullet}OH$ generates from $O_2^{\bullet -}$ and H_2O_2 in presence of metal ions through Fenton reaction (except exercise), and as a by-product of immune action especially by the macrophages and microglia when exposed to certain bacteria. • In reaction with aromatic compounds $^{\bullet}OH$ is responsible for generation of hydroxycyclohexadienyl radical, which in reaction with oxygen can produce peroxyl radical. • $OH^{\bullet}$ can induce the conversion of many fatty acid side chains into lipid hydroxyl peroxides • Catalase (CAT) causes dismutation of $^{\bullet}OH$ to H_2O and O_2, reduced glutathione (GSH) is also scavenge $^{\bullet}OH$.
	Peroxyl radical ($ROO^{\bullet}$) Alkoxyl radical ($RO^{\bullet}$)	• $ROO^{\bullet}$ generates through a direct reaction of oxygen with alkyl radicals ($R^{\bullet}$). Decomposition of alkyl peroxides (ROOH) also responsible for formation of $ROO^{\bullet}$ and $RO^{\bullet}$. • Hydroperoxyl radical ($HOO^{\bullet}$) is the simplest peroxyl radical, which is the protonated form of $O_2^{\bullet -}$. • Several enzymatic reactions (i.e. cycloxygenases, oxidases, lipoxygenases, peroxidases, and NADPH-cyt P_{450} reductases) and non-enzymatic reactions (LOOH-derived Fenton reaction, a reductive cleavage, or combination of two peroxyl radicals) can trigger the formation of $RO^{\bullet}$. • $HOO^{\bullet}$ along with $^{\bullet}OH$ can affect the lipids profoundly. • Lipid alkoxyl radical can induce damage of DNA or other surrounding organic molecules. • Both the peroxyl and alkoxyl radicals are good oxidizing agents.
Non-radicals	Hydrogen peroxide (H_2O_2)	• H_2O_2 produced through a dismutation reaction from $O_2^{\bullet -}$ induced by SOD. • Several oxidase enzymes like amino acid oxidases, xanthine oxidase in cell are involve in the production of H_2O_2. • H_2O_2 is weak oxidizing and reducing agent, and it is considered as least reactive molecule. • H_2O_2 involve in the production of thyroid hormones, and also may act as intracellular signal molecule. • Under physiological pH and in absence of metal ion H_2O_2 is stable. • H_2O_2 can induce cell toxicity by inducing DNA damage, membrane disruption and release calcium ions within cell which is responsible for activation of calcium dependent proteolytic enzyme. • H_2O_2 is responsible for generation of $^{\bullet}OH$, $O_2^{\bullet -}$.
	Hypochlorous acid (HOCl)	• HOCl is generated by the enzyme myeloperoxidase in activated neutrophils and initiates the deactivation of antiproteases and activation of latent proteases which is responsible for tissue damage. • HOCl can cause damage of biomolecules, directly and also decomposes to liberate toxic chlorine. • During inflammation activated neutrophils and eosinophils can generate several ROS including HOCl and HOBr. • HOCl and HOBr contribute to the generation of ROS and radicals through different secondary reactions. • HOCl and HOBr causes the formation of advanced oxidation products (AOPPs) which alter the cell structure and physiology by targeting thiols, thioethers, disulfides, amines and amides
	Hypobromous acid (HOBr)	
	Ozone (O_3)	• It is not generated *in vivo*, but considered as an unwanted oxidant and very toxic air pollutant. On exposure to lung ozone cause tissue damage. O_3 directly or via free radical can induced oxidation or peroxidation of biomolecules.
	Singlet oxygen ($^1O_2$)	• Singlet oxygen is an excited status, mild and nontoxic for mammalian tissue compare to other ROS. • It involved in cholesterol oxidation. • $^1O_2$ can be generated from H_2O_2, which reacts with $O_2^{\bullet -}$ or with HOCl or chloroamines in cells and tissues.

continued on following page

Table 1. Continued

Reactive Nitrogen Species (RNS)		
Radicals	Nitric oxide ($NO^{\bullet}$)	• $NO^{\bullet}$ is formed from the amino acid L-arginine by NO synthase in vascular endothelial cells, phagocytes, and many other cell types. • NO• in low concentration act as biological signaling molecule and involved in regulation of several biological functions like neurotransmission, regulation of blood pressure, defense mechanisms, smooth muscle relaxation and immune function. • It is as such not a highly reactive free radical, but ischemia reperfusion, neurodegenerative and chronic inflammatory diseases can be caused by the overproduction of $NO^{\bullet}$. • NO after exposed in plasma can reduce the level of ascorbic acid and uric acid, and can initiate lipid peroxidation. • NO• can react with oxygen and water to generate nitrate and nitrite anions.
	Nitrogen dioxide ($NO_2^{\bullet}$)	• $NO_2^{\bullet}$ is generated from the reaction between peroxyl radical and NO, polluted air and smoking. • $NO_2^{\bullet}$ can initiate lipid peroxidation and responsible for generation of other free radicals. • It involve in the oxidation of ascorbic acid.
Non-radicals	Peroxynitrite ($ONOO^-$)	• $ONOO^-$ can be formed by the reaction of $NO^{\bullet}$ and superoxide anion. • Peroxynitrite is a cytotoxic molecule and good oxidizing agent, which can oxidizes LDL and cause tissue injury. It also involved in the direct protein and DNA base oxidation, modification of DNA base. • Peroxynitrite also involved in the pathogenesis of several disorders like neurodegenerative and kidney diseases. • Peroxynitrite-mediated reactions are responsible for formation of nitrotyrosine.
	Nitrous acid (HNO_2)	• Nitrous oxide acts as a precursor of HNO_2. It encourages the deamination of DNA bases (cytosine, adenine and guanine) containing free NH_2 groups.
	Dinitrogen trioxide(N_2O_3)	• N_2O_3 is the anhydride of nitrous acid, which is generated through the reaction of $NO^{\bullet}$ and $NO_2^{\bullet}$. N_2O_3 is a strong oxidizing agent and responsible for nitrosylation of phenols.
	Peroxynitrous acid (ONOOH)	• ONOOH can induce a cycle of events leading to the generation of highly reactive and damaging radicals like $CO_3^{\bullet-}$, NO_2^+, NO_2, $O_2^{\bullet-}$, $OH^{\bullet}$, which can lead to significant damage in biological milieu.
Other reactive nitrogen species includes alkyl peroxynitrites (ROONO), nitronium (nitryl) cation (NO_2^+), Nitrosyl cation (NO^+), Nitroxyl anion (NO^-), Dinitrogen tetroxide (N_2O_4)		

Halliwell and Gutteridge (1999); Jiang, Zhang, and Dusting (2011); Lee, Koo, and Min (2004); Marcinkiewicz (2010); Sen and Chakraborty (2011); Soneja, Drews, and Malinski (2005); Valko et al. (2007)

is preserved towards more negative redox potential values. Level of ROS and RNS produced inside the cell tightly regulated by the different endogenous antioxidants. Though, augment in ROS production or reduction in antioxidant protection within cells responsible for less negative redox potential values, which in turn results the oxidizing environment. This change from reducing status to oxidizing status is explained as oxidative stress (Kunwar & Priyadarsini, 2011). Oxidative stress is responsible for the damage of biomolecules like lipids, proteins, carbohydrates and nucleic acids, and such oxidative modification of biomolecules due to toxic concentration of ROS and RNS lead to deleterious consequences such as loss of cell function and diseases state. Due to high elevation of ROS/RNS level, mitochondria lose its function which in turn responsible for ATP depletion and necrotic cell death, while moderate oxidation can induce apoptosis (Kunwar & Priyadarsini, 2011; Sen & Chakraborty, 2011). Reactive species are responsible for change of cell function and alteration of signal pathway. Oxidative stress causes damage to lipid present in membrane of subcellular organelles, alters enzyme activity, and modifies function & structure of protein. Reactive species also leads to DNA fragmentation, mutation, damage, and apoptosis through the activation of the poly (ADP-ribose) syntheses (Sen & Chakraborty, 2011; Valko et al., 2007).

'Oxidative stress' is a basic phenomenon which is used to describe the relation between free radicals and molecular damage. Long time exposure to reactive species, even at a low concentration may cause tissue injury through the damage of biomolecules. Recent researches identified oxidative stress as a key underlying cause of different diseases and aging process. Majorly, four key processes in oxidative stress involve in the pathogenesis of numerous diseases, (1) membrane lipid peroxidation, (2) protein oxidation, (3) DNA damage and (4) disturbance in reducing equivalents of the cell (Sen & Chakraborty, 2011; Valko et al., 2007).

ANTIOXIDANTS AND PROXIDANTS

Antioxidants and Their Effect on Health

Antioxidants are the molecule which essential to maintain structural and tissue integrity. Antioxidants scavenge free radicals, stabilize the level of reactive species and thus play a key role in maintenance of optimal cellular and systemic health. Antioxidants include diverse substances like enzyme, vitamins, minerals, phytoconstituents etc. They generally retard the process of oxidative degeneration or oxidative damage. Level of antioxidant and free radical influenced by several factors like production/destruction rate of reactive species, potency and concentration of antioxidant, gene expression, diet, stress, hormones, smoking, drugs intake, pollution and lifestyle condition, pathological condition etc (Hegde, Rai, & Padmanabhan, 2009; Van't Veer, Jansen, Klerk, & Kok, 2000; Sen & Chakraborty, 2011). Antioxidant system can be classified majorly in three groups. (1) Primary antioxidant defense: these are also known as chain breaking antioxidants which can neutralize free radicals by giving one of their own electron, and thus end the electron "stealing" reaction. (2) Secondary antioxidant defense: antioxidants under these classes are called as preventive antioxidants, which act through number of mechanism including sequestration of transition metal ions, removal of peroxides by antioxidant enzyme, removal of ROS. (3) Tertiary antioxidant defenses: they mainly involve in repair mechanism. Though, antioxidants can be classified in several way based on origin, nature/structure, chemical-physical properties, and mechanism (Vertuani, Angusti, & Manfredini, 2004; Tandaon, Verma, Singh, & Mahajan, 2005).

Based on the origin and nature the antioxidants can be classified as,

1. Natural antioxidants
    a. Endogenous antioxidants
        i. **Enzymatic antioxidants:** Superoxide dismutase (SOD), Catalase (CAT), Glutathione peroxidase (GPx), Glutathione reductase (GR), Glutathione-*S*-transferase (GST)
        ii. **Non-enzymatic antioxidants:** Glutathione (GSH), bilirubin, albumin, vitamin C, vitamin E, β-carotene, ferritin, uric acid, transferring, ubiquinone.
    b. Natural exogenous antioxidants
        i. **Vitamins:** Vitamin C, Vitamin A (ß-carotene)
        ii. **Minerals:** Selenium, Copper, Iron, Zinc and Manganese.
        iii. **Phytochemicals:** Phenols, Flavonoids, Alkaloids,
2. Synthetic antioxidant: Butylated hydroxyl anisole (BHA), Butylated hydroxy toluene (BHT), Tertiary butylated hydroxy quinine (TBHQ)

In nature, antioxidants confer protective effect in living organisms from oxidative damage. Antioxidant system is essential for protection and integrity of cell structure and function. Foods like fruits, vegetable,

Table 2. Different types of endogenous antioxidants & their function

Antioxidant	Location and Importance
Superoxide dismutase (SOD).	There are three isomer of SOD in human. SOD1 located on cytoplasm, SOD2 in mitochondria, and SOD3 present in extracellular area Superoxide dismutase (SOD) is an important endogenous antioxidant enzyme. SOD scavenge $O_2^{\bullet-}$ to H_2O_2 and O_2.
Catalase (CAT)	Located in intracellular area and decomposes H_2O_2 to water and oxygen.
Glutathione peroxidase (GPx)	Present in plasma and intracellular area. GPx remove H_2O_2 and inhibit the formation of hydroxyl radical. It inactivates hydroperoxides.
Glutathione reductase (GR)	GR a key intracellular antioxidant enzyme require for the conversion of GSH from glutathione disulphide.
Glutathione-*S*-transferase (GST)	Present intracellularlly, conjugates xenobiotics and alkylating substances for excretion with GSH.
Glutathione (GSH)	Located in plasma, cytosol, nuclei and mitochondria. Maintain redox potential and –SH groups in other biomolecules. GSH scavenge $OH^{\bullet}$, singlet oxygen directly. GSH involved in the detoxification of H_2O_2 and lipid peroxides, regeneration of some antioxidants like vitamins C and vitamin E.
Bilirubin	Present is plasma. It is a free radical scavenger. Nonconjugated bilirubin acts as endogenous lipid antioxidant.
Albumin	Present in plasma. Act by binding with metal ions such as Fe, Cu.
Ascorbic acid	Present in extracellular fluid. Neutralize ROS in aqueous phase before the initiation of lipid peroxidation. It induces the regeneration of α-tocopherol.
Vitamin E	Present in plasma. Act as electron donor, H^+ donor and quencher of $^1O_2$. It acts as chain-breaking antioxidant within the cell membrane and protects membrane fatty acids from lipid peroxidation
β-carotene	Located in plasma and in cell membrane. Act as electron donor and quencher of $^1O_2$.
Ferritin	Present in plasma. Act by binding with Fe ions
Uric acid	Present in plasma. Act by binding with free Fe ions, and also scavenge $^1O_2$and $OH^{\bullet}$.
Transferrin	Present in plasma. It act by binding with free Fe ions, and inhibits iron-catalyzed radical formation.
Ubiquinone	Present in plasma. It can prevent the initiation and/or propagation of lipid peroxidation.

Yuan and Kitts (1997); Sies, Stahl, and Sundquist (1992); Halliwell and Gutteridge (1999)

food grains are essential for health. Current understanding reveled that they contain abundant antioxidant in addition to the other numerous biomolecule. The favorable effect of vegetables, fruits, and other foods against degenerative diseases has been credited, in part, to the antioxidants they provide. Consumption of food rich in antioxidant believed to confer benefit by protecting the body's cells.

Antioxidants eliminate free radicals that damage cells and also involve in damage cell repair mechanism, promotion of cell growth, protection of cells against premature and abnormal ageing, prevention of diseases. Antioxidants also offer excellent support for our immune system (Sen & Chakraborty, 2011). Current researches have confirmed that free radical induced oxidative stress has been implicated in several diseases like cancer, cardiovascular diseases (hypertension, atherosclerosis, ischemic heart disease, cardiomyopathies and congestive heart failure), neurological disorders (Parkinson's disease, Alzheimer's disease, Multiple Sclerosis and amyolotrophic lateral sclerosis), gastrointestinal diseases (peptic ulcers, gastrointestinal cancers, and inflammatory bowel disease), kidney disease (urolithiasis, diabetic nephropathy), diseases of premature infants (bronchopulmonary, dysplasia, periventricular leukomalacia), lung disease (asthma, pulmonary fibrosis), eye disease (cataract, age related macular degeneration, diabetic retinopathy), joint disorder, diabetes, malaria, chronic fatigue syndrome, lichen planus, vitiligo, autism, infection and aging (Gupta et al., 2014; Adly, 2010; Sen et al., 2010). Thus numerous researches devote to exploring and utilizing antioxidants in the prevention and treatment of such diseases. However, synthetic antioxidants showed several toxic effects to some extents, thus utilization of natural antioxidants could be the best way to defend oxidative stress (Li et al., 2014). Due to the beneficial effect of antioxidants the use of antioxidant dietary supplements are in rise.

Pro-Oxidants and Health

Prooxidants are any endobiotic or xenobiotic substances/molecule that results generation of ROS or inhibition of antioxidant system and thus induce oxidative stress. Overproduction of pro-oxidants can induce significant damage to cell or cell death. Pro-oxidant capable to induce the damage of mitochondria, genetic material and thus leads to reduced adaptability, disease and aging. Chemically, pro-oxidants have an electron-imbalance – they have chemically very unstable unpaired electron. Thus pro-oxidants aggressively want to receive an electron from another molecule around them. All ROS/RNS, drugs, and pesticides even some cases popular antioxidants also reported to act as prooxidant in specific environment. Different pro-oxidants includes, (1) Drugs, chemicals and pesticide – drugs like NSAIDS or anticancer drugs, pesticide such as DDT can induce organ damage by inducing the generation of ROS, alteration of antioxidant defence mechanism and lipid peroxidation. (2) Transition metals (i.e. magnesium, copper iron etc) which can induce diseases like chronic magnesium, Wilson disease, and hemochromatosis. These metal cause generation of free radicals through Fenton reaction and Haber-Weiss reaction. (3) Excessive physical exercise and mental stress/anxiety also responsible for oxidative stress. (4) Diseases - disease condition like local ischemia can enhance ROS generation. (5) Environmental factor i.e. heat, cold, pollution increase ROS production through the disruption of electron transfer caused by decreased membrane fluidity of mitochondria. (6) Antioxidants – under specific condition, well known antioxidants like ascorbic acid, vitamin E, polyphenols can behave like pro-oxidants (Rahal et al., 2014).

It is also true that pro-oxidants are not essentially “bad” in-and-of themselves. They of course play a key role in our health and survival by helping to generate the inflammatory responses that protect us. Several molecules can serve as either antioxidants or pro-oxidants, depending on environment. A number of studies indicated that exogenous antioxidants may act as pro-oxidant and may cause damage of health, though results are controversial. Some studies mostly *in vitro* have shown that exogenous antioxidants, under certain conditions, like high doses or presence of metal ions can act as pro-oxidant, and may responsible for damage of biomolecules, and the consequent cellular death. (Teeguarden, 2007; Yordi, Pérez, Matos & Villares, 2012)

ANTIOXIDANT POTENTIAL OF FOOD AND HEALTH

Exogenous Antioxidant and their Health Benefit

Food from plant contains diverse phytochemicals like dietary fiber, antioxidants, detoxifying substances, immunity-boosting chemicals and neuropharmacological substances, which have disease-preventing functions. Polyphenolic compounds, carotenoids, flavonoids, anthocyanidines and isothiocyanates are the major antioxidant constituents present in the food. Several vitamins (i.e. vitamin E, vitamin C), minerals (i.e. zinc, selenium) are also present in food and exert free radical scavenging activity. Foods rich in antioxidant molecule are exhibiting disease-protecting and health promotion effect. Foods like cereals, pulses, fruits, oils, spices, and vegetable are the good sources of antioxidant constituents. Majority of the plant foods contain phenolic and flavonoids as antioxidant. Green leafy vegetables, fruits and yellow vegetables are the rich source of carotenoids, flavonoids and vitamin C. These phytochemicals inhibit lipid peroxidation and also support the endogenous antioxidants. In general, total antioxidant potential of a food is estimated by considering its capacity to prevent lipid peroxidation in an *in vitro* system. However, the effectiveness of antioxidants or activity of antioxidant containing foods are not only depend on the level of antioxidant present in foods but also on their bioavailability, that is, the level to which the of antioxidants in active forms are released from the food and absorbed through the gut. It was observed that few flavonoids and phenolic antioxidants are rather poorly absorbed; they usually form insoluble complexes with metals. The level of oxidants in food is a determinant factor of antioxidant potency of a diet, for example, high PUFA content can decrease the antioxidant potency of food as PUFA is prone to formation of lipid peroxide (Rao, 2003).

Recent studies have proved the positive association between polyphenolic compounds and disease prevention. Consumption of food and beverages rich in polyphenolic compounds increases the antioxidative capacity of plasma. Several clinical trials have indicated that consumption of food containing polyphenolic compounds reduces the incidence of cardiovascular disease, cancer and other oxidative induce diseases. Polyphenols are powerful inhibitors of LDL oxidation and showed their potent effect as cardioprotective agents. Beneficial effect of quercetin and resveratrol in coronary heart disease, flavonol-rich dark chocolate in reduction blood pressure was studied. Flavonol cocoa drink consumption is associated in arterial dilation in people with smoking-related endothelial dysfunction was reported. Anticancer activity of different polyphenol (like, theaflavins and thearubigins, soy isoflavones, quercetin, catechins, isoflavones, lignans, flavanones ellagic acid, red wine polyphenols, resveratrol and curcumin) against different types of cancer like mouth, stomach, duodenum, colon, liver, lung, renal, breast, prostate and skin have been observed through clinical trials and *in vivo* or *in vitro* studies. Potential benefit of (+) catechin, (-)epicatechin, (-)epigallocatechin, epicatechin gallate, quercetin, soyabeans isoflavones, tannic acid, glycyrrhizin, chlorogenic acid, curcumin and ferulic acid were observed in diabetes or in diabetic complications. Curcumin also found to boost immunity. Epidemiological observations indicated positive association between polyphenols and obstructive lung disease, osteoporosis. Soy isoflavone, genistein promotes lung function in asthmatic people; while genistein, daidzein helpful to prevents the loss of bone mineral density and trabecular volume due to ovariectomy. Polyphenols also protect skin damages induced by sunlight. Polyphenols present in the tea may protect the skin from UV light. Polyphenols like theaflavin 3 3' digallate, and theaflavin 3' gallateare reported to possess antiviral activity. Consumption of fruit and with high levels of flavonoids may exert anti-aging effect. Tea catechins, resveratrol a grape polyphenol emerged as potent anti-aging substance. Daidzein and genistein investigated for their hepatoprotective effect. Another key effect of polyphenol is their beneficial effect against different degenerative diseases and also helpful in maintaining central nervous system health (Pandey & Rizvi, 2009; Stevenson & Hurst, 2007; Han, Shen & Lou, 2007).

Mode of Action of Antioxidants

Vitamin E

Vitamin E denotes a group of potent, lipid-soluble antioxidants. Naturally occurring different form of vitamin E includes tocopherols (α, β, γ, δ) and tocotrienols (α, β, γ, δ). Vitamin E is chain-breaking antioxidants which avert the propagation of free radical reactions. Vitamin E terminates free radical chain reactions by interacting with lipid peroxyl radical, and thus inhibits the generation of new radical. Vitamin E also promote endogenous antioxidant defense like up-regulation of GPX, CAT from liver, SOD, GST, GR and NAD(P)H, along with its direct ROD scavenging activity. Vitamin E can be recycled back to its previous unoxidized state after oxidation by several antioxidants like vitamin C and ubiquinol. This process averts the gathering of vitamin E radicals and their subsequent peroxidation of lipids which can be crucial for its antioxidant effect. α-tocopherol is the most abundant form found in nature and has the potent biological activity. A number of research confirmed that vitamin E could be beneficial in cancer, cardiovascular diseases, coronary artery diseases, diabetes etc. *In vitro* studies also found that vitamin E may exert anti- and pro-oxidative effects depending on the environment (Brigelius-flohe & Traber, 1999; Farbstein, Kozak-Blickstein & Levy, 2010; Vertuani et al., 2004)

Vitamin C

Vitamin C is an electron donor and powerful water-soluble antioxidant. Ascorbic acid is widely distributed in fresh fruits especially citrus fruit. Green leafy vegetable also have high level of vitamin C. Now a days, synthetic ascorbic acid which is identical to natural ascorbic acid available as tablets, capsules, chewable tablets, crystalline powder. Average daily intake of ascorbic acid which is essential to meet the nutritional requirement or recommended dietary allowances (RDA) for adults are 90 mg/day (man) and 75 mg/day (women). Ascorbic acid can react with radicals and terminate the reaction, thus protects the cell from oxidative stress. Vitamin C gives two electrons from a double bond between the second and third carbons of six-carbon molecule. Ascorbic acid prevents other substances from being oxidized by donating its electrons. Vitamin C scavenges ROS and RNS and thus protects the biological macromolecules from oxidative damage. It also involves in many enzymatic reactions as co-factor, and acts as plasma localized anti-oxidant. Once oxidized, ascorbate generates ascorbate free radical, although this free radical can donate another electron but does not undergo further oxidation. L-ascorbate radical can increase redox reactions in presence of transition metals, therefore some investigations suggested that vitamin C might serve as a pro-oxidant depends on physiological environment. For example, in atherosclerotic plaque where ferric iron is present, vitamin C could act as a pro-oxidant rather than as an anti-oxidant. But majority of *in vivo* studies fails to establish the pro-oxidant of vitamin C (Farbstein et al, 2010; Padayatty et al., 2003; Carr & Frei, 1999).

Polyphenolic Compounds

Polyphenolic compounds are the largest group of phytochemicals widely distributed in different plant based food. Polyphenolic phytochemicals emerged as source of potent therapeutic for diverse diseases. Intake of large amount of food with a high level of such compounds may promote health by reducing the risk of a number of diseases due to their antioxidant potential, among other factors. Over 8000 phenolic compounds are currently known, of which more than 4000 flavonoids have been discovered. Fruits, vegetables, grains, beverages like tea, chocolate are rich sources of polyphenols. Polyphenols are the group of natural substances that is highly diverse and can be categorized as several sub-groups, such as, flavonoids, phenolic acid, tannins, simple phenol, stilbenes, lignans, xanthones, coumarins (Tsao, 2010). Polyphenols mainly exhibit the antioxidant and free radical scavenging effect by several mechanisms. (1) They act as primary antioxidant and scavenge free radicals by donating hydrogen atom. Some cases these reactions can leads to the generation of another radical but this is less reactive compare to previous one. O–H group in phenolic compound is most important for this effect. (2) Polyphenols also act by chelating transition metals ions, leading to stable complexed compounds (Leopoldini, Russo & Toscano, 2011). Several researchers have found that several polyphenol antioxidants may act as pro-oxidant under certain conditions like high doses or presence of metal ions. Though, most of the investigations determining pro-oxidant effect of antioxidants are inconclusive and sometimes contradictory. Polyphenols, particularly different flavonoids and phenolic acid showed such dual behavior, but mostly in *in vitro* studies. Pro-oxidant activity of quercetin, myricetin, kaempferol and phenolic acids (i.e. caffeic, coumaric, salicylic, vanillic, hydroxybenzoic, vanillic, syringic, protocatechuic, gallic, ellagic, chlorogenic and ferulic acids) have been investigated. Therefore safety aspects, structure-activity, bioavailability and metabolism of such antioxidant compounds need to be investigate properly. Current research also indicated that pro-oxidant effect of natural antioxidant polyphenols could be useful in prevention of certain types of cancer. Pro-oxidant activity of certain dietary polyphenols can cause mitochondrial dysfunction, apoptosis and could mobilize endogenous copper in humans which may contribute in anti-cancer mechanism of such agents (Yordi et al., 2012).

Flavonoids are a group of ubiquitous polyphenolic compounds readily found in plant with variable phenolic structures. Flavonoids as a dietary component have health-promoting activity, which largely due to their high antioxidant activity. Flavonoids cannot be synthesized by humans and animals. Depending on chemical structure flavonoid can be divided into several classes, i.e. flavanols (catechin, epicatechin, epigallocatechin), flavones (apigenin, rutin, luteolin), flavonols (kaempferol, quercitrin, myricetin, quercetin), flavanones (hesperidin, naringenin), isoflavones (genistin, daidzin), anthocyanins (apigenidin, cyanidin), flavanonols (dihydroquercetin) and chalcones (phloretin, arbutin). Flavonoids are the most potent antioxidants available in plants. Potent antioxidant effect of flavonoids is due to the presence of hydroxyl groups in positions 3' and 4' of the B ring, which exert increased stability to the formed radical by joining in the displacement of the electron. Double bond present between carbons C2 and C3 (ring C) together with carbonyl group at C4 position helps in an electron displacement from ring B. Free hydroxyl groups in 3rd position of ring C and 5th position of ring A, together with the carbonyl group in 4th position, are also significant for the antioxidant activity of flavonoids. However, the efficiency of flavonoids reduces with the substitution of hydroxyl groups for sugars, as glycosides possess less antioxidant capacity compare to their corresponding aglycons. Flavonoids can suppress the formation of ROS either by enzymes (i.e. microsomal monooxygenase, glutathione S-transferase, mitochondrial succinoxidase, NADH oxidase) inhibition or by chelating trace elements involved in the generation of radicals, scavenging of ROS, and upregulation of antioxidant defenses. Flavonoids can inhibit lipid peroxidation, and significantly scavenge superoxide, hydroxyl, alkoxyl, and peroxyl radicals by donation of hydrogen atom, and thus protect biomolecule from oxidative damage. Different flavonoids have shown antimicrobial, hepatoprotective, anti-inflammatory, nephroprotective, anticancer, antiallergic, antimutagenic, antiviral, anti-thrombotic, and vasodilatory actions (Kumar & Pandey, 2013; Giada, 2013).

Phenolic acids are another non-flavonoid polyphenolic compounds that can be subdivided into two major classes, benzoic acid (protocatechuic acids, vanillic acids, syringic acid, gentisic acid, salicylic acid, p-hydroxybenzoic acid and gallic acid)and cinnamic acid derivatives (*p*-coumaric, ferulic, caffeic and sinapic acids). It was observed that phenolic acid and their esters have potent antioxidant effect, especially hydroxybenzoic acid, hydroxycinnamic acid, caffeic acid and chlorogenic acid, and although the number of hydroxyl groups found in constituent also detrimental for antioxidant activity. Usually, hydroxylated cinnamic acids exert better effect than benzoic acids derivatives (Tsao, 2010; Giada, 2013).

Stilbenes are relatively small group of non-flavonoid phenolic substance found in a large number of plant sources. Resveratrol, a key stilbene mainly found in grapes skin showed beneficial effect against cancer, diabetes, obesity, cardiovascular, neurodegenerative diseases. Currently, pterostilbene and pinosylvin have also been attracted the interest of scientist due to their beneficial effect on health. Stilbenes exert cellular defence against oxidative stress which is mediated through the nuclear factor-erythroid-2-related factor-2 (Nrf2). These agents also have potential roles in SQSTM1/p62 protein in Nrf2/Keap1 signaling and autophagy (Reinisalo, Karlund, Koskela, Kaarniranta & Karjalainen, 2015). Lignans, xanthones are also representing important class of polyphenolic compounds. *Xanthones* like 8-hydroxycudraxanthone G, gartanin, α-mangostin, γ-mangostin, smeathxanthone A showed potent antioxidant activity (Jung, Su, Keller, Mehta & Kinghorn, 2006). *Lignans* are a group of the polyphenoic compound, that have phenylpropane dimer linkage with a 1,4-diarylbutane structure by β-β bonds (MacRae & Towers, 1984). They possess good antioxidant and anticancer activity. Example of lignans includes secoisolariciresinol, mataisoresinol, and pinoresinol. Few polyphenols may contain N-containing functional substituents. Two such groups of polyphenolic amides are capsaicinoids in chili peppers and avenanthramides in oats (Tsao, 2010)

Tannins are phenolic compounds, which denoted as antinutrients of plant origin as tannin precipitate proteins, inhibit digestive enzymes, and reduces the consumption of vitamins and minerals. Although, tannins also been recorded for their health-promoting effect. Tannins acknowledged widely for antioxidant, antiradical, anticarcinogenic, antimutagenic, antimicrobial activities. Tannins are mainly divided into two groups: hydrolysable tannins (i.e. ellagitannins, gallotannins) and non-hydrolysable or condensed tannins (i.e. polymers of catechin and/or leucoanthocyanidin). Tannin act as both primary and secondary antioxidant, as they donate hydrogen atom or electrons to terminate free radical chain reaction and also to chelate metal ions such as iron by interfering the steps involve Fenton reaction. Tannins also inhibit the lipid peroxidation. Some research also found that extract rich in tannins i.e. extracts of hazelnuts (prepared from green leafy cover) has better antioxidant effect than those of extracts contain less tannins i.e. extract prepared from hazelnut kernels (Amarowicz, 2007; Ghosh, 2015).

Coumarins are the secondary metabolites widely distributed in plants. Coumarins are present in nature as free form or as glycosides. Over 300 coumarins have been discovered from nature particularly from green plants. Some coumarins constituents include aesculin and esculetin (simple hydroxycoumarins), psoralen and isopsoralen (furocoumarins and isofurocoumarin), xanthyletin, xanthoxyletin, seselin, khellactone and praeuptorin A (pyranocoumarins), biscoumarins, bergenin (dihydroisocoumarins) etc. Beneficial effects of coumarins include in different diseases like cancer, inflammation, diabetes, cardiovascular and brain diseases, and these activity of coumarins related with their strong antioxidant effect may be in part (Kostova, et al., 20111; Bubols et al., 2013).

Carotenoids are a group of more than 600 fat-soluble plant pigments that provide color. Apart from the aesthetic role of carotenoids, they are found abundantly in foods and considered to be beneficial in treatment/prevention of several ailments. Nearly fifty different carotenoids have been found in the human diet and approximately twenty have been present in plasma and tissues. Major carotenoids available in diet include β-carotene, α-carotene, lycopene, β-cryptoxanthin, lutein and zeaxanthin. Carotenoids can efficiently quenche singlet oxygen and other ROS. Carotenoids also serve as chemical quenchers undergoing irreversible oxygenation. Though, exact molecular mechanisms underlying antioxidant and pro-oxidant activity of carotenoids are not fully understood. But numerous studies suggested that antioxidant activity of carotenoids have great impact on human health, by preventing oxidative stress situation. β-carotene and α-tocopherol can act synergistically as an effective "radical-trapping antioxidant" in biological membranes. The inhibition of lipid peroxidation by a combination of the two fat-soluble antioxidants was shown to be greater than the sum of the individual inhibitions. β-carotene, zeaxanthin, cryptoxanthin, α-carotene is the strong quencher of singlet molecular oxygen. Carotenoids also deactivate peroxyl radical efficiently (Fiedor & Burda, 2014; Krinsky and Johnson, 2005; Patrick, 2000; Stahl & Sies, 2003).

Primarily physical quenching takes place between carotenoids with $^1O_2$, which involves direct energy transfer between both molecules. Singlet molecular oxygen transferred the energy to carotenoid molecule and thus ground state oxygen and a triplet excited carotene molecule formed. Carotenoids are beck to ground state dissipating the energy, instead of any other chemical reactions. In comparison to physical quenching, chemical reactions between $^1O_2$ and carotenoids are of minor importance (Stahl & Sies, 2003).

β-carotene is the major source of vitamin A. Major source of β-carotene includes apricot, carrots, spinach, green collard, cantaloupe, beet green, broccoli, tomato. β-carotene was established as an antioxidant that can prevent cancer, heart disease, macular degeneration, ageing etc and also act as immunomodulator. In both observational and case control studies found that intake of fruits and vegetables rich in β-carotene can reduce the risk for cardiovascular disease. Protective effect of β-carotene supplementation on sunburn and other disorder was investigated, but the effect of β-carotene supplementation on cancer risk is controcertial (Burri, 1997; Patrick, 2000; Rao and Rao, 2007; Sen and Chakraborty, 2015).

Various investigations also showed that other phytochemicals like saponin, alkaloids, steroids from different plant are the produce strong antioxidant activities.

Food as Potential Source of Antioxidants

Fruits and vegetables are the rich source of diverse free phenolic acids. Phenolic acid in bound form present in grains and seeds, particularly in bran or hull. Hydroxycinnamic acids found in bluberry, cranberry, pear, sweet cherry, apple, orange, grape, apple juice, lemon, peach, potato, lettuce, spinach, coffee beans, tea, coffee, cider; while strawberry, raspberry, grape juice, longan seed, pomegranate juice contain hydroxybenzoic acids. Capsaicin (a capsaicinoids), main component responsible for chili hotness has also strong antioxidant effect. Tannins present in number of fruits, vegetables and beverages like bananas, sorghum, grapes, apple, strawberries, raspberries, pomegranate, blackberry, olive, plum walnuts, chick pea, black-eyed peas, lentils, curry leaves spinach, red wine, persimmons, chocolate, tea and coffee. Red and bluish-red cherries contain high percentage of anthocyanidins, while proanthocyanidins are available in grape, red wine. Other source of anthocyanidin includes black and blue berries, black grape, strawberries, cherries, plums, cranberry, pomegranate, raspberry and red wine. Vegetables (like celery, onions, dock leaves, fennel, hot peppers, tomatoes, spinach, lettuce, broccoli, kale), cereal (i.e. buckwheat, green/yellow beans), fruits (apples, apricots, grapes, plums, berries, currants, cherries, black currant juice, apple juice, ginkgo biloba), red wine, green and black tea, cocoa are rich source of flavonols. Quercetin, a important antioxidant molecule found in fruits and vegetables like green-yellow onions, apples, broccoli, cherries, grapes and red cabbage. Citrus fruits and juice, peppermint contains flavanones. Flavones are available in celery, olives, hot peppers, celery hearts, fresh parsley, oregano, rosemary, dry parsley, thyme. Different fruits (i.e. apples, apricots, grapes, pears, plums, raspberries, cherries, blackberries, blueberries, cranberries), red and white wine, green and black tea, chocolate, wine, cocoa contain different flavanols. Isoflavones i.e. genistein and daidzein are available in beans, tofu, soy milk, grape, flour, miso, tea, coffee, spinach and potato. Hesperidin is available in oranges and lemons peels, narangin is found in many fruits such as orange, lemon and grapefruit. Grapes and vegetables are the good source of ellagic acid, on the other hand kaempferol is abundant in vegetables like broccoli, beets. Green and black tea is considered as rich sources of catechins. Grapes, peanut, red wine contain resveratrol and trans-resveratrol (Ghosh, 2015; Yordi et al., 2012; Tsao, 2010; Han et al. 2007). Flaxseed and grains like wheat are the great source of lignans. Content of polyphenolic substance in foods are largely affected by environmental factors, soil, sunlight, rainfall etc. Stage of ripeness also affects the proportions of various antioxidants present in fruit. For example, content of phenolic acid reduces during ripening, whereas anthocyanin level increases (Pande & Rizvi, 2009). The major source of coumarin includes green plants, fruits (e.g. bilberry, cloudberry), olive oil, and beverages (coffee, wine, and tea) (Kostova et al., 20111; Bubols et al., 2013). Green leafy vegetables, orange and yellow fruits are the major source of β-carotene. Dietary lycopene is predominately found from tomatoes and tomato products, while lutein and zeaxanthin is more in spinach and kale (Krinsky & Johnson, 2005).

Cereals and millets are the popular food grain consumed as main food around the world. Wheat, rice, maize, barley, oat, rye etc. confer nutritional benefits and helpful to promote the health. They contain a large variety of health promoting phytochemicals, including antioxidants. Generally cereals are rich in phenolic acids which are found as free, soluble conjugates or as bound forms in endosperm, germ, and bran fractions of grains (Goufo & Trindade, 2014). Rice (*Oryza sativa*) is the major food in different Asian countries like India, Bangladesh. Several epidemiological researches have suggested that rice-consuming regions of the world have low incidence of certain chronic diseases, which might be due to the presence of antioxidant molecules in rice (Goufo & Trindade, 2014). Wheat is one of the most important cereals and considered as an important source of nutrients. It was observed that among the 4 fractions (seed capsule, aleurone layer, outer endosperm and inner endosperm) of wheat (surface layer to the centre of a grain), total phenolic content and antioxidant activity of ethanol extract is as high in aleurone layer than those of other fractions (Shi, Tian, Ru & Guo, 2011). Pearl millet a key cereal of India, an investigation has found that bran rich fraction of millet contains high tannin, phytic acid and flavonoid. Pearl millet is a rich source of antioxidant molecule thus it could possible that pearl millet could confer beneficial effect in cancer, hyperlipedemia, and in prevention of liposome oxidation, proliferation of HT-29 adenocarcinoma (Daniel et al., 2012). Different varieties of rice, wheat, ragi, maize, jowar, barley, oats, rye have been investigated for antioxidant activity and showed moderate to strong antioxidant effect. A number of studies found that regular intake of wheat whole grains and whole grain products responsible for reduced risk of cardiovascular disease, stroke, diabetes, some cancers (El-Baky, 2009). A number of reports observed the beneficial effect of maize on obesity, diabetes, cancer, immunity, kidney and urinary tract infection, gout, inflammation etc. (Pedreschi & Cisneros-Zevallos, 2007; Escudero et al, 2012), antioxidant phytochemicals present in maize may responsible for their beneficial effect. Available epidemiological surveys have shown that sorghum intake lower the risk of certain types of human cancer compared to other cereals. Sorghum phytochemicals are also helpful to promote cardiovascular health and reduce obesity. High level of antioxidant phytochemicals present in sorghum may be partly responsible for its health beneficial effect (Awika & Rooney, 2004; Mathangi, 2012). Pharmacological screenings showed that oats possesses antioxidant, immunomodulatory, antidiabetic, anticholesterolaemic, antiinflammatory, wound healing activities. Phytoconstituents of oats found to protect LDL during oxidation, cardiovascular and coronary artery diseases (Singh, De, & Belkheir, 2013). Health benefit of barley, rye also reported in several epidemiological and scientific investigations. Cereals & millets are very good source of dietary phenolic and other antioxidants which may have potential health promotive and diseases preventive effects.

Table 3. Antioxidant/pro-oxidant molecules in food (by focusing on common food)

Food		Phytoconstituents (mainly antioxidant/pro-oxidant molecules)
Cereals & Millets	Rice (*Oryza sativa*)	phenolic acids (gallic, protocatechuic, *p*-hydroxybenzoic, vanillic, syringic acids, *p*-coumaric, ferulic, caffeic, sinapic, chlorogenic, and cinnamic, ellagic acids), flavonoids (tricin, luteolin, apigenin, quercetin, isorhamnetin, kaempferol, myricetin, tricin 4′-*O*-(*erythro-β* guaiacylglyceryl) ether, tricin 4′-*O*-(*threo-β* guaiacylglyceryl) ether, isovitexin, naringenin, hesperidin, rutin, luteolin-7-*O*-glucoside, apigenin-7-*O*-glucoside, qrcetin-3-*O*-glucoside, quercetin-3-*O*-rutinoside, isorhamnetin-3-*O*-glucoside, isorhamnetin-3-*O*-acetylglucoside, isorhamnetin-7-*O*-rutinoside, taxifolin-7-*O*-glucoside, 5,3′,4′,5′-tetrahydroxyflavanone-7-*O*-glucoside, myricetin-7-*O*-glucoside, 5,6,3′,4′,5-′pentahydroxyflavone-7-*O*-glucoside, apigenin-6-*C*-glucoside-8-*C*-arabinoside, (+)-3′-*O*-methyltaxifolin, brassicin, isorhamnetin-4′-*O*-glucoside, 3′-*O*-methyltaxifolin-5-*O*-glucoside, 3′-*O*-methyltaxifolin-7-*O*-glucoside, 3′-*O*-methyltaxifolin-4′-*O*-glucoside, isorhamnetin-7-*O*-cellobioside, and brassicin-4′-*O*-glucoside), anthocyanins (cyaniding-3-*O*-glucoside, peonidin-3-*O*-glucoside, cyaniding-3-*O*-rutinoside, cyaniding-3-*O*-galactoside, cyaniding-3-*O*-sophoroside, peonidin-3-*O*-rutinoside, cyaniding-3,5-*O*-diglucoside, peonidin-3,5-*O*-diglucoside, pelargonidin-3-*O*-glucoside, delphinidin-3-*O*-glucoside, petunidin-3-*O*-glucoside, petunidin-3-*O*-galactoside, petunidin-3-*O*-arabinoside, delphinidin-3-*O*-galactoside, delphinidin-3-*O*-arabinoside, malvidin-3-*O*-galactoside, malvidin-3-*O*-glucoside, pelargonidin-3,5-*O*-diglucoside), proanthocyanidins (catechin, epicatechin), Vitamin E (*α,β,γ,δ*-tocotrienol, *α,β,γ,δ*-tocopherol), *γ*-oryzanol, and phytic acid (Goufo & Trindade, 2014).
	Pearl millet (*Pennisetum typhoideum*)	Flavonoids likes tricin, 7-OMe luteolin, acacetin, glucosyl orientin, glucosyl vitexin, and phenolic acids (i.e. vanillic, syringic, ferulic p-hydroxy benzoic acid, *cis/trans* pcoumaric acids). It is also rich source several antioxidants minerals like zinc, copper etc and omega 3-fatty acid (Daniel, Denni & Chauhan, 2012; Nambiar, Dhaduk, Sareen, Shahu & Desai, 2011)
	Wheat (*Triticum aestivum*)	Phenolic compounds (phenolic acids, anthocyanidins, quinones, flavonoids and amino phenolic compounds), several tocopherols and tocotrienols like α-tocopherol, β-tocopherol, α-tocotrienol, and β-tocotrienol, carotenoid like *trans* lutein were found in different wheat species. Flavonoids (cyanidin 3-galactoside, cyanidin 3-glucoside, cyanidin 3-rutinoside, delphinidin 3-glucoside, delphinidin 3-rutinoside, peonidin-3-glucoside, petunidin-3-glucoside, petunidin-3-rutinoside, apigenin glycosides, tricin), lignans. Level of ferulic acid and diferulates are found in significant level in wheat (Abdel-Aal & Rabalski, 2008; El-Baky, 2009; Dykes & Roonwy, 2007).
	Finger millet or ragi (*Eleusine coracana*)	A number of phenolics like benzoic acid and cinnamic acid derivatives (i.e. gallic, protocatechuic, *p*-hydroxybenzoic, vanillic, ferulic, syringic, *trans*-cinnamic, gentisic, sinapic and *p*-coumaric acids) identified in ragi. Several tannins, flavonoid like quercetin, orientin, isoorientin, vitexin, isovitexin, saponarin, violanthin, lucenin-1, and tricin are present in finger millet (Mathangi & Sudha, 2012; Banerjee, Sanjay, Chethan, & Malleshi, 2012).
	Purple corn or maize (*Zea mays*)	Phenolic compounds like chlorogenic acid, caffeic acid, rutin, ferulic acid, morin, quercetin, naringenin, kaempferol, anthocyanins, cyanidin-3-glucoside, pelargonidin-3-glucoside, peonidin-3-glucoside, cyaniding-3-(6′′-malonylglucoside), pelargonidin-3-(6′′-malonylglucoside), peonidin-3-(6′′-malonylglucoside), cyaniding-3-(6′′-ethylmalonylglucoside), pelargonidin-3-(6′′-ethylmalonylglucoside), peonidin-3-(6′′-ethylmalonylglucoside). Flavanol anthocyanins like catechin-(4,8)-cyanidin-3-glucoside, catechin-(4,8)-cyanidin-3-malonylglucoside, epicatechin-(4,8)-cyanidin-3-malonylglucoside, catechin-(4,8)-peonidin-3-glucoside, epicatechin-(4,8)-peonidin-3-glucoside, catechin-(4,8)-pelargonidin-3-glucoside, catechin-(4,8)-cyanidin-3,5-diglucoside, catechin-(4,8)-cyanidin-3-malonylglucoside-5-glucoside, epicatechin-(4,8)-cyanidin-3-malonylglucoside-5-glucoside. Phenolic acids i.e. *p*-coumaric acid, vanillic acid, protocatechuic acid, ferulic acid, *p*-hydroxybenzoic acid, *p*-hydroxyphenyl acetic acid, syringic acid, caffeic, sinapic acid. Derivatives of hesperitin and quercetin (Pedreschi & Cisneros-Zevallos, 2007; Escudero, Munoz, Alvarado-Ortiz, Alvarado & Yanez, 2012).
	Great millet or jowar (*Sorghum vulgare*)	Phenolic acid (gallic, protecatechuic, *p*-hydroxybenzoic, gentisic, salicylic, vanillic, syringic, ferulic, caffeic, *p*-coumaric, cinnamic and sinapic acid), flavonoids (apigeninidin, apigeninidin-5-glucoside, luteolinidine, luteolinidine 5-glucoside, 5-glucoside, 5-methoxyapigeninidin, 7-methoxyapigeninidin, 7-methoxyapigeninidin 5-methoxyluteolinidin, 5-methoxyluteolinidin 7-glucoside, 7-methoxyluteolinidin, luteolin, apigenin, eriodictyol, eriodictyol 5-glucoside, naringenin, kaempferol 3-rutinoside-7-glucuronide, taxifolin, taxifolin 7-glucoside, apiforol, luteoforol, catechin and its derivatives, procyanidin, proluteolinidin, procyanidin B-1, fisetinidin, cyanidin, pelargonidin, peonidin, 3-deoxyanthocyanidins, 7-*O*-methyl luteolin), condensed tannin (Dykes & Roonwy, 2007; Awika & Rooney, 2004).
	Barley (*Hordeum vulgare*)	A number of phenolic antioxidants like benzoic and cinnamic acid derivative, proanthocyanidine, flavonols, chalcones, flavones etc present in barley. Phenolic acid (protecatechuic, salicylic, vanillic, syringic, ferulic, *o*-coumaric, *m*-coumaric, *p*-coumaric, and sinapic acid), Anthocyanins (apigeninidin, apigeninidin-5-glucoside, cyanidin, cyanidin-3-galactoside, cyanidin-3-glucoside, cyanidin 3-rutinoside), flavonoids (cyanidin, cyanidin-3-glucoside, delphinidin, pelargonidin, pelargonidin glycosides, petunidin 3-glucoside, chrysoeriol, catechin, leucocyanidin, leucopelargonidin, procyanidin B-3, prodelphinidin B-3), lignans (Dykes & Roonwy, 2007; Gamel & Abdel-Aal, 2012).
	Rye or sarsoo (*Secale cereale*)	Phenolic acid (protecatechuic, *p*-hydroxybenzoic, vanillic, syringic, ferulic, caffeic, *p*-coumaric and sinapic acid), flavonoids (cyanidin-3-glucoside, peonidin-3-glucoside, delphinidin 3-rutinoside), alkylresorsinols, lignans, tannin (Dykes & Roonwy, 2007).
	Oats (*Avena sativa*)	A number of phytoconstituents like avenanthramides, an indole alkaloidgramine, flavonoids, flavonolignans, triterpenoid saponins, sterols (β-sitosterol, Δ^5-avenasterol, Δ^7-avenasterol) and tocols present in oats. Phenolic acid (gallic, protecatechuic, *p*-hydroxybenzoic, *p*-hydroxyphenylacetic, vanillic, syringic, ferulic, caffeic, *p*-coumaric, *o*-coumaric and sinapic acid), flavonoids (tricin, apigenin, apigenin-6-C-glucoside, apigenin-8-C-glucoside luteolin, isovitexin, tricin, vitexin, homoeriodictyol, kaempferol, kaempferol 3-*O*-rutinoside, kaempferol 3-rutinoside-7-glucuronide, quercetin, quercerin 3-*O*-rutinoside, catechol,), lignans, tocol (α-tocotrienol, α-tocopherol), phytic acid (Dykes & Roonwy, 2007; Paterson, 2001)

continued on following page

Table 3. Continued

Food		Phytoconstituents (mainly antioxidant/pro-oxidant molecules)
Pulses and Legumes	Black gram, Urad dal (*Vigna mungo*)	β-carotene, ascorbic acid, various tocopherols, phenolic compounds, flavonoids, condensed tannins, minerals like zinc, iron, copper. Phenolic acid (gallic, protocatechuic, gentisic, vanillic, syringic, caffeic and ferulic acids), apigenin, 7-methoxy apigenin (Luthria, Singh & D'souza, 2014; Soris, Kala, Mohan & Vadivel, 2010; Girish, Pratape & Rao, 2012)
	Bengal gram or Chana (*Cicer arietinum*)	Flavonoids like (+)-catechin, (–)-epicatechin, naringenin, naringenin-7- *O* -β-D-glucopyranoside, (epi)afzelechin, epicatechin, epicatechin 3-gallate, epigallocatechin, epigallocatechin 3-gallate, catechin, gallocatechin, daidzein, genistein, matairesinol, secoisolariciresinol, kaempferol, kaempferol 3-*O*-β-D-glucopyranoside, kaempferol 3-*O*-rutinoside, kaempferide, quercetin 3-*O*- β-D-glucopyranoside, rutin, kaempferol and quercetin derivatives, including methylated such as isorhamnetin (3-*O*-methoxyquercetin) and myricetin-*O*-methyl ethers and glycosides; aromadendrin, apigenin and their derivatives. Isoflavones (like biochanin A, genistein, formononetin, orobol and two isomers of dalpanin), *α*-resorcylic acid, biochanin glucoside, antioxidant minerals, carotenoids (β-carotene, lutein, zeaxanthin, β-cryptoxanthin, lycopene and α-carotene), sterols (β-sitosterol, Δ^5-avenasterol, Δ^7-avenasterol), cajaninstilbene acid, pinostrobin, vitexin and orientin, phenolic acid (gallic, p-hydroxybenzoic and caffeoylquinic, sinapic, ferulic, *p*-coumaric, vanillic acids and their derivatives), saponins (Bhagwat, Haytowitz & Holden, 2011; Jukanti, Gaur, Gowda & Chibbar, 2012; Wu et al., 2009; Mekky et al., 2015).
	Green gram, mug dal *(Vigna radiata)*	Luteolin, kaempferol, myricetin, quercetin, aureol, coumestrol, cyclokievitone, dalbergioidin, 2,3-dehydrokievitone, 5-deoxykievitone, genistein, 2'-hydroxygenistein, isovitexin, kievitone, myrtillin, phaseol, phaseollidin, vitexin, ß-sitosterol, stigmasterol, soyasapogenol C (Battu, Male, Haripriya, Malleswari & Reeshma, 2011).
	Peas green *(Pisium sativum)*	Phenolic acids (protocatechuic, gentisic, sinapic, *m*-hydroxybenzoic, vanillic, syringic, caffeic, *o*-coumaric, *p*-coumaric, ferrulic, veratric and 2,3-dihydroxybenzoic acid), kaempferol, quercetin, daidzein, formononetin, isoformononetin, prunetin (Troszynska & Ciska, 2002; Amarowicz, Karamac & Weidner, 2001).
	Rajmah *(Phaseolus vulgaris)*	Anthocyanidins (pelargonidin, malvidin, petunidin, cyanidin, delphinidin, peonidin), catechin, catechol, saponin, and phenolic acids (gallic, vanillic, caffeic, coumaric, sinapic, chlorogenic, caffeine, cholchecien, *p*-hydroxybenzoic, chrysin, p-coumaric, protocatechuic and ferrulic acid), quercetin 3-*O*-glucoside and protoanthocyanidins (condensed tannins), vitamin C, vitamin E, kaempferol 3-*O*-glucoside, kaempferol 3-*O*-acetyl-glucoside (Bhagwat et al., 2011; Nyau, 2014; Camara, Urrea & Schlegel, 2013; Hassan & Youssef, 2012).
	Soya bean *(Glycine max)*	Simple phenols, benzoic acid derivatives, flavonoids, tannins, lignans, isoflavones, anthocyanins, saponin. Phytic acid (phytate), saponins, plant sterols (phytosterols), vitamins (γ-tocopherol) and minerals. Luteolin, kaempferol, myricetin, quercetin, phenolic acid (chlorogenic acid, caffeic acid, ferulic acid, and *p*-coumaric acid), anthocyanins (delphinidin-3-glucoside, cyanidin-3-galactoside, cyanidin-3-glucoside, petunidin-3-glucoside, peonidin-3-glucoside, and malvidin-3-glucoside), aroma compounds (1-octen-3-ol, maltol, phenylethyl alcohol, hexanol) isoflavones (glucosides, i.e., daidzin, genistin and glycitin; acetylglucosides, i.e. acetyldaidzin, acetylgenistin and acetylglycitin; malonylglucosides, i.e. malonyldadzin, malonylgenistin and malonylglycitin; and structure unconjugated aglycone, like daidzein, genistein and glycitein) (Bhagwat et al., 2011; Zhang et al., 2011; Lee, & Shibamoto, 2000; Cheng, 2009; Martino et al., 2011; Reynoso-Camacho, Ramos-Gomez & Loarca-Pina, 2006).
	Lentil, massor dal (*Lens esculenta,* syn. *Lens culinaris)*	Phenolic acids, flavanols, flavonols, soyasaponins, phytic acid, hydroxycinnamates, procyanidins, gallates, flavonols, dihydroflavonols, dihydrochalcones and condensed tannins. catechin and epicatechin derivatives, epicatechin, epicatechin 3-gallate, epigallocatechin, epigallocatechin 3-gallate, catechin, gallocatechin, kaempferol glycosides, 3′,5′-di-*c*-*β*-glucopyranosyl phloretin, catechin-3-*o*-glucoside, β-sitosteryl-3-(2′-n-eicosanyloxy)-benzoate, n-octadec-9-enoyl-1-β-d-glucurano-pyranoside, α-d-galactopyranosyl-(6→1′)-α-d-galactopyranosyl-(6′→1″)-α-d-galactopyranosyl-(6″→1‴)-α-d-galactopyranoside, benzoyl-o-α-d-glucopyranosyl-(2a→1b)-o-α-d-glucopyranosyl-(2b→1c)-o-α-d-glucopyranosyl-(6c→1d)-o-α-d-glucopyranosyl-(6d→1e)-o-α-d-gluco-pyranoside, n-heptadecanyl n-octadec-9-enoate, β-sitosterol, cis-n-docos-15-enoic acid, n-dodecanoyl-*O*-ß-D-glucuranopyranoside, n-tetradecanoyl-*O*-ß-D–arabinopyranoside, n-eicosanoyl-*O*-ß-D–arabinopyranoside, epicatechin glucosides, procyanidin dimers, quercetin diglycoside, *trans-p*-coumaric acid (Bhagwat et al., 2011; Zou, Chang, Gu & Qian, 2011; Jameel, Ali & Ali, 2015a,b)
Edible Oils	Coconut oil	Virgin coconut oil contain tocopherol and phenolic compounds like protocatechuic acid, vanillic acid, syringic acid, p-coumaric acid, caffeic acid and ferulic acid. Presence of catechin is reported in commercial and traditional coconut oil (Marina, Man, Nazimah & Amin, 2009; Arlee, Suanphairoch & Pakdeechanuan, 2013).
	Rice bran oil	Gamma oryzanol and other phytosterols like β-sitosterol, squalene. Sterol esters, triterpene, tocopherols, tocotrienols, ferulic acid and other phenolic compounds (Patel & Naik, 2004)
	Olive oil	Oleic acid (i.e. omega-6 fatty acid, linoleic acid), Phenolic compounds (hydroxytyrosol, tyrosol, oleuropein, ligstroside, hydroxytyrosol, tyrosol, oleuropein), squalene, tocopherols. Extra virgin/virgin olive oil contain phenolic acids like caffeic, vanillic, syringic, *p*-coumaric, *o*-coumaric, protocatechuic, sinapic, *p*-hydroxybenzoic, ferulic, cinnamic and gallic acid; falvonoids (taxifolin, luteolin and apigenin); phenolic alcohols like 3,4-dihydroxyphenyl ethanol and *p*-hydroxyphenyl ethanol; lignans like (+)-1-acetoxypinoresinol and (+)-pinoresinol (Servili et al., 2014; Waterman & Lockwood, 2007; Bendini et al., 2007; Bulotta et al., 2014).
	Palm oil	Vitamin E (tocotrienol, tocopherol, tocotrie), 5-avenasterol, carotenoids (different carotene including beta carotene, lycopene), coenzyme Q10, polyphenols, squalene. Major phenolics in palm includes cinnamic acid, ferulic acid, caumaric acid (Sundram, 2015)

continued on following page

Table 3. Continued

Food		Phytoconstituents (mainly antioxidant/pro-oxidant molecules)
	Mustard oil	Vitamin E omega alpha 3 and omega alpha 6 fatty acid, selenium and magnesium, phenolic compounds (Khan, Sankhyan & Kumar, 2013; Sarwar, Rahman, Raza, Rouf & Rahman, 2014).
	Sunflower oil	α/β/γ/δ tocopherol, α/γ/δ tocotrienol, sterols (β-sitosterol, Δ^5-avenasterol, Δ^7-avenasterol, Δ^7-stigmasterol), minerals (like: iron, copper, zinc, selenium), omega 3 and omega 6 fatty acid (Khan, Choudhary, Pandey, Khan & Thomas, 2015; Warner, Vick, Kleingartner, Isaak & Doroff, 2015).
	Peanut/ groundnut oil	Resveratrol, α/β/γ/δ tocopherol, tocotrienol, sterols (β-sitosterol, Δ^5-avenasterol, Δ^7-avenasterol, Δ^7-stigmasterol), squalene, β-carotene, *p*-coumaric acid (Akhtar, Khalid, Ahmed, Shahzad, Suleria, 2014).
Spices and Herb	Nutmeg (*Myristica fragrans*)	Essential oil contain α-pinenes, camphene, p-cymene, sabinene, β-phellandrene, γ-terpinene, limonene, myrcene, (linalool, geraniol, terpineol, myristicin, elemicin, safrole. Saponin, tannins, epicatechin, cyanidin, carotene (Latha et al., 2005)
	Curry leaf (*Murraya koenigii*)	alkaloids (mahanine, koenine, koenigine, koenidine, girinimbiol, girinimibine, koenimbine, *O*-methyl murrayamine A, isomahanine), Vitamin C, carotene, 5,8-dimethyl furanocoumarin, β-sitosterol, coumarin glycoside like scopotin, murrayanine. Essential oil from leaves contain di- α-phellandrene, D-sabinene, D-α-pinene, dipentene, D-α-terpinol and caryophyllene (Ajay et al., 2011).
	Clove (*Syzygium aromaticum*)	Eugenol, eugenol acetate, limonin, ferulic aldehyde, tamarixetin 3-*O*-b-D-glucopyranoside, ombuin 3-*O*-b-D-glucopyranoside, quercetin, D-glucopyranoside, biflorin, kaempferol, rhamnocitrin, myricetin, gallic acid, ellagic acid, oleanolic acid, orsellinic acid (Nassar et al., 2007).
	Aniseed (*Pimpinella anisum*)	*trans* and *cis*-anethole, palmitic and oleic acids, eugenol *trans*-anethole, methylchavicol, anisaldehyde, estragole, scopoletin, umbelliferone, estrols, terpene hydrocarbons, estragole, (E)-methyleugenol, *α*-cuparene, *α* and *γ* - himachalene, *β*-bisabolene, *p*-anisaldehyde, carvone, *β*-caryophyllene, dihydrocarvyl acetate, limonene, coumarins, *cis*-pseudoisoeugenyl 2-methylbutyrate, *trans*-pseudoisoeugenyl 2-methylbutyrate, 4-(*β*-d-glucopyranosyloxy) benzoic acid, (E)-3-hydroxy-anethole *β*-d-glucopyranoside, (E)-10-(2-hydroxy-5-methoxyphenyl) propane *β*-d-glucopyranoside, 3-hydroxyestragole *β*-d-glucopyranoside, methyl syringate 4-*O*-*β*-d-glucopyranoside, hexane-1,5-diol 1-*O*-*β*-d-glucopyranoside, 1-deoxy-l-erythritol 3-*O*-*β*-dglucopyranoside, quercetin 3-glucuronide, rutin, luteolin 7-glucoside, isoorientin, isovitexin, apigenin 7-glucoside, luteolin glycoside (Shojaii & Fard, 2012).
	Saffron (*Crocus sativus*)	Carotenoids (zeaxanthin, lycopene, α and β carotenes), carotenes, crocetin, picrocrocin, rutin, quercetin, luteolin, hesperidin, and bioflavonoids, terpenes, terpene alcohols and their esters, safranal. 3,5-β-diglucosides of delphinidin and petunidin, 3-β-rutinosides, delphinidin 3-*O*-(β-d-glucopyranoside)-5-*O*-(6-*O*-malonyl-β-d-glucopyranoside), petudin 3,7-di-*O*-(β-d-glucopyranoside). 3,7 di-*O*-β-d-glucoside and 3,5 di-*O*-β-d-glucosides of delphinidin, petunidin, kaempferol 3-*O*-α-(2,3-di-*O*-β-d-glucopyranosyl) rhamnopyranoside and 3,8 dihydroxy1methylanthroquinone-2-carboxylic (Srivastava, Ahmed, Dixit, Dharamveer & Saraf, 2010; Gohari, Saeidnia & Mahmoodabadi, 2013).
	Rose mary (*Rosmarinus officinalis*)	Carnosic acid, carnosol, carnosol isomer, cirsimaritin, epiisorosmanol, epirosmanol, epirosmanol methyl ether, gallocatechin, genkwanin, hesperidin, homoplantaginin, luteolin 3'-*o*-(*o*-acetyl)-β-d-glucuronide isomer I, luteolin 3'-*o*-(*o*-acetyl)-β-d-glucuronide isomer II, luteolin-3'-glucuronide, micromeric acid, nepetrin, quinic acid, rosmadial, rosmanol, rosmaridiphenol, rosmarinic acid, rosmarinic acid-3-*O*-glucoside, siringic acid, ursolic acid, [9]-shogaol, [9]-shogaol isomer, 12-metoxy-carnosic acid, 6-hydroxyluteolin 7-glucoside, naringenin, apigenin, luteolin, isorhamnetin, kaempferol, quercetin, anemosapogenin, asiatic acid, augustic acid, benthamic acid, betulinic acid, and 2,3,4,4a,10,10a-hexahidro-5,6-dihydroxy-1,1-dimethyl-7- (1-methylethyl)-9(1h)-phenantrenone (Bhagwat et al., 2011; Borras-Linares et al., 2014).
	Cumin (*Cuminum cyminum*)	Cuminaldehyde, limonene, α- and β-pinene, 1,8-cineole, *o*- and *p*-cymene, α- and γ-terpinene, safranal, linalool, myrcene, limonene, *p*-mentha-1, 3-dien-7-ol, caryophyllene, β-bisabolene, β-phellandrene, D-terpinene, cuminyl alcohol, β-farnesene, α-phellandrene, cis and trans sabinene, myrtenol, α-terpineol, phellandral, quercitrin (Nadeem & Riaz, 2012; Johri, 2011).
	Caraway (*Carum carvi*)	Carvacrol, carvone, α and β-pinene, limonene, γ-terpinene, linalool, carvenone, *p*-cymene, β-myrcene, thujone, anethole, sabinene, β-selinene, β-cyclolavandulal, quercetin 3-methyl ether, isoquercetin, quercetin 3-*O*-glucuronide, quercetin 3-*O*-caffeyl-glucoside, kaempferol 3-glucoside, isorhamnetin glycoside (Agrahari & Singh, 2014; Johri, 2011).
	Fenugreek (*Trigonella foenum-graecum*)	Trimethylamine, neurin, trigonelline, gentianine, carpaine, betain, graecunins, fenugrin, fenugreekine, trigofoenosides, yamogenin, diosgenin, smilagenin, sarsasapogenin, tigogenin, neotigogenin, gitogenin, neogitogenin, yuccagenin, saponaretin, coumarin, anethol, 4-hydroxyisoleucin, arginine, piperidine, trigonelloside C, yamogenin tetroside B and C, tenugrin B, tigogenin, yuccagenin, lilagenin, quercetin, luteolin, vitexin, isovitexin, homoerietin, vicenin-1, vicenin-2, coumarin acid, scopoletin acid, chlorogenic acid, caffeic acid and *p*-coumaric acid (Yadav & Kaushik, 2011; Patil & Jain, 2014).
	Ginger, (*Zingiber officinale*)	Gingerol, camphene, betaphellandrene, curcumene, cineole, geranyl acetate, terphineol, terpenes, borneol, geraniol, limonene, linalool, α-zingiberene, β-sesquiphellandrene, betabisabolene, α-farmesene, (-)-zingiberene, β-sesquiphellandrene, bisabolene, farnesene, β-phelladrene, cineol, amadaldehyde, paradols, gingerdiols, gingerdiacetates, gingerdiones, 6-gingersulfonic acid, gingerenones, gingerglycolipids A-C, diaryleheptanonesgingerenones A-C, isogingerenone B, methylegingediol, gingediacetates, methylegingediacetates (Ghosh, Banerjee, Mullick & Banerjee, 2011).

continued on following page

Table 3. Continued

Food		Phytoconstituents (mainly antioxidant/pro-oxidant molecules)
	Fennel *(Foeniculum vulgare)*	Vitamin C, trans-anethole, fenchone, estragol, α-phellandrene, (+) fenchone, p-anisaldehyde, 3-*O*-caffeoylquinic acid, 4-*O*-caffeoylquinic acid, 5-*O*-caffeoylquinic acid, 1,3-*O*-di-caffeoylquinic acid, 1,4-*O*-di-caffeoylquinic acid, 1,5-*O*-di-caffeoylquinic acid, eriodictyol-7-rutinoside, quercetin-3-rutinoside, rosmarinic acid, quercetin-3-*O*-galactoside, kaempferol-3-*O*-rutinoside, kaempferol-3-*O*-glucoside, quercitin-3-*O*-glucuronide, kampferol-3-*O*-glucuronide, isoquercitin, isorhamnetin-3-*O*-glucoside, cis and trans-miyabenol C, trans-resveratrol-3-*O*-β-D-glucopyranoside, sinapyl glucoside, syringin-4-O-b-glucoside, oleanolic acid, 7-α-hydroxycampesterol, (3b,5a,8a,22E) 5,8-epidioxy-ergosta-6,22-dien-3-ol, and 2,3-dihydropropylheptadec-5-onoate (Rather, Dar, Sofi, Bhat & Qurishi, 2012).
	Turmeric *(Curcuma longa)*	Curcumin I-III, diketones demethoxycurcumin, bis-demethoxycurcumin, tumerones (a and b), curdione, curzerenone, mono and di demethoxycurcumin, α-phellandrene, sabinene, cineol, borneol, zingiberene, sesquiterpines, (6S)-2-methyl-6-(4-hydroxyphenyl-3-methyl)-2-hepten-4-one, bisabolane sesquiterpenes, calebin derivatives (Yadav, Yadav, Khar, Mujeeb, & Akhtar, 2013).
	Tulsi *(Ocimum sanctum)*	Euginal, urosolic acid, linalool, limatrol, caryophyllene, methyl carvicol, estragol, rosmarinic acid, apigenin, cirsimaritin, isothymusin, isothymonin, orientin, vicenin (Rahaman, Islam, Kamruzzaman, Alam & Jamal, 2011).
Beverages	Tea	Alkaloids (caffeine, theophylline, and theobromine), amino acids, carbohydrates, proteins, chlorophyll, volatile compounds, fluoride, mineral (Se, Zn). Phenolic compounds in tea includes (-)-epigallocatechin gallate, (-)-epigallocatechin, (-)-epicatechin gallate, (-)-epicatechin, gallic acid, (-)-epicatechin (Cabrera, Gimeanez & Loapez, 2003).
	Green tea	Proteins, amino acids, carbohydrates, lipids, acids; sterols as stigmasterol, vitamins (vitamin B, C, E); alkaloids (caffeine and theophyllin), chlorophyll, carotenoids, volatile compounds, minerals and (like, Mg, Cr, Mn, Fe, Cu, Zn, Se, etc.), flavonoids like catechins are (-)-epigallocatechin-3-gallate, (-)-epigallocatechin, (-)-epicatechin-3-gallate, (-)-epicatechin, gallic acid, kaempferol, myricetin, quercetin and phenolic acids such as chlorogenic acid, caffeic acid (Cabrera, Artacho & Gimeanez, 2006).
	Coffee	3,4-dicaffeoylquinic acid, 3,5-dicaffeoylquinic acid, 3-caffeoylquinic acid, 3-feruloylquinic acid, 4,5-dicaffeoylquinic acid, 4-caffeoylqunic acid, 5-feruloylquinicacid, 5-caffeoylquinicacid, 5-feruloylquinicacid, caffeic acid, 4-ethylguaiacol, 4-vinylguaiacol, 3-methylcatechol, 4-ethylcatechol, 4-methylcatechol, guaiacol, catechol, pyrogallol (Tresserra-Rimbau, Medina-Remon, Estruch & Lamuela-Raventos, 2014).
	Beer	4-hydroxy benzoic acid, protocatechuic acid, vanillic acid, gallic acid, syringic acid, *o*-vanillin, (+)-catechin, (-)-epicatechin, gallocatechin, catechin gallate, 3′-*O*-methylcatechin, cinnamic acid, *p*-coumaric acid, caffeic acid, ferulic acid, sinapic acid, procyanidin, prodelphinidin, apigenin, tricin, vitexin, saponarin, saponaretin, isoxanthohumol, naringerin, taxifolin, kaempferol, myricetin, myticitrin, quercetin, quercitrin, rutin, isoquercitrin, kaempferol-3-rhamnosid (Saura-Calixto, Serrano, Perez-Jimemez, 2008)
Fruits & Vegetable	Kiwi *(Actinidia deliciosa planch)*	Phenolic acids (protocatechuic, vanillic, chlorogenic, catechol, caffeine, catechin and cinnamic acid), pyrogallol, coumarin, flavonoids like rosmarinic acid, narengnin, hespererctin (Shehata & Soltan, 2013).
	Avocado *(Persea americana)*	Phenolic acids (protocatechuic, vanillic, catechol, catechin, ferulic, coumarin and ellagic acid), pyrogallol, flavonoids like rosmarinic, hespererctin, rutin, quercitrinic, quercitin, kampferol (Shehata & Soltan, 2013).
	Amla *(Emblica officinalis)*	Vitamin C, gallic acid, ellagic acid, quercetin, 1-*O*-galloyl-beta-D-glucose, 3,6-di-*O*-galloyl-D-glucose, chebulinic acid, quercetin, chebulagic acid, 1,6-di-*O*-galloyl beta-D-glucose, 3-ethylgallic acid, isostrictinin, kaempferol-3-O-alpha L-(6''-methyl) rhamnopyranoside, kaempferol-3-*O*-α-L(6''-ethyl) rhamnopyranoside (Dasaroju & Gottumukkala, 2014).
	Lichi *(Litchi chinensis)*	Anthocyanins (i.e., cyanidin-3-glucoside, cyanidin-3-rutinoside, malvidin-3-glucoside), epicatechin, quercetin glycosides, 2-(2-hydroxyl-5-(methoxycarbonyl) phenoxy benzoic acid, kaempferol, isolariciresinol, stigmasterol, butylated hydroxytoluene, 3,4-dihydroxyl benzoate, methyl shikimate and ethyl shikimate, 3,4-dihydroxybenzoic acid, (+)-catechin, vanillic acid, caffeic acid, syringic acid, (-)-epicatechin, 4-methylcatechol, ferulic acid, rutin and quercetin (Li et al., 2012; Jiang et al., 2013; Su et al., 2014).
	Apple *(Malus x domestica)*	Quercetin, quercetin-3-galactoside, quercetin-3-glucoside, quercetin-3-rhamnoside, catechin, epicatechin, cyanidin, procyanidin, cyanidin-3-galactoside, coumaric acid, chlorogenic acid, gallic acid, and phloridzin, hydroxycinnamates, vitamin C (Francini & Sebastiani, 2013; Boyer & Liu, 2004).
	Guava *(Psidium guajava)*	Vitamin C, vitamin E, carotenoids (lycopene), polyphenols (gallic acid, myricetin, apigenin, elagic acid), saponin combined with oleanolic acid, morin-3-*O*-α-L-lyxopyranoside, morin-3-*O*-α-L-arabopyranoside, flavonoids like guaijavarin and quercetin (Rueda, 2005; Dweck & Data, 2015)
	Watermelon *(Citrullus lanatus)*	Vitamin C, vitamin E, zinc, carotene-alpha, crypto-xanthin-beta, lutein-zeaxanthin, lycopene, flavonoids, tannins and catechin. Vanillic acid, *p*-coumaric acid glucoside, protocatechuic acid glycoside, sinapic acid glucoside, taxifolin-*O*-hexoside, rutin, dihydrophilonotisflavone, rutin, naringenin, quercetin rhamnoside, isovitexin, ferulic acid hexoside, calodendroside A, dihydrokaempferol 7-glycoside, luteolin-*O*-hexoside, apigenin-*O*-hexoside, dihydrophilonotisflavone, cyanidin, delphinidin, malvidin (Reidah, 2013; Bhagwat et al., 2011).

continued on following page

Table 3. Continued

Food		Phytoconstituents (mainly antioxidant/pro-oxidant molecules)
	Date palm (*Phoenix dactylifera*)	Phenolic acids (protocatechuic, vanillic, syringic, ferulic, gallic, protocatechuic, p-hydroxybenzoic, vanillic, caffeic syringic, sinapic, p-coumaric and o-coumaric acid), quercetin, chlorogenic acids, proanthocyanidins, β-carotene, apigenin and luteolin. Different glycosides of luteolin, quercetin, and apigenin (Al-Orf et al., 2012; Hong, Tomas-Barberan, Kader & Mitchell, 2006).
	Grapes (*Vitis vinifera*	Phenolic acids (gallic, protocatechuic, p-hydroxybenzoic, vanillic, caffeic, p-coumaric, salicylic, ferulic, anisic and sinapic acid), stilbene derivatives (resveratrol), flavan-3-ols (catechin, epicatechin), flavonols (kaempferol, quercetin, myricetin), anthocyanins, proanthocyanidins, ellagic acid, kaempferol, trans-resveratrol, flavanones (didymin, eriocitrin, hesperidin, naringin, narirutin, neoeriocitrin, neohesperidin, poncirin) (Gorinstein et al., 2004; Chiou et al., 2007; Peterson et al., 2006).
	Strawberry (*Arbutus unedo*)	Vitamin C, carotenoid, quercetin, ellagic acid, kaempferol-3-glucuronide, quercetin-3-glucuronide, quercetin-3-glucoside, pelargonidin-3-glucoside, pelargonidin-3-rutinoside, cyanidin-3-glucoside, catechin, apiginin, silybin, fisetine and naringin, tocopherol, triterpenoids, arbutin, β-D-glucogalline. Gallic acid, gallic acid 4-*O*-β-D-glucopyranoside, 3-*O*-galloylquinic acid, 5-*O*-galloylquinic acid, 3-*O*-galloylshikimic acid, and 5-*O*-galloylshikimic acid. Phenolic acids (gallic, protocatechuic, gentisic, p-hydroxibenzoic, vanillic and m-anisic acid), delphinidin-3-galactoside, cyanidin-3-galactoside, cyanidin-3-arabinoside, delphinidin, cyanidin, ellagic acid diglucoside, ellagic acid glucoside, myricetin-3-xyloside, methylellagic acid rhamnoside, ellagic acid arabinoside, ellagic acid xyloside, quercetin-3-rutinoside, quercetin-3-xyloside, quercetin-3-rhamnoside, ellagic acid, myricetin, quercetin, gallocatechin, theogallin (3-*O*-galloylquinic acid), gallocatechin-4,8-catechin, epicatechin-4,8-catechin, catechin-4,8-catechin, epicatechin-4,8-epicatechin-4,8-catechin, catechin, epicatechin-4,8-epicatechin, epicatechin, epicatechin-4,8-epicatechin-4,8-epicatechin, epicatechin-4,6-catechin, epicatechin-4,6-catechin (Pawlowska, Leo & Braca, 2006; Pallauf, Rivas-Gonzalo, del Castillo, Cano & de Pascual-Teresa, 2008; Bouzid et al., 2015; Xie et al., 2015).
	Jamun (*Syzygium cumini*)	Ellagitannins, condensed tannins (B-type oligomers of epiafzelechin), kaempferol 7-*O*-methylether, γ-sitosterol, *β*-sitosterol, corilagin, ellagitannins, ellagic acid, galloyl-galactoside, gallic acid, oleanolic acid, quercetin, myricetin, kaempferol, anthocyanins (3,5-diglucosides of delphinidin, petunidin and malvidin), carotenoids (Faria, Marques & Mercadante, 2011; Swami, Thakor, Patil & Haldankar, 2012; Afify, Fayed, Shalaby & El-Shemy, 2011; Zhang & Lin, 2009).
	Cucumber (*Cucumis sativus*)	Glycosides of salicylic acid, vanillic acid, *p*-coumaric acid, saponarin. Chlorogenic acid, sinapic acid hexoside, rutin, luteolin and apigenin derivatives, kaempherol-*O*-glycoside, quercetin-3-*O*-pentosyl-rutinoside, kaempferol derivatives, quercetin derivatives, naringenin-*O*-glucoside, theaflavanoside (Reidah, 2013).
	Mango (*Mangifera indica*)	Mangiferin, isomangiferin, quercetin 3-*O*-galactoside, quercetin-3-*O*-glucoside, quercetin-3-*O*-xyloside, quercetin-3-*O*-arabinopyranoside, quercetin-3-*O*-arabinofuranoside, quercetin 3-*O*-rhamnoside, kaempferol 3-*O*-glucoside, quercetin, rhamnetin and its glycoside (Masibo & He, 2008).
	Indian date/palm (*Ziziphus jujube*)	Anthocyanins, delphinidin, petunidin, malvidin-diglucosides, rutin, quercetin, quercitrin, phlorizin, catechol, gallic acid, catechin, chlorogenic acid, caffeic acid, epicatechin, *p*-coumaric acid, ferulic acid, quinic acid, sinapic acid, kaempferol, *p*-hydroxy benzoic acid, protocatechuic acid, rutin, vitamin C, vitamin E, zinc, selenium, beta-catotene, triterpenoic acids (Zhao, Zhang & Yang, 2014; Wu, Gao, Kjelgren, Guo & Wang, 2013; Swami et al., 2012)
	Pomegranate (*Punica granatum*)	Ellagic acid, gallic acid, catechin, catechol, cyanidin 3-*O*-glucoside, cyanidin 3,5-di-*O*-glucoside, delphinidin 3-*O*-glucoside, delphinidin 3,5-di-*O*-glucoside, epicatechin, epigallocatechin 3-gallate, isoquercetin, pelargonidin 3-*O*-glucoside, pelargonidin 3,5-di-*O*-glucoside, procyanidin, quercetin, tryptamine, melatonin (Wang, Ding, Liu, Xiang & Du, 2010).
	Cabbage (*Brassica oleracea* var capitata)	Vitamin C, β-carotene, lutein, DL-α-tocopherol, phenolics compounds [quercetin-3-*O*-sophoroside-7-*O*-glucoside, quercetin-3,7-di-*O*-glucoside, quercetin-3-*O*-sophoroside, quercetin-3-*O*-(caffeoyl)-sophoroside-7-*O*-glucoside, quercetin-3-*O*-(methoxycaffeoyl)-sophoroside-7-*O*-glucoside, quercetin-3-*O*-(sinapoyl)-sophoroside-7-*O*-glucoside, quercetin-3-*O*-(feruloyl)-sophoroside, kaempferol-3-*O*-sophorotrioside-7-*O*-sophoroside, kaempferol-3,7-di-*O*-glucoside, kaempferol-3-*O*-sophoroside, kaempferol-7-*O*-glucoside, kaempferol-3-*O*-(caffeoyl)sophoroside-7-*O*-glucoside, kaempferol-3-*O*-(methoxycaffeoyl)sophoroside-7-*O*-glucoside, kaempferol-3-*O*-(sinapoyl)-sophoroside-7-*O*-glucoside, kaempferol-3-*O*-(feruloyl)-sophoroside-7-*O*-glucoside, kaempferol-3-*O*-(*p*-coumaroyl)-sophoroside-7-*O*glucoside, kaempferol-3-*O*-(methoxycaffeoyl)-sophoroside, kaempferol-3-*O*-(sinapoyl)-sophoroside, kaempferol-3-*O*-(feruloyl)-sophoroside, kaempferol-3-*O*-(*p*-coumaroyl)-sophoroside, 3-caffeoyl quinic acid, 3-*p*-coumaroyl quinic acid, 4-caffeoyl quinic acid, sinapylglucoside, 4-feruloyl quinic acid, sinapic acid (Cartea, Francisco, Soengas & Velasco, 2011; Singh et al., 2006).
	Ivy gourd (*Coccinia indica*)	Taraxerone, taraxerol, and (24R)-24- ethylcholest- 5-en- 3β-ol glucoside, β- carotene, lycopene, cryptoxanthin, apo-6'-lycopenal, β-sitosterol, taraxerol (Deokate & Khadabadi, 2012)
	Bottle gourd (*Lagenaria siceraria*)	Ascorbic acid, β-carotene, 22-deoxocurcubitacin-d, 22-deoxoisocurcubitacin-d, 7-*O*-glucosyl-6-C-glucoside apigenin, 6-C-glucoside apigenin, 6-C-glucoside luteolin, and 7,4′-*O*-diglucosyl-6-C-glucoside apigenin. Flavonoids like isovitexin, isoorientin, saponarin, and saponarin 4′-*O*-glucoside. Triterpenes such as 3 b-*O*-(*E*)-feruloyl D:*C*-friedooleana-7,9(11)-dien-29-ol, 3b-*O*-(*E*)-coumaroyl-D:*C*-friedooleana-7,9(11)-dien-29-ol, 3b-*O*-(*E*) coumaroyl-d:*C*-friedooleana-7,9(11)-dien-29-oic acid, methyl 2b,3b-dihydroxy-D:C-friedoolean-8-en-29-oate, 3-epikarounidiol, 3-oxo-d:C-friedoolena-7,9 (11)-dien-29-oic acid, bryonolol, bryononic acid, 20-epibryonolic acid. Volatile essential oil (Prajapati, Kalariya, Parmar & Sheth, 2010).

continued on following page

Table 3. Continued

Food		Phytoconstituents (mainly antioxidant/pro-oxidant molecules)
	Tamato (*Lycopersicon esculentum)*	Vitamins C, vitamin E, selenium, zinc, quercetin, kaempferol, lycopene, gallic acid, catechin, chlorogenic acid, caffeic acid, coumarin, rutin, quercitrin, luteolin, β-carotene. cis *p*-coumaric acid derivative, caffeic acid hexoside, 4-*O*-caffeolyquinic acid, 5-*O*-caffeolyquinic acid, trans *p*-coumaric acid hexoside, cis *p*-coumaric acid hexoside, ferulic acid hexoside, 4-*O*-*p*-coumarolyquinic acid, caffeic acid, 5-*O*-*p*-coumarolyquinic acid, syringic acid hexoside derivative, quercetin pentosylrutinoside, trans-*p*-coumaric acid, quercetin-3-*O*-rutinoside, kaempferol pentosylrutinoside, kaempferol-3-*O*-rutinoside (Barros et al., 2012; Akomolafe & Oboh, 2015)
	Papaya (*Carica papaya)*	Vitamin C, volatile compounds (linalol, benzylisothiocynate, cis and trans 2, 6-dimethyl-3,6 expoxy-7 octen-2-ol), α-carpaine, benzyl-β-d glucoside, 2-phenylethl-β-D-glucoside, 4-hydroxyl -phenyl-2 ethyl-B-D glucoside. Myristic, palmitic, stearic, linoleic, linolenic acids-vaccenic acid and oleic acids. β carotene, crytoxanthin, violaxanthin, zeaxanthin (Karunamoorthi, Kim, Jegajeevanram, Xavier & Vijayalakshmi, 2014; Krishna, Paridhavi & Patel, 2008).
	Bitter gourd (*Momordica charantia)*	Momordicin, charantin, cryptoxanthin, cucurbitins, cucurbitacins, cucurbitanes, cycloartenols, diosgenin, gentisic acid, goyaglycosides, goyasaponins, karounidiols, lanosterol, lauric acid, linoleic acid, linolenic acid, momorcharasides, momorcharins, momordenol, momordicillin, momordicinin, momordicosides, momordin, momordolo, multiflorenol, myristic acid, nerolidol, oleanolic acid, oleic acid, rosmarinic acid, rubixanthin, spinasterol, steroidal glycosides, stigmastadiols, stigmasterol, taraxerol, trehalose, verbascoside, zeatin, zeatinriboside, zeaxanthin, zeinoxanthin, β-sistosterol-d-glucicide, citruline, elasterol, flavochrome, lutein, lycopene, curbitacin B, catechin, vitamin C, zinc (Gupta, Sharma, Gautam & Bhadauria, 2011).
	Centella (*Centella asiatica)*	Hydrocotylin, asiaticoside A and B, madecassoside, centelloside, indocentelloside, brahmoside, brahminoside, thankuniside, iso-thankuniside, 3-glucosylquercetin, 3-glucosylkaempferol, 7-glucosylkaempferol, kaempferol, quercetin, stigmasterol, sitosterol, carotenoids, vitamin C, ursolic acid, triterpene acids (asiatic, madecassic, terminolic, centic, centellic, madasiatic acid), centellasaponin B, C and D (Jamil, Nizami & Salam, 2007).
	Sponse gourd (*Luffa cylindrical)*	*p*-coumaric acid, 1-*O*-feruloyl-β-D-glucose, 1-*O*-*p*-coumaroyl-β-D-glucose, 1-*O*-caffeoyl- β-D-glucose, 1-*O*-(4-hydroxybenzoyl)glucose, diosmetin-7-*O*-β-D-glucuronide methyl ester, apigenin-7-*O*- β-D-glucuronide methyl ester, luteolin-7-*O*-β-D-glucuronide methyl ester (Du et al., 2011).
	Potato (*Solanum tuberosum)*	catechin, epicatechin, erodictyol, kaempeferol, naringenin, rutin, lutein, zeaxanthin, violaxanthin, neoxanthin, β-carotene, vitamins C and E, cyanidin,pelargonidin, malvidin (Ezekiel, Singh, Sharma & Kaur, 2013)
	Broccoli (*Brassica oleracea* var *botrytis italica*)	Ferulic acid, caffeic acid, sinapinic acid, kaempferol, quercetin, and isorhamnetin. Quercetin derivatives like quercetin -3-*O*-sophorotrioside-7-*O*-sophoroside, quercetin -3-*O*-sophorotrioside-7-glucoside, quercetin -3-*O*-sophoroside-7-*O*-glucoside, quercetin -3,7-di-*O*-glucoside, quercetin-3-*O*-sophoroside, quercetin -3-*O*-glucoside, quercetin-3-*O*-(caffeoyl)-sophorotrioside-7-*O*-glucoside, quercetin-3-*O*-(sinapoyl)-sophorotrioside-7-*O*-glucoside, quercetin-3-*O*-(feruloyl)-sophorotrioside-7-*O*-glucosid, quercetin-3-*O*-(*p*-coumaroyl)-sophorotrioside-7-*O*glucoside, quercetin-3-*O*-(caffeoyl)-sophoroside-7-*O*-glucoside, quercetin-3-*O*-(*p*-coumaroyl)-sophoroside-7-*O*-glucoside, quercetin-3-*O*-(feruloyl)-sophoroside). Kaempferol derivatives like K-3-*O*-sophorotrioside-7-*O*-sophoroside, kaempferol-3-*O*-sohorotrioside-7-*O*-glucoside, kaempferol-3-*O*-sophoroside-7-*O*-diglucoside, kaempferol-3-*O*-sophoroside-7-*O*-glucoside, kaempferol-3,7-di-*O*-glucoside, kaempferol-3-*O*-sophoroside, kaempferol-3-*O*-sophoroside-7-*O*-glucoside, kaempferol-3,7-di-*O*-glucoside, kaempferol-3-*O*-sophoroside, kaempferol-3-*O*-glucoside, kaempferol-3-*O*-(caffeoyl)-sophorotrioside-7-*O*sophoroside, kaempferol-3-*O*-(methoxycaffeoyl)-sophorotrioside-7-*O*-sophoroside, kaempferol-*O*-(sinapoyl)-sophorotrioside-7-*O*-sophoroside, kaempferol-*O*-(feruloyl)-sophorotrioside-7-*O*-sophoroside, kaempferol-3-*O*-(*p*-coumaroyl)-sophorotrioside-7-*O*-sophoroside, kaempferol-3-*O*-(caffeoyl)-sophorotrioside-7-*O*-glucoside, kaempferol-3-*O*-(methoxycaffeoyl)-sophorotrioside-7-*O*glucoside, kaempferol-*O*-(sinapoyl)-sophorotrioside-7-*O*-glucoside, kaempferol-*O*-(feruloyl)-sophorotrioside-7-*O*-glucoside, kaempferol-3-*O*-(caffeoyl)sophoroside-7-*O*-glucoside. 1,2-disinapoylgentiobiose, 1-sinapoyl-2-feruloylgentiobiose, 1,2,2'-trisinapoylgentiobiose, 1,2'-disinapoyl-2-feruloylgentiobiose (Gawlik-Dziki, 2008; Cartea et al., 2011).
	Indian spinach (*Basella alba)*	Vitamins A and C, thaimine, betacyanin, oxalic acid, acacetin, 4,7- dihydroxy kempferol, 4'-methoxyisovitexin, vanilla, syringic and ferulic acid, betacyanins and gomphrenin (Kumar, Prasad, Iyer & Vaidya, 2013)
	Spinach (*Spinacia oleracea)*	β-carotene, violaxanthin, 9'-(Z)-neoxanhin, vitamin A, vitaminE, vitamin C, iron, zinc, copper, querecetin, myricetin, kampeferol, apigenin, luteolin, patuletin, spinacetin, jaceidin, 4´-glu-curonide, 5,3´,4´-trihydroxy-3-methoxy-6:7-methylenedioxyflavone-4´-glucuronide, 5,4'-dihydroxy-3.3´-dimethoxy-6:7-methylene dioxyflavone-4´-glu-curonide, 5,4´-dihydroxi-3,3´-dimithoxi-6,7-methylene-dioxi-flavone, 3,5,7,3´,4´-pentahydroxi-6-methoxiflavone, *p*-coumaric acid, ferulic acid, *o*-coumaric acid (Subhash, Virbhadrappa & Vasanth, 2010).

*Antioxidant present in the grain, friut, vegitables etc. can be vary with environment, soli types etc.

Legumes belong to the most important family leguminosae, which include 700 genera and 20,000 species. They are the second most significant source of food and fodder. Legumes can be divided into two groups: (*i*) oil seeds like soybeans and peanuts, and (*ii*) grain legumes, including common beans, lentils, lima beans, and common peas. Grain legumes are commonly recognized as pulses. Legumes are rich in nutrient content, and contain starch, protein, dietary fibre, oligosaccharides, phytochemicals and minerals. In addition, legumes are also the rich sources numerous bioactive phytochemicals which possess antioxidant activity. Different bioactive compounds such as simple phenols, phytosterols, saponins, phenyl propanoids, phenolic acids, flavonoids, stilbenes, tannins, lignans and lignins are present in legumes which have been acknowledged to promote good health and have therapeutic potential. Proanthocyanidines (i.e. condensed tannins) are also the key phenolic substances found in legume seeds, which mainly found in seed coats (hulls). Some studies also correlate the antioxidant activity of different legumes with their protein content and suggested that proteins of different legume seeds might have antioxidant potential. Legumes have been used as therapeutic medicine since ancient time in old traditional medicine. Current researches and observational studies found that legumes confer significant health benefit and beneficial to improve serum lipid profiles, platelet activity, and inflammation and in the treatment of cardiovascular disease, coronary artery diseases, cancer. A number of investigational studies also confirmed that different extract/parts of legumes have free radical and antioxidant effect. Natural polyphenols possess antioxidant and free radical scavenging activities and thus confer miscellaneous therapeutic effects for disease prevention and health promotion. Phytochemicals like saponins, tannin, phenolic acid, flavonoid, sterol etc. found in legumes possess antioxidant activity, which inpart or fully responsible for their protective or therapeutic effect (Venter & van Eyssen, 2011; Kappor, 2015; Petchiammal & Hopper, 2014).

Edible oils are used as important cooking ingredients, and as salad dressing, margarine spreads, and dips around the world. These oils are extracted from different sources like plants (e.g., soybean, canola), seeds (e.g., sunflower) and husk (e.g., rice bran), nuts (e.g., walnut) and fruits (e.g., olive, coconut). Several phenolic antioxidants are also used as edible oil preservatives to prevent rancidity (Dauqan, Abdullah & Sani, 2011; Pantsi, Bester, Esterhuyse & Aboua, 2014). Intake of virgin coconut oil found beneficial in reducing lipid profile and LDL oxidation by physiological oxidants. This effect may be due to presence of polyphenol components in virgin coconut oil. Another study showed that virgin coconut oil supplemented diet increases antioxidant level in experimental animals (Nevin & Rajamohan, 2006, 2014). Olive oil is important vegetable oil believed to produce its beneficial effect majorly via antioxidant constituents. Although the composition of olive oil is complex, but majority of its compounds likes oleic acid, phenolics, and squalene can inhibit oxidative stress. Olive oil consumption found useful in several diseases conditions like cancer, coronary heart disease, blood pressure, high lipid content etc (Waterman & Lockwood, 2007). Vitamin E in different isomer form, coenzyme Q10 and squalene present in palm oil possess strong antioxidant effect and found beneficial in several oxidative stress induced diseases (Loganathan, Selvaduray, Radhakrishnan, & Nesaretnam, 2010). Gamma-oryzanol is a mixture of sterol esters of ferulic acid and triterpene alcohols. Rice bran oil showed very potent antioxidant activity and reduces triglyceride level. Rice bran oil also contains omega-3, omega-6 and omega-9 fatty acid. It is also rich in essential vitamin E complex (α, β, γ, δ tocopherols and α, β, γ, δ tocotrienols). Gamma-oryzanol showed antioxidant, antihyperlipedemic, antidiabetic, anti-inflammatory and anticancer effect. It reduces platelet aggregation, increase the muscle mass and used to treat the disorders of menopause (Vorarat, Managit, Iamthanakul, Soparat & Kamkaen, 2010; Patel & Naik, 2004). Sunflower oil contain several components including antioxidant substance which responsible for several curative effect of the oil such as anti-inflammatory, anti-bacterial, anti-fungal, anti-cancer, cardioprotective and dermoprotective (Warner et al., 2015; Khan et al., 2015). Peanut has been acknowledged as a functional food due to its role in a health promoting effect. Several fatty acid and antioxidant found in peanut oil which provide protection against oxidative stress. Phenolic compound resveratrol present is peanut oil that exhibits antiplatelet, anti-inflammatory, anticancer, antimutagenic, antifungal effect, and reduces lipid peroxidation. Peanut oil also contain vitamin E, squalene, β-carotene which also known well for their curative effect (Akhtar et al., 2014).

Herbs and spices are traditionally used as flavor-enhancement substance in food and considered to have low nutritional value. Though, the spices are used as medicine since encient time. Recent investigations showed that herbs and spices contain various phytochemicals, many of which possess powerful antioxidant activity. They inhibit lipid peoxidation, promote antioxidant defence mechanism, protect LDL cholesterol from oxidation, inhibit cyclooxygenase and lipoxygenase enzymes, and produce anticancer or antimicrobial effect. Epidemiological and preclinical evidence indicated that herbs and spices though used as minor dietary constituents but possess anticancer activity. Herb and spice and their chemical constituents are poved effective in the treatment of neurodegenerative disorders (e.g. Alzheimer's disease, Parkinson's disease and multiple sclerosis), cardiovascular diseases i.e. stroke. Herb and spice also exert immune enhancing effect. Ginsenosides, a active principal of Ginseng species, curcumin from turmeric and other phytoconstituent are reported for diverse beneficial effect on health (Kaefer & Milner, 2008; Dharmananda, 2005; Craig, 1999).

Tea is the most common beverage with antioxidant potency. Tea is rich in natural antioxidants, and reported to be used in management of different types of cancer, stone, dental caries, and other diseases. Wide number of research found that green tea is useful in variety of implications, including cancer, heart disease, liver disease, diabetes, inflammatory bowel disease, skin disorders, hair loss, weight loss etc. Flavonoids present in green tea mainly responsible for such effects (Sinija & Mishra, 2008). Several epidemiological studies have suggested that moderate coffee consumption may helpful to prevent diseases, like diabetes mellitus, Parkinson's disease and liver diseases. Though, some studies have indicated revrese association between coffee consumption and cardiovascular diseases (Higdon & Frei, 2006). Little to moderate beer consumption could helpful in prevention of cardiovascular diseases, coronary artery diseases, risk of developing gallstones, risk of osteoporosis etc. (Anonymous, 2002)

Fruits and vegetable are the key source of diverse antioxidant molecules. Consumption of fruits and vegetables in proper quantity has been associated with protection against various diseases and aging. Though, role of diet is complex in describing their action against chronic and acute diseases. It was estimated that a typical diet may supply more than 25,000 bioactive food constituents, and several of them can alter magnitude of diseases through the multitude of processes. Due to such complexity it is essential to understand the role of these bioactive substances in prevention, cure or development of disease. Majority of bioactive constituents from diet mainly from plant sources are redox active molecules and therefore identified as antioxidants (Carlsen et al., 2010). Fruits and vegetable contain several well characterized antioxidant substances, including vitamins C, vitamin E, phenolic substances, β-carotene and minerals (zinc, selenium), which showed prominent beneficial effect against oxidative stress induced diseases. A study has investigated the antioxidant activity of more than 3100 foods, beverages, spices, herbs and supplements used around the world, and reported that different foods possess moderate to high antioxidant activity. Spices, herbs, fruits like berries, nuts, chocolate, and vegetables showed potent antioxidant activity (Carlsen et al., 2010). In last few decade the usefulness of antioxidant substances are in spotlight and thus number of researches are going on in this regard. Huge numbers of epidemiological studies are conducted or going on and majority of such studies found that consumption of fruit and vegetable which has high polyphenolic antioxidants showed beneficial effect on health. Antioxidant potency of fruits and vegetables may be influenced genetics and environmental factors. Cooking also may alter the antioxidant activity of a food. Several chemical and biological properties of antioxidant molecule such as absorption, cellular uptake, biotransformation, transport and excretion may eventually modify the action antioxidant substance containing diet. A number of epidemiological survey and researchers have suggested the inverse association of fruit and vegetable intake with the risk of cardiovascular disease, diabetes, cancer, neurodegenerative diseases etc. (Bazzano et al., 2002; Hu et al., 2013, Key, 2011; Isao et al., 2013; Patrice et al., 2010).

Of cource, diet from animal sources also confers strong antioxidant activity. Milk, dairy products, fish, meat also contain numerous antioxidant molecule. Milk contains vitamin A, E which may contribute the antioxidant capacity of milk (Tijerina-Saenz, Innis & Kitts, 2009). Several molecules like ascorbic acid, tocopherols, omega-3 fatty acids are available in fish, beneficial effect of these compounds already been reported by the researchers.

PRO-OXIDANT EFFECT OF ANTIOXIDANTS

Some flavonoids have shown prooxidant activity provided a transition metal is available. The OH substitution is essential for antioxidant activity of flavonoids. If OH substitution is absents in then the molecule will not produce neither antioxidant nor transition metal initiated prooxidant activities. Copper induced prooxidant effect of a flavonoid largely depends on number of free OH substitutions present in molecule, if the number of OH substitutions is more than the prooxidant activity will be stronger. Flavonoids from foods usually present as *O*-glycosides with sugars bound at the C3 position. Methylation or glycosidic alteration of OH substitutions causes the inactivation of transition metal-induced prooxidant activity of a flavonoid. Mostly *in vitro* studies found that flavonoids like quercetin and kaempferol can cause nuclear DNA damage and lipid peroxidation if transition metals are present. Though, *in vivo* studies didn't found significant transition metal-initiated prooxidant actions of flavonoids, ascorbic acid and vitamin E. It is possible that result of *in vivo* studies are negative as in normal condition (except metal toxicity case) transition metal like copper ion will be mostly sequestered in the tissues. Several researches also confirmed that quercetin, a flavonoid can prevent ion-induced lipid peroxidation in liver cells (Rahal et al., 2014). An *in vitro* study concluded that phenolic compounds like quercetin, rutin, protocatechuic acid with low oxidation potentials (Epa lower than 0.45) confer antioxidant activity, whereas compounds (i.e. vanillic acid, syringic acid, coumaric acid) with high Epa values (>0.45) produce prooxidant activity (Simic, Manojlovic, Segan & Todorovic, 2007).

ANTIOXIDANT SUPPLEMENTS VS. FOOD RICH IN ANTIOXIDANT MOLECULE

In recent years the role of oxidative stress in different diseases came in focus and thus use of antioxidant supplements have increased significantly among the general people with the hope to prevent diseases. A number of researches mainly epidemiological and observational studies reported the positive effect of antioxidant supplements. Similar beneficial effect of antioxidant supplements are also confirmed by different several randomized controlled trials (RCTs). However, the reports are not consistent and several of the RCTs also reported null/negative effect when antioxidant supplements consumed for long time and in high dose. For example, a clinical study on 47 street workers (who exposed to high level of ozone) found beneficial effect of vitamin E (75 mg), vitamin C (650 mg) and β-carotene (15 mg) supplement given for the period of 6 months. A study in US, Canada, and Puerto Rico found that vitamin E produces negative effect on incidence of prostate cancer. Though most of the clinical trial showed null effect, like long term supplementation of vitamin C (500 mg/day), vitamin E (600 IU every other day), β-carotene (50 mg every other day) in different combinations did not show any effect on the outcome of cancer risk, diabetes and secondary cardiovascular diseases. High doses of isolated compounds also may cause toxic, or prooxidative effects. Exogenous antioxidants may exibit diuble-edged phenomenon in cellular redox states depends upon physiological environment and dose (Sen & Chakraborty, 2015; Bouayed & Bohn, 2010). Thus potential clinical benefit deriving from antioxidant supplements for the general population is still under wide debate.

Fruits and vegetables contain antioxidant molecules, vitamins, micronutrients and macronutrients which act through different mechanisms. Thus a diet rich in fruit and vegetables is vital for optimum health. It was observed that reduce intake of nutritional and antioxidant food may increase the chance of oxidative stress which may leads to cell damage. Thus intake of fruit, vegetable, beverages and natural antioxidant containing product may confer protective effect against free radical induced diseases through diverse mechanism. Experimental study also shown that rice, different food grains, vegetables, fruits, animal products, tea, and other beverages exert significant antioxidant activity and a number of bioactive antioxidant molecules isolated from those. Thus it is essential to have food containing antioxidant molecule in proper rationally a better health (Sen & Chakraborty, 2015).

CONCLUSION

Maintenance of redox balance is believed to be critical in maintaining disease free good health. However, in modern era change in life style, less consumption of health food, stress, pollutions etc make us more prone to oxidative stress. Thus it is required to consume endogenous antioxidant for maintenance of health. Of course excessive intake of exogenous antioxidants especially isolated compounds may exert prooxidative effects or can disrupt redox balance, which intern responsible for harmful effect. But food like fruit, vegetables, food grain etc contain numerous vitamin, minerals, nutrient and phytochemicals, among them several substances are greatly acknowledged for antioxidant property. It is evident that consumption of natural food are associated with health promotive and disease preventive effect which may fully/partly associate related with antioxidant molecule presents such food. Thus it is truly essential consumption of a healthy and antioxidant rich natural diet for better and healthy life.

REFERENCES

Abdel-Aal, E. M., & Rabalski, I. (2008). Bioactive compounds and their antioxidant capacity in selected primitive and modern wheat species. *The Open Agriculture Journal*, *2*(1), 7–14. doi:10.2174/1874331500802010007

Adly, A. A. M. (2010). Oxidative stress and disease: An updated review. *Research Journal of Immunology*, *3*, 129–145. doi:10.3923/rji.2010.129.145

Afify, A. E. M. R., Fayed, S. A., Shalaby, E. A., & El-Shemy, H. A. (2011). *Syzygium cumini* (pomposia) active principles exhibit potent anticancer and antioxidant activities. *African Journal of Pharmacy and Pharmacology*, *5*(7), 948–956.

Agrahari, P., & Singh, D. K. (2014). A review on the pharmacological aspects of *Carum carvi*. *Journal of Biology and Earth Sciences*, *4*, M1–M13.

Ajay, S., Rahul, S., Sumit, G., Paras, M., Mishra, A., & Gaurav, A. (2011). Comprehensive review: *Murraya koenigii Linn*. *Asian Journal of Pharmacy and Life Science*, *1*(4), 417–425.

Akhtar, S., Khalid, N., Ahmed, I., Shahzad, A., & Suleria, H. A. R. (2014). Physicochemical characteristics, functional properties, and nutritional benefits of peanut oil: A review. *Critical Reviews in Food Science and Nutrition*, *54*(12), 1562–1575. doi:10.1080/10408398.2011.644353 PMID:24580558

Akomolafe, S. F., & Oboh, G. (2015). Characterization of polyphenolic constituents and radical scavenging ability of ripe tomato and red pepper fruits. *Journal of Experimental and Integrative Medicine*, *5*(1), 61–67. doi:10.5455/jeim.080215.or.123

Al-Orf, S. M., Ahmed, M. H. M., Al-Atwai, N., Zaidi, H. A., Dehwah, A., & Dehwah, S. (2012). Review: Nutritional properties and benefits of the date fruits (*Phoenix dactylifera L.*). *Bulletin of the National Nutrition Institute of the Arab Republic of Egypt*, *39*, 98–129.

Amarowicz, R. (2007). Tannins: The new natural antioxidants? *European Journal of Lipid Science and Technology*, *109*(6), 549–551. doi:10.1002/ejlt.200700145

Amarowicz, R., Karamac, M., & Weidner, S. (2001). Antioxidant activity of phenolic fraction of pea (*Pisum sativum*). *Czech Journal Food Science*, *19*, 139–142.

Anonymous. (2002). The benefits of moderate beer consumption. CBMC – The Brewers of Europe.

Arlee, R., Suanphairoch, S., & Pakdeechanuan, P. (2013). Differences in chemical components and antioxidant-related substances in virgin coconut oil from coconut hybrids and their parents. *International Food Research Journal*, *20*(5), 2103–2109.

Awika, J. M., & Rooney, L. W. (2004). Sorghum phytochemicals and their potential impact on human health. *Phytochemistry*, *65*(9), 1199–1221. doi:10.1016/j.phytochem.2004.04.001 PMID:15184005

Banerjee, S., Sanjay, K. R., Chethan, S., & Malleshi, N. G. (2012). Finger millet (*Eleusine coracana*) polyphenols: Investigation of their antioxidant capacity and antimicrobial activity. *African Journal of Food Science*, *6*(13), 362–374. doi:10.5897/AJFS12.031

Barros, L., Duenas, M., Pinela, J., Carvalho, A. M., Buelga, C. S., & Ferreira, I. C. (2012). Characterization and quantification of phenolic compounds in four tomato (*Lycopersicon esculentum* L.) farmers' varieties in northeastern Portugal homegardens. *Plant Foods for Human Nutrition (Dordrecht, Netherlands)*, *67*(3), 229–234. doi:10.1007/s11130-012-0307-z PMID:22922837

Battu, G., Male, C. K. V. L. S. N. A., Haripriya, T., Malleswari, V. N., & Reeshma, S. (2011). A phytopharmacological review on vigna species. *Pharmanest*, *2*, 62–67.

Bazzano, L. A., He, J., Ogden, L. G., Loria, C. M., Vupputuri, S., Myers, L., & Whelton, P. K. (2002). Fruit and vegetable intake and risk of cardiovascular disease in us adults: The first national health and nutrition examination survey epidemiologic follow-up study. *The American Journal of Clinical Nutrition*, *76*, 93–99. PMID:12081821

Bendini, A., Cerretani, L., Carrasco-Pancorbo, A., Gomez-Caravaca, A. M., Segura-Carretero, A., Fernandez-Gutierrez, A., & Lercker, G. (2007). Phenolic molecules in virgin olive oils: A survey of their sensory properties, health effects, antioxidant activity and analytical methods. An overview of the last decade. *Molecules (Basel, Switzerland)*, *12*(8), 1679–1719. doi:10.3390/12081679 PMID:17960082

Bhagwat, S., Haytowitz, D. B., & Holden, J. M. (2011). USDA database for the flavonoid content of selected foods Release 3. U.S. Department of Agriculture. Retrieved from http://www.ars.usda.gov/nutrientdata

Borras-Linares, I., Stojanovic, Z., Quirantes-Pine, R., Arraez-Roman, D., Svarc-Gajic, J., Fernandez-Gutierrez, A., & Segura-Carretero, A. (2014). *Rosmarinus officinalis* leaves as a natural source of bioactive compounds. *International Journal of Molecular Sciences*, *15*(11), 20585–20606. doi:10.3390/ijms151120585 PMID:25391044

Bouayed, J., & Bohn, T. (2010). Exogenous antioxidants— double-edged swords in cellular redox state. *Oxidative Medicine and Cellular Longevity*, *3*(4), 228–237. doi:10.4161/oxim.3.4.12858 PMID:20972369

Bouzid, K., Benali, F. T., Chadli, R., Bouzouina, M., Bouzid, A., Benchohra, A., & Bouzid, S. et al. (2015). Extraction, identification and quantitative HPLC analysis of flavonoids from fruit extracts of *Arbutus unedo* L. from Tiaret area (Western Algeria). *Basic Research Journal of Agricultural Science and Review*, *4*(1), 24–30.

Boyer, J., & Liu, R. H. (2004). Apple phytochemicals and their health benefits. *Nutrition Journal*, *3*(1), 5. doi:10.1186/1475-2891-3-5 PMID:15140261

Brigelius-flohe, R., & Traber, M. G. (1999). Vitamin E: Function and metabolism. *The FASEB Journal*, *13*, 1145–1155. PMID:10385606

Bubols, G. B., Viann, D. R., Medina-Remónd, A., Poser, G., Lamuela-Raventos, R. M., Eifler-Lim, V. L., & Garcia, S. C. (2013). The antioxidant activity of coumarins and flavonoids. *Mini Reviews in Medicinal Chemistry*, *13*, 1–17. PMID:22876957

Bulotta, S., Celano, M., Lepore, S. M., Montalcini, T., Pujia, A., & Russo, D. (2014). Beneficial effects of the olive oil phenolic components oleuropein and hydroxytyrosol: Focus on protection against cardiovascular and metabolic diseases. *Journal of Translational Medicine*, *12*(1), 219. doi:10.1186/s12967-014-0219-9 PMID:25086598

Burri, B. J. (1997). Beta-carotene and human health: A review of current research. *Nunition Research*, *1*(17), 547–580. doi:10.1016/S0271-5317(97)00011-0

Cabrera, C., Artacho, R., & Gimeanez, R. (2006). Beneficial effects of green tea - A review. *Journal of the American College of Nutrition*, *25*(2), 79–99. doi:10.1080/07315724.2006.10719518 PMID:16582024

Cabrera, C., Gimeanez, R., & Loapez, M. C. (2003). Determination of tea components with antioxidant activity. *Journal of Agricultural and Food Chemistry*, *51*(15), 4427–4435. doi:10.1021/jf0300801 PMID:12848521

Camara, C. R. S., Urrea, C. A., & Schlegel, V. (2013). Pinto beans (*Phaseolus vulgaris* L.) as a functional food: Implications on human health. *Agriculture*, *3*(1), 90–111. doi:10.3390/agriculture3010090

Carlsen, M. H., Halvorsen, B. L., Holte, K., Bøhn, S. K., Dragland, S., Sampson, L., & Blomhoff, R. et al. (2010). The total antioxidant content of more than 3100 foods, beverages, spices, herbs and supplements used worldwide. *Nutrition Journal*, *9*(1), 3. doi:10.1186/1475-2891-9-3 PMID:20096093

Carr, A., & Frei, B. (1999). Does vitamin C act as a pro-oxidant under physiological conditions? *The FASEB Journal*, *13*, 1007–1024. PMID:10336883

Cartea, M. E., Francisco, M., Soengas, P., & Velasco, P. (2011). Phenolic compounds in *Brassica* vegetables. *Molecules (Basel, Switzerland)*, *16*(1), 251–280. doi:10.3390/molecules16010251 PMID:21193847

Chiou, A., Karathanos, V. T., Mylona, A., Salta, F. N., Preventi, F., & Andrikopoulos, N. K. (2007). Currants (*Vitis vinifera* L.) content of simple phenolics and antioxidant activity. *Food Chemistry*, *102*(2), 516–522. doi:10.1016/j.foodchem.2006.06.009

Chung, H. (2009). *Characterization of antioxidant activities of soybeans and assessment of their bioaccessibility after in vitro digestion. Ph.D thesis*. Virginia Polytechnic Institute and State University. Retrieved from http://vtechworks.lib.vt.edu/handle/10919/29638?show=full

Craig, W. J. (1999). Health-promoting properties of common herbs. *The American Journal of Clinical Nutrition*, *70*, 491s–499s. PMID:10479221

Daniel, M., Denni, M., & Chauhan, D. (2012). Polyphenols, phospholipids and fixed oil composition of pearl millet. *International Journal of Pharmacy & Life Sciences*, *3*(11), 2098–2102.

Dasaroju, S., & Gottumukkala, K. M. (2014). Current trends in the research of *emblica officinalis (amla):* A pharmacological perspective. *International Journal of Pharmaceutical Sciences Review and Research*, *24*(2), 150–159.

Dauqan, E. M. A., Abdullah, A., & Sani, H. A. (2011). Natural antioxidants, lipid profile, lipid peroxidation, antioxidant enzymes of different vegetable oils. *Advance Journal of Food Science and Technology*, *3*(4), 308–316.

Deokate, U. A., & Khadabadi, S. S. (2012). Pharmacology and phytochemistry of *Coccinia indica. Pharmacophore*, *3*, 179–185.

Dharmananda, S. (2005). *Neuroprotective herbs and active constituents approaches to preventing degenerative diseases*. Retreated from: http://www.itmonline.org/arts/neuro.htm

Du, Q., Xu, Y., Li, L., Zhao, Y., Jerz, G., & Winterhalter, P. (2011). Antioxidant constituents in the fruits of *Luffa cylindrica* (L.) Roem. *Food Chemistry*, *127*, 609–614. PMID:23140707

Dweck, A. C., & Data, D. (2015). *A review of Guava (*Psidium guajava*)*. Retreated from: www.dweck-data.co.uk/Published_papers/Psidium_guajava.pdf

Dykes, L. & Roonwy, L.W. (2007). *Phenolic compounds in cereals grains and their health benefit.* Cereal Foods World, AACC International Inc. doi:10.1094/CFW-52-3-0105

El-Baky, H. H. (2009). Enhancing antioxidant availability in grains of wheat plants grown under seawater-stress in response to microalgae extracts treatments. *African Journal of Biochemistry Research*, *3*(4), 77–83.

Escudero, F. E., Munoz, A. M., Alvarado-Ortiz, C., Alvarado, A., & Yanez, J. A. (2012). Purple corn (*Zea mays* L.). Phenolic compounds profile and its assessment as an agent against oxidative stress in isolated mouse organs. *Journal of Medicinal Food*, *15*(2), 206–215. doi:10.1089/jmf.2010.0342 PMID:22082063

Ezekiel, R., Singh, N., Sharma, S., & Kaur, A. (2013). Beneficial phytochemicals in potato — a review. *Food Research International*, *50*(2), 487–496. doi:10.1016/j.foodres.2011.04.025

Farbstein, D., Kozak-Blickstein, A., & Levy, A. P. (2010). Antioxidant vitamins and their use in preventing cardiovascular disease. *Molecules (Basel, Switzerland)*, *15*(11), 8098–8110. doi:10.3390/molecules15118098 PMID:21063272

Faria, A. F., Marques, M. C., & Mercadante, A. Z. (2011). Identification of bioactive compounds from jambolao (*Syzygium cumini*) and antioxidant capacity evaluation in different pH conditions. *Food Chemistry*, *126*(4), 1571–1578. doi:10.1016/j.foodchem.2010.12.007 PMID:25213929

Fiedor, J., & Burda, K. (2014). Potential role of carotenoids as antioxidants in human health and disease. *Nutrients*, *6*(2), 466–488. doi:10.3390/nu6020466 PMID:24473231

Francini, A., & Sebastiani, L. (2013). phenolic compounds in apple (Malus X domestica Borkh.): Compounds characterization and stability during postharvest and after processing. *Antioxidants*, *2*(3), 181–193. doi:10.3390/antiox2030181 PMID:26784345

Gamel, T., & Abdel-Aal, E.-S. (2012). Phenolic acid and antioxidant properties of barley wholegrain and pearling fractions. *Agricultural and Food Science*, *21*, 118–131.

Gawlik-Dziki, U. (2008). Effect of hydrothermal treatment on the antioxidant properties of broccoli (*Brassica oleracea* var. botrytis italica) florets. *Food Chemistry*, *109*(2), 393–401. doi:10.1016/j.foodchem.2007.12.058 PMID:26003363

Ghosh, A. K., Banerjee, S., Mullick, H. I., & Banerjee, J. (2011). Zingiber officinale: A natural gold. *International Journal of Pharma and Bio Sciences*, *2*, 283–294.

Ghosh, D. (2015). Tannins from foods to combat diseases. *International Journal of Pharma Research & Review*, *4*(5), 40–44.

Giada, M. L. R. (2013). Food phenolic compounds: Main classes, sources and their antioxidant power, oxidative stress and chronic degenerative diseases - a role for antioxidants. In Oxidative stress and chronic degenerative diseases - A role for antioxidants (pp. 87-112). IntTech Publisher.

Girish, T. K., Pratape, V. M., & Rao, U. J. S. P. (2012). Nutrient distribution, phenolic acid composition, antioxidant and alphaglucosidase inhibitory potentials of black gram (*Vigna mungo* L.) and its milled byproducts. *Food Research International*, *46*(1), 370–377. doi:10.1016/j.foodres.2011.12.026

Gohari, A. R., Saeidnia, S., & Mahmoodabadi, M. K. (2013). An overview on saffron, phytochemicals, and medicinal properties. *Pharmacognocy Reviews*, *7*(13), 61–66. doi:10.4103/0973-7847.112850 PMID:23922458

Gorinstein, S., Cvikrov, M., Machackova, I., Haruenkit, R., Park, Y., Junge, S., & Trakhtenberg, S. et al. (2004). Characterization of antioxidant compounds in Jaffa sweeties and white grapefruits. *Food Chemistry*, *84*(4), 503–510. doi:10.1016/S0308-8146(03)00127-4

Goufo, P., & Trindade, H. (2014). Rice antioxidants: Phenolic acids, flavonoids, anthocyanins, proanthocyanidins, tocopherols, tocotrienols, γ-oryzanol, and phytic acid. *Food Science Nutrition*, *2*(2), 75–104. doi:10.1002/fsn3.86 PMID:24804068

Gupta, M., Sharma, S., Gautam, A. K., & Bhadauria, R. (2011). *Momordica charantia* Linn. (karela): Nature's silent healer. *International Journal of Pharmaceutical Sciences Review and Research*, *11*, 32–37.

Gupta, R. K., Patel, A. K., Shah, N., Choudhary, A. K., Jha, U. K., Yadav, U. C., & Pakuwal, U. et al. (2014). Oxidative stress and antioxidants in disease and cancer: A review. *Asian Pacific Journal of Cancer Prevention*, *15*(11), 4405–4409. doi:10.7314/APJCP.2014.15.11.4405 PMID:24969860

Halliwell, B., & Gutteridge, J. M. C. (1999). *Free radicals in biology and medicine* (2nd ed.). Oxford, UK: Clarendon Press.

Han, X., Shen, T., & Lou, H. (2007). Dietary polyphenols and their biological significance. *International Journal of Molecular Sciences*, *8*(9), 950–988. doi:10.3390/i8090950

Hassan, M. A. M., & Youssef, A. M. K. (2012). Effect of toasting and microwaving on gross chemical composition, total phenolics, antioxidant activity and phenolic acids fractionation of white beans flour (*Phaseolus vulgaris* L.). *World Applied Sciences Journal*, *18*, 731–736.

Hegde, A. M., Rai, K., & Padmanabhan, V. (2009). Total antioxidant capacity of saliva and its relation with early childhood caries and rampant caries. *The Journal of Clinical Pediatric Dentistry*, *33*(3), 231–234. doi:10.17796/jcpd.33.3.c730518021m56077 PMID:19476096

Higdon, J. V., & Frei, B. (2006). Coffee and health: A review of recent human research. *Critical Reviews in Food Science and Nutrition*, *46*(2), 101–123. doi:10.1080/10408390500400009 PMID:16507475

Hong, Y. J., Tomas-Barberan, F. A., Kader, A. A., & Mitchell, A. E. (2006). The flavonoid glycosides and procyanidin composition of deglet noor dates (*Phoenix dactylifera*). *Journal of Agricultural and Food Chemistry*, *54*(6), 2405–2411. doi:10.1021/jf0581776 PMID:16536626

Hu, N., Yu, J., Tan, L., Wang, Y., Sun, Y., Sun, L., & Tan, L. (2013). Nutrition and the risk of Alzheimer's disease. *Biomed Research International*, *2013*, 1–12. PMID:23865055

Isao, M., Fumiaki, I., Manson, J. E., Frank, H. B., Walter, W. C., & Rob, D. M. et al.. (2013). Fruit consumption and risk of type 2 diabetes: Results from three prospective longitudinal cohort studies. *British Medical Journal*, *347*(1), f5001. doi:10.1136/bmj.f5001 PMID:23990623

Jameel, M., Ali, A., & Ali, M. (2015a). Isolation of antioxidant phytoconstituents from the seeds of *Lens culinaris* Medik. *Food Chemistry*, *175*, 358–365. doi:10.1016/j.foodchem.2014.11.130 PMID:25577092

Jameel, M., Ali, A., & Ali, M. (2015b). New fatty acid and glycosides from the seeds of *Lens culinaris* Medik. *International Journal of Advances in Pharmacy Medicine and Bioallied Sciences*, *3*, 50–54.

Jamil, S. S., Nizami, Q., & Salam, M. (2007). *Centella asiatica* (Linn.) urban oA review. *Natural Product Radiance*, *6*, 158–170.

Jiang, F., Zhang, Y., & Dusting, G. J. (2011). NADPH oxidase-mediated redox signaling: Roles in cellular stress response, stress tolerance, and tissue repair. *Pharmacological Reviews*, *63*(1), 218–242. doi:10.1124/pr.110.002980 PMID:21228261

Jiang, G., Lin, S., Wen, L., Jiang, Y., Zhao, M., Chen, F., & Yang, B. et al. (2013). Identification of a novel phenolic compound in litchi (Litchi chinensis Sonn.) pericarp and bioactivity evaluation. *Food Chemistry*, *136*(2), 563–568. doi:10.1016/j.foodchem.2012.08.089 PMID:23122098

Johri, R. K. (2011). *Cuminum cyminum* and *Carum carvi*: An update. *Pharmacognosy Review*, *5*(9), 63–72. doi:10.4103/0973-7847.79101 PMID:22096320

Jukanti, A. K., Gaur, P. M., Gowda, C. L. L., & Chibbar, R. N. (2012). Nutritional quality and health benefits of chickpea (*Cicer arietinum* L.): A review. *The British Journal of Nutrition*, *108*(S1), S11–S26. doi:10.1017/S0007114512000797 PMID:22916806

Jung, H. A., Su, B. N., Keller, W. J., Mehta, R. G., & Kinghorn, A. D. (2006). Antioxidant xanthones from the pericarp of *Garcinia mangostana* (Mangosteen). *Journal of Agricultural and Food Chemistry*, *54*(6), 2077–2082. doi:10.1021/jf052649z PMID:16536578

Kaefer, C. M., & Milner, J. A. (2008). The role of herbs and spices in cancer prevention. *The Journal of Nutritional Biochemistry*, *19*(6), 347–361. doi:10.1016/j.jnutbio.2007.11.003 PMID:18499033

Kapoor, S. (2015). Bioactives and therapeutic potential of legumes: A review. *International Journal of Pharmacy and Biological Sciences*, *5*, 65–74.

Karunamoorthi, K., Kim, H., Jegajeevanram, K., Xavier, J., & Vijayalakshmi, J. (2014). Papaya: Agifted nutraceutical plant -acritical review of recent human health research. *TANG*, *4*, 1–17.

Key, T. J. (2011). Fruit and vegetables and cancer risk. *British Journal of Cancer*, *104*(1), 6–11. doi:10.1038/sj.bjc.6606032 PMID:21119663

Khan, A., Sankhyan, P., & Kumar, S. (2013). Biochemical characterization of mustard oil (*Brassica campestris* L.) with special reference to its fatty acid composition. *Asian Journal of Advances in Basic Sciences*, *1*, 1–9.

Khan, S., Choudhary, S., Pandey, A., Khan, M. K., & Thomas, G. (2015). Sunflower oil: Efficient oil source for human consumption. *Emer Life Science Research*, *1*, 1–3.

Kostova, I., Bhatia, S., Grigorov, P., Balkansky, S., Parmar, V. S., Prasad, A. K., & Saso, L. (2011). Coumarins as antioxidants. *Current Medicinal Chemistry*, *18*, 3929–3951. doi:10.2174/092986711803414395 PMID:21824098

Krinsky, N. I., & Johnson, E. J. (2005). Carotenoid actions and their relation to health and disease. *Molecular Aspects of Medicine*, *26*(6), 459–516. doi:10.1016/j.mam.2005.10.001 PMID:16309738

Krishna, K. L., Paridhavi, M., & Patel, J. A. (2008). Review on nutritional, medicinal and pharmacological properties of papaya (*Carica papaya* Linn.). *Natural Product Radiance*, *7*, 364–373.

Kumar, S., & Pandey, A. K. (2013). Chemistry and biological activities of flavonoids: An overview. *TheScientificWorldJournal*, *2013*, 1–16. PMID:24470791

Kumar, S., Prasad, A. K., Iyer, S. V., & Vaidya, S. K. (2013). Systematic pharmacognostical, phytochemical and pharmacological review on an ethno medicinal plant, *Basella alba* L. *Journal of Pharmacognosy and Phytotherapy*, *5*, 53–58.

Kunwar, A., & Priyadarsini, K. I. (2011). Free radicals, oxidative stress and importance of antioxidants in human health. *Journal of Medical & Allide Science*, *1*(2), 53–60.

Latha, G., Sindhu, P. G., Suja, S. R., Geetha, B. S., Pushpangadan, P., & Rajasekharan, S. (2005). Pharmacology and chemistry of Myristica fragrans Houtt. A review. *Journal of Spices and Aromatic Crops*, *14*(2), 94–101.

Lee, J., Koo, N., & Min, D. B. (2004). Reactive oxygen species, aging, and antioxidative nutraceuticals. *Comprehensive Reviews in Food Science and Food Safety*, *3*(1), 21–33. doi:10.1111/j.1541-4337.2004.tb00058.x

Lee, K. G., & Shibamoto, T. (2000). Antioxidant properties of aroma compounds isolated from soybeans and mung beans. *Journal of Agricultural and Food Chemistry*, *48*(9), 4290–4293. doi:10.1021/jf000442u PMID:10995351

Leopoldini, M., Russo, N., & Toscano, M. (2011). The molecular basis of working mechanism of natural polyphenolic antioxidants. *Food Chemistry*, *125*(2), 288–306. doi:10.1016/j.foodchem.2010.08.012

Li, S., Chen, G., Zhang, C., Wu, M., Wu, S., & Liu, Q. (2014). Research progress of natural antioxidants in foods for thetreatment of diseases. *Food Science and Human Wellness*, *3*, 110–116.

Li, W., Liang, H., Zhang, M., Zhang, R., Deng, Y., Wei, Z., & Tang, X. et al. (2012). Phenolic profiles and antioxidant activity of litchi (*Litchi chinensis* Sonn.) fruit pericarp from different commercially available cultivars. *Molecules (Basel, Switzerland)*, *17*(12), 14954–14967. doi:10.3390/molecules171214954 PMID:23247368

Loganathan, R., Selvaduray, K. R., Radhakrishnan, A., & Nesaretnam, K. (2010). Palm oil: Risch in health promoting phytonutrients. *Palm Oil Developments*, *50*, 16–25.

Luthria, A., Singh, K., & D'souza, M. (2014). *In vitro* antioxidant activity of black gram, cowpea, desi chickpea and yellow mustard as affected by sprouting. *Journal of Global Biosciences*, *3*(1), 385–389.

MacRae, W. D., & Towers, G. H. N. (1984). Biological activities of lignans. *Phytochemistry*, *23*(6), 1207–1220. doi:10.1016/S0031-9422(00)80428-8

Marcinkiewicz, J. (2010). Taurine bromamine (TauBr) - its role in immunity and new perspectives for clinical use. *Journal of Biomedical Science*, *17*(Suppl 1), S3. doi:10.1186/1423-0127-17-S1-S3 PMID:20804605

Marina, A. M., Man, Y. B., Nazimah, S. A., & Amin, I. (2009). Antioxidant capacity and phenolic acids of virgin coconut oil. *International Journal of Food Sciences and Nutrition*, *60*(sup2Suppl 2), 114–123. doi:10.1080/09637480802549127 PMID:19115123

Martino, H. S. D. M., Cardoso, L. M., Ribeiro, S. M. R., Dantas, M. I. S., Piovesan, N. D., & Mejia, E. D. (2011). Nutritional and bioactive compounds of soybean: benefits on human health, soybean and health. InTech Publisher.

Masibo, M., & He, Q. (2008). Major mango polyphenols and their potential significance to human health. *Comprehensive Reviews in Food Science and Food Safety*, *7*(4), 309–319. doi:10.1111/j.1541-4337.2008.00047.x

Mathangi, S. K. (2012). Nutraceutical properties of great millet – *Sorghum vulgare*. *International Journal of Food. Agriculture and Veterinary Sciences*, *2*, 40–45.

Mathangi, S. K., & Sudha, K. (2012). Functional and phytochemical properties of finger millet (*Eleusine coracana* L.) for health. *International Journal of Pharmaceutical Chemical and Biological Sciences*, *2*, 431–438.

Mekky, R. H., Contreras, M. M., El-Gindi, M. R., Abdel-Monem, A. R., Abdel-Sattar, E., & Segura-Carretero, A. (2015). Profiling of phenolic and other compounds from Egyptian cultivars of chickpea (*Cicer arietinum* L.) and antioxidant activity: A comparative study. *RSC Advances*, *5*(23), 17751–17767. doi:10.1039/C4RA13155J

Nadeem, M., & Riaz, A. (2012). Cumin (*Cuminum cyminum*) as a potential source of antioxidants. *Pakistan Journal of Food Science*, *22*, 101–107.

Nambiar, V. S., Dhaduk, J. J., Sareen, N., Shahu, T., & Desai, R. (2011). Potential functional implications of pearl millet (*Pennisetum glaucum*) in health and disease. *Journal of Applied Pharmaceutical Science*, *1*, 62–67.

Nevin, K. G., & Rajamohan, T. (2006). Virgin coconut oil supplemented diet increases the antioxidant status in rats. *Food Chemistry*, *99*(2), 206–266. doi:10.1016/j.foodchem.2005.06.056

Nevin, K. G., & Rajamohan, T. (2014). Beneficial effects of virgin coconut oil on lipid parameters and *in vitro* LDL oxidation. *Clinical Biochemistry*, *37*(9), 830–835. doi:10.1016/j.clinbiochem.2004.04.010 PMID:15329324

Nyau, V. (2014). Nutraceutical perspectives and utilization of common beans (*Phaseolus Vulgaris* L.): A review. *African Journal of Food Agriculture Nutrition and Development*, *14*, 9483–9496.

Padayatty, S. J., Katz, A., Wang, Y., Eck, P., Kwon, O., Lee, J., & Levine, M. et al. (2003). Vitamin C as an antioxidant: Evaluation of its role in disease prevention. *Journal of the American College of Nutrition*, *22*(1), 18–35. doi:10.1080/07315724.2003.10719272 PMID:12569111

Pallauf, K., Rivas-Gonzalo, J. C., del Castillo, M. D., Cano, M. P., & de Pascual-Teresa, S. (2008). Characterization of the antioxidant composition of strawberry tree (*Arbutus unedo* L.) fruits. *Journal of Food Composition and Analysis*, *21*(4), 273–281. doi:10.1016/j.jfca.2007.11.006

Pandey, K. B., & Rizvi, S. I. (2009). Plant polyphenols as dietary antioxidants in human health and disease. *Oxidative Medicine and Cellular Longevity*, *2*(5), 270–278. doi:10.4161/oxim.2.5.9498 PMID:20716914

Pantsi, W. G., Bester, D. J., Esterhuyse, A. J., & Aboua, G. (2014). Dietary antioxidant properties of vegetable oils and nuts – the race against cardiovascular disease progression. In Antioxidant-antidiabetic agents and human health (pp. 209-238). InTech Publisher.

Patel, M., & Naik, S. N. (2004). Gamma-oryzanol from rice bran oil – A review. *Journal of Scientific and Industrial Research*, *63*, 569–578.

Paterson, D. M. (2001). Oat antioxidants. *Journal of Cereal Science*, *33*(2), 115–129. doi:10.1006/jcrs.2000.0349

Patil, S., & Jain, G. (2014). Holistic approach of *Trigonella foenum-graecum* in phytochemistry and pharmacology- A review. *Current Trends in Technology and Science*, *3*, 34–48.

Patrice, C., Laura, G. J., Jacqui, T., Kamlesh, K., & Melanie, D. J. (2010). Fruit and vegetable intake and incidence of type 2 diabetes mellitus: Systematic review and meta-analysis. *British Medical Journal*, *341*(4), c4229. doi:10.1136/bmj.c4229 PMID:20724400

Patrick, L. (2000). Beta-carotene: The controversy continues. *Alternative Medicine Review*, *5*(6), 530–545. PMID:11134976

Pawlowska, A. M., Leo, M. D., & Braca, A. (2006). Phenolics of *Arbutus unedo* L. (Ericaceae) fruits: Identification of anthocyanins and gallic acid derivatives. *Journal of Agricultural and Food Chemistry*, *54*(26), 10234–10238. doi:10.1021/jf062230o PMID:17177565

Pedreschi, R., & Cisneros-Zevallos, L. (2007). Phenolic profiles of Andean purple corn (*Zea mays* L.). *Food Chemistry*, *100*(3), 956–963. doi:10.1016/j.foodchem.2005.11.004

Petchiammal, C., & Hopper, W. (2014). Antioxidant activity of proteins from fifteen varieties of legume seeds commonly consumed in India. *International Journal of Pharmacy and Pharmaceutical Sciences*, *6*, 476–479.

Peterson, J. J., Beecher, G. R., Bhagwat, S. A., Dwyer, J. T., Gebhardt, S. E., Haytowitz, D. B., & Holden, J. M. (2006). Flavanones in grapefruit, lemons, and limes: A compilation and review of the data from the analytical literature. *Journal of Food Composition and Analysis*, *19*, S74–S80. doi:10.1016/j.jfca.2005.12.009

Prajapati, R. P., Kalariya, M., Parmar, S. K., & Sheth, N. R. (2010). Phytochemical and pharmacological review of *Lagenaria sicereria. J Ayurveda Integr Med*, *1*(4), 266–272. doi:10.4103/0975-9476.74431 PMID:21731373

Rahal, A., Kumar, A., Singh, V., Yadav, B., Tiwari, R., Chakraborty, S., & Dhama, K. (2014). Oxidative stress, prooxidants, and antioxidants: The interplay. *BioMed Research International*, *2014*, 1–19. doi:10.1155/2014/761264 PMID:24587990

Rahaman, S., Islam, R., Kamruzzaman, M., Alam, K., & Jamal, A.H.M. (2011). *Ocimum sanctum* L.: A review of phytochemical and pharmacological profile. *American Journal of Drug Discovery and Development*, 1-15.

Rao, A. V., & Rao, L. G. (2007). Carotenoids and human health. *Pharmacological Research*, *55*(3), 207–216. doi:10.1016/j.phrs.2007.01.012 PMID:17349800

Rao, B. S. N. (2003). Bioactive phytochemicals in Indian foods and their potential in health promotion and disease prevention. *Asia Pacific Journal of Clinical Nutrition*, *12*(1), 9–22. PMID:12737006

Rather, M.A., Dar, B.A., Sofi, S.N., Bhat, B.A., & Qurishi, M.A. (2012). Foeniculum vulgare*: A comprehensive review of its traditional use, phytochemistry, pharmacology, and safety*. Doi: 10.1016/j.arabjc.2012.04.011

Reidah, I. M. (2013). *Characterization of phenolic compounds in highly-consumed vegetable matrices by using advanced analytical technique*. (Ph.D thesis). University of Granada.

Reinisalo, M., Karlund, A., Koskela, A., Kaarniranta, K., & Karjalainen, R. O. (2015). Polyphenol stilbenes: Molecular mechanisms of defence against oxidative stress and aging-related diseases. *Oxidative Medicine and Cellular Longevity*, *2015*, 1–24. doi:10.1155/2015/340520 PMID:26180583

Reynoso-Camacho, R., Ramos-Gomez, M., & Loarca-Pina, G. (2006). Bioactive components in common beans (Phaseolus vulgaris L.). In R. G. Guevara-Gonzalez & I. Torres-Pacheco (Eds.), Advances in Agricultural and Food Biotechnology (pp. 217–236). Academic Press.

Rueda, F. D. M. N. (2005). *Guava (*Psidium guajava *l.) fruit phytochemicals, antioxidant properties and overall quality as influenced by postharvest treatments*. (M.Sc Thesis). University of Florida.

Sarwar, M. T., Rahman, M. H., Raza, M. S., Rouf, S. M. A., & Rahman, M. N. (2014). Determination of Erucic acid content in traditional and commercial mustard oils of Bangladesh by gas- liquid chromatography. *Advances in Biochemistry*, *2*(1), 9–13. doi:10.11648/j.ab.20140201.12

Saura-Calixto, F., Serrano, J., & Perez-Jimemez, J. (2008). What constribution is beer to the intake of antioxidant in diet. In V. Preedy (Ed.), *Beer in health and disease prevention*. London: Academic Press.

Sen, S., & Chakraborty, R. (2011). The role of antioxidants in human health. In A. Silvana & M. Hepel (Eds.), *Oxidative stress: Diagnostics, prevention, and therapy* (pp. 1–37). Washington, DC: American Chemical Society. doi:10.1021/bk-2011-1083.ch001

Sen, S., & Chakraborty, R. (2015). Antioxidant supplements: Friend or foe? In V. Rani & U. C. S. Yadav (Eds.), *Free radicals in human disease and health* (pp. 293–322). New Delhi: Springer Publication.

Sen, S., Chakraborty, R., Sridhar, C., Reddy, Y. S. R., & De, B. (2010). Free radicals, antioxidants, diseases and phytomedicines: Current status and future prospect. *International Journal of Pharmaceutical Sciences Review and Research*, *3*(1), 91–100.

Servili, M., Sordini, B., Esposto, S., Urbani, S., Zeneziani, G., Maio, I. D., & Taticchi, A. et al. (2014). Biological activities of phenolic compounds of extra virgin olive oil. *Antioxidants*, *3*(1), 1–23. doi:10.3390/antiox3010001 PMID:26784660

Shehata, M. S. M., & Soltan, S. S. A. (2013). Effects of bioactive component of kiwi fruit and avocado (fruit and seed) on hypercholesterolemic rats. *World Journal of Dairy & Food Sciences*, *8*(1), 82–93.

Shi, Y., Tian, F., Ru, Z., & Guo, L. (2011). Antioxidant activity of different fractions of wheat grains. *Advances in Biomedical Engineering*, *1-2*, 107–109.

Shojaii, A., & Fard, M. A. (2012). Review of pharmacological properties and chemical constituents of *Pimpinella anisum*. *International Scholarly Research Network*, *2012*, 1–8. PMID:22848853

Sies, H., Stahl, W., & Sundquist, A. R. (1992). Antioxidant functions of vitamins. Vitamins E and C, beta-carotene, and other carotenoids. *Annals of the New York Academy of Sciences*, *669*(1), 7–20. doi:10.1111/j.1749-6632.1992.tb17085.x PMID:1444060

Simic, A., Manojlovic, D., Segan, D., & Todorovic, M. (2007). Electrochemical behavior and antioxidant and prooxidant activity of natural phenolics. *Molecules (Basel, Switzerland)*, *12*(10), 2327–2340. doi:10.3390/12102327 PMID:17978760

Singh, J., Upadhyay, A. K., Bahadur, A., Singh, B., Singh, K. P., & Rai, M. (2006). Antioxidant phytochemicals in cabbage (*Brassica oleracea* L. var. capitata). *Scientia Horticulturae*, *108*(3), 233–237. doi:10.1016/j.scienta.2006.01.017

Singh, R., De, S., & Belkheir, A. (2013). *Avena sativa* (Oat), a potential neutraceutical and therapeutic agent: An overview. *Critical Reviews in Food Science and Nutrition*, *53*(2), 126–244. doi:10.1080/10408398.2010.526725 PMID:23072529

Sinija, V. R., & Mishra, H. N. (2008). Green tea: Health benefit. *Journal of Nutritional & Environmental Medicine*, *17*(4), 232–242. doi:10.1080/13590840802518785

Soneja, A., Drews, M., & Malinski, T. (2005). Role of nitric oxide, nitroxidative and oxidative stress in wound healing. *Pharmacological Reports*, *57*(Suppl), 108–119. PMID:16415491

Soris, T. P., Kala, K. B., Mohan, V. R., & Vadivel, V. (2010). The biochemical composition and nutritional potential of three varieties of *Vigna mungo* (L.) Hepper. *Advances in Bioresearch*, *1*, 6–16.

Srivastava, R., Ahmed, H., Dixit, R. K., Dharamveer, , & Saraf, S. A. (2010). *Crocus sativus* L.: A comprehensive review. *Pharmacognosy Review*, *4*(8), 200–208. doi:10.4103/0973-7847.70919 PMID:22228962

Stahl, W., & Sies, H. (2003). Antioxidant activity of carotenoids. *Molecular Aspects of Medicine*, *24*(6), 345–351. doi:10.1016/S0098-2997(03)00030-X PMID:14585305

Stevenson, D. E., & Hurst, R. D. (2007). Polyphenolic phytochemicals – just antioxidants or much more? *Cellular and Molecular Life Sciences*, *64*(22), 2900–2916. doi:10.1007/s00018-007-7237-1 PMID:17726576

Su, D., Zhang, R., Hou, F., Zhang, M., Guo, J., Huang, F., & Wei, Z. et al. (2014). Comparison of the free and bound phenolic profiles and cellular antioxidant activities of litchi pulp extracts from different solvents. *BMC Complementary and Alternative Medicine*, *14*(1), 9. doi:10.1186/1472-6882-14-9 PMID:24405977

Subhash, G. P., Virbhadrappa, S. R., & Vasanth, O. K. (2010). *Spinacia oleracea* Linn: A pharmacognostic and pharmacological overview. *International Journal of Research in Ayurveda & Pharmacy*, *1*, 78–84.

Sundram, K. (2015). *Palm oil: Chemistry and nutrition updates*. Retreated from: www.americanpalmoil.com/pdf/DR%20Sundram.pdf

Swami, S. B., Thakor, N. S. J., Patil, M. M., & Haldankar, P. M. (2012). Jamun (*Syzygium cumini* L.): A review of its food and medicinal uses. *Food and Nutrition Sciences*, *3*(08), 1100–1117. doi:10.4236/fns.2012.38146

Tandaon, V. R., Verma, S., Singh, J. B., & Mahajan, A. (2005). Antioxidants and cardiovascular health. *Drug Review*, *7*(2), 61–64.

Teeguarden, R. (2007). *The pro-oxidant/antioxidant dance of life. dragon time — summer 2007*. Retrieved from http://www.bluetoad.com/article/The+Pro-OxidantAntioxidant+Dance+of+Life/10364/0/article.html

Tijerina-Saenz, A., Innis, S. M., & Kitts, D. D. (2009). Antioxidant capacity of human milk and its association with vitamins A and E and fatty acid composition. *Acta Paediatrica (Oslo, Norway)*, *98*(11), 1793–1798. doi:10.1111/j.1651-2227.2009.01437.x PMID:19807706

Trachootham, D., Lu, W., Ogasawara, M. A., Valle, N. R., & Huang, P. (2008). Redox regulation of cell survival. *Antioxidants & Redox Signalling*, *10*(8), 13430–1374. doi:10.1089/ars.2007.1957 PMID:18522489

Tresserra-Rimbau, A., Medina-Remon, A., Estruch, R., & Lamuela-Raventos, R. M. (2014). Coffee polyphenol and high cardiovascular risk parameters. In V. Preedy (Ed.), *Coffee in health and disease prevention* (p. 388). London: Academic Press.

Troszynska, A., & Ciska, E. (2002). Phenolic compounds of seed coats of white and coloured varieties of pea (*Pisum sativum* L.) and their total antioxidant activity. *Czech Journal Food Science*, *20*, 15–22.

Tsao, R. (2010). Chemistry and biochemistry of dietary polyphenols. *Nutrients*, *2*(12), 1231–1246. doi:10.3390/nu2121231 PMID:22254006

Valko, M., Leibfritz, D., Moncol, J., Cronin, M. T. D., Mazur, M., & Telser, J. (2007). Free radicals and antioxidants in normal physiological functions and human disease. *The International Journal of Biochemistry & Cell Biology*, *39*(1), 44–84. doi:10.1016/j.biocel.2006.07.001 PMID:16978905

Van't Veer, P., Jansen, M. C., Klerk, M., & Kok, F. J. (2000). Fruits and vegetables in the prevention of cancer and cardiovascular disease. *Public Health Nutrition*, *3*(1), 103–107. PMID:10786730

Venter, C. S., & van Eyssen, E. (2011). More legumes for better overall health. *South African Journal of Clinical Nutritional*, *14*(suppl), S32–S38.

Vertuani, S., Angusti, A., & Manfredini, S. (2004). The antioxidants and pro-antioxidants network: An overview. *Current Pharmaceutical Design*, *10*(14), 1677–1694. doi:10.2174/1381612043384655 PMID:15134565

Vorarat, S., Managit, C., Iamthanakul, L., Soparat, W., & Kamkaen, N. (2010). Examination of antioxidant activity and development of rice bran oil and gamma-oryzanol microemulsion. *Journal of Health Research*, *24*(2), 67–72.

Wahlqvist, M. L. (2013). Antioxidant relevance to human health. *Asia Pacific Journal of Clinical Nutrition*, *22*(2), 117–176. PMID:23635359

Wang, R., Ding, Y., Liu, R., Xiang, L., & Du, L. (2010). Pomegranate: Constituents, bioactivities and pharmacokinetics. *Fruits. Vegetable and Cereal Science and Biotechnology*, *4*(2), 77–87.

Warner, K., Vick, B., Kleingartner, L., Isaak, R., & Doroff, K. (2015). *Compositions of sunflower, nusun (mid-oleic sunflower) and high-oleic sunflower oils*. Retreated from: https://www.sunflowernsa.com/uploads/resources/51/warner_.pdf

Waterman, E., & Lockwood, B. (2007). Active components and clinical applications of olive oil. *Alternative Medicine Review*, *12*, 331–342. PMID:18069902

Wu, C., Gao, Q., Kjelgren, R. K., Guo, X., & Wang, M. (2013). Yields, phenolic profiles and antioxidant activities of *Ziziphus jujube* mill. in response to different fertilization treatments. *Molecules (Basel, Switzerland)*, *18*(10), 12029–12040. doi:10.3390/molecules181012029 PMID:24084012

Wu, N., Fu, K., Fu, Y., Zu, Y., Chang, F., Chen, Y., & Gu, C. et al. (2009). Antioxidant activities of extracts and main components of pigeonpea [*Cajanus cajan* (L.) Millsp.] leaves. *Molecules (Basel, Switzerland)*, *14*(3), 1032–1043. doi:10.3390/molecules14031032 PMID:19305357

Xie, Z., Fan, J., Charlebois, D., Roussel, D., Dube, C., Charles, M. T., & Khanizadeh, S. (2014). Agronomic characteristics and phytochemical profiles of advanced june-bearing strawberry lines for the northern Candian climate. *Agricultural and Food Science*, *23*, 38–47.

Yadav, D., Yadav, S. K., Khar, R. K., Mujeeb, M., & Akhtar, M. (2013). Turmeric (*Curcuma longa* L.): A promising spice for phytochemical and pharmacological activities. *International Journal of Green Pharmacy*, *7*(2), 82–89. doi:10.4103/0973-8258.116375

Yadav, R., & Kaushik, R. (2011). A study of phytochemical constituents and pharmacological actions of *Trigonella foenum-graecum*: A review. *International Journal of Pharmacy & Technology*, *3*, 1022–1028.

Yordi, E. G., Pérez, E. M., Matos, M. J., & Villares, E. U. (2012). Antioxidant and pro-oxidant effects of polyphenolic compounds and structure-activity relationship evidence. In Nutrition, well-being and health (pp. 2-48). InTech Publisher.

Yuan, Y. V., & Kitts, D. D. (1997). Endogenous antioxidants: role of antioxidant enzyme in biological systems. In F. Shahidi (Ed.), *Natural antioxidants- Chemistry, health effects, and applications* (pp. 258–270). Champaign, IL: Amer Oil Chemists Society.

Zhang, L. L., & Lin, Y. M. (2009). Antioxidant tannins from *Syzygium cumini* fruit. *African Journal of Biotechnology*, *8*, 2301–2309.

Zhang, R. F., Zhang, F. X., Zhang, M. W., Wei, Z. C., Yang, C. Y., Zhang, Y., & Chi, J. W. et al. (2011). Phenolic composition and antioxidant activity in seed coats of 60 Chinese black soybean (*Glycine max* L. Merr.) varieties. *Journal of Agricultural and Food Chemistry*, *59*(11), 593–544. doi:10.1021/jf201593n PMID:21548651

Zhao, H., Zhang, H., & Yang, S. (2014). Phenolic compounds and its antioxidant activities in ethanolicextracts from seven cultivars of Chinese jujube. *Food Science and Human Wellness*, *3*(3-4), 183–190. doi:10.1016/j.fshw.2014.12.005

Zorov, D. B., Bannikova, S. Y., Belousov, V. V., Vyssokikh, M. Y., Zorova, L. D., Isaev, N. K., & Plotnikov, E. Y. et al. (2005). Reactive oxygen and nitrogen species: Friends or foes? *Biochemistry (Moscow)*, *70*(2), 215–221. doi:10.1007/s10541-005-0103-6 PMID:15807661

Zou, Y., Chang, S. K. C., Gu, Y., & Qian, S. Y. (2011). Antioxidant activity and phenolic compositions of lentil (*Lens culinaris* var. Morton) extract and its fractions. *Journal of Agricultural and Food Chemistry*, *59*(6), 2268–2276. doi:10.1021/jf104640k PMID:21332205

Chapter 14
Antimicrobial Edible Films and Coatings for Fruits and Vegetables

Amrita Poonia
Banaras Hindu University, India

ABSTRACT

Non-degradable packaging materials are doing much damage to the environment. So the interest has been developed in biodegradable films and coatings these days. Use of edible films and coatings is eco-friendly technology used for enhancing the shelf life of the fruits and vegetables. The use of antimicrobial compounds in edible coatings of proteins, starch, cellulose derivatives, chitosan, alginate, fruit puree, and egg albumin has been successfully added to the edible films and coatings. This chapter focuses on the development of edible films and coatings with antimicrobial activity, effect of these coatings on the target microorganisms, the influence of these antimicrobial agents on mechanical & barrier properties and application of antimicrobial edible coatings on the quality of fresh fruits and vegetables.

INTRODUCTION

The demand for minimally processed, easily prepared and ready-to-eat (RTE) 'fresh' food products, globalization of food trade, and distribution from centralized processing pose major challenges for food safety and quality. Recent food-borne microbial outbreaks are driving a search for innovative ways to inhibit microbial growth in the foods while maintaining quality, freshness and safety. One option is to use packaging to provide an increased margin of safety and quality. These packaging technologies could play a vital role in extending shelf-life of food(s) and reduce the risk from pathogens. Antimicrobial polymers may find use in other food contact applications as well (Rooney, 1995). It acts to reduce, inhibit or retard the growth of pathogen microorganisms in packed foods and packaging material (Vermeiren, *et al.* 1999).

Most food consumed comes directly from nature, some of them eaten directly after harvesting from the tree, vine or ground. With increased transportation distribution systems, storage needs and advent of ever larger supermarkets and warehouse stores, foods are not consumed just in the orchard, on the

DOI: 10.4018/978-1-5225-0591-4.ch014

field, in the farmhouse, or close to processing facilities. It takes much time for a food product to reach the table of the consumer. During this whole process time-consuming steps are involved in handling, storage and transportation, the food product start to dehydrate, deteriorate and lose loose appearance, flavor and nutritional value. If no special care is provided, damage can occur within hours or days, even if this damage is not immediately visible. Today various modern methods, including combinations of these such as refrigeration, controlled atmosphere storage, and sterilization by both UV and gamma radiation are used to keep food safe. Nevertheless, for many kinds of food, coating with edible film continues to be one of the most cost effective ways to maintain their quality and safety.

Edible films and coatings made by use of agricultural commodities and wastes of food products have gained considerable attention in last few years. The biopolymers i.e. polysaccharides, proteins and their blends plays an important role as a carrier for different additives like antimicrobial, antioxidants, nutraceuticals and flavouring agents. Organic acids, chitosan, nisin and lactoperoxidase system and plant extracts & essential oils are the most commonly used antimicrobials. The main objectives of this chapter are to discuss the use of edible films and coatings, the applications and legislations concerning edible films and coatings. The information provided in this chapter helps to improve the design, development, applicability of edible films and coatings, their safety aspects that might be important while planning the future trends and better functionality of edible films as a preservation technique to enhance the shelf life of the food products.

BACKGROUND

Edible films and coatings like wax have been used for long time to prevent moisture loss and to stop the respiration process. These practices are still carried out in the present time. The association of edible fruits and vegetables are 50 years old. In 1967, edible films had very little use and were limited to wax layers only. A good business came out from this concept and by 1996, numbers grew to 600 companies. In twelfth century citrus fruits were preserved by placing them in box and pouring molten wax on them to preserve them for Emperor's table. Later in fifteenth century edible films made up of boiled soy milk were used in Japan for maintaining the food quality and appearance. In the nineteenth century, a US patent was used for preservation of various meat products by gelatin. But these days, many other methods and combination of these methods are used to keep the food safe. Use of edible films and coatings continues as one of the most cost effective method of food preservation.

HISTORY OF EDIBLE FILMS AND COATINGS

The use of wax coating of fruits by dipping is one of the old methods that became into vogue in the early 12th century (Krochta & Mulder-Johnston 1997). This was practiced in China, essentially to retard water transpiration loss in lemons and oranges. Application of lipid-based coatings to meats to prevent shrinkage has been a traditional practice since the sixteenth century, while later in the last century, meat and other foodstuffs were preserved by coating them with gelatin films. Yuba, a protein edible film obtained from the skin of boiled soymilk, was traditionally used in Asia to improve appearance and help preservation of foods since the fifteenth century. In the nineteenth century, sucrose solution was applied as an edible protective coating on nuts, almonds and hazelnuts to prevent their oxidation and rancidity during storage.

One of the most important advancements in edible film and coating technology since the 1930s involves use of an emulsion made of wax, oil and water. Such emulsions are applied to fruits to improve appearance (gloss and color) and to prevent softening and onset of mealiness. They are also used for delivery of fruits against fungicides, to control ripening, and retard moisture loss in fruit. A number of edible polysaccharide coatings including alginates, carrageenans, cellulose ethers, pectin and starch derivatives have been used to improve stored meat quality. Over the last forty years, a great number of studies have investigated formulation, application and characterization of edible films and coatings; evidence of such efforts can be found in both the scientific and patent literature (Debeaufort, *et al.* 1998).

DEFINITION

Edible films are defined as thin layers of material which can be eaten by the consumer and provide a barrier to moisture, oxygen and solute movement in the food. The material can be used as complete food coating or it can be disposed as a continuous layer between food components (Guilbert, 1986). A film or coating also provide surface sterility and prevent loss of other important components. Generally, its thickness is less than 0.3 mm. Items which are edible or are in contact with food should be generally recognized by qualified experts as being safe under conditions of its intended use, with amount applied in accordance with good manufacturing practices (GMPs). These food-safe materials must typically have approval of the Food and Drug Administration (FDA). Since it is impractical for FDA to have an all-inclusive list of every potential food ingredient, there are also other opportunities to acquire Generally Recognized as Safe (GRAS) status – i.e., manufacturers can petition for approval of an ingredient or food composite provided that this petition is supported by considerable studies. However, GRAS status does not guarantee complete product safety, especially for consumers who have food allergies or sensitivities, such as lactose intolerance (milk) and Celiac disease (wheat gluten).

COMPOSITION AND CLASSIFICATION OF EDIBLE FILMS AND COATINGS

Edible films and coatings are composed of hydrocolloids, which consist of either proteins or hydrophobic compounds (e.g., lipids or waxes). Edible films may also be a mixture of hydrocolloids and hydrophobic compounds (composite films or coatings). Figure 1 illustrates the most common compounds used in edible films and coatings.

Prerequisites of Edible Films and Coatings

Ideal edible film should have the following characteristics:

- Contain no toxic, allergic and non-digestible components
- Provide structural stability and prevent mechanical damage during transportation, handling and display
- Have good adhesion to surface of food to be protected providing uniform coverage
- Control water migration both in and out of protected food to maintain desired moisture content

Figure 1. Classification of edible films and coatings applied in food according to their components

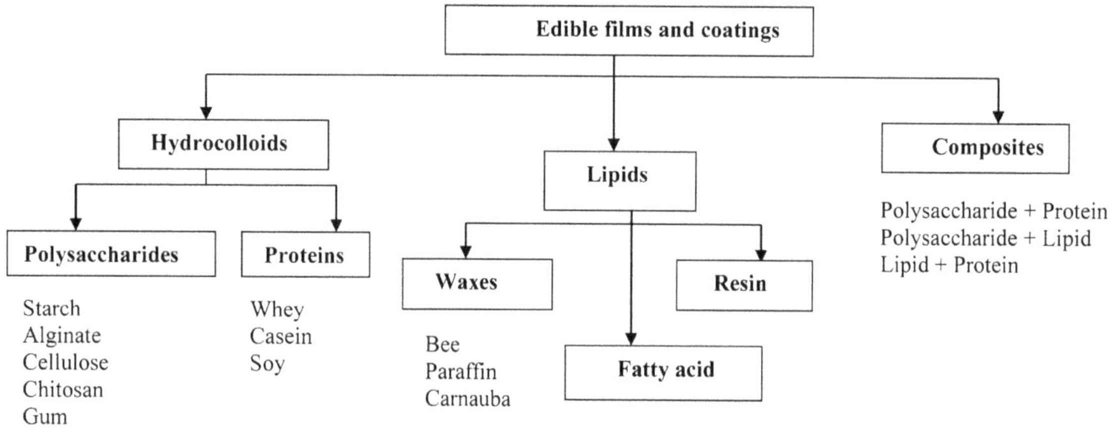

- Provide semi-permeability to maintain internal equilibrium of gases involved in aerobic and anaerobic respiration, thus retarding senescence
- Prevent loss or uptake of components that stabilize aroma, flavor, nutritional and organoleptic characteristics necessary for consumer acceptance while not adversely altering the taste or appearance
- Provide biochemical and microbial surface stability while protecting against contamination, pest infestation, microbe proliferation and other types of decay
- Film must retain flavor during the drying process to provide the whole range of desired notes during consumption
- The film has to protect flavor compounds from oxygen during storage; the flavor release must occur very slowly with water contact or with heating.
- Low cost of raw materials; and
- Simple technology for production

Advantages Microbial Films and Coatings

Advantages of edible coatings (Park, *et al.* 1994; Sothornvit & Krochta, 2000) include:

- Improves external appearance by giving additional shine to the fruit surface.
- Reduces weight loss and keep the fruit firm, so that its fresh look can be maintained.
- Reduces rate of respiration and ethylene production, thus delaying senescence.
- Prevents fruits and vegetables against chilling injuries and storage disorders.
- Act as barrier to free gas exchange.
- Provides a carrier for postharvest chemical treatments.
- Encapsulates aroma compounds, antioxidants, pigments, ions that stop browning reactions and Nutritional substances such as vitamins.
- Reduces the use of synthetic packaging material.
- In some countries, taxes levied on the shipment of packaging material can be saved by use of edible coatings and films.

ACTIONS OF MICROBIAL FILMS AND COATINGS

Fruits and vegetables continue to respire even after harvesting and use up all the oxygen within the produce, which is not replaced as quickly as by edible coating and produce carbon dioxide, which accumulates within the produce because it cannot escape as easily through coating.

Avoid Water Loss

A barrier is formed on the surface of fruits and/or vegetables by edible films/coatings, which decrease water vapor transmission rate. This barrier prevents texture decay, since water is essential for preservation of cell turgor (Garcia & Barret, 2002). Metabolic alterations that can cause accelerated rate of senescence due to water loss can also be avoided with their use. Ability of films and coatings to function as barriers to water vapor relies on external conditions, which include (1) temperature and relative humidity, (2) characteristics of commodity such as type of product, variety, maturity and water activity, and (3) characteristics of film such as composition, concentration of solids, viscosity, chemical structure, polymer morphology, degree of crosslinking, solvents used in casting the film, and type of plasticizer used (Olivas & Barbosa-Canovas 2005). In minimally-processed fruits, there is usually very high water activity present at the surface, making it difficult to develop a coating that delays water loss, since capacity of films to work as barriers to water vapor decreases as water activity increases in the commodity (or relative humidity of the environment) (Hagenmaier & Shaw 1990).

Enhance Texture

The action of pectic enzymes during storage causes dramatic loss of firmness in fruit tissues. The most common way of controlling softening phenomenon in fresh fruits is the use of treatments with calcium salts. Calcium ions interact with pectic polymers to form a cross linked network that increases mechanical strength, thus delaying senescence and controlling physiological disorders in fruits and vegetables. Texture enhancers can be into the formulation of edible coatings to minimize softening phenomena of produce. Hernandez-Munoz et al. (2006) observed that the addition of calcium gluconate to the chitosan (1%) coating formulation increased the firmness of strawberries during refrigerated storage.

Reduce Respiration

Respiration can be reduced by edible films or coatings and hence increase shelf life of a commodity. In selection of a coating, several considerations should be addressed to avoid extremely low oxygen concentration inside the commodity. Low oxygen concentration in the product could lead to anaerobic respiration, which can result in deterioration of product due to production of off-flavors and accelerated senescence (Kays & Paull 2004).

Decreased Ethylene Production

A well selected edible coating will produce a modified atmosphere inside the fruit, reducing levels of internal oxygen. If oxygen concentration inside the commodity drops below 8%, there will be a decrease in ethylene production (Kader, 1986) and the commodity's quality will be preserved longer.

Improve Colour

Color is one of the most important attributes of fruits and vegetables (Kays 1999). For some minimally-processed fruits and vegetables, browning is a big problem that can be controlled by use of films or coatings as carriers of anti-browning agents. The most common antioxidant used on fruits and vegetables is ascorbic acid; however other compounds have been successfully used such as cysteine, 4-hexylresorcinol, citric acid and calcium chloride (Olivas, *et al.* 2007). Baldwin et al. (1996) coated apple slices and potato cores with Nature Seal™ and found that ascorbic acid delayed browning more effectively when applied in edible coating than in aqueous solution. Depending on coating formulation, appearance of fruit can be affected positively or negatively by selected coating. For instance, candelilla wax gives a natural, non coated appearance to apples, whereas shellac or carnauba coating (when in contact with water) will give whitish color to apples (Bai, *et al.* 2003).

Preserve Flavor

Consumers may buy the commodity based on its appearance when first purchased, but if the flavor is not acceptable, they will avoid buying the product a second time. Flavor can be preserved or modified with edible films or coatings by two different means: (1) as a barrier to aroma volatiles, and (2) as a carrier of flavors. Baldwin, *et al.* (1999) found that a polysaccharide coating worked as a barrier to aroma volatiles on whole mango. Edible coatings can also modify internal atmosphere of the commodity, causing low oxygen and high carbon dioxide concentration. This is not beneficial to flavor, since it could lead to a decrease in production of characteristic flavor compounds (Fellman, *et al.* 2003). Some works have even suggested the possibility that edible coatings on cut fruits can supply fruits with volatile precursors (Olivas *et al.* 2003). Pear wedges coated with a methylcellulose-stearic acid formulation contained higher amounts of hexyl acetate throughout storage, probably due to synthesis in wounded tissue from the stearic acid contained in the coating (Olivas, *et al.* 2003). Higher production of hexanol was observed in apples coated with alginate-linoleic acid.

Minimization of Microbial Contamination

In case of minimally-processed fruits and vegetables, where natural protection (skin) has been eliminated, opportunity for microorganisms to invade and grow on the surface of the fruit is present. Incorporating antimicrobial compounds into edible films or coatings will preserve quality of fresh-cut fruits and vegetables. Since antimicrobials are needed just on the surface of the product, their application as part of a coating will help minimize antimicrobial usage. Retention of antimicrobial compounds on coated produce surface will depend on coating attributes (composition, hydrophilic characteristics and manufacturing procedure) and type (pH and water activity), as well as storage conditions (temperature and duration) (Cagri, *et al.* 2004). Antimicrobials most commonly used include potassium sorbate, sodium benzoate, sorbic acid, benzoic acid and propionic acid; other natural antimicrobials such as lemongrass, oregano oil and vanillin have also been used (Rojas-Grau, *et al.* 2007) .

Antimicrobial Food Additives

A wide variety of antimicrobials have been added to edible films and coatings to control microbiological growth and extend produce shelf-life. Antimicrobials used for the formulation of edible films and coatings must be classified as food-grade additives or compounds generally recognized as safe (GRAS) by the relevant regulations. International regulatory agencies are in charge of approving antimicrobials for the use on foods. In the European Union (EU), those compounds are regulated by the EU Framework Directive 89/107 (EU, 1989) and in the United States (US) by the part 21CFR172 enacted by the US Food and Drug Administration (US FDA 2009). Table 1 shows antimicrobial agents used on edible films and coatings and their code numbers for food additives approved by the EU (E-Code) or the regulation numbers established by the US FDA (RegNum).

ANTIMICROBIAL SYNTHETIC CHEMICAL AGENTS

Organic acids are the most common synthetic antimicrobial agents and include acetic, benzoic, citric, fumaric, lactic, malic, propionic, sorbic, succinic, and tartaric acid, among others. These acids typically inhibit the outgrowth of bacterial and fungal cells. Potassium sorbate and sodium benzoate are the two organic acid salts more widely used as antimicrobial food additives. Benzoic acid is also called phenyl-formic acid or benzene-carboxylic acid. The antimicrobial activity of benzoic acid and SB is related to pH, and the most effective are the undissociated forms. Therefore, the use of these preservatives has been limited to those products that are acid in nature (Chipley, 2005). Sorbic acid is a straight-chain unsaturated fatty acid. The carboxyl group of sorbic acid is highly reactive with calcium, sodium or potassium, and results in the formation of various salts and esters (Stopforth, *et al.* 2005b). PS, the most soluble form of sorbate is well known for its potent antifungal activity. Major mold species inhibited by PS belong to the genera *Alternaria, Penicillium*, and others. Propionic acid is a naturally-occurring monocarboxylic acid. Salts of the acid have a slight cheese like flavor. The antimicrobial activity of propionate salts is pH dependent, being also more effective at low pH because of the higher activity of the undissociated form. Propionic acid is primarily inhibitory to molds; however, some yeasts and bacteria have also been satisfactorily controlled (Doores, 2005).

Parabens are the alkyl esters of *para*-hydroxybenzoic acid. The alkyl chain length of parabens determines their water solubility. The shorter the alkyl chain length, the higher the water solubility of parabens. Parabens are inhibitory to either several gram-positive and gram-negative bacteria or molds, although fungi are generally more susceptible to parabens than bacteria (Davidson 2005). For both bacteria and fungi, the inhibitory activity generally increases as the alkyl chain length of parabens also increases. The optimum pH for effective antimicrobial activity of parabens is in the range 3.0–8.0.

NATURAL ANTIMICROBIAL AGENTS

Chitosan

Chitosan is a high-molecular-weight cationic polysaccharide composed of (1→4)-linked 2-acetamido-2-deoxy- β -D-glucopyranosyl and 2-amino- 2-deoxy- β-D-glucopyranosyl units (Sebti et al. 2005), and

Table 1. Antimicrobial compounds used on edible films and coatings

Food Preservatives			
Chemical Compounds	**E-Code[a]**	**Natural Compounds**	**E-Code/Reg.Num[b]**
Organic acids		*Polypeptides*	
Acetic		Lysozyme	E-1105
Benzoic	E-210	Peroxidase	____
Citric	E-330	Lactoperoxidase	____
Lactic	E-270	Lactoferrin	____
Malic	E-296	Nisin	E-234
Propionic	E-280	Natamycin	E-235
Tartaric	E-334		
Organic acid salts		*Plant extract esessential oils, spices*	
Sodium acetate	E-262(I)	Cinnamon	182.10
Sodium diacetate	E-262(II)	Capsicum	182.10
Sodium benzoate	E-211	Lemongrass	182.20
Sodium citrate	E-331(I)	Oregano	182.10
Sodium formate	E-237	Rosemary	182.20
Calcium formate	E-238	Garlic	184.1317
Sodium L-lactate	E-325	Vanilla	182.10
Sodium propionate	E-281	Carvacrol	172.515
Calcium propionate	E-282	Citral	182.60
Potassium sorbate	E-202	Cinnamaldehyde	182.60
Sodium L-tartrate	E-335(I)	Vanillin Grape seed extracts	182.60 ____
Parabens			
Methyl paraben	E-218		
Ethyl paraben	E-214		
Propyl paraben	E-216		
Sodium salt of methyl paraben	E-219		
Sodium salt of ethyl paraben	E-215		
Sodium salt of propyl paraben	E-217		
Mineral salts			
Sodium bicarbonate	E-500(I)		
Ammonium bicarbonate	E-237		
Sodium bicarbonate	E-500(II)		
Others			
EDTA-$CaNa_2$[c]	E-385		

Silvia, *et al.* (2011)

[a]E-Code = code number for food additives approved by the European Union.

[b]RegNum = Regulation number in Title 21 of the U.S. Code of Federal Regulations where the chemical appears.

cEDTA-CaNa2 = disodium calcium ethylenediaminetetraacetate.

produces transparent films. Chitosan is not water-soluble, so a coating solution comprised of weak organic acid (acetic acid) must be used. Chitosan has been shown to be a natural food preservative, though the antimicrobial mechanism involved is not well elucidated.

It is believed that positively charged chitosan molecules interact with negatively charged microbial cell membranes, causing change in microbial cell permeability that leads to leakage of cell constituents (No, *et al.* 2007). Chitosan films or coatings can increase shelf life and preserve quality of fruits and vegetables by decreasing respiration rates, inhibiting microbial development and delaying ripening. They have been used on fruits and vegetables with good results, showing antimicrobial activity against *Bacillus cereus, Brochothrix thermosphacta, Lactobacillus curvatus, Lactobacillus sakey, Listeria monocytogenes, Pediococcus acidilactici, Photobacterium phosphoreum, Pseudomona fluorescens, Candida lambica, Cryptococcus humiculus,* and *Botrytis cinerea* (Devlieghere, *et al.* 2004 ; Romanazzi, *et al.* 2002). Chitosan is considered ideal coating for fruits and vegetables, mainly because it can form a good film on the commodity's surface and can control microbial growth (Muzzarelli 1986; No, *et al.* 2007).

Nisin

Nisin is a small antimicrobial peptide produced by lactic acid bacteria; it inhibits gram positive bacteria such as *L. monocytogenes* and *Staphylococcus aureus* and gram negative bacteria, when the bacteria cell wall was previously weakened by a permeabilising agent such as EDTA or lysozime. Nisin is generally recognized as safe and is permitted for use in over 50 countries (Thomas & Delves- Broughtonmedia 2005; Ko, *et al.* (2001) found that nisin in whey protein films was more effective in reducing *Listeria* growth than in wheat gluten films, suggesting that antilisterial activity of nisin was enhanced in hydrophobic films. Also, a greater inhibitory activity against *Listeria* was verified under acidic conditions. The commented results demonstrated that nisin effectiveness is strongly dependent on system characteristics and environmental conditions.

Natamycin

Natamycin is a tetraene polyene macrolide. It is a natural antifungal agent produced by *Streptomyces natalensis*. Natamycin has no effect on bacteria, but it is active against nearly all molds and yeasts. Natamycin is usually applied as a surface treatment for hard cheese and dry or ripened sausages.

Lactoperoxidase

The lactoperoxidase system (LPS) is a natural antimicrobial present in milk and in mammalians saliva and tears. It presents a broad antimicrobial spectrum since it shows bactericidal effect on gram (–) bacteria, bacteriostatic effect on gram (+) bacteria, and antifungal activity (Naidu 2000). The LPS system consists of three components: LPS, thiocyanate, and hydrogen peroxide (H_2O_2). The enzyme catalyzes the oxidation of thiocyanate (SCN–) by the use of H_2O_2 and produces hypothiocyanite (OSCN–) and hypothiocyanous acid (HOSCN). These products inhibit microorganisms by the oxidation of sulphydryl (–SH) groups in their enzyme systems and proteins (Seifu, *et al.* 2005). From another point of view, the incorporation of the LPS to alginate films did not modify significantly the mechanical and barrier properties of evaluated films (Yener, *et al.* 2009). However, in a whey protein film, incorporation of LPS promoted a significant reduction in elastic modulus and in tensile strength when LPS concentration was equal to or higher than 0.15 g of LPS per gram of film (Min, *et al.* 2005).

Lactoferrin

Lactoferrin is an iron-binding, bioactive glycoprotein of the transferrin family that contributes to the control of iron in biological fluids. Lactoferrin inhibits microorganisms by binding iron and making it unavailable for microbial development (Stopforth, *et al.* 2005a).

Lysozyme

Lysozyme is an enzyme comprising 129 amino acids crosslinked by disulfide bonds (Cagri, *et al.* 2004). Lysozyme exhibits antimicrobial activity against vegetative cells of a wide variety of organisms, including numerous food borne pathogens and spoilage microorganisms. Gram-negative bacteria are generally less sensitive than Gram-positive bacteria to lysozyme, mainly as a result of protection of the cell wall by the outer membrane (Johnson and Larson 2005). The rate of cell catalysis by lysozyme depends upon the pH of the medium, showing a bell-shape with a maximum at pH 5.0 and inflections at pH 3.8 and 6.7 (Naidu 2003).

Plant and Herbs Essential Oils

Essential oils (EOs) are aromatic oily liquids obtained from individual or integrated plant material: flowers, buds, seeds, leaves, twigs, bark, herbs, wood, fruits, and roots (Burt 2004). EOs are commonly obtained by steam distillation of plants. Chemical composition of EOs is complex and strongly dependent on the part of the plant considered (e.g., seed vs. leaves), the moment of the harvest (before, during, or after flowering), the harvesting season and the geographical sources. Major components in EOs are phenolic substances, which are thought as the responsible of the antimicrobial properties, and many of them are classified as GRAS. However, it has been reported that other minor components have a critical influence in the antimicrobial and antioxidant activity, acting synergistically with other components (Zheng, *et al.* 2009). There is abundant scientific evidence in relation to the effectiveness of EOs fractions of many spices and herbs and their components as antimicrobial, antifungal, and antiviral compounds (Burt 2004; Valero & Francs 2006; Hoque, *et al.* 2006, Hoque, *et al.* 2008; Taniya, *et al.* 2016). Examples of such plants are cassia, clove, garlic, cinnamon, sage, oregano, pimento, thyme, rosemary, lemongrass, scutellaria, and forsythia suspense. The antimicrobial activity of the EOs can be attributed to their content of monoterpenes that, due to their lipophilic character, act by disrupting the integrity of microbial cytoplasmic membrane, which thus loses its high impermeability for protons and bigger ions. Lipophilic compounds accumulate in the lipid bilayer according to its specific partition coefficient, leading to disruption of the membrane structure (Zhang, *et al.* 2009). Then, membrane functions are compromised, not only as a barrier but also as a matrix for enzymes and as an energy transducer (Liolios, *et al.* 2009). Some disadvantages of EOs are their biological and chemical instability, reduced solubility in water and poor distribution to target sites.

ANTIMICROBIAL EDIBLE COMPOSITE COATINGS APPLIED TO FRUITS AND VEGETABLES

Antimicrobial edible films and coatings can potentially serve as active food packaging materials by altering permeability of a product to water vapor and oxygen, as well as by minimizing growth of surface contaminants during refrigerated storage, providing an alternative to post process pasteurization for inactivation of surface contaminants.

Some of the more commonly used preservatives and antimicrobials in edible films and coatings include benzoates, proprionates, sorbates, parabens, acidifying agents (e.g., acetic and lactic acids), curing agents (e.g., sodium chloride and sodium nitrite) bacteriocins, and natural preservatives (e.g., natural oils, lysozyme, liquid smoke) (Cagri, *et al.* 2004). Antifungal compounds, organic acids, potassium sorbate, or the bacteriocin, nisin, were reported to be more effective in reducing levels of food borne microorganisms when immobilized or incorporated into edible gels (i.e. starch, carrageenan, waxes, cellulose ethers, or alginate). Incorporation of essential oils has also been investigated in production of antimicrobial edible films and coatings. Although antimicrobial properties of essential oils have been recognized for centuries, there has been renewed interest in their use because of consumer demand for natural ingredients and additives. Table 2 summarizes relevant applications of an antimicrobial external edible films or coatings to prevent microbial spoilage.

EFFECT OF EDIBLE COATINGS ON SENSORY QUALITY

Thick coating on fruits and vegetables surface becomes an undesirable barrier between the external and internal atmosphere and restricts exchange of respiratory gases (CO_2 and O_2) (Cisneros-Zevallos & Krochta, 2003). This may result in anaerobic respiration, which produces much more carbon dioxide, acetaldehyde and ethanol. The acetaldehyde and ethanol result in fermentation and give off-flavor to the product, which are detrimental to the perceived quality. It is therefore necessary to adjust the thickness of the wax coat according to the variety and storage and marketing temperatures. Park, *et al.* (1994) reported that tomatoes coated with 2.6 mm zein film produced alcohol and off-flavors internally which is due to low oxygen and high carbon dioxide concentration. Smith, *et al.* (1987) summarized that use of coatings results disorders like core flush, flesh breakdown, accumulation of ethanol, and alcoholic off-flavors, which is due to modification of internal atmosphere. Edible coatings are usually consumed with the coated products. Therefore, the incorporation of compounds such as antimicrobials, antioxidants and nutraceuticals should not affect consumer acceptance. Some authors have indicated that the incorporation of antimicrobial agents into edible coatings could impart undesirable sensorial modifications in foods, especially when EOs are used (Burt 2004). Sometimes the incorporation of certain anti-browning agents into edible coatings can yield an unpleasant odor, particularly when high concentrations of sulfur-containing compounds such as N-acetylcysteine and glutathione are used as dipping agents (Richard, *et al.* 1992; Iyidogan & Bayindirli 2004; Rojas-Grau, *et al.* 2006). Not many studies have been reported on the sensory characteristics of coated fruits when nutraceutical ingredients are incorporated. The addition of nutraceutical compounds to edible coatings may impart bitter taste, astringent or off-flavor (Drewnowski & Gomez-Carneros 2000) that can lead to rejection of the product by consumers (Le Clair 2000).

Table 2. Application of antimicrobial edible films and coatings to improve the quality of fruits and vegetables

Hydrocolloid	Antimicrobial	Fruit/Vegetable	Effect	Reference
Starch/chitosan	Chitosan	Carrot slices	Inhibition of total viable count, lactic acid bacteria, psicrotrophic total coliforms and yeast and moldduring storage at 10 °C	Durango, *et al.* 2006
Cassava starch	Potassium sorbate	Pumpkin cylinders	Aerobic mesophiles, lactic acid bacteria, yeasts, and molds growth was prevented	Garcia, *et al.* 2008
Starch or MC/ HPMC	Propolis extract	Fresh noodle	Total microorganism count was reduced during 4 weeks at 10 °C	Kim, *et al.* 2005
Alginate	Potassium sorbate	Potato cylinders	Initial microbial load was decrease during refrigerated storage at 5 °C	Mitrakas, *et al.* 2008
Chitosan Casein CMC	Chitosan	Butternut squash	Coating reduced the counts of mesophilic aerobic bacteria	Moreira *et al.*2009
Chitosan, carboxymethyl cellulose, and Casein	Natural plant extracts	Butternut	Coatings enriched with rosemary and olive oleoresins produced a slight antimicrobial effect against native microflora and Listeria monocytogenes	Ponce, *et al.* 2008
Alginate	Cinnamon, palmarosa, and lemongrass	Fresh-cut melon	Native flora growth and S. enteritidis population was reduced extending shelf life by more than 21 days	Raybaudi-Massilia, *et al.* 2008
Agar-agar	Chitosan and acetic acid	Garlic	Filamentous fungi and aerobic mesophilic were inhibited during 6 days storage, at 25 °C	Robson, *et al.* 2008
Chitosan	Chitosan	Carrots slices	Native microbial populations were maintained very low	Simoes, *et al.* 2009
Hydroxypropyl methylcellulose-lipid	Organic acid salts, parabens	Mandarins	Antifungal action of the coatings was fungistatic rather than fungicidal	Valencia-Chamorro, *et al.* 2009
Chitosan/cassava starch/ gelatin	Chitosan	Mango slices	Inhibition of Botryodiplodia theobromae was reduced on fruit surface was observed	Zhong and Xia 2008

EFFECT OF EDIBLE COATINGS ON NUTRITIONAL ASPECTS

Edible films and coatings can affect nutritional quality of fruits and vegetables. They can be used as carriers of nutrients. On the other hand, they can produce abiotic stress, which could modify metabolism of the commodity, affecting production of nutrients. Some works have determined effects of coatings on nutritional quality, and on phenolics and other phytochemicals. Han, *et al.* (2004) found higher amounts of vitamin E and calcium on strawberries coated with chitosan, containing calcium and vitamin E in the formulation, due to diffusion of these nutrients into the fruit. Romanazi, *et al.* (2002) observed an increase in phenylalanine ammonia–lyase activity, a key enzyme for synthesis of phenolic compounds, on grapes coated with chitosan. Edible coatings have also been used as carriers of probiotics. *Bacillus lactis* was maintained for 10 days on fresh-cut fruits under refrigeration, when applied on alginate- and gellan based edible coatings (Tapia, *et al.* 2007).

LEGISLATION RELATED TO EDIBLE FILMS AND COATINGS

Edible films supporting antimicrobials can be considered as an active film. Definitions stated in Regulation 1935/2004/ EC and in Regulation 450/2009/EC consider that "active materials and articles are intended to extend the shelf life or to maintain or improve the condition of packaged food". They are designed to deliberately incorporate components that would release or absorb substances into or from the packaged food or the environment surrounding the food (Restuccia, *et al.* 2010). According to legislation and labeling in the USA, edible coatings and films are considered part of the food; as a consequence, their ingredients must comply with the Code of Federal Regulations and be declared on the label under the Federal Food, Drug, and Cosmetic Act (Franssen & Krochta 2003). The EU considers that an edible film is a special active part of the food and, seen from a legal point of view, it is to be regarded as a foodstuff, along with the food packed in the film, having to fulfill the general requirements for food (Fabec, *et al.* 2000). According to Rojas-Grau, *et al.* (2009), another important issue within regulatory status is the presence of allergens because many edible films and coatings are made with or can contain ingredients that could cause allergic reactions such as wheat protein (gluten) or peanut protein. Therefore, the presence of a known allergen on a film or coating on a food must be also clearly stated in the label.

CONCLUSION

Antimicrobial edible films and coatings are used for improving the shelf life of food products without impairing consumer acceptability. They are designed as a stress factor in order to prevent surface contamination and/or providing a gradual release of the active substance. The edible film formulation proposed must be adapted in order to ensure a content of the food that nisin accordance with maximum values allowed by food legislation of the country of application. Characteristics of edible films depend greatly on hydrocolloid used. Polysaccharides rend transparent and homogeneous edible films with moderate mechanical properties. However, the application of these films is limited by their water solubility and poor water vapor permeability. Protein based films could have impressive gas barrier properties and mechanical properties compared with those prepared from polysaccharides; however, the poor water vapor resistance limits their application. To solve this shortcoming, the blending with different biopolymers, the addition of hydrophobic materials such as oils or waxes or chemical and/or enzymatic modification of polymer can be performed. There is a trend to select the antimicrobials from natural sources and to use generally recognized as safe (GRAS) compounds so as to satisfy consumer demands for healthy foods free of chemical additives. The more commonly antimicrobials used are organic acids, the polysaccharide chitosan, some polypeptides as nisin, the system, and some plant extracts and its essential oils among others. It must be remarked that the release of the from a film or coating exerts a great influence on its effectiveness. As a consequence, the evaluation of the rate of release together with the evaluation of antimicrobial activity through the time will help to optimize the development of films and coatings for lengthening the shelf life of food products.

CHALLENGES AND FUTURE RESEARCH

Most work in this area has dealt with changes in quality due to application of coating. But very less work has been done to identify the relationship between the internal atmosphere caused by the coating and velocity of physiological ripening processes, such as respiration, tissue softening, metabolic reactions, production of metabolites and secondary compounds generated during storage.

To preserve quality of fruits by means of decreasing oxygen in the internal atmosphere, special care should be taken not to minimize oxygen concentration to a point where anaerobic respiration may occur. Thus, for each fruit, it is necessary to know the optimum oxygen concentration at which rate of consumption is minimized without promoting development of anaerobic respiration. Future research should be focused on the following aspects:

- Properties of coating solution: composition, concentration, viscosity and density
- Properties of film: mechanical, gas and vapor barrier properties
- Properties of coating: thickness, temperature, and atmospheric conditions
- Properties of the produce (fresh or minimally-processed): respiration rate, water activity, composition, etc.
- Variation in chemical and physical conditions (e.g., pH, temperature, time, etc.) could affect these properties.
- To understand possible changes to properties of a film when chemical and physical conditions are modified, simulating likely events a commodity could face during actual handling and storage.
- Study of metabolic reactions occurring within commodities and the extent to which they can be modified with coatings.
- Study of internal gas composition of coated commodities and relationships between internal atmosphere and velocity of physiological ripening processes, such as respiration, metabolic reactions and production of secondary compounds during storage.
- To study of impact of coatings on quality and shelf life of commodities, taking into account all possible conditions they could face during handling and storage.
- Determination of optimal methods of applying coatings most conducive to obtaining high quality product at lowest possible cost.
- Study of consumer acceptability of coatings.
- Study of impact of edible coatings on final cost of commodities.
- Studies should focus on commercial viability of edible film and coating technology for fruits and vegetables.

REFERENCES

Bai, J., Hagenmaier, R. D., & Baldwin, E. A. (2003). Coating selection for "Delicious" and other apples. *Postharvest Biology and Technology*, *28*(3), 381–390. doi:10.1016/S0925-5214(02)00201-6

Baldwin, E. A., Burns, J. K., Kazokas, W., Brecht, J. K., Hagenmaier, R. D., Bender, R. J., & Pesis, D. E. (1999). Effect of two edible coatings with different permeability characteristics on mango (*Mangifera indica* L.) ripening during storage. *Postharvest Biology and Technology*, *17*(3), 215–226. doi:10.1016/S0925-5214(99)00053-8

Burt, S. (2004). Essential oils: Their antibacterial properties and potential applications in foods—A review. *International Journal of Food Microbiology*, *94*(3), 223–253. doi:10.1016/j.ijfoodmicro.2004.03.022 PMID:15246235

Cagri, A., Ustunol, Z., & Ryser, E. T. (2004). Antimicrobial edible films and coatings. *Journal of Food Protection*, *67*(4), 833–848. PMID:15083740

Chanes, & Arias, P. (Eds.). (2008). *Food Engineering: Integrated Approaches*. New York: Springer.

Chipley, J. (2005). Sodium benzoate and benzoic acid. In P. M. Davidson, J. N. Sofos, & A. L. Branen (Eds.), *Antimicrobials in Food* (pp. 11–48). Boca Raton, FL: CRC Press.

Cisneros-Zevallos, L., & Krochta, J. M. (2003). Dependence of coating thickness on viscosity of coating solution applied to fruits and vegetables by dipping method. *Journal of Food Science*, *68*(2), 503–510. doi:10.1111/j.1365-2621.2003.tb05702.x

Davidson, P. M. (2005). Parabens. In P. M. Davidson, J. N. Sofos, & A. L. Branen (Eds.), *Antimicrobials in Foods* (pp. 291–303). Boca Raton, FL: CRC Press.

Debeufort, F., Quezada-Gallo, J. A., & Voilley, A. (1998). Edible films and coatings: Tomorrow's packaging: A review. *Critical Reviews in Food Science and Nutrition*, *38*(4), 299–313. doi:10.1080/10408699891274219 PMID:9626488

Devlieghere, F., Vermeulen, A., & Debevere, J. (2004). Chitosan: Antimicrobial activity, interactions with food components and applicability as a coating on fruit and vegetables. *Food Microbiology*, *21*(6), 703–714. doi:10.1016/j.fm.2004.02.008

Doores, S. (1993). Organic acids. In Antimicrobials in Food (pp. 95–136). Marcel Dekker, Inc.

Drewnowski, A., & Gomez-Carneros, C. (2000). Bitter taste, phytonutrients and the consumer: A review. *Amarican journal of Clinical. Nutrition (Burbank, Los Angeles County, Calif.)*, *72*, 1424–1435.

Fabec, B., Hellstrom, T., Henrysdotter, G., Hjulmand-Lassen, M., Nilsson, J., Rudinger, L., . . . Tuomala, V. (2000). *Active and intelligent food Packaging. A Nordic report on the legislative aspects*. Retrieved from www.norden.org/ pub/ebook/2000-584.pdf

Fellman, J. K., Rudell, D. R., Mattinson, D. S., & Mattheis, J. P. (2003). Relationship of harvest maturity to Flavor regeneratin after CA storage of 'Delicious' apples. *Postharvest Biology and Technology*, *27*(1), 39–51. doi:10.1016/S0925-5214(02)00193-X

Franssen, L. R., & Krochta, J. M. (2003). Edible Coatings containing natural antimicrobials for processed foods. In S. Roller (Ed.), Naturals antimicrobials for the minimal processing of foods (pp. 120-132). Boca Raton, FL: CRC Press. doi:10.1533/9781855737037.250

Garcia, E., & Barret, D. M. (2002). Preservative treatments for fresh cut fruits and vegetables. In O. Lamikanra (Ed.), *Fresh-Cut Fruits and Vegetables* (pp. 267–304). Boca Raton, FL: CRC Press.

Guilbert, S. (1986). Technology and application of edible protective films. In M. Mathlouthi (Ed.), *Food packaging and preservation: Theory and practice* (pp. 371–393). London: Elsevier Applied Science Publishing Co.

Hagenmaier, R. D., & Shaw, P. E. (1990). Moisture permeability of edible films made with fatty acid and (hydroxypropyl) methylcellulose. *Journal of Agricultural and Food Chemistry*, *38*(9), 1799–1803. doi:10.1021/jf00099a004

Han, C., Zhao, Y., Leonard, S. W., & Traber, M. G. (2004). Edible coatings to improve storability and enhance nutritional value of fresh and frozen strawberries *Fragaria ananassa*) and raspberries (*Rubus ideaus*). *Postharvest Biology and Technology*, *33*(1), 67–78. doi:10.1016/j.postharvbio.2004.01.008

Hernandez-Munoz, P., Almenar, E., Ocio, M. J., & Gavara, R. (2006). Effect of calcium dips and chitosan coatings on postharvest life of strawberries (Fragaria × Ananassa). *Postharvest Biology and Technology*, *39*(3), 247–253. doi:10.1016/j.postharvbio.2005.11.006

Hoque, M. M., Bari, I. M. L., Inatsu, Y., & Kawamoto, S. (2006). Antibacterial activity of some Asian Spices and Herbs against Selected Potent Food Borne Pathogens and Spoilage Bacteria. In *Proceeding of the Japan-Bangladesh Joint International Conference on Microbiology Education and the Prospect of Japanese Collaboration in Education and Research* (*vol. 2*, pp. 22-30). Academic Press.

Hoque, M. M., Bari, I. M. L., Vijay, Y. K. J., & Kawampto, S. (2008). Antibacterial activity of cloves and cinnamon extracts against food borne pathogens and spoilage bacteria and inactivation of *Listeria monocytogenes* in ground chicken meat with their essential oils. *Rep. Natural Food Researh*, *72*, 9–21.

Iyidogan, N. F., & Bayindirli, A. (2004). Effect of L-cysteine, kojic acid and 4- hexylresorcinol combination on inhibition of enzymatic browning in Amasya apple juice. *Journal of Food Engineering*, *62*(3), 299–304. doi:10.1016/S0260-8774(03)00243-7

Johnson, E. A., & Larson, A. E. (2005). Lysozyme. In M. P. Davidson, J. N. Sofos, & A. L. Branen (Eds.), *Antimicrobials in Food* (pp. 361–387). Boca Raton, FL: CRC Press.

Kader, A. A. (1986). Biochemical and physiological basis for effects of controlled and modified atmospheres on fruits and vegetables. *Food Technology*, *40*(5), 99–104.

Kays, S. J. (1999). Preharvest factors affecting appearance. *Postharvest Biology and Technology*, *15*(3), 233–247. doi:10.1016/S0925-5214(98)00088-X

Kays, S. J., & Paull, R. E. (2004). Stress in harvested products. In Postharvest Biology (pp. 355-414). Athens, GA: Exon Press.

Ko, S., Janes, M. E., Hettiarachchy, N. S., & Johnson, M. G. (2001). Physical and chemical properties of edible films containing nisin and their action against Listeria monocytogenes. *Journal of Food Science*, *66*(7), 1006–1011. doi:10.1111/j.1365-2621.2001.tb08226.x

Krochta, J. M., & Mulder-Johnston, C. D. (1997). Edible and biodegradable polymer films: Challenges and opportunities. *Food Technology*, *51*, 61–74.

LeClair, K. (2000). Breaking the sensory barrier for functional foods. *Food Product Design*, *7*, 59–63.

Liolios, C. C., Gortzi, O., Lalas, S., Tsaknis, J., & Chinou, I. (2009). Liposomal incorporation of carvacrol and thymol isolated from the essential oil of *Origanum dictamnus* L. and in vitro antimicrobial activity. *Food Chemistry*, *112*(1), 77–83. doi:10.1016/j.foodchem.2008.05.060

Min, S., Harris, L., & Krochta, J. (2005). Antimicrobial effects of lactoferrin, lysozyme, and the lactoperoxidase system and edible whey protein films incorporating the lactoperoxidase system against Salmonella enterica and *Eschericchia coli* O157:H7. *Journal of Food Science*, *70*(7), 332–338. doi:10.1111/j.1365-2621.2005.tb11476.x

Moreira, M. R., Ponce, A., Del Valle, C. E., & Roura, S. I. (2009). Edible coatings on fresh squash slices: Effect of film drying temperature on the nutritional and microbiological quality. *Journal of Food Processing and Preservation*, *33*, 226–236. doi:10.1111/j.1745-4549.2008.00295.x

Muzzarelli, R. A. A. (1986). Filmogenic properties of chitin/chitosan. In R. A. A. Muzzarelli, C. Jeuniaux, & G. W. Gooday (Eds.), *Chitin in Nature and Technology* (pp. 389–396). New York: Plenum Press. doi:10.1007/978-1-4613-2167-5_48

Naidu, A. S. (2000). Lactoferrin, lactoperoxidase. In Natural food antimicrobial systems (pp. 17–132). New York: CRC Press.

No, H. K., Meyers, S. P., Prinyawiwatkul, W., & Xu, Z. (2007). Applications of chitosan for improvement of quality and shelf life of Foods: A Review. *Journal of Food Science*, *72*(5), 87–100. doi:10.1111/j.1750-3841.2007.00383.x PMID:17995743

Olivas, G. I., & Barbosa-Canovas, G. V. (2005). Edible coatings for fresh cut fruits. *Critical Reviews in Food Science and Nutrition*, *45*(7-8), 657–670. doi:10.1080/10408690490911837 PMID:16371333

Olivas, G. I., Mattinson, D. S., & Barbosa-Canovas, G. V. (2007). Alginate coatings for preservation of minimally processed "Gala" apples. *Postharvest Biology and Technology*, *45*(1), 89–96. doi:10.1016/j.postharvbio.2006.11.018

Olivas, G. I., Rodriguez, J. J., & Barbosa-Cánovas, G. V. (2003). Edible coatings composed of methylcellulose stearic acid, and additives to preserve quality of pear wedges. *Journal of Food Processing and Preservation*, *27*(4), 299–320. doi:10.1111/j.1745-4549.2003.tb00519.x

Park, H. J., Chinnan, M. S., & Shewfelt, R. L. (1994). Edible corn-zein film coatings to extend storage life of tomatoes. *J. Food Process*, *18*(4), 317–331. doi:10.1111/j.1745-4549.1994.tb00255.x

Restuccia, D., & Spizzirri, U.G., Parisi, O.I., Cirillo, G., Curcio, M., Iemma, F., Puoci, F., … Picci, N. (2010). New EU regulation aspects and global market of active and intelligent packaging for food industry applications. *Food Control*.

Richard, F. C., Goupy, P. M., & Nicolas, J. J. (1992). Cysteine as an inhibitor of enzymatic browning. 2. Kinetic studies. *Journal of Agricultural and Food Chemistry*, *40*(11), 2108–2114. doi:10.1021/jf00023a014

Rojas-Grau, M., Raybaudi-Massilia, R. M., Soliva-Fortuny, R. C., Avena-Bustillos, R. J., McHugh, T. H., & Martín-Belloso, O. (2007). Apple puree-alginate edible coating as carrier of antimicrobial agents to prolong shelf-life of fresh-cut apples. *Postharvest Biology and Technology*, *45*(2), 254–264. doi:10.1016/j.postharvbio.2007.01.017

Rojas-Grau, M. A., Sobrino-Lopez, A., Tapia, M. S., & Martın-Belloso, O. (2006). Browning inhibition in fresh-cut 'Fuji' apple slices by natural anti-browning agents. *Journal of Food Science*, *71*(1), S59–S65. doi:10.1111/j.1365-2621.2006.tb12407.x

Rojas-Grau, M. A., Soliva-Fortuny, R., & Martin-Belloso, O. (2009). Edible coatings to incorporate active ingredients to fresh cut fruits: A review. *Trends in Food Science & Technology*, *20*(10), 438–447. doi:10.1016/j.tifs.2009.05.002

Romanazzi, G., Nigro, F., Ippolito, A., Di Venere, D., & Salerno, M. (2002). Effects of pre- and post-harvest chitosan treatments to control storage grey mold of table grapes. *Journal of Food Science*, *67*(5), 1862–1867. doi:10.1111/j.1365-2621.2002.tb08737.x

Rooney, M. L. (1995). Active packaging in polymer films. In *Active Food Packaging* (pp. 74–110). Glasgow, UK: Blackie Academic & Professional. doi:10.1007/978-1-4615-2175-4_4

Sebti, I., Martial-Gros, A., Carnet-Pantiez, A., Grelier, S., & Coma, V. (2005). Chitosan polymer as bioactive coating and film against *Aspergillus niger* contamination. *Journal of Food Science*, *70*(2), 100–104. doi:10.1111/j.1365-2621.2005.tb07098.x

Seifu, E., Buys, E. M., & Donkin, E. F. (2005). Significance of the lactoperoxidase system in the dairy industry and its potential applications: A review. *Trends in Food Science & Technology*, *16*(4), 1–18. doi:10.1016/j.tifs.2004.11.002

Silvia, A., Valencia-Chamorro, L., Palou, L., Miguel, A., Del R´Io, L., & Mari, A B. (2011). Antimicrobial Edible Films & Coatings for Fresh and Minimally Processed Fruits And Vegetables: A Review. *Critical Reviews in Food Science & Nutrition*, *51*, 872–900.

Smith, S., Geeson, J., & Stow, J. (1987). Production of modified atmospheres in deciduous fruits by the use of films and coatings. *Horticulture Science*, *22*, 772–776.

Sothornvit, R., & Krochta, J. M. (2000). Oxygen permeability and mechanical properties of films from hydrolyzed whey protein. *Journal of Agricultural and Food Chemistry*, *48*(9), 3913–3916. doi:10.1021/jf000161m PMID:10995290

Stopforth, J. D., Skandamis, P. N., Davidson, P. M., & Sofos, J. N. (2005a). Naturally ocurring compounds: Animal sources. In Antimicrobials in Food (pp. 453–505). Boca Raton, FL: CRC Press.

Stopforth, J. D., Sofos, J. N., & Busta, F. F. (2005b). Sorbic acid and sorbates. In Antimicrobials in Food (pp. 49–90). Boca Raton, FL: CRC Press.

Taniya, A. J., Kabir, Y., & Hoque, M. M. (2015). *Occurrence of emerging food borne pathogens in common fast foods and inactivation of pathogens with essential oil.* (Unpublished M. Phil Dissertation). University of Dhaka, Bangladesh.

Tapia, M., Rojas-Grau, M., Rodriguez, F., Ramirez, J., Carmona, A., & Martin-Belloso, O. (2007). Alginate- and gellan-based edible films for probiotic coatings on fresh-cut fruits. *Journal of Food Science*, *72*(4), 190–196. doi:10.1111/j.1750-3841.2007.00318.x PMID:17995771

Thomas, L. V., & Delves-Broughton, J. (2005). Nisin. In P. M. Davidson, J. N. Sofos, & A. L. Branen (Eds.), *Antimicrobials in Food* (pp. 237–274). Boca Raton, FL: CRC Press.

Valero, M., & Frances, E. (2006). Synergistic bactericidal effect of carvacrol, cinnamaldehyde or thymol and refrigeration to inhibit Bacillus cereus in carrot broth. *Food Microbiology*, *23*(1), 68–73. doi:10.1016/j.fm.2005.01.016 PMID:16942988

Vermeiren, L., Devlieghere, F., Beest, M., de Kruijf, N., & Debevere, J. (1999). Developments in the active packaging of foods. *Trends in Food Science & Technology*, *10*(3), 77–86. doi:10.1016/S0924-2244(99)00032-1

Yener, F. Y. G., Korel, F., & Yemenicioglu, A. (2009). Antimicrobial activity of lactoperoxidase system into crosslinked alginate films. *Journal of Food Science*, *74*(2), 73–79. doi:10.1111/j.1750-3841.2009.01057.x PMID:19323761

Zhang, H., Kong, B., Xiong, Y. L., & Sun, X. (2009). Antimicrobial activities of spice extracts against pathogenic and spoilage bacteria in modified atmosphere packaged fresh pork and vacuum packaged ham slices stored at 4°C. *Meat Science*, *8*(4), 686–692. doi:10.1016/j.meatsci.2008.11.011 PMID:20416570

Chapter 15
Traditional African Foods and Their Potential to Contribute to Health and Nutrition:
Traditional African Foods

John H. Muyonga
Makerere University, Uganda

Ilona Steenkamp
Stellenbosch University, South Africa

Sophie Nansereko
Makerere University, Uganda

Marena Manley
Stellenbosch University, South Africa

Judith Kanensi Okoth
Jomo Kenyatta University of Agriculture and Technology, Kenya

ABSTRACT

The nutritional state of large segments of the African population remains alarming despite the positive socio-economic development that is taking place. The most significant nutritional problems include undernutrition, iron deficiency and vitamin A deficiency. Malnutrition and deficiencies also exacerbate a number of other diseases and health conditions. Besides undernutrition, the prevalence of overnutrition and obesity on the African continent are rising, as are the associated health conditions such as diabetes and coronary heart diseases. This chapter outlines the unique nutritional and bioactive properties of Traditional African Foods (TAFs) and their potential to contribute to the alleviation of undernutrition, overnutrition and associated health problems. Special emphasis is placed on vegetables, fruits, cereals, edible insects, small fish species, mushrooms, legumes, sesame, tuber and root crops. Some of the identified health benefits of these TAFs include lowering of serum cholesterol, anti-carcinogenic, anti-diabetic and anti-inflammatory, cardiovascular disease prevention and anti-hypertensive properties.

DOI: 10.4018/978-1-5225-0591-4.ch015

INTRODUCTION

The traditional African diet has always been rather unique, as it comprises a wide variety of African crops and food products, prepared using traditional African methods that are generally not consumed in other parts of the world. However, significant dietary changes are taking place, not only in Africa, but in most developing countries, resulting in substantial changes in the traditional diets of large segments of the population. The impact of the "Western" influence on the traditional African diet is growing rapidly and many elements of African diets have already been replaced by more convenient and conventional alternatives. Against the backdrop of malnutrition and nutrient deficiencies that are still widespread throughout Africa, the question is whether these shifts in dietary patterns are beneficial or detrimental to the general health status of the African population. To answer this question, the nature of these dietary changes and their associated health implications are analysed, followed by a review of the nutritional value and functional benefits of various traditional African foods. Food safety aspects related to dietary changes as well as constraints limiting the consumption of traditional African foods are also reviewed.

BACKGROUND

Dietary Changes in Africa

Over the last decades it has been observed that significant dietary changes are taking place in developing countries at an ever-increasing rate. The general pattern seems to be a transition towards a more "westernized" diet at the expense of traditional diets and common staples. The changes include a reduction in the intake of traditional cereals, complex carbohydrates, vegetables and fibre, with an increased consumption of energy dense foods containing higher levels of saturated fats, added sugars and salt (Uusitalo et al., 2002; Stamoulis et al., 2004). The traditional African diet was largely plant-based, comprising various small grain cereals, mainly millet and sorghum, dark green leafy vegetables, tropical fruits, legumes, starchy stems and root tubers. Animal products that dominated African diets included fish, fermented milk, and to a small extent game meat, poultry, beef and mutton. One of the most evident dietary shifts has been the significant increase in maize, rice and wheat consumption, replacing the traditional staple cereals and roots and tubers (Uusitalo et al., 2002; Lopriore & Muehlhoff, 2003). Introduced vegetables and fruits, e.g. cabbage and oranges, have largely replaced traditional ones and general consumption of fruits and vegetables seem to be on the decline. A number of contributing factors that have played a part in such dietary shifts include higher levels of income, demographic changes, urbanization and an increase in the spread of supermarkets, and thereby an increase in the availability of convenient and affordable prepared or semi-prepared foods (Stamoulis et al., 2004). Consequently, there is a decrease in the consumption of traditional foods, which mostly require time- and labour-intensive home-based preparation. Such changes in diets can give rise to an increased incidence of diet-related non-communicable diseases resulting from a high intake of fats, sugars and salt, and a sedentary lifestyle. Some developing countries are already experiencing a rise in these chronic diet-related diseases associated with dietary changes (Stamoulis et al., 2004). Such diseases include cardiovascular disorders, various forms of cancer, diabetes, hypertension, obesity and osteoporosis (Uusitalo et al., 2002). This places a double burden on the African healthcare system, since under-nutrition and micronutrient deficiencies, as well as problems related to obesity and overnutrition need to be addressed.

Malnutrition and Disease Burden in Africa

Malnutrition is still a major problem in Africa and the continent's progress towards its eradication is slowest in comparison with other regions. The African continent claims the highest level of prevalence of undernourishment, currently at 20.5%, and although Sub-Saharan Africa accounts for only 12.5% of the world population, 26.6% of undernutrition cases are found in this region (FAO et al., 2014). Micronutrient deficiencies are wide-spread and the World Health Organisation estimates for prevalence of iron deficiency (67.6% among pre-school children and 57.1% among women of child bearing age), vitamin A deficiency (44.4% among school age children, 13.5% among women of child bearing age), and iodine deficiency (42.3% among children aged 6-12 years, 42.6% among entire population) on the continent reveal unacceptably high levels (WHO, 2004; 2008; 2009). Iron deficiency anaemia not only has a negative impact on child development, but also increases risk of maternal mortality, perinatal mortality and malaria associated morbidity and mortality (Stoltzfus et al., 2004). Vitamin A deficiency, the global leading cause of blindness, has been linked to increased maternal mortality and higher child mortality from measles, diarrhoea and malaria (Rice et al., 2004), whereas zinc deficiency (with a prevalence of 37-62% in Central and Southern Africa) has been shown to increase the incidence of diarrhoeal disease, malaria and pneumonia and mortality from these conditions among children less than 5 years old (Caulifield & Black, 2004).

Undernutrition acts as an underlying factor of mortality for about half of children whose lives are claimed by the most prevalent diseases of low income countries, which include acute respiratory infections, diarrhoea, measles, malaria, HIV and perinatal cases (Rice et al., 2000). Malnutrition has been shown to increase morbidity and mortality from common ailments, as the effect of diseases is exacerbated and immune systems are weakened. Addressing the issue of malnutrition is therefore essential for public health improvement in Africa.

Health issues arising from overnutrition are placing additional pressure on public health in Africa. The prevalence of obesity and overnutrition on the continent is on the rise, having jumped from 18% in 1980 to 30% in 2008 (Finucane et al., 2011). Many countries have even reached the point where the number of overweight cases has surpassed that of underweight cases. It can therefore be expected that the dominant health threat in Africa will shift from infectious diseases and diseases related to malnutrition, to non-communicable diseases associated with obesity and overnutrition. Furthermore, evidence has indicated that childhood undernutrition increases the risk of adult obesity (Fung, 2009), suggesting that the potential magnitude of the burden of overnutrition could be greater than expected, especially against the backdrop of underdeveloped healthcare systems and disproportionately high healthcare costs in comparison to incomes. Currently the capacity to effectively manage non-communicable chronic diseases in Africa is rather low, and prospects for raising this capacity in the near future are bleak. Maintenance of healthy diets in order to prevent rather than treat such chronic diseases would naturally be the most economical and reasonable option for the continent.

In light of the critical role foods play in health and nutrition, the nutritional and nutraceutical properties of traditional African foods are reviewed to analyse their potential of contributing to the sustenance of nutrition and health for Africa's population.

TRADITIONAL AFRICAN FOOD PRODUCTS AND THEIR NUTRITIONAL VALUE

Description of the Main Groups of Traditional African Foods

1. Traditional African Vegetables (TAVs)

A large variety of vegetables have always formed an important part of the traditional African diet as they represent inexpensive, high-quality nutrition sources for the poorer population segments (MacCalla, 1994; Abukutsa-Onyango, 2003; ICRAF, 2004; Odhav et al., 2007). Most of these vegetables, many of which are green leafy vegetables, grow readily in African soil under harsh conditions, and often do not require formal cultivation. Several of these traditional vegetables have long been known to exhibit health-protecting properties and have been used for generations for their prophylactic and therapeutic effects (Smith & Eyzaguirre, 2007). A number of publications have emphasised the outstanding nutritional value of many of these vegetables (Nesamvuni et al., 2001; Steyn et al., 2001; Jansen van Rensburg et al., 2004), concluding that they may be key in the fight against malnutrition and micronutrient deficiencies on the African continent. It has even been found that some TAVs are superior to introduced vegetables like spinach (*Spanacia oleracea*), kale (*Brassica oleracea var. acephala*) and cabbage (*Brassica oleracea var. capitata*) with regard to nutritional value (Orech et al., 2007). Amaranth and pumpkin leaves, for instance, contain higher levels of the carotenoids compared to most of the introduced vegetables (Tiwari & Cummins, 2013).

Numerous studies on a number of different TAVs have shown that they are good sources of fibre, minerals, vitamins and bioactive phytochemicals (Odhav et al., 2007; Uusiku et al., 2010; Kamga et al., 2013; Hamzah et al., 2013; Oulai et al., 2014b). Table 1 shows a number of TAVs that are good sources of iron, zinc, calcium or vitamin A. Considering the high prevalence of iron and vitamin A deficiencies in Africa, the great value of such vegetables in prevention of such deficiencies becomes apparent.

Their nutritional value is not the only benefit of such traditional vegetables. A number of studies have reported health effects and medicinal properties of certain African vegetables (Table 2). Such health benefits are linked to a range of bioactive compounds, such as polyphenols, carotenoids, glucosinolates, alkaloids, betalains and vitamin E (Tiwari & Cummins, 2013). Phenolic compounds are also responsible for the high level of antioxidant activity that is associated with many vegetables (Andabati & Muyonga, 2014). Numerous studies have analysed the antioxidant activities of various African vegetables, as reviewed by Hamzah et al. (2013). Some TAVs, reported to exhibit high antioxidant activities, include *Portulaca olecae* and *Justicia flavia* from South Africa (Odhav et al., 2007), *Solanum nigrum, Acalypha bipartite, Corchorusolitorius* L.,*Acalypha bipartite, Ipomeaeriocarpa, Corchorustrilocularis* and *Ocimum suave* from Uganda (Andabati & Muyonga, 2014) and *Pterocarpus mildbraedi* and *Sesasum radiatum* from Nigeria (Hamzah et al., 2014). Stangeland *et al.* (2009) showed that vegetables make an important contribution to the antioxidant activity of meals consumed in different parts of Uganda. The level of bioactive compounds and the antioxidant activity of meals is also affected by preparation methods used (Uusiku et al., 2010; Mwanri et al, 2011; Olumakaiye, 2011; Tumwet et al, 2013; Oulai et al., 2014a).

Generally, consumption of traditional African vegetables seems an effective means of preventing and protecting against a variety of diseases associated with oxidative stress, for example cardiovascular diseases, diabetes, inflammatory diseases, cancer other adverse consequences of nutrition in transition (Hamzah et al., 2013; Johns and Sthapit, 2004).

Table 1. Some traditional African vegetables that are good sources of iron, zinc, calcium or vitamin A

Scientific Name	English Name	Source of	Concentration	Country	Reference
Adansonia digitata	Baobab	Iron	38.4 mg/100g	CóteD'Ivoire	Oulai et al. (2014b)
Amaranthus (species not specified)	Amaranth leaves	Iron	45.8 mg/100g	Kenya	Kunyanga et al. (2013)
Amaranthus cruetus	Amaranth leaves	Iron	50.8 mg/100g	Ghana	Kwenin et al. (2011)
Ceiba patendra	Kapok tree	Iron	80 mg/100g	CóteD'Ivoire	Oulai et al. (2014b)
Solanum nigrum	Black nightshade	Iron	85 mg/100g	South Africa	Odhav et al. (2007)
Vigna unguculata	Cowpea	Iron	48.5 mg/100	CóteD'Ivoire	Oulai et al. (2014b)
Chenopodium album	Fat hen	Zinc	109 mg/100g	South Africa	Odhav et al. (2007)
Amaranthus hybridus	Cockscomb	Calcium	2363 mg/100g	South Africa	Odhav et al. (2007)
Ama ranthus spinosus	Spiny pigweed	Calcium	3931 mg/100g	South Africa	Odhav et al. (2007)
Asystasia gangetica	Hunter's spinach	Calcium	2566 mg/100g	South Africa	Odhav et al. (2007)
Cleome monophylla	Spindle-pod	Calcium	3203 mg/100g	South Africa	Odhav et al. (2007)
Cucumis metuliferus	Jelly melon	Calcium	2974 mg/100g	South Africa	Odhav et al. (2007)
Justicia flava	Yellow justicia	Calcium	2073 mg/100g	South Africa	Odhav et al. (2007)
Momordica balsamina	Balsam apple	Calcium	2688 mg/100g	South Africa	Odhav et al. (2007)
Senna occidentalis	Coffee senna	Calcium	2230 mg/100g	South Africa	Odhav et al. (2007)
Telfaria accidentalis	Fluted pumpkin	Vitamin A	610 IU	Nigeria	Olaiya & Adebisi, (2009)
Basella alba	Malabar spinach	Vitamin A	8100 IU	Nigeria	Olaiya & Adebisi (2009)
Manihot esculenta	Cassava leaves	Beta carotene	1970 µg vit A equivalents/100g	Western, Central, Eastern and Southern Africa	Uusiku et al. (2010)

2. Traditional African Fruits

Like vegetables, fruits are good sources of health promoting phytochemicals (Tiwari & Cummins, 2013). Some of the African traditional fruits with nutritional and economic potential include jackfruit (*Artocarpusheterophyllus*), sumac (*Rhusnatalensis*), guava (*Psidium guajava*), tamarind (*Tamarindusindica*), bush mango (*Irvingia gabonensis),* African plum (*Dacryodes edulis),* bitter cola (*Garcinia kola*) and white star apple (*Chrysophyllum albidum)* (Abukutsa-Onyango, 2011). Guava is a good source of both minerals (iron, calcium, phosphorus) as well as vitamins (vitamin C, pantothenic acid, vitamin A, niacin). In fact, its vitamin C content is four times that of an orange (Hamzah et al., 2013). Both the seed and the pulp of tamarind fruit have been shown to contain high levels of phenolics and to exhibit high antioxidant activity (Andabati & Muyonga, 2014). Tamarind is traditionally used in Uganda and Nigeria for treatment of a number of ailments, including measles, abdominal pain, diarrhoea and dysentery, malaria and fever (Table 2, Andabati & Muyonga, 2014; Bhadoriya et al., 2011). The African bread fruit (*Treculia africana*) has been found to contain high levels of zinc (8.5mg/100g) and substantial levels of flavonoids, polyphenols, anthraquinones, saponins and glycosides (Osabor et al., 2009). African elemi (*Canariumscheinfurthii*) and pomegranate (*Punicagranatum*) have also been reported to have very high antioxidant activities, much higher than those of conventional fruits (Stangeland et al., 2009). The fruit

Table 2. Reported medicinal properties of traditional African fruits and vegetables

Scientific Name	Common Name	Ascribed Medicinal Value	Country	Reference
*Adansonia digitata*L	Baobab	Anti-asthmatic, antihistamine and anti-tension properties Leaves used to treat insect bites, guinea worm and internal pains, dysentery, diseases of the urinary tract, opthalmia and otitis Used medicinally as a diaphoretic, an astringent, an expectorant and as a prophylactic against fever Show antiviral activity against influenza virus, herpes simplex virus and respiratory syncytial virus and polio	Nigeria,Kenya, Mali, Senegal	Hamzah et al. (2013)
Amaranthus cruentus	Blood amaranth, red amaranth, purple amaranth	Tapeworm, expellant, relief of respiratory disease	Nigeria	Mensah et al. (2008)
Basellarubra	Climbing Ceylon spinach, Red vine spinach, Spinach vine	Fertility enhancement in women	Nigeria	Mensah et al. (2008)
Celosia argentea	Plumed cockscomb, or the silver cock's comb	Diuretic, cough, diarrhoea	Nigeria	Mensah et al. (2008)
Cleome rutidosperma	Fringed spider flower	Ear cure for inflammation Anti-helminthic and carminative	Nigeria	Edeoga et al. (2005)
Corchorusolitorius (Linn).	Jute mallow	Treatment of gonorrhoea, pain, fever and tumour Treating iron deficiency, folic acid deficiency, anaemia Leaves act as blood purifier and against heart troubles and to restore appetite and strength Leaves used for treatment of ascites, pains, piles, tumours, gonorrhoea and fever	Egypt, Sudan, Ghana, Nigeria and Sierra Leone	Hamzah et al. (2013)
Corchorustrilocularis L.	Threeloculecorchorus	Improves heart health, and reduces blood sugar	Uganda	Andabati (2014)
Gnetnumafricanum	Eru	Treatment of enlarged spleen, sore throat and as a cathartic Provides relief from nausea and neutralizes poison Applied externally to manage boils and warts; used to reduce child birth pain	Cameroon, Gabon, Congo, Angola, Nigeria	Hamzah et al. (2013)
Gongronemalatifolium	Amaranth globe	Cough, intestinal worms, dysentery, dyspepsia and malaria. Taken as a tonic to treat loss of appetite, colic, stomach-ache diabetes and high blood pressure Controlling weight gain in lactating women and overall health management Asthma patients chew fresh leaves to relieve wheezing	Sierra Leone Senegal and Ghana	Hamzah et al. (2013)
Hibiscus sabdariffa	Roselle	Treats blood pressure, after effect of drunkenness, coughs, feet cracks and boils, sores on camels, dysuria, mild cases of dyspepsia and debility	West Africa	Shei (2008)
Ipomeaeriocarpa R.Br	Morning glory	Headache, ulcers, diabetes	Uganda	Andabati (2014)
Moringa oleifera	Moringa, drumstick tree	Diabetes	Senegal	Mathieu & Meissa, (2007)

continued on following page

Table 2. Continued

Scientific Name	Common Name	Ascribed Medicinal Value	Country	Reference
Ocimumgratissimum	Clove Basil, African Basil	Upper respiratory tract infection, diarrhoea, headache, skin disease, pneumonia, fever, and conjunctivitis	Nigeria	Hamzah et al.(2013)
Piper guineense	West African black pepper	Stomach ache, gonorrhoea, and fertility enhancement in women	Nigeria	Mensah et al.(2008)
Piper umbellatum	Cow-foot leaf, wild pepper	Stomach ache, edema, malaria, urinary and kidney problems, venereal infections, menstrual and stomach problems Used in treatment of wounds and inflamed tumours The root is diuretic, stimulant and promotes the flow of bile	Nigeria	Nwauzoma et al. (2013), Mensah et al. (2008)
Solanumaethiopicum L.	Ethiopian nightshade	Hypertension, poor eye sight	Uganda	Andabati (2014)
Solanumanguivi Lam	African eggplant	Hypertension, ulcers, diabetes, low breast milk secretion, malaria	Uganda	Andabati (2014)
Solanumnigrum L.	Black night-shade	Heart burn, inflamed throats, eye inflammations, ringworm, ulcers, testicular swelling, gout and ear pains, convulsions, insomnia, antiseptic and anti-dysenteric	Uganda, Cameroon, Ghana, Kenya,Madagascar, Nigeria	Andabati (2014)
Talinumtriangulare	Waterleaf Philippine spinach, Ceylon spinach	Diuretic, gastro-intestinal disorder	Nigeria	Mensah et al. (2008)
Tamarindusindica L	Tamarind	Measles, abdominal pain, diarrhoea and dysentery, helminthes infections, wound healing, malaria and fever, constipation, inflammation, cell cytotoxicity, gonorrhoea, and eye diseases	Uganda Nigeria	Andabati, (2014) Bhadoriya et al. (2011)
*Telfairiaoccidentalis*Hook f.	Fluted pumpkin	Convulsion, gastrointestinal disorders, malaria, anaemia, liver damage	Benin, Nigeria and Cameroon	Hamzah et al. (2013), Kayode & Kayode, (2010)
Vernoniaamygdalina	Bitter leaf	Antihelminthic, antimalarial, cough remedy and as a laxative, aids post-partum uterine contraction, induces lactation and controls postpartum haemorrhage	Guinea, Ghana Malawi and Uganda	Hamzah et al.(2013)
Vignaunguiculata L.	Cowpea	Hypertension, diabetes, **prevent vitamin deficiency and malnutrition**	Uganda	Andabati (2014), Mathieu & Meissa, (2007)

of the African baobab is said to exhibit antioxidant activity and be an excellent source of vitamin; with levels as high as ten times that of orange fruits (Bamalli et al, 2014).

The coconut fruit is the source of three different products, namely coconut water, coconut oil and coconut flour. Coconut water is gaining popularity in the world, and has been considered to be a 'natural sports drink' which is rich in sugars, amino acids and some aromatic compounds (Prades et al, 2012). It also contains cytokins with anticancer and antithrombotic activities as well as peptides with antibiotic activity (Prades et al, 2012). Virgin coconut oil is of nutraceutical value due to the presence of medium chain fatty acids and polyphenols which contribute to reduced weight gain, anti-inflammatory and antiatherogenic activities (Babu et al, 2014). Coconut flour is rich in dietary fiber and contributes to reduction in serum triglycerides and low density lipoporotein (LDL) cholesterol.

3. Traditional African Cereals

Cereals have formed the basis of African diets for centuries, and a number of these traditional staples are still consumed in large quantities in different parts of the continent. These include mainly sorghum (*Sorghum bicolor*), pearl millet (*Pennisetum glaucum*), finger millet (*Eleucine corocana*), teff (*Eragrostis tef*), fonio (*Digitaria spp*) and African rice (*Oryza glaberrima*). However, introduced cereals like maize, rice and wheat are starting to replace the traditional African cereals (TACs) to a large extent, resulting in a decrease in both their production and consumption (FAOSTAT, 2013). Worldwide production of sorghum and millet is minuscule compared to that of the major cereals and reflects the contribution of Africa to global cereal production. Africa generates 100%, 42% and 51% of the total production of fonio, sorghum and millet, respectively, whereas the contribution towards maize, rice and wheat production lies at 7%, 4% and 4%, respectively. These data reveal the high relative importance of the traditional cereals to Africa, showing that these crops are still major sources of energy, protein, vitamins and minerals for millions of the poorest people in Africa. Also, traditional cereals have a high agronomic resilience and can be grown in semi-arid areas and marginal soils, which increases their significance in terms of food security in Africa (FAO, 1995).

A comparison of the nutritional information between TACs and the major cereals indicates that these African cereals generally have better nutritional profiles. Protein content of TACs depends on the type of cereal, but tends to be higher than that of the major cereals (FAO, 2010). Also, compared to rice, maize and refined wheat, the proteins of TACs generally have higher proportions of lysine, which is the most limiting essential amino acid among cereals (Lukmanji et al., 2008). Fonio, which has been named one of the most nutritious of all grains, is rich in important amino acids (e.g. methionine and cystine) not present in wheat, rice or maize (Stone et al., 2011). Finger millet has also been considered to be superior to wheat in terms of its protein digestibility (Stone et al., 2011). Compared to maize (3.2-4.1 mg/100g), rice (0.7-2.5 mg/100g) and wheat (2 mg/100g), finger millet (10-20.7 mg/100g), pearl millet (97.6-20.9 mg/100g), fonio (9.4-10 mg/100g) and sorghum (3.4-8.7 mg/100g) contain higher levels of iron (FAO, 2010), one of the minerals with high deficiency prevalence in Africa. Fonio and some sorghum and millet varieties are also excellent sources of calcium, whereas sorghum and millet are rich sources of B-complex vitamins (Obilana and Manyasa, 2002) while teff is high in calcium and iron (FAO, 2015; Gebremariam et al, 2012). Among the B-group vitamins, concentrations of thiamin, riboflavin and niacin in sorghum are comparable to those in maize.

Numerous studies on the health benefits of sorghum and millet have shown that these two cereals are good sources of health-promoting bioactive compounds, such as phenolic acids, flavonoids, condensed tannins, anthocyanins, phytosterols and policosanols (Taylor et al., 2014; Shahidi & Chandrasekara, 2013; Mathanghi & Sudha, 2012; Dykes & Rooney, 2006; Awika et al., 2005; Awika & Rooney, 2004). Such phytochemicals have been shown to exhibit antioxidant activity and bioactivity against several pathophysiological conditions (Shahidi &Chandrasekara, 2013). They have been found to lower serum cholesterol, inhibit cataracts and prevent cardiovascular disease, as well as having anti-carcinogenic, anti-diabetic, anti-inflammatory, and anti-hypertensive properties (Taylor et al., 2014; Dykes & Rooney, 2006). According to Borneo and Leon (2012), the main chemical components of whole grains with health enhancing properties are dietary fiber, inulin, beta-glucan, resistant starch, carotenoids, phenolics, tocotrienols, and tocopherols and these could aid in disease prevention of cardiovascular diseases and strokes, hypertension, metabolic syndrome, type 2 diabetes mellitus, obesity, as well as different forms of cancer. Sorghum and millet are usually consumed as whole grains compared to wheat and maize that undergo various milling degrees of extraction.

One of the major drawbacks of TACs is the relatively high level of tannins and phytates, which bind to proteins, carbohydrates and minerals, thereby reducing digestibility and bioavailability of these nutrients. Various methods of reducing such tannin binding can be used, some of which form part of traditional processing methods, for example decortication, fermentation and germination/malting (Dykes & Rooney, 2006; El Hag, 2013). However, it has been shown that such processes may lead to a reduction in antioxidant activity (Shahidi & Chandrasekara, 2013). Alternatively, through genetic modification sorghum and millet accessions with lower tannin and phytate levels can be produced, which would result in improved bioavailability and protein digestibility (Taylor et al., 2014).

Compared to the major cereals, TACs are also better adapted to growing in semi-arid regions because of their greater resistance to pests and diseases, shorter growing seasons, and their ability to grow in less fertile soils under conditions of heat and drought (FAO, 1995). Furthermore, TACs are less prone to rot and insect damage during storage, which is an important aspect in terms of food security for small scale farmers with largely inadequate storage facilities. It has also been shown that millet is less prone to mycotoxin contamination (unpublished data).

4. Edible Insects

Edible insects form a part of the traditional African diet of many African populations and up to 250 insect species are used as a food source in Africa, including caterpillars, ants, grasshoppers, locusts, crickets, termites, beetles and cicadas (Van Huis, 2003). It has been estimated that in Southern Africa alone about 9.5 billion caterpillars, worth approximately US$85 million, are harvested annually.

The nutritional composition of various insects has been analysed, indicating that edible insects generally represent rich sources of energy, protein, unsaturated fatty acids and micronutrients such as copper, iron, magnesium, manganese, phosphorus, selenium and zinc, as well as riboflavin, pantothenic, biotin and folic acids (FAO, 2013). The protein content of insects can range from 13% up to 77% (Xiaoming et al., 2010), which can make them a significant source of protein in the African diet, which is largely comprised of plant-based foods with low levels of protein. In some African countries 5 to10% of protein consumed is derived from edible insects (Ayieko & Ariaro, 2008). Furthermore, insect protein generally has a good balance of essential amino acids, which complements the amino acid intake of African staple diets that are often deficient in certain essential amino acids. Certain edible insects, like caterpillars and grasshoppers, also contain substantial levels of polyunsaturated fatty acids and health-promoting omega-3 fatty acids (Womeni et al., 2009). Edible grasshoppers (*Ruspolia differens*) consumed in East Africa, in addition to containing high levels of protein and fat, also supply substantial levels of macro minerals, especially potassium, as well as trace minerals, like iron, and various vitamins (Table 3). Evidently, these grasshoppers represent an excellent nutritional source that can be exploited in the fight

Table 3. Nutritional composition of East African grasshoppers (Ruspolia differens)

Nutrient	Green Grasshopper	Brown Grasshopper
Protein	37.1%	35.3%
Fat	48.2%	46.2%
Ash	2.8%	2.6%
Potassium	370.6 mg/100 g	259.7 mg/100 g
Phosphorus	140.9 mg/100 g	121.0 mg/100 g
Calcium	27.4 mg/100 g	24.5 mg/100 g
Iron	16.6 mg/100 g	13.0 mg/100 g
Zinc	17.3 mg/100 g	12.4 mg/100 g
Retinol	2.1 µg/g	2.8 µg/g
α-tocopherol	201.0 µg/g	152.0 µg/g
Riboflavin	1.2 mg/100 g	1.4 mg/100 g
Niacin	2.1 mg/100 g	2.4 mg/100 g

Source: Kinyuru at al. (2010)

against nutritional deficiencies on the African continent. The same is true for edible termites (e.g. *Macrotermes subhylanus, Pseudacanthotermes militaris, Macrotermes bellicosus* and *Pseudacanthotermes spinigertermite)*, which are frequently consumed in western Kenya, and are high in fat and protein, as well as iron and zinc (Kinyuru et al., 2013).

5. African Cichlid Fish Species

Fish consumption in sub-Saharan Africa is currently the lowest in the world (Kawarazuka, 2010). Nevertheless, in some African countries, fish is still an important source of protein. In Uganda, Nigeria, Cote d'Ivoire, Malawi, Cameroon and the Congo, fish contributes between 34% and 42% of the total animal protein consumption. In Sierra Leone this figure is as high as 75% (Kawarazuka, 2010).

African cichlid species, including *Rastrineobola argentea* (silver cyprinid) and *Haplochromines cichlids,* make an important contribution to the diets of poor people in Africa because they are relatively inexpensive and accessible. As they are eaten whole, small fish species generally have a higher concentration of many essential nutrients, including calcium, omega-3 fatty acids and vitamin A, iron and zinc (Kawarazuka, 2010; Kawarazuka N. & Be´ne´, C. 2010). This makes them a cost-effective choice for complementation of diets for the poor. *Rastrineobola argentea* has been shown to exhibit antioxidant properties (Mbatia et al., 2014). Small cichlid species are also good dietary sources of protein, especially for the poor. *Haplochromines cichlids* is traditionally used in Uganda for the management of measles, possibly because of its high vitamin A content (Magala-Nyago et al., 2005).

6. Mushrooms

A variety of mushrooms form part of the traditional African diet, and although little data is available on the composition of African mushrooms, it has been determined that mushrooms are good sources of protein, fibre and minerals (Mshandete & Cuff, 2007; Sadler, 2003). Mushrooms also contain various bioactive compounds, particularly polysaccharides and phenolics, which are associated with a wide variety of health effects, as reviewed by Hamzah et al. (2013). These include activity against diarrhoea, renal infections, epilepsy, headaches, colds, fever, cardiovascular diseases, high blood pressure and arthritis, as well as anti-oxidant, anti-mutagenic, anti-tumour, anti-cholesterol, anti-allergic, anti-aging, anti-viral, anti-fungal, anti-inflammatory and anti-diabetic activities. Oyetayo (2011) analysed the medicinal uses of 12 mushroom species in Nigeria that are used in the traditional treatment of various ailments, and found that some of the species exhibited significant anti-oxidant and anti-microbial properties. This was also the case for *Cantharellus cibarius*, a Nigerian mushroom species (Aina, 2012), whereas two species from Ghana (*Pheurotus tuber-regium* and *Termmitomyces robustus*) had a substantial protein content and antioxidant activity (Obodai et al., 2014). Another study on a mushroom grown in East Africa (*Termitomyces microcarpus*) showed that it exhibited hypolipidemic and hypoglycaemic properties (Nabubuya et al., 2010).

7. Sesame

Sesame is an oil seed which has been traditionally consumed in parts of Africa, in the form of spreads, as part of traditional sauces, or as snack-type popped grains, bars or balls. The continent is also responsible for a large part of the global production of sesame. Of the global annual production of 4,756,752 tonnes, 2,117,585 tonnes were produced in Africa, with the greatest contributing countries being Sudan (former), Tanzania, Ethiopia, Uganda and Nigeria (FAOSTAT, 2013).

Sesame is a rich source of protein and energy and also contains high levels of iron (14.56 mg/100 g) and zinc (7.75 mg/100 g), as well as phosphorous (629 mg/100 g) and magnesium (351 mg/100 g). Sesame oil, which makes up 47-49% of the seed (Bahkali et al., 1998), consists of *ca.* 50% unsaturated fatty acids, dominated by linoleic acid (Were et al., 2006). Sesame is important as a functional food, being rich in lignans such as sesamin, sesamolin, and sesaminol that are associated with high antioxidant activity and activity against physiological disorders such as hypertension, hypercholesterolemia, cancer and aging (Kanu et al, 2010).

8. Legumes

A number of legumes are traditionally consumed in Africa. Like other legumes traditional African legumes are not only good dietary sources of proteins but also confer agronomic advantages, as they are well adapted to the different soils and climatic conditions of Africa, in particular drought and low nutrients (Sprent et al., 2009). The consumption of legumes has been linked to a reduction in the risk of diabetes, obesity and coronary heart diseases (Bazzano et al., 2001).

African legumes include marama beans (*Tylosema esulantum*), cowpeas (*Vigna unguiculata* (L.) *Walp.*), groundnut beans (*Vigna subterranean*) and chick peas (*Cicer arietinum*). Marama beans, a perennial, tuberous, drought-resistant legume which grows in Southern Africa, have a protein content of 29-38% while also containing high levels of fibre (18.5-25.8%), vitamin E (21.4-67.1 α-tocopherol equivalents), zinc (12-40 mg/100 g) and iron (31-39 mg/100 g) (Holse et al., 2010). The cowpea is an important crop in Africa since an estimated 200 million people subsist on a diet comprised mainly of this legume (Stone et al., 2011). It therefore represents a major source of protein and nutrients for many African communities. It has also been found to improve the body's absorption and breakdown of other staple foods (Stone et al., 2011). Phenolic compounds in cowpeas have been shown to be potent antioxidant sources (Siddhuraju & Becker, 2007). Groundnut beans have high levels of methionine, which makes its essential amino acid content more complete than other legumes. It also has the highest concentration of soluble fibre, which has been linked to reduction of heart disease and cancer (Stone et al., 2011).

9. Roots and Tubers

Tuber and root crops, especially cassava, yams and sweet potatoes form an important component of diets in Africa. With respect to nutritional value the now less grown traditional African tuber crops, including wild yam species (*Dioscorea species*), African potato (*Plectranthus esculentus*), *Disa species, Habenaria walleri* and *Satyrium species,* are superior to the commonly grown roots and tuber crops like cassava (*Manihot esculenta*), potato (*Solarium tuberosome*) and sweet potato (*Ipomea batatas*) (Maliro, 2001). The African potato, for example, contains twice the protein of common potatoes, and is a rich source of calcium, vitamin A and iron (Stone et al., 2011).

Food Fermentations and Their Benefits

A wide variety of traditional fermented food and beverage products are produced throughout the African continent. The large variety of these products arises from the different types of raw materials that are used for fermentation. These include various cereals, dairy products, root/tuber products (e.g. cassava) and legumes, meat products and some fruit and vegetable products (Franz et al., 2014; Chelule et al., 2010a). The benefits of food fermentation have been well documented and reviewed (Mensah, 1997; Caplice & Fitzgerald, 1999; Anukam & Reid, 2009; Saranraj et al., 2013). Fermentation leads to flavour enhancement, an improvement in the nutritional quality and digestibility, and an extension of the shelf life of the fermented product (Chelule et al., 2010a). Fermentation is also an excellent means of improving food safety of certain products as it has been shown to lead to de-toxification of certain food substrates, as well as resulting in antibiotic and anti-diarrheal activities (Chelule et al., 2010a). Since fermentation is a low-cost way of reducing food spoilage and improving food safety it may be one of the most useful food processing technologies for the African continent. This is particularly important given the high prevalence of diarrheal diseases and their contribution to morbidity and mortality.

The most accepted and widely used type of fermentation used in African countries is lactic acid fermentation (Franz et al., 2014). One of the most significant advantages of lactic acid bacteria (LAB) involved in this fermentation process is their protective role against infection and colonization of pathogenic microorganisms in the digestive tract (Saranraj et al., 2013). It has been found that certain lactic acid bacteria also shorten periods of diarrhoea (Isolauri et al. 1991; Raza et al. 1995; Pochapin 2000; Saavedra 2000; Rosenfeldt et al. 2002). The regulation of intestinal disorders, and particularly diarrhoea, can be a very meaningful advantage of consumption of traditional African fermented foods, as 37% of childhood deaths in sub-Saharan Africa are caused by diarrhoea (Franz et al., 2014). A number of studies have indicated that the typical diet of African children, which is high in fibre and carbohydrates, selects for a highly diverse microbiota which protects against infection and inflammation (De Filippo et al., 2010; Grzeskowiak et al., 2012). Consumption of various fermented cereal and plant food products, such as millet porridge (Lei & Jakobsen, 2004), could therefore promote a beneficial microbiota in African children which would boost gut health and overall well-being. There is also evidence suggesting that certain probiotics could improve the general well-being of HIV patients by alleviating gastrointestinal symptoms and by improving the nutritional intake tolerance to antiretroviral treatment (Irvine et al., 2011). In addition to such intestinal effects, some lactic acid bacteria (LAB) are capable of producing bacteriocins, compounds that exhibit antibacterial activity. These substances may prevent the growth of harmful pathogens on the food substrate (Saranraj et al., 2013), thereby improving food safety of fermented, traditionally produced products. Anti-bacterial properties were observed for certain African fermented foods, such as Nigerian dairy products or West-African fermented cassava products (Anukam & Reid, 2009).

Fermentation has also been associated with detoxification of specific harmful compounds in certain food products. Cassava, for example, is a popular traditional staple food in many African countries. However, its shelf life after harvesting is rather short (Oyewole, 1997). Also, one of the food safety risks associated with this tuber-based product is the residual cyanide level that may still be present if the product is not adequately processed (Iwuoha & Eke, 1996; Iwuoha et al., 2013). Fermentation and processing of cassava into products such as fufu (fermented cassava paste) can significantly prolong its shelf life, while simultaneously acting as an effective, inexpensive means of naturally detoxifying cassava tubers (Oyewole, 1997; Chelule et al., 2010a; Iwuoha et al., 2013).

It has also been shown that LAB fermentation leads to detoxification of mycotoxins (Mokoena et al., 2005; Mokoena et al., 2006; Chelule et al., 2010b). Several physical and chemical methods for the removal of mycotoxins from foods have been suggested in literature. However, many of these methods affect the nutritive value and flavour of the food product, may have undesirable health effects or may be simply impractical or ineffective (Peltonen et al., 2000). The reduction of mycotoxins by probiotic LAB would therefore be an effective natural way of increasing food safety of products frequently contaminated with mycotoxins. A number of studies have shown that LAB can bind certain mutagens and carcinogens, including aflatoxins and fumonisins, thereby removing them from the food product and preventing the harmful effects associated with these toxins (Peltonen et al., 2000; Dalié et al., 2010). Chelule et al. (2010b), for example, have investigated the effect of lactic acid fermentation on the levels of mycotoxins in a traditional maize-based porridge and observed a drastic reduction of up to 100% of myctoxins following fermentation. In addition, LAB can prevent or limit the growth of mycotoxigenic moulds and thereby improve the shelf life of such fermented products (Dalié et al., 2010).

All of the above mentioned advantages of fermented products indicate that the potential benefits of various traditional African fermented food and beverage products could be manifold and meaningful in the context of African food security and food safety. A number of studies (Oyewole, 1997; Anukam & Reid, 2009; Franz et al., 2014) have pointed out that although there may be several traditional African products with probiotic potential, there is not yet enough scientific evidence to ascertain which products do indeed exhibit probiotic effects and to which extent. Furthermore, processing of traditional African fermented foods often takes place under variable conditions, which would lead to large differences in product quality and attributes. The type, load and mixture of microorganisms on such fermented foods could therefore vary widely, leading to large differences in probiotic potential. Literature agrees that much work remains to be done before the potential of traditional African fermented foods can be fully developed and the possible health-benefits of such products be fully utilized.

Safety Considerations Associated with Traditional African Foods

One of the greatest food-associated health threats that has emerged on the African continent is mycotoxin intoxication (Williams et al., 2004). It has been well substantiated that mycotoxin exposure throughout many African countries is alarmingly high, especially in countries which have a tropical climate with high ambient temperatures and relative humidity (Bankole & Adebanjo, 2003). The presence and levels of these secondary fungal metabolites on a variety of African food and beverage products has been a topic of interest that has received much attention, revealing that mycotoxins remain a major African food safety issue that urgently needs to be addressed.

The two mycotoxins that are of gravest concern on the African continent are aflatoxins and fumonisins, as they are widespread in major dietary staples (Wagacha & Muthomi, 2008). Maize and groundnuts have been shown to be the most frequently contaminated food products, as both are highly suitable substrates for mould growth (Bankole & Adebanjo, 2003). A recent study (Probst et al., 2014) found detectable levels of aflatoxins and/or fumonisins in maize samples from 18 sub-Saharan African countries; 47% and 49% of samples exceeded the US regulatory limits for aflatoxins and fumonisins, respectively. The greatest proportion of samples contaminated with aflatoxin concentrations of more than 100 µg/kg originated from Kenya. It was also in Kenya that the most severe case of an aflatoxin-poisoning outbreak took place in 2004, resulting in 317 case-patients and 125 deaths, followed by smaller outbreaks in the subsequent years (Wagacha & Muthomi, 2008). Numerous other studies have confirmed the presence of mycotoxins on maize in other African countries like Nigeria (Adetunji et al., 2014), South Africa (Chilaka et al., 2012), Senegal (Diedhiou et al., 2011), Zambia (Kankolongo et al., 2009), Tanzania and the Republic of Congo (Manjula et al., 2009).

Mycotoxins have also been found in a variety of other cereal-based products, including fermented African beverages like maize-based or sorghum-based traditional beer (Matumba et al., 2011; Matumba et al., 2014). Since a large proportion of Africans often consume large volumes of beer, mycotoxin intake may greatly exceed the maximum tolerable daily intake, even if the mycotoxin levels are relatively low.

A recent study tested for mycotoxins in traditional Nigerian maize- and sorghum-based beverages (Ezekiel et al., 2015). Twelve different mycotoxins were identified, but it was found that processing of these beverages significantly reduced the concentrations of mycotoxins so that the drinks were considered safe for consumption. The reduction of mycotoxin levels during processing was in line with the findings of various other authors (Fandohan et al., 2005; Inoue et al., 2013). Fandohan et al. (2005), for instance, have analysed the fate of aflatoxins in fermented and processed African maize-based products and found that processing resulted in a significant reduction of both aflatoxin and fumonisin by up to 93%. Such processing methods included steps such as simple sorting and washing of maize grains, crushing and dehulling. Fermentation and cooking steps did not significantly affect the level of toxins in the final maize products. Traditional processing of cereal-based food and beverages could therefore be an effective way of reducing exposure to mycotoxins through consumption of African food and beverage products.

Other frequently consumed African food commodities that have been associated with mycotoxin contamination include groundnuts/nuts and traditional nut-based products, soybeans (Abia et al., 2013; Ezekiel et al., 2013), yam and cassava chips (Bassa et al., 2001; Mestres et al., 2004; Bankole & Mabekoje, 2004; Wareing et al., 2001), melon seeds (Bankole et al., 2004) and peanut cake (Ezekiel et al., 2012). However, as mycotoxin contamination has been associated most frequently with maize and maize-based products, which are consumed in large quantities, the risk of mycotoxin contamination through maize-based products will far outweigh the risk associated with other traditional African food and beverage products. The dietary changes in Africa may therefore have resulted in an increase in mycotoxin exposure of certain segments of the population.

Constraints to Consumption of Traditional African Foods

During the course of socio-economic development, dietary changes are, to a large extent, inevitable and natural, and should not necessarily be prevented since not all changes in dietary patterns are detrimental. Nevertheless, the exclusion of traditional foods from the African diet would be tragic, as these foods have the potential to make a significant contribution to the nutritional wellbeing and food security of the people in Africa.

One of the constraints that may limit the consumption of TAFs is the fact that they are not readily available and that their supply is limited. This is an especially important factor in light of increasing levels of urbanisation and the continuous spread of supermarkets. Furthermore, knowledge on production and processing of TAFs is mostly passed from generation to generation by means of word of mouth. As increasing numbers of the younger generation resettle in urban areas, the knowledge transfer is interrupted, bringing an end to the traditional production and processing methods. In conjunction with this is the fact that word of mouth knowledge transfer will lead to products which are of inconsistent quality, since processing and preparation largely depends on the person completing these tasks. Product quality may thus differ from batch to batch, from family to family, and from community to community depending on the production and processing methods that were applied. This can be coupled to the lack of research on optimizing production and processing parameters of TAFs in order to improve product quality, consistency and safety. Such research could be of great value for the promotion of TAFs, as it would provide scientific production and processing guidelines. Research on improving seeds for African crops and guidelines for their production are also still lacking, which greatly reduces the potential value of such traditional crops.

Another major constraint is the fact that TAFs often require time- and labour intensive preparation before they can be consumed. Making TAFs available in more convenient forms could therefore be a key element in promoting their consumption. This has been attempted for specific African foods, such as *bushera*, a packaged fermented millet drink from Uganda, dry packaged dark leafy vegetables in Kenya, and preserved and packaged *Rastrineobolaargentea* fish in Uganda.

To an extent, TAFs are viewed by some as food for the poor, a perception which negatively affects their acceptability, especially among the youth (Taruvinga & Nengovhela, 2015). The negative perception is re-inforced by agricultural extension agents and researchers who consider some of the traditional African crops as weeds which need to be eliminated in order to foster productivity of conventional crops (Vorster et al., 2007; Taruvinga & Nengovhela, 2015).

SUGGESTIONS FOR PROMOTING UTILISATION OF TAFs

There is need for further research on the less studied TAFs, especially with respect to their functional properties to elucidate the link between their consumption and associated health benefits. Results from such studies would provide strong evidence for promotion of TAFs. There is also need to improve production technology and presentation of TAFs to fit in the modern food supply systems. Development of recipes for the utilisation of TAFs would also help promote consumption, especially among communities not exposed to the traditional cuisines.

CONCLUSION

Inevitable dietary changes, ignited by socio-economic transformation on the African continent, are changing the composition of traditional diets, resulting in a decrease in the consumption of traditional African foods and a concomitant increase in more conventional, and often nutritionally poor, food choices. These changes are paired with a detrimental impact on the general health of the population, as many TAFs are valuable sources of nutrients, often having superior nutritional profiles compared to conventional or introduced foods. Furthermore, a large number of TAFs have been associated with numerous functional properties that can prevent or treat a wide variety of ailments. TAFs therefore hold great potential, not only in the fight against malnutrition and deficiencies, but also in the prevention of health conditions, particularly those linked to overnutrition and obesity which are on the rise in Africa.

Various ways of promoting the consumption of TAFs must be implemented in order to prevent their complete loss from traditional African diets. To achieve this successfully would require the cooperation of policy makers, nutrition, food science, agriculture and health researchers, practitioners and entrepreneurs. Investment in the development and production of traditional African foods paves a way for tapping of their potential to contribute to the general health of the people in Africa through preventative measures, rather than treatment.

REFERENCES

Abia, W. A., Warth, B., Sulyok, M., Krska, R., Tchana, A. N., Njobeh, P. B., & Moundipa, P. F. et al. (2013). Determination of multi-mycotoxin occurrence in cereals, nuts and their products in Cameroon by liquid chromatography tandem mass spectrometry (LC-MS/MS). *Food Control*, *31*(2), 438–453. doi:10.1016/j.foodcont.2012.10.006

Abukutsa-Onyango, M. O. (2003). Unexploited potential of indigenous African vegetables in Western Kenya. *Maseno Journal of Education. Arts and Science*, *4*(2), 103–122.

Abukutsa-Onyango, M. O. (2011). *Researching African indigenous fruits and vegetables – Why?* Retrieved July 30, 2015 from http://knowledge.cta.int/Dossiers/Commodities/Fruits/Feature-articles/Researching-African-Indigenous-Fruits-and-Vegetables-Why

Adetunji, M., Atanda, O., Ezekiel, C. N., Sulyok, M., Warth, B., Beltrán, E., & Chilaka, C. A. et al. (2014). Fungal and bacterial metabolites of stored maize (*Zea mays,* L.) from five agro-ecological zones of Nigeria. *Mycotoxin Research*, *30*(2), 89–102. doi:10.1007/s12550-014-0194-2 PMID:24643458

Aina, D. A., Jonathan, S. G., Olawuyi, O. J., & Durowoju, B. M. (2012). Antioxidant, antimicrobial and phytochemical properties of alcoholic extracts of *Cantharellus cibarius* – a Nigerian mushroom. *New York Science Journal*, *5*, 114–120.

Andabati, A. (2014). *Nutraceutical potential of selected Ugandan traditional foods*. (Unpublished Master's Thesis). Makerere University, Uganda.

Andabati, A., & Muyonga, J. (2014). Phenolic content and antioxidant activity of selected Ugandan traditional medicinal foods. *African Journal of Food Science*, *8*(8), 427–434. doi:10.5897/AJFS2014.1136

Anukam, K. C., & Reid, G. (2009). African traditional fermented foods and probiotics. *Journal of Medicinal Food*, *12*(6), 1177–1184. doi:10.1089/jmf.2008.0163 PMID:20041769

Awika, J. M., McDonough, C. M., & Rooney, L. W. (2005). Decorticating sorghum to concentrate healthy phytochemicals. *Journal of Agricultural and Food Chemistry*, *53*(16), 6230–6234. doi:10.1021/jf0510384 PMID:16076098

Awika, J. M., & Rooney, L. W. (2004). Sorghum phytochemicals and their potential impact on human health. *Phytochemistry*, *65*(9), 1199–1221. doi:10.1016/j.phytochem.2004.04.001 PMID:15184005

Ayieko, M. A., & Ariaro, V. (2008). Consumption, indigeneous knowledge and cultural values of the lakefly species within the Lake Victoria region. *African Journal of Environmental Science and Technology*, *10*, 282–286.

Babu, A. S., Veluswami, S. K., Arena, R., Guazzi, M., & Lavie, C. J. (2014). Virgin coconut oil and its potential cardioprotective effects. *Postgraduate Medicine*, *126*(7), 76–83. doi:10.3810/pgm.2014.11.2835 PMID:25387216

Bahkali, A.H., Hussain, M.A., & Basahy, A.Y. (1998). Protein and oil composition of sesame seeds (*Sesamum indicum*, L.) grown in the Gizan area of Saudi Arabia. *International Journal of Food Sciences and Nutrition*, *49*, 409-414.

Bamalli, Z., Mohammed, A. S., Ghazali, H. M., & Karim, R. (2014). Baobab tree (*Adansonia digitata L*) parts: Nutrition, applications in food and uses in ethno-medicine – A Review. *Annals of Nutritional Disorders and Therapy*, *1*, 1011.

Bankole, S. A., & Adebanjo, A. (2003). Mycotoxins in food in West Africa: Current situation and possibilities of controlling it. *African Journal of Biotechnology*, *2*(9), 254–263. doi:10.5897/AJB2003.000-1053

Bankole, S. A., & Mabekoje, O. O. (2004). Mycoflora and occurrence of aflatoxin B1 in dried yam chips from markets in Ogun and Oyo States, Nigeria. *Mycopathologia*, *157*(1), 111–115. doi:10.1023/B:MYCO.0000012211.31618.18 PMID:15008353

Bankole, S. A., Ogunsanwo, B. M., & Mabekoje, O. O. (2004). Natural occurrence of moulds and aflatoxin B1 in melon seeds from markets in Nigeria. *Food and Chemical Toxicology*, *42*(8), 1309–1314. doi:10.1016/j.fct.2004.03.015 PMID:15207382

Bassa, S., Mestre, C., Hell, K., Vervia, P., & Cardwell, K. (2001). First report of aflatoxin in dried yam chips in Benin. *Plant Disease*, *85*(9), 1032. doi:10.1094/PDIS.2001.85.9.1032A

Bazzano, L., He, J., Ogden, L. G., Loria, C., Vuputuri, S., & Myers, L. et al.. (2001). Legume consumption and risk of coronary heart disease in US men and women. *Archives of Internal Medicine*, *161*(21), 2573–2578. doi:10.1001/archinte.161.21.2573 PMID:11718588

Bhadoriya, S. S., Ganeshpurkar, A., Narwaria, J., Rai, G., & Jain, A. P. (2011). *Tamarindus indica*: Extent of explored potential. *Pharmacognosy Review*, *5*(9), 73–81. doi:10.4103/0973-7847.79102 PMID:22096321

Borneo, R., & Leon, A.E. (2012). Whole grain cereals: functional components and health benefits. *Food and Function*, *3*, 110-119.

Caplice, E., & Fitzgerald, G. F. (1999). Food fermentations: Role of microorganisms in food production and preservation. *International Journal of Food Microbiology*, *50*(1-2), 131–149. doi:10.1016/S0168-1605(99)00082-3 PMID:10488849

Caulifield, L. E., & Black, R. E. (2004). Zinc Deficiency. In Comparative quantification of health risks: Global and regional burden of disease attributable to selected major risk factors (vol. 1, pp. 257-279). Geneva, Switzerland: World Health Organisation.

Chelule, P. K., Mbongwa, H. P., Carries, S., & Gqaleni, N. (2010b). Lactic acid fermentation improves the quality of amahewu, a traditional South African maize-based porridge. *Food Chemistry*, *122*(3), 656–661. doi:10.1016/j.foodchem.2010.03.026

Chelule, P. K., Mokoena, M. P., & Gqaleni, N. (2010a). Advantages of traditional lactic acid bacteria fermentation of food in Africa. In A. Méndez-Vilas (Ed.), *Current Research, Technology and Education Topics in Applied Microbiology and Microbial Biotechnology* (pp. 1160–1167). Badajoz: Formatex Research Center.

Chilaka, C. A., De Kock, S., Phoku, J. Z., Mwanza, M., Egbuta, M. A., & Dutton, M. F. (2012). Fungal and mycotoxin contamination of South African comercial maize. *Journal of Food Agriculture and Environment*, *10*, 296–303.

Dalié, D. K. D., Deschamps, A. M., & Richard-Forget, F. (2010). Lactic acid bacteria - Potential for control of mould growth and mycotoxins: A review. *Food Control*, *21*(4), 370–380. doi:10.1016/j.foodcont.2009.07.011

De Filippo, C., Cavalieri, D., Di Paola, M., Ramazzotti, M., Poullet, J. B., Massart, S., & Lionetti, P. et al. (2010). Impact of diet in shaping gut microbiota revealed by a comparative study in children from Europe and rural Africa. *Proceedings of the National Academy of Sciences of the United States of America*, *107*(33), 14691–14696. doi:10.1073/pnas.1005963107 PMID:20679230

Diedhiou, P. M., Bandyopadhyay, R., Atehnkeng, J., & Ojiambo, P. S. (2011). Aspergillus colonization and aflatoxin contamination of maize and sesame kernels in two agroecological zones in Senegal. *Journal of Phytopathology*, *159*(4), 268–275. doi:10.1111/j.1439-0434.2010.01761.x

Dykes, L., & Rooney, L. W. (2006). Sorghum and millet phenols and antioxidants. *Journal of Cereal Science*, *44*(3), 236–251. doi:10.1016/j.jcs.2006.06.007

Edeoga, H. O., Okwu, D. E., & Mbaebie, B. O. (2005). Phytochemical constituents of some Nigerian medicinal plants. *African Journal of Biotechnology*, *4*(7), 685–688. doi:10.5897/AJB2005.000-3127

El Hag, I. M. N., Ahmed, I. A. M., Ahmed, S. O., Eltayeb, M. M., & Babiker, E. E. (2013). Effect of processing methods on antinutritional factors, protein digestibility and minerals extractability of winter sorghum cultivars. *Australian Journal of Basic and Applied Sciences*, *7*(12), 229–237.

Ezekiel, C. N., Abia, W. A., Ogara, I. M., Sulyok, M., Warth, B., & Krska, R. (2015). Fate of mycotoxins in two popular traditional cereal-based beverages (*kunu-zaki and pito*) from rural Nigeria. *LWT -. Food Science and Technology (Campinas.)*, *60*, 137–141.

Ezekiel, C. N., Sulyok, M., Babalola, D. A., Warth, A., Ezekiel, V. C., & Krska, R. (2013). Incidence and consumer awareness of toxigenic *Aspergillus* section Flavi and aflatoxin B1 in peanut cake from Nigeria. *Food Control*, *30*(2), 596–601. doi:10.1016/j.foodcont.2012.07.048

Ezekiel, C. N., Sulyok, M., Warth, B., Odebode, A. C., & Krska, R. (2012). Natural occurrence of mycotoxins in peanut cake from Nigeria. *Food Control*, *27*(2), 338–342. doi:10.1016/j.foodcont.2012.04.010

Fandohan, P., Zoumenou, D., Hounhouigan, D. J., Marasas, W. F. O., Wingfield, M. J., & Hell, K. (2005). Fate of aflatoxins and fumonisins during the processing of maize into food products in Benin. *International Journal of Food Microbiology*, *98*(3), 249–259. doi:10.1016/j.ijfoodmicro.2004.07.007 PMID:15698686

FAO. (1995). *Sorghum and millets in human nutrition*. Retrieved April 20, 2015, from http://www.fao.org/docrep/t0818e/t0818e00.htm

FAO. (2010). *Composition of selected foods from West Africa*. Rome: Food and Agriculture Organisation.

FAO. (2013). *Edible insects: Future prospects for food and feed security*. Rome: Food and Agriculture Organisation.

FAO, IFAD, & WFP. (2014). *The State of Food Insecurity in the World 2014. Strengthening the enabling environment for food security and nutrition*. Rome: FAO.

FAO. (2015). *A resource book for teachers of agriculture*. Retrieved March 25, 2015 from http://www.fao.org/docrep/w0078e/w0078e06.htm

FAOSTAT. (2013). Retrieved March 25, 2015 from http://faostat.fao.org/site/567/DesktopDefault.aspx?PageID=567#ancor

Finucane, M.M., Stevens, G.A., Cowan, M.J., Danaei, G., Lin, J.K., Paciorek, C.J., … Ezzati, M. (2011). Global Burden of Metabolic Risk Factors of Chronic Diseases Collaborating Group (Body Mass Index). National, regional, and global trends in body-mass index since 1980: systematic analysis of health examination surveys and epidemiological studies with 960 country-years and 9·1 million participants. *Lancet, 377*(9765), 557-67.

Franz, C. M. A. P., Hucha, M., Mathara, J. M., Abriouel, H., Benomar, N., Reid, G., & Holzapfel, W. H. et al. (2014). African fermented foods and probiotics. *International Journal of Food Microbiology*, *190*, 84–96. doi:10.1016/j.ijfoodmicro.2014.08.033 PMID:25203619

Fung, W. (2009). *Early childhood malnutrition and adult obesity: Evidence from the 1959-61 China famine*. Retrieved March 25, 2015 from http://www.cpc.unc.edu/projects/china/ publications/1219

Gebremariam, M. M., Zarnkow, M., & Becker, T. (2012). Teff (*Eragrostis tef*) as a raw material for malting, brewing and manufacturing of gluten-free foods and beverages: a review. *Journal of Food Science & Technology*. DOI 10.1007/s13197-012-0745-5

Grzeskowiak, L., Collado, M. C., Mangani, C., Maleta, K., Laitinen, K., Ashorn, P., & Salminen, S. et al. (2012). Distinct gut microbiota in southeastern African and northern European infants. *Journal of Pediatric Gastroenterology and Nutrition*, *54*(6), 812–816. doi:10.1097/MPG.0b013e318249039c PMID:22228076

Haggblade, S., Duodu, G., Kabasa, J. D., Minnaar, A., Ojijo, N., & Taylor, J. R. N. (2014). *Bending the curve in Africa's nutrition transition*. Retrieved July 20, 2015 from http://www.ifama.org/files/conf/2014%20Conference/T1Bending%281%29.pdf

Hamzah, R. U., Jagam, A. A., Makun, H. A., & Engwin, E. C. (2013). *Antioxidant properties of selected African vegetables, fruits and mushrooms: A review*. Retrieved March 25, 2015 from

Hamzah, R. U., Jigam, A. A., Makun, H. A., & Egwim, E. C. (2014). Phytochemical screening and in-vitro antioxidant activity of methanolic extract of selected Nigerian vegetables. *Asian Journal of Basis and Applied Sciences*, *1*(1), 1–14.

Holse, M., Husted, S., & Hansen, A. (2010). Chemical composition of Marama beans (*Tylosema esculentum*): A wild African bean with unexploited potential. *Journal of Food Composition and Analysis*, *23*(6), 648–657. doi:10.1016/j.jfca.2010.03.006

ICRAF. (2004). *Agroforestry Database, a tree species reference and selection guide*. Nairobi: ICRAF.

Inoue, T., Nagatomi, Y., Uyama, A., & Mochizuki, N. (2013). Fate of mycotoxins during beer brewing and fermentation. *Bioscience, Biotechnology, and Biochemistry*, *77*(7), 1410–1415. doi:10.1271/bbb.130027 PMID:23832360

Irvine, S. L., Hummelen, R., & Hekmat, S. (2011). Probiotic yogurt consumption may improve gastrointestinal symptoms,productivity, and nutritional intake of people living with humanimmunodeficiency virus in Mwanza, Tanzania. *Nutrition Research (New York, N.Y.)*, *31*(12), 875–881. doi:10.1016/j.nutres.2011.10.005 PMID:22153512

Isolauri, E., Juntunen, M., Rautanen, T., Sillanaukee, P., & Koivula, T. (1991). A human *Lactobacillus*strain (*Lactobacillus casei*sp. strain GG) promotes recovery from acute diarrhea in children. *Pediatrics*, *88*, 90–97. PMID:1905394

Iwuoha, C. I., & Eke, O. S. (1996). Nigerian Indigenous Fermented foods: Their traditional process operations, inherent problems, improvements and current status. *Food Research International*, *29*(5-6), 527–540. doi:10.1016/0963-9969(95)00045-3

Iwuoha, G. N., Ubeng, G. G., & Onwuachu, U. I. (2013). Detoxification effect of fermentation on cyanide content of cassava tuber. *Journal of Applied Sciences and Environmental Management*, *17*(4), 567–570.

Jansen van Rensburg, W. S., Venter, S. L., Netshiluuhi, T. R., Van der Heever, E., Vorster, H. J., & De Rorde, J. A. (2004). Role of indigenous leafy vegetables in combating hunger and malnutrition. *South African Journal of Botany*, *70*(1), 116–123. doi:10.1016/S0254-6299(15)30268-4

Johns, T., & Sthapit, B. (2004). Biocultural diversity in the sustainability of developing country food systems. *Food and Nutrition Bulletin*, *25*(2), 143–155. doi:10.1177/156482650402500207 PMID:15214260

Kamga, R. T., Kouame, C., Atangana, A. R., Chagomoka, T., & Ndango, R. (2013). Nutritional Evaluation of Five African Indigenous Vegetables. *Journal of Horticultural Research*, *21*(1), 99–106. doi:10.2478/johr-2013-0014

Kankolongo, M. A., Hell, K., & Nawa, I. N. (2009). Assessment for fungal, mycotoxin and insect spoilage in maize stored for human consumption in Zambia. *Journal of the Science of Food and Agriculture*, *89*(8), 1366–1375. doi:10.1002/jsfa.3596

Kanu, P. J., Bahsoon, J. Z., Kanu, J. B., & Kandeh, J. B. A. (2010). Nutraceutical Importance of Sesame Seed and Oil: A Review of the Contribution of their Lignans. Sierra Leone. *Journal of Biomedical Research*, *2*, 4–16.

Kawarazuka, N. (2010). *The contribution offish intake, aquaculture, and small-scale fisheries to improving nutrition: A literature review*. The World Fish Center Working Paper No.2106. The World Fish Center.

Kawarazuka, N., & Be'ne´, C. (2010). The potential role of small fish species in improving micronutrient deficiencies in developing countries: Building evidence. *Public Health Nutrition*, *14*(11), 1927–1938. doi:10.1017/S1368980011000814 PMID:21729489

Kayode, A.A., & Kayode, O.T. (2010). Some medicinal values of *Telfairia occidentalis:* A review. *American Journal of Biochemistry and Molecular Biology*, *1*(1), 30-38.

Kinyuru, J. N., Kenji, G. M., Muhoho, S. N., & Ayieko, M. (2010). Nutritional potential of longhorn grasshopper (*Ruspolia differens*) consumed in Siaya District. *Journal of Agriculture, Science and Technology*, *12*, 32–47.

Kinyuru, J. N., Konyole, S. O., Roos, N., Onyango, C. A., Owino, V. O., Owuor, B. O., & Kenji, G. M. et al. (2013). Nutrient composition of four species of winged termites consumed in western Kenya. *Journal of Food Composition and Analysis*, *30*(2), 120–124. doi:10.1016/j.jfca.2013.02.008

Kunyanga, C. N., Imungi, J. K., & Vellingiri, V. (2013). Nutritional evaluation of indigenous foods with potential food-based solution to alleviate hunger and malnutrition in Kenya. *Journal of Applied Biosciences*, *67*(0), 5277–5288. doi:10.4314/jab.v67i0.95049

Kwenin, W. K. J., Wolli, M., & Dzomeku, B. M. (2011). Assessing the nutritional value of some African indigenous green Leafy Vegetables in Ghana. *Journal of Animal & Plant Sciences*, *10*, 1300–1305.

Lei, V., & Jakobsen, M. (2004). Microbiological characterization and probiotic potentialof *koko* and *kokosourwater*, African spontaneously fermented millet porridge and drink. *Journal of Applied Microbiology*, *96*(2), 384–397. doi:10.1046/j.1365-2672.2004.02162.x PMID:14723700

Lopriore, C., & Muehlhoff, E. (2003). *Food security and nutrition trends in West Africa - Challenges and the way forward*. Retrieved April 15, 2015 from ftp://ftp.fao.org/es/esn/nutrition/ouagafinal.pdf

Lukmanji, Z., Hertzmark, E., Mlingi, N., Assey, V., & Ndossi, G. et al.. (2008). *Tanzania food composition Tables. MUHAS-TFNC*. Dar es Salaam, Tanzania: HSPH.

MacCalla, A. F. (1994). *Agriculture and Food Need to 2025, Why we should be concerned.* Washington, DC: CGIAR.

Magala-Nyago, C. M., Kikafunda, J.K., Mwasaru, M.A., Kenji, G.M., & Connely, R.K. (2005). Evaluation of nutritional value of malted and extruded finger millet based complementary foods. In *Proceedings of African Crop Science Conference* (*vol. 7*, pp 677-686). Kampala, Uganda: ACSJ.

Maliro, M. F. A. (2001). The role and potential of traditional tuber crops in Malawi. In D. Pasternak & A. Schlissel (Eds.), *Combating Desertification with Plants* (pp. 55–64). Kluwer Academic Press. doi:10.1007/978-1-4615-1327-8_5

Manjula, K., Hell, K., Fandohan, P., Abass, A., & Bandyopadhyay, R. (2009). Aflatoxin and fumonisin contamination of cassava products and maize grain from markets in Tanzania and Republic of Congo. *Toxin Reviews*, *28*(2-3), 63–69. doi:10.1080/15569540802462214

Mathanghi, S. K., & Sudha, K. (2012). Functional properties of finger millet (*Eleusine coracana L.*) for health. *International Journal of Pharmaceutical. Chemical and Biological Sciences*, *2*(4), 431–438.

Mathieu, G., & Meissa, D. (2007). Traditional leafy vegetables in Senegal: Diversity and Medicinal Uses. *African Journal of Traditional, Complementary, and Alternative Medicines*, *4*(4), 469–475. doi:10.4314/ajtcam.v4i4.31239 PMID:20161914

Matumba, L., Monjerezi, M., Khonga, E. B., & Lakudzala, D. D. (2011). Aflatoxins in sorghum, sorghum malt and traditional opaque beer in southern Malawi. *Food Control*, *22*(2), 266–268. doi:10.1016/j.foodcont.2010.07.008

Matumba, L., Van Poucke, C., Biswick, T., Monjerezi, M., Mwatseteza, J., & De Saeger, S. (2014). A limited survey of mycotoxins in traditional maize based opaque beers in Malawi. *Food Control*, *36*(1), 253–256. doi:10.1016/j.foodcont.2013.08.032

Mbatia, B., Awuor, O. L., Kirwa, M. E., & Kackim, M. F. (2014). Antioxidative and functional properties of *Rastrineobola argentea* (dagaa) fish protein hydrolysate. *Discourse Journal of Agriculture and Food Sciences*, *2*, 180–189.

Mensah, J. K., Okoli, R. I., Ohaju-Obodo, J. O., & Eifediyi, K. (2008). Phytochemical, nutritional and medical properties of some leafy vegetables consumed by Edo people of Nigeria. *African Journal of Biotechnology*, *7*, 2305–2309.

Mensah, P. (1997). Fermentation - the key to food safety assurance in Africa? *Food Control*, *8*(5-6), 271–278. doi:10.1016/S0956-7135(97)00020-0

Mestres, C., Bassa, S., Fagbohoun, E., Nogo, M., Hell, K., Vernier, P., & Cardwell, K. F. et al. (2004). Yam chip food subsector: Hazardous practices and presence of aflatoxins in Benin. *Journal of Stored Products Research*, *40*(5), 575–585. doi:10.1016/j.jspr.2003.11.003

Mokoena, M. P., Chelule, P. K., & Ggaleni, N. (2005). Reduction of fumonisin B1 and zearalenone by lactic acid bacteria in fermented maize meal. *Journal of Food Protection*, *68*, 2095–2099. PMID:16245712

Mokoena, M. P., Chelule, P. K., & Gqaleni, N. (2006). The toxicity and decreased concentration of aflatoxin B1 in natural lactic acid fermented maize meal. *Journal of Applied Microbiology*, *100*(4), 773–777. doi:10.1111/j.1365-2672.2006.02881.x PMID:16553732

Mshandete, A. M., & Cuff, J. (2007). Proximate and nutrient composition of three types of indigenous edible wild mushrooms grown in Tanzania and their utilization prospects. *African Journal of Food Agriculture Nutrition and Development*, *7*(6), 1–16.

Mwanri, A. W., Kogi-Makau, W., & Laswai, H. S. (2011). Nutrients and antinutrients composition of raw, cooked and sun- dried sweetpotato leaves. *African Journal of Food, Agriculture. Nutrition and Development*, *11*(5), 5142–5156.

Nabubuya, A., Muyonga, J. H., & Kabasa, J. D. (2010). Nutritional and hypocholesterolemic properties of *Termitomyces microcarpus* Mushrooms. *African Journal of Food, Agriculture, Nutrition and Development*, *10*(3), 2235–2257.

Nesamvuni, C., Steyn, N. P., & Potgieter, M. J. (2001). Nutritional value of wild, leafy plants consumed by the Vhavenda. *South African Journal of Science*, *97*, 51–54.

Nwauzoma, A. B., & Dawari, S. L. (2013). Study on the phytochemical properties and proximate analysis of *Piper Umbellatum* (LINN) from Nigeria. *American Journal of Research Communication*, *1*(7), 164–177.

Obodai, M., Ferreira, I. C. R. R., Fernandes, A., Barros, L., Mensah, D. L., Dzomeku, M., & Takli, R. et al. (2014). Evaluation of the chemical and antioxidant properties of wild and cultivated mushrooms in Ghana. *Molecules (Basel, Switzerland)*, *19*(12), 19532–19548. doi:10.3390/molecules191219532 PMID:25432007

Odhav, B., Beekrun, S., Akula, U., & Baijnath, H. (2007). Preliminary assessment of nutritional value of traditional leafy vegetables in KwaZulu-Natal, South Africa. *Journal of Food Composition and Analysis*, *20*(5), 430–435. doi:10.1016/j.jfca.2006.04.015

Olaiya, C., & Adebisi, J. (2009). Phytoevaluation of the nutritional values of ten green leafy vegetables in South -Western Nigeria. *The Internet Journal of Nutrition and Wellness*, *9*, 2.

Olumakaiye, M. F. (2011). Evaluation of nutrient contents of amaranth leaves prepared using different cooking methods. *Food and Nutrition Sciences*, *2*(04), 249–252. doi:10.4236/fns.2011.24035

Orech, F. O., Christensen, D. L., Larsen, T., Friis, H., Aagaard-Hansen, J., & Estambale, B. A. (2007). Mineral content of traditional leafy vegetables from western Kenya. *International Journal of Food Sciences and Nutrition*, *58*(8), 595–602. doi:10.1080/09637480701350288 PMID:17852510

Osabor, V. N., Ogar, D. A., Okafor, P. C., & Egbung, G. E. (2009). Profile of the African Bread Fruit (*Treculia africana*). *Pakistan Journal of Nutrition*, *8*(7), 1005–1008. doi:10.3923/pjn.2009.1005.1008

Oulai, P., Zoue, L., Megnanou, R., Doue, R., & Niamke, S. (2014b). Value of leafy vegetables consumed in Northern Cöte D'ivoire. *European Scientific Journal*, *10*, 212–227.

Oulai, P. D., Zoue, L. T., Bedikou, M. E., Rose-Monde, M., & Niamke, L. S. (2014a). Impact of cooking on nutritive and antioxidant characteristics of leafy vegetables consumed in Northern Côte d'Ivoire. *International Journal of Plant. Animal and Environmental Sciences*, *4*, 576–583.

Oyetayo, O. V. (2011). Medicinal Uses of Mushrooms in Nigeria: Towards Full and Sustainable Exploitation. *African Journal of Traditional, Complementary, and Alternative Medicines*, *8*(3), 267–274. doi:10.4314/ajtcam.v8i3.65289 PMID:22468005

Oyewole, O. B. (1997). Lactic fermented foods in Africa and their benefits. *Food Control*, *8*(5-6), 289–297. doi:10.1016/S0956-7135(97)00075-3

Peltonen, K. D., El-Nezami, H. S., Salminen, S. J., & Ahokas, J. T. (2000). Binding of aflatoxin B1 by probiotic bacteria. *Journal of the Science of Food and Agriculture*, *80*(13), 1942–1945. doi:10.1002/1097-0010(200010)80:13<1942::AID-JSFA741>3.0.CO;2-7

Pochapin, M. (2000). The effect of probiotics on *Clostridium difficile* diarrhea. *The American Journal of Gastroenterology*, *95*(1), S11–S13. doi:10.1016/S0002-9270(99)00809-6 PMID:10634221

Prades, A., Dornier, M., Diop, N., & Pain, J.-P. (2012). Coconut water uses, composition and properties: A review. *Fruits*, *67*(2), 87–107. doi:10.1051/fruits/2012002

Probst, C., Bandyopadhyay, R., & Cotty, P. J. (2014). Diversity of aflatoxin-producing fungi and their impact on food safety in sub-Saharan Africa. *International Journal of Food Microbiology*, *174*, 113–122. doi:10.1016/j.ijfoodmicro.2013.12.010 PMID:24480188

Raza, S., Graham, S. M., Allen, S. J., Sultana, S., Cuevas, L., & Hart, C. A. (1995). Lactobacillus GG promotes recovery from acute non-bloody diarrhea in Pakistan. *The Pediatric Infectious Disease Journal*, *14*(2), 107–111. doi:10.1097/00006454-199502000-00005 PMID:7746691

Rice, A. L., Sacco, L., Hyder, A., & Black, R. E. (2000). Malnutrition as an underlying cause of childhood deaths associated with infectious diseases in developing countries. *Bulletin of the World Health Organization*, *78*, 1207–1221. PMID:11100616

Rice, A. L., West, K. P., & Black, R. (2004). Vitamin A deficiency. In Comparative quantification of health risks: Global and regional burden of disease attributable to selected major risk factors (vol. 1, pp. 212-256). World Health Organisation.

Rosenfeldt, V., Michaelsen, K. F., Jakobsen, M., Larsen, C. N., Møller, P. L., Pedersen, P., & Pærregaard, A. et al. (2002). Effect of *Lactobacillus* strains in young children hospitalized with acute diarrhea. *The Pediatric Infectious Disease Journal*, *21*(5), 411–416. doi:10.1097/00006454-200205000-00012 PMID:12150178

Saavedra, J. (2000). Probiotics and infectious diarrhea. *The American Journal of Gastroenterology*, *95*(1), S16–S18. doi:10.1016/S0002-9270(99)00811-4 PMID:10634223

Sadler, M. (2003). Nutritional properties of edible fungi. *British Nutrition Foundation Nutrition Bulletin*, *28*(3), 305–308. doi:10.1046/j.1467-3010.2003.00354.x

Saranraj, P., Naidu, M. A., & Sivasakthivelan, P. (2013). Lactic acid bacteria and its antimicrobial properties: A review. *International Journal of Pharmaceutical & Biological Archives*, *4*(6), 1124–1133.

Shahidi, F., & Chandrasekara, A. (2013). Millet grain phenolics and their role in disease risk reduction and promotion: A review. *Journal of Functional Foods*, *5*(2), 570–581. doi:10.1016/j.jff.2013.02.004

Shei, L. C. (2008). *An Evaluation of Native West African Vegetables.* Paper presented at Conference on International Research on Food Security, Natural Resource Management and Rural Development, Tropentag, Germany.

Siddhuraju, P., & Becker, K. (2007). The antioxidant and free radical scavenging activities of processed cowpea (*Vigna unguiculata* (L.) Walp.) seed extracts. *Food Chemistry*, *101*(1), 10–19. doi:10.1016/j.foodchem.2006.01.004

Smith, F. I., & Eyzaguirre, P. (2007). African leafy vegetables: Their role in the World Health Organisation's global fruit and vegetable initiative. *African Journal of Food Agriculture Nutrition and Development*, *7*(3), 1–17.

Sprent, J. I., Odee, D. W., & Dakora, F. D. (2009). Chemical composition of Marama bean (*Tylosema esculentum*) – A wild African bean with unexploited potential. *Journal of Experimental Botany*. doi:10.1093/jxb/erp342

Stamoulis, K.G., Pingali, P., & Shetty, P. (2004). Emerging challenges for food and nutrition policy in developing countries. *e-Journal of Agricultural and Development Economics*, *1*(2), 154–167.

Stangeland, T., Remberg, S. F., & Lye, K. A. (2009). Total antioxidant activity in 35 Ugandan fruits and vegetables. *Food Chemistry*, *113*(1), 85–91. doi:10.1016/j.foodchem.2008.07.026

Steyn, N. P., Olivier, J., Wirter, P., Burger, S., & Nesamvuni, C. (2001). A survey of wild, green, leafy vegetables and their potential in combating micronutrient deficiencies in rural populations. *South African Journal of Science*, *97*, 276–278.

Stoltzfus, R., Mullany, L., & Black, R. E. (2004). Iron deficiency Anaemia. In Comparative quantification of health risks: Global and regional burden of disease attributable to selected major risk factors (vol. 1, pp. 163-209). World Health Organisation.

Stone, A., Massey, A., Theobald, M., Styslinger, M., Kane, D., Kandy, D., . . . Davert, E. (2011). *Africa's indigenous crops.* Retrieved April 20, 2015 from http://www.worldwatch.org/system/files/NtP-Africa%27s-Indigenous-Crops.pdf

Taruvinga, A., & Nengovhela, R. (2015). *Consumer perceptions and consumption dynamics of African leafy vegetables(ALVs): Evidence from Feni communal area, Eastern Cape Province, South Africa.* Paper presented at the 5th International Conference on Biomedical Engineering and Technology, Seoul, Korea. Doi doi:10.773/IPCBEE.2015.V81.16

Taylor, J. R. N., Belton, P. S., Beta, T., & Duodu, C. K. (2014). Increasing the utilization of sorghum, millets and pseudocereals: Developments in science of their phenolic phytochemicals, biofortification and protein functionality. *Cereal Science*, *59*(3), 257–275. doi:10.1016/j.jcs.2013.10.009

Tiwari, U., & Cummins, E. (2013). Fruits and vegetables. In B. K. Tiwari, N. P. Brunton, & C. S. Brennan (Eds.), *Handbook of plant food phytochemicals: Sources, stability and extraction* (pp. 107–137). Oxford, UK: John Wiley & Sons Ltd. doi:10.1002/9781118464717.ch5

Tumwet, T. N., Mwangi, A. M., Kogi-makau, W., & Kang, E. K. (2013). Effect of different cooking methods on the nutritional value of some African indigenous leafy vegetables in Kenya. In *Proceedings of African Crop Science Conference* (vol. 11, pp 441 - 443). Kampala, Uganda: ACSJ.

Uusiku, N. P., Olefose, A., Duodu, K. G., Bester, M. J., & Faber, M. (2010). Nutritional value of leafy vegetables of sub-Saharan Africa and the potential contribution to human health: A review. *Journal of Food Composition and Analysis*, *23*(6), 499–509. doi:10.1016/j.jfca.2010.05.002

Uusitalo, U., Pietinen, P., & Puska, P. (2002). *Dietary transition in developing countries: Challenges for chronic disease prevention.* Retrieved April 20, 2015 from http://whqlibdoc.who.int/publications/9241590416.pdf

van Huis, A. (2003). Insects as food in sub-Saharan Africa. *Insect Science and Its Application*, *23*, 163–185.

Vorster, I. H. L., van Rensburg, W. J., van Zijl, J. J. B., & Venter, S. L. (2007). The importance of traditional leafy vegetables in South Africa. *African Journal of Food, Agriculture. Nutrition and Development*, *7*, 49–54.

Wagacha, J. M., & Muthomi, J. W. (2008). Mycotoxin problem in Africa: Current status, implications to food safety and health and possible management strategies. *International Journal of Food Microbiology*, *124*(1), 1–12. doi:10.1016/j.ijfoodmicro.2008.01.008 PMID:18258326

Wareing, P. W., Westby, A., Gibbs, J. A., Allotey, L. T., & Halm, M. (2001). Consumer preferences and fungal and mycotoxin contamination of dried cassava products from Ghana. *International Journal of Food Science & Technology*, *36*(1), 1–10. doi:10.1046/j.1365-2621.2001.00419.x

Were, B. A., Okware, A. O., Gudu, S., Welander, M., & Carlsson, A. S. (2006). Seed oil content and fatty acid composition in East African sesame (*Sesamum indicum L.*) accessions evaluated over 3 years. *Field Crops Research*, *97*(2-3), 254–260. doi:10.1016/j.fcr.2005.10.009

WHO. (2004). *Iodine status worldwide: WHO Global Database on Iodine Deficiency*. Retrieved July 15, 2015, from http://www.who.int/nutrition/publications/micronutrients/iodine_deficiency/9241592001/en/

WHO. (2008). *Worldwide prevalence of anaemia 1993–2005: WHO global database on anaemia*. Retrieved July 15, 2015 from http://www.who.int/vmnis/anaemia/prevalence/en/

WHO. (2009). *Global prevalence of vitamin A deficiency in populations at risk 1995–2005. WHO Global Database on Vitamin A Deficiency*. Retrieved July 15, 2015 from http://www.who.int/vmnis/database/vitamina/x/en/

Williams, J. H., Phillips, T. D., Jolly, P. E., Stiles, J. K., Jolly, C. M., & Aggarwal, D. (2004). Human aflatoxicosis in developing countries: A review of toxicology, exposure, potential health consequences, and interventions. *The American Journal of Clinical Nutrition*, *80*, 1106–1122. PMID:15531656

Womeni, H. M., Linder, M., Tiencheu, B., Mbiapo, F. T., Villeneuve, P., Fanni, J., & Parmentier, M. (2009). Oils of insects and larvae consumed in Africa: Potential sources of polyunsaturated fatty acids. *Oilseeds and Fats Crops Lipids*, *16*, 230–235.

Xiaoming, C., Ying, F., Hong, Z., & Zhiyonga, C. (2010). Review of the nutritive value of edible insects. In *Proceedings of a workshop on Asia-Pacific resources and their potential for development* (pp 85-92), Bangkok, Thailand: Food and Agriculture Organisation.

Chapter 16
Functional Foods of the Indian Subcontinent

Jiwan S. Sidhu
Kuwait University, Kuwait

Tasleem A. Zafar
Kuwait University, Kuwait

ABSTRACT

The medicinal effects of food have been recognized on the Indian subcontinent since many centuries. The current thinking on functional foods can easily be applied to many traditional Indian subcontinent foods as these are based on whole grains, legumes, oilseeds, nuts, vegetables, fruits, spices, condiments, and many fermented milk products. Consumption of such foods on a regular basis not only provides most of nutrients in adequate quantities but also improve gastrointestinal health, boost immune functions, improve bone health, lower cholesterol, oxidative stress, reduce the risk of cardiovascular diseases, various types of cancers, neurodegenerative diseases, ill-effects of obesity, and metabolic syndrome. Various chemical and biological components present in Indian subcontinent traditional foods, such as phytochemicals, dietary fiber, oligosaccharides, lignins, omega-3 fatty acids, phenolics, flavonoids, carotenoids, and probiotic bacteria play an important role in improving the health of consumers of these foods. The history of Indian traditional foods has been adequately reviewed by Srinivasan (2011). The traditional food habits of each specific area of the Indian subcontinent have been influenced by the culture and the availability of locally grown food materials. Some of the important functional foods of India subcontinent will be briefly discussed in this chapter.

FUNCTIONAL FOODS FROM VARIOUS COMMODITIES

Under this section, functional foods based on cereals, legumes, milk and milk products, oilseeds, herbs and condiments, fruits, vegetables, nuts and some miscellaneous commodities will be briefly discussed.

Cereals

The food industry is focused on producing functional foods based on various cereals due to consumer demands for healthier foods. Some of the major cereals such as wheat, barley, and oats being rich in

DOI: 10.4018/978-1-5225-0591-4.ch016

many phytochemicals and other nutrients, thus offer an excellent opportunity for the production of functional foods (Sidhu et al. 1989; Seibel et al. 1990; Singh et al. 1993; Sidhu, 1995). Whole grain wheat is rich in dietary fiber which has association with cardiovascular diseases, type-2 diabetes, bowl function and colon cancer; vitamins and provitamins such as vitamin E, B-group vitamins, carotenoids; minerals like magnesium and selenium; other bio-actives, such as, polyphenols, phenolic acids, ferulic acid, alkylresorcinols, flavonoids, phytosterols, lignins (Dalton et al. 2012; Zhu et al. 2015; Lu et al. 2015a). Bran, aleurone and germ are the components of whole grains that are rich in above mentioned nutritional compounds (Table 1 and Figure 1) providing high health benefits (Chhabra & Sidhu 1988; Bajaj et al. 1991; Sidhu et al. 1999; Al-Hooti et al. 2000; Al-Saqer et al. 2000; Sidhu et al. 2001; Al-Hooti et al. 2001; Adom et al. 2005; Chen et al. 2015; Rosa-Sibakov et al. 2015; Levent et al. 2015). With reduction in particle size of bran as well as during fermentation of wheat dough, a significant increase in extraction of anthocyanins, carotenoids and antioxidant properties has been reported (Chhabra & Sidhu 1988; Brewer et al. 2014; Pekkinen et al. 2014; Savolainen et al. 2015).

Genotype, growing environment and their interaction have been shown to significantly affect the selected health components and antioxidant properties of soft wheat bran (Lu et al. 2015b). Sprouting of different grains (durum, spelt, einkorn, emmer and soft wheat) into wheatgrass produced increased amounts of phytochemicals and other high value nutrients, which might potentially be valuable for the development of functional foods (Zilic et al. 2014; Benincasa et al. 2015). Cereal grains are also known to be an important source of fructans, a kind of carbohydrate that has health promoting potential not only as a dietary fiber source but also serves as a prebiotic (Verspreet et al. 2015). Dietary fiber is one of the major phytochemicals present in cereals and is of two categories according to their water solubility. Water-soluble fraction (soluble fiber) is mainly of nonstarchy polysaccharides such as β-glucans and pentosans. This fraction is known to decrease serum cholesterol, postprandial blood glucose, and insulin levels in humans (Edge et al. 2005). Water-insoluble fraction (insoluble fiber) consists of lignin, cellulose,

Table 1. Principal components and phytochemicals (g/100g) in wheat grain fractions

Constituents	Whole Grain	Bran	Aleurone
Arabinoxylan	6.5	22-30	24.3
β-glucans	0.7	2.2-2.6	3.9
Lignin	1.9	5.6	-
Cellulose	2.1	6.5-9.9	3.0
Ferulic acid monomer	0.02-0.21	0.5-0.7	0.66-.82
Ferulic acid dimer	0.01	0.8-1.0	0.03-0.1
Sinapic acid	0.06	0.02	0.03
p-Coumaric acid	0.00	0.01	0.02
Flavonoids (in µg)	37	28	8
Lignans (in µg)	0.2-0.7	5	7
Phytic acid	0.90	4.20	15-20
Minerals	1.1	3.4	12.0
Alkylresorcinols	0.07	0.27	0.17
Betaine	0.02	0.87	1.50

Adapted from: Rosa-Sibakov et al. (2015)

Figure 1. Nutritionally important technological fractions of wheat grain
Source: Rosa-Sibakov et al. (2015)

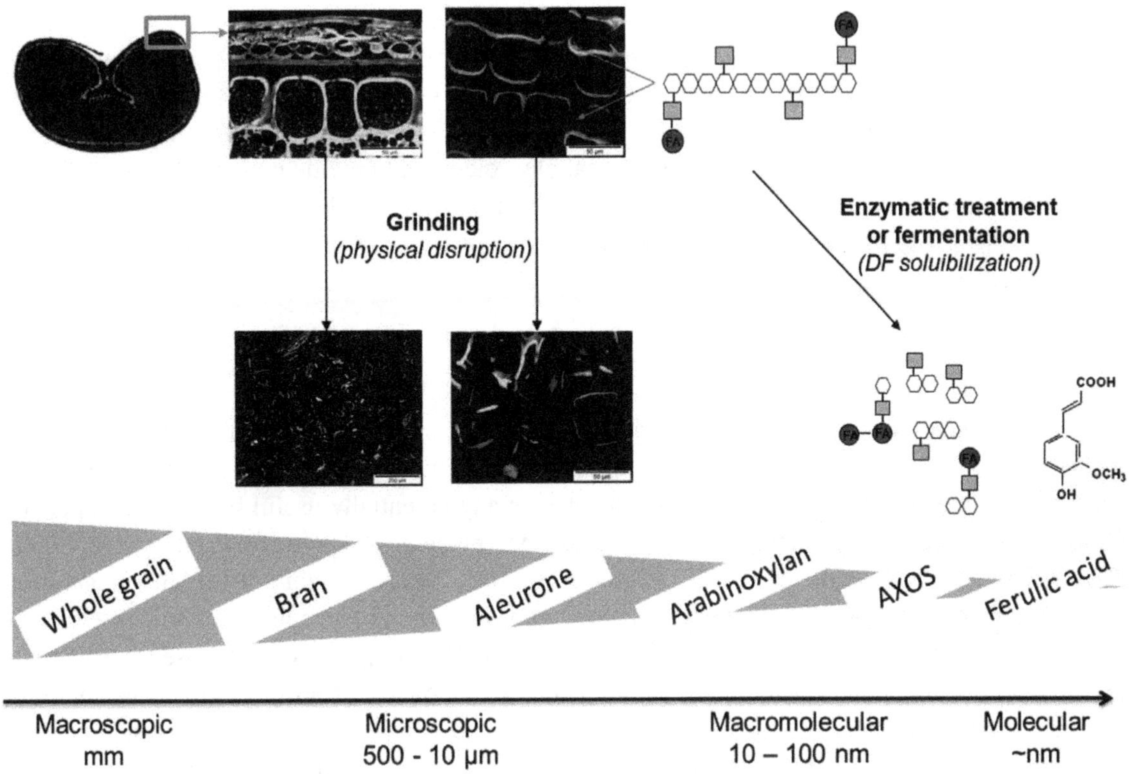

hemicelluloses and prevents constipation. The average values for the total dietary fiber in barley, wheat and oats have been reported to be 10, 12 and 14% (dry basis), respectively (Charalampopoulos et al. 2002).

Because of their phytochemicals and nutritional potential, there has been a considerable increase in interest in the utilization of sorghum, millets and pseudo-cereals for developing gluten-free food products. Enhanced nutritional traits such as higher amylopectin, higher lysine, improved protein digestibility and utilization, higher provitamin A, higher iron and zinc contents, and improved mineral bioavailability thru phytate reduction, are being explored using traditional breeding and recombinant DNA technology (Taylor et al. 2014). Anthocyanins and other phytochemicals in purple wheat have been measured using HPLC techniques by Hosscinian et al (2008). In addition to anthocyanins, they also reported the presence of a lignin (secoisolariciresinol diglucoside) and melatonin, which may contribute to the health benefits associated with the consumption of purple wheat or other colored cereal grains.

Resistant starch (not digested by salivary amylases) has been shown to provide benefits for the production of short-chain fatty acids (SCFA) in the large intestine. This resistant starch in the large intestine can serve as prebiotics for growth of probiotic bacteria which are known to decrease the risk of bowel diseases (Yue & Waring 1998). Phytic acid, a natural plant antioxidant present in wheat bran in relatively high amounts (4.8%) has been shown to suppress iron-catalyzed oxidative reactions. The bran layers of cereal grains are relatively rich in antioxidants. The antioxidants present in bran layers are either water- or fat-soluble and nearly one half are insoluble. Soluble antioxidants in oats include phenolic acids, flavonoids, tocopherols, tocotrienols, and avenanthramides (Slavin, 2004). Ferulic acid present in bran may provide health benefits because of its antioxidant properties (Thompson 1994). In addition, ferulic acid has been shown to have nitrite scavenging effect as efficient as that of ascorbic acid under acidic conditions (Moller et al. 1998). Wheat, barley and oats are also known to contain many other bioactive compounds, namely, lignans, phytosterols, isoflavones, resorcyclic acid lactones, coumestans, unsaturated fatty acids, lutein, cryptoxanthin, zeaxanthin, tocopherols, tocotrienols, glutathione, melatonin. These compounds may affect gastrointestinal physiology and provide protection against chronic diseases like coronary heart disease and some cancers (Jacobs et al. 2002; Zielinski 2002; Slavin 2003; Zhou et al. 2004). The phytochemicals present in cereal grains have also been extensively reviewed by Sidhu et al (2007).

Legumes (Pulses)

Legumes have been staple food and are important source of proteins, several vitamins, minerals, dietary fiber and many phytochemicals throughout the history of mankind. In addition to their low fat and higher dietary fiber contents, pulses are important sources of many potentially useful bioactive compounds, such as enzyme inhibitors, lectins, phytates, oxalates, polyphenolics, saponins and phytosterols (Dilis & Trihopoulou 2009; Marathe et al. 2011; Faris et al. 2013; Nasir & Sidhu, 2013; Vila-Donat et al. 2015). As the awareness of the potential of legumes consumption to reduce many chronic diseases has increased during the last decade, it is expected that legume consumption will increase tremendously. The consumption of dry beans having low glycemic index is known to improve the glycemic control in case of hyperglycemic patients, lowers blood cholesterol, and reduces body fat (Anderson et al 2004; Bazzano et al 2011a, b; Tucker & Thomas, 2009). Dry beans are natural sources of both the soluble and insoluble dietary fiber and produces lower glycemic response compared to carbohydrates from food sources (Livesey et al. 2008). Low GI legume consumption also reduces all the metabolic syndrome risks associated with obesity such as high blood pressure, insulin resistance, and hypertriglyceridemia.

The only one study that specifically examined the relationship between one serving of bean consumption and the risk of CVD found 38% lower risk of myocardial infarction compared with individuals who rarely consumed beans (Kabagambe et al. 2005). Compared with a calorie-restricted legume-free diet, the obese subjects when fed a calorie-restricted legume-based diet consisting of beans, chickpeas, lentils or peas, lost more weight and had a significant reduction in plasma C-reactive protein (Hermsdorff et al. 2011). The nutritional quality of legumes and their potential contribution in cardiometabolic risk prevention has recently been reviewed by Bouchenak & Lamri-Senhadji, 2013). The health potential of pulses and the bioactivity of their isoflavones, phytosterols, resistant starch, bioactive carbohydrates, alkaloids and saponins, as well as the effect of processing and cooking on these potentially beneficial bioactive compounds has been discussed by Rochfort and Panozzo (2007).

Black soybean is reported to have the highest saponin and phytic acid contents, peroxyl radical scavenging capacity and the strongest cellular antioxidant activity, thus can serve as an excellent dietary source of natural antioxidants for health promotion and cancer prevention (Xu & Chang 2012). Sprouting of various pulses has been shown to enhance the folate, vitamin C, total phenolics and total antioxidant activities and these values varied among various cultivars (Shohag et al. 2012). According to their results, folate content was the highest in soybean (815.2 μg/100g, fresh wt.) and mung bean (675.4 μg/100g, fresh wt.) on 4th day of germination. The vitamin C (not detected in raw seeds) increased rapidly in sprouts of soybean and mung bean on the 4th day of germination (29 and 27.7 mg/100g fresh wt., respectively).

Total phenolics and total antioxidant capacity were also the highest on the 4th day of germination thus providing maximum health-promoting properties by these pulses.

Oilseeds

Oilseeds are extremely popular edible grains that are often added to cereal flours to enhance their nutritional and sensory qualities. Soybean (Glycine max) is one of the most widely cultivated oilseeds in the world, because of its higher protein (40-50%) and oil (20-30%) contents. Various bioactive components, such as, isoflavones, saponins, phytic acid, phytosterols, trypsin inhibitors, peptides, and stilbenoids, present in oilseeds have become the subject of extensive scientific research, especially due to their functionality in disease prevention and treatment (Isanga and Zhang, 2008; Kisbenedek et al. 2014). Soy foods have been suggested to provide protection against breast, intestine, bladder, liver, prostate, skin and stomach cancer. Consumption of soybean based products is also known to reduce the risk of osteoporosis, lowers LDL cholesterol, increases HDL cholesterol, helps in chronic renal disease, lowers the risk of coronary heart disease, and shows antiatherosclerotic activity (Messina et al. 1994; Ranich et al. 2001). A number of studies have been reported on the beneficial effect of fermentation of soy products. In fermented soy products (soy milk, soy sauce, soy meal), the enhanced amounts of bioactive components and their antioxidant capacities confers health-promoting effects (Duenas et al. 2012; Ma & Huang 2014; Xu et al. 2015; Silva & Perrone, 2015).

Peanuts are grown in a number of countries and it makes a multibillion US$ industry in the world. The dibble part of peanuts is the kernel and the protective skin. The skin has pinkish-red color and astringent taste, because of which it is usually discarded. Peanuts are known to be rich in proteins, trans-fatty acids-free lipids, monounsaturated fatty acids, vitamin E, folate, potassium, magnesium, zinc, dietary fiber and many health-promoting phytochemicals (resveratrol, flavonoids, isoflavones, flavonols, phenolic acids, phytosterols). Peanut skins, a byproduct of processing, have been reported to be a good source of antioxidant phenolics, such as phenolic acids, flavonoids, and stilbene (Yu et al. 2005; Isanga & Zhang 2007; Chukwumah et al. 2007; Ressureccion et al. 2009; Camargo et al. 2012).

Sunflower is another oilseed crop where health-promoting phenolic compounds are present in abundance. These phenolics get bound to the sunflower proteins during oil extraction, thus their antioxidant properties are preserved in the meals (Salgado et al. 2012). Safflower (*Carthamus tinctorius* L.) is another oilseed that has also been reported to be valuable source of bioactive compounds that can impart functional food and natural antioxidant properties (Yu et al. 2013). Members of the Brassica family (e.g., mustard, Brussels sprouts, broccoli, cabbage, cauliflower, kale, chard) are known as dietary sources of glucosinolates, which are a large group of organic compounds containing sulfur and nitrogen. Glucosinolates and their breakdown products during chopping/cooking/processing are largely responsible for their bitter/astringent taste and characteristic aroma that limits the consumer acceptability of these vegetables. The seeds as well as leaves of the Brassica family are reported to be a good source of many bioactive compounds that have antioxidant, chemoprotective and anti-carcinogenic properties (Bala et al. 2012; Ghawi et al. 2014).

Bioactive Compounds from Milk and Milk Products

Milk is one of the nature's best gifts for feeding the off-springs after birth. Milk proteins have attracted extensive interest from the food scientists and nutritionists because of the various bioactive peptides generated during their digestion. Both human milk and infant formulae based on bovine's milk have been found to be the potential sources of bioactive peptides which have multiple health-promoting properties (Raikos & Dassios 2014). Some of the natural bioactive compounds, such as, β-lactoglobulin, α-lactalbumin, immunoglobulins, cytokines, lactoferrin, sphingolipids, conjugated linoleic acid, phospholipids, lactoperoxidase system and lysozyme in milk have been identified (Kavaz & Bakirci 2009). The bioactive peptides produced from both casein and whey proteins during enzymic digestion or microbial fermentation have been presented in Figure 2 (Ricci-Cabello et al. 2012). Depending upon the number and/or sequence of amino acids in the food-derived bioactive peptides, diverse activities, such as, enhancement of mineral bioavailability, opoid activity, boosting of immune system, anticancinogenic activity, and antihypertensive activity have been exhibited (Mills et al. 2011; Koliwer-Brandl et al. 2011; Mallik et al. 2013; Tan et al. 2014; Wada & Lonnerdal 2014; Nongonierma & Fitzgerald 2015a; Irshad et al. 2015). Using whey proteins (a by-product of cheese industry), Brandelli et al (2015) have produced bioactive peptides having all the above mentioned health-promoting properties.

Tryptophan is one of the essential amino acid present in milk proteins that serves as a precursor for certain biomolecules important for human health. Some of these are: serotonin, melatonin, tryptamine, niacin, adenine dinucleotide (NAD), phosphorylated NAD (NADP), quinolinic acid and kynureric acid.

Figure 2. Release of bioactive peptides from milk proteins by lactic acid bacteria
Source: Ricci-Cabello et al. (2012)

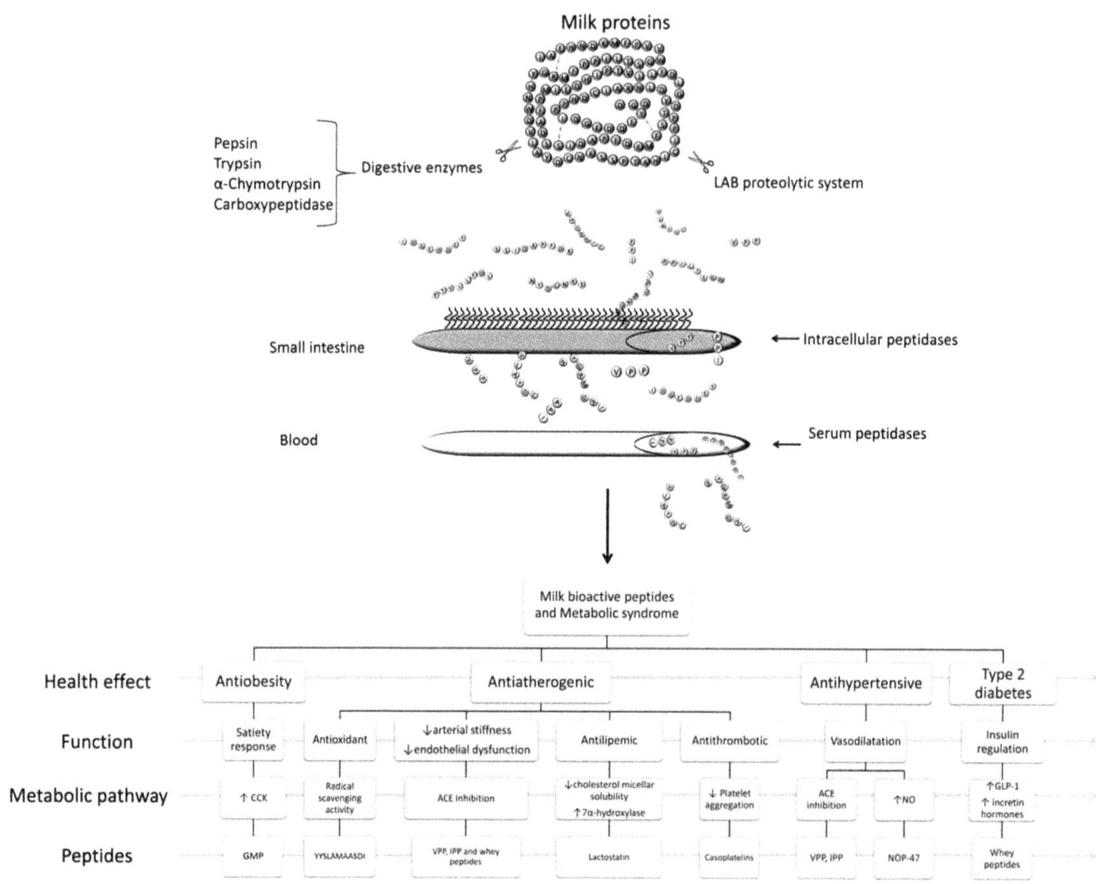

Free tryptophan is also shown to have some effect on cognition and hypotensive properties, however, higher bioactive potency has been observed with specific tryptophan-containing peptides than the free tryptophan (Nongonierma & FitzGerald 2015b). Cow milk has also been reported to contain bioactive secondary phenolic compounds which are formed by gut bacterial flora from plant phenolic compounds (Tsen et al. 2014). Equol and total phenolic compounds correlated positively with the milk lipid concentrations, and these were distributed to a large extent in the lipid fraction than in the aqueous fraction of cow milk. Evidently, skim milk will be of lower overall nutritive value and functional properties than the full cream milk.

Goat milk lactoferrin is a good candidate for use in infant foods because of its high homology with its human counterpart (Parc et al. 2014). Their results showed that among the N-glycans, 37% were sialylated and 34% were fucosylated. They demonstrated the existence of similar glycans in human and goat milk and also identified some novel glycan in goat milk which were never found in human milk. Goat milk is a good source of antioxidant bioactive compounds (including lactoferrin) and can be used in food products beneficial to human nutrition (Ahmad et al. 2015). Kiss et al (2014) have developed suitable packaging materials for sheep and goat milk yogurt which preserved the bioactive compounds throughout the 35 days of storage without any significant loss in nutritional value.

The composition of bioactive compounds in fermented dairy products depends on their content in raw milk and the processing conditions employed for the production of such products. Cais- Sokolinska et al (2015) have produced kefir from goat milk after feeding these animals with flax cake in their diet. Milk and kefir produced from these goats contained higher amounts of bioactive compounds (PUFA including CLA, omega-3 fatty acids). Higher amounts of bioactive lipids (MUFA, PUFA) in milk have also been reported from cows fed with flax seed and fresh forage (Guerra et al. 2015). The daily intake of yogurt enriched with bioactive components has been suggested to manage the stress in a double-blinded randomized controlled trial (Jaatinen et al. 2014). Garcia-Tejedor et al (2015) have used casein and the yeast, *Debaryomyces hansenii*, to produce bioactive peptides having antihypertensive properties. Colostrum is known to be a rich source of high quality proteins, minerals, vitamins and bioactive compounds (e.g., immunoglobulins, lactoferrin, etc.) which exert positive health effects on human health. Hyrslova et al (2014) have produced yogurt from colostrum without influencing sensory quality of the final product.

Herbs and Condiments

On the Indian subcontinent, spices are integral part of any cooking and these spices are used mainly to enhance the flavor of a dish. The most common spices used are turmeric, chilli pepper, cumin, coriander, fenugreek, garlic, ginger, onion, mustard seeds, saffron, cinnamon, cloves, cardamom and asafetida. Some of these spices such as ginger, turmeric, garlic, onions, fenugreek seeds and saffron are known to contain many antioxidant and certain bioactive compounds such as curcumin, alliin, flavonoids, carotenoids and essential oils. Besides contributing flavor, color to the diet, these spices and condiments possess chemical constituents having beneficial physiological health effects. With a long history of use of spices and condiments in Indian subcontinent cooking dating back to 5000 years BC, these spices as functional foods have significantly contributed to the human health by supplying many health-promoting bioactive compounds in the diet.

Historically, ginger has been used in treating various ailments such as alleviating symptoms of nausea, vomiting, reduction of inflammation and pain, and is also known for its antioxidant, antimicrobial activities, and its possible beneficial effects against CVD due to its action against inflammation, platelet aggregation and hypertension (Singletary 2010: Gundala et al. 2014). The anticancer activities of ginger extract (GE) due to its phytochemicals, 6-gingerol, 8-gingerol, 10-gingerol and 6-shogaol and their effect on cytochrome P450 enzyme activity have been investigated by Mukkavilli et al (2014).Ginger has also been shown to protect live again the toxic effects of xenobiotic compounds and inhibits prostate cancer cell proliferation (Haniadka et al. 2013: Brahmbhatt et al. 2013).

Onion (*Allium cepa*) is a vegetable widely sued all over the world not only for its culinary properties but also for its medicinal values. The flavonoids present in onions have been reported to have a range of health benefits such as anticancer properties, antiplatelet activity, antithrombotic activity, antiasthmatic and anti-microbial activity (Jan et al. 2010; Joung & Jung 2014; Suleria et al. 2015; Lee et al. 2015: Sidhu et al. 2015). Onion extract has been shown to ameliorate high blood sugar and cholesterol in women with gestational diabetes (Anon 2015). Storage of fresh-cut onions at 0°C has been shown to preserve phenolics, anthocyanin and quercetin contents (Berno et al. 2014).

Garlic (*Allium sativum*) has long been used both for culinary as well as medicinal purposes in Asian countries. Preliminary investigations have suggested various health benefits of garlic consumption such as lowered risk of esophageal, stomach and prostate cancers, lowering of blood cholesterol, antiplatelet aggregation properties, antimicrobial, antioxidant, immune boosting, antidiabetic, hepatoprotective, antifibrinolytic, and its potential role in preventing cardiovascular diseases (Santhosha et al. 2013; Akan 2014; Trio et al. 2014; Matysiak et al. 2015; Seham et al. 2015; Suru & Ugwu 2015).

Turmeric (Curcuma longa) is a spice used extensively as one of the important components of curry powder in Asia for centuries. It is used as a natural coloring agent in culinary preparations has found many applications in functional foods (Pathak et al. 2015; Siruguri and Bhat 2015). The major chemical constituents of turmeric, curcumin, demethoxycurcumin, and bisdemethoxycurcumin) are commonly known as curcuminoids. Many benefits of turmeric, such as, anticarcinogenic, hepatoprotective, thrombo-suppressive, cardioprotective, antiarthritic, antimicrobial, antioxidative, lowering of plasma triglycerides (TG), lowering of plasma β-amyloid, protective against neurodegenerative diseases, improvement in life span, have been reported (Vankar 2008; Singletary 2010; DiSilvestro et al. 2012;Monray et al. 2013). However, some of the limitations of curcumin are its poor solubility, low absorption from the GI tract, rapid metabolism and rapid systemic elimination from the body. Use of hydrophilic carrier, cellulosic derivatives and natural antioxidants has been reported to significantly increase the absorption from the gut into the blood (Jager et al. 2015).

Fenugreek (*Trigonella foenum-graecum*) seeds have been used as a condiment in Asia for thousands of years in the culinary preparations as well as for medicinal uses. Fenugreek seeds are rich in many bioactive compounds, such as, flavonoids, isoflavones, saponins, oil, proteins insoluble and soluble dietary fiber. Fenugreek seeds have been shown to provide many health benefits, including, hypolipaemic activity, lowering of TG, LDL, amelioration of abnormalities in lipid homeostasis (Ramulu & Udayasekhararao 2006; Losso et al. 2010; Vijay Kumar et al. 2010).

Since ancient times, saffron (*Crocus sativus* L.) is being used as a flavoring and coloring agent in many culinary preparations, but the chemical, biological, nutritional value and health benefits of the world's most expensive spice have been reviewed in detail by Melnyk et al (2010). Saffron obtained from the stigmas and styles of the blue-purple saffron flower. Due to the presence of proteins, vitamins, minerals, carbohydrates, carotenoids and phytochemicals has been found to provide health-promoting properties as an antioxidant, antitumor, memory enhancer, antidepressant, anxiolytic, aphrodisiac, but has no toxicity. One of the carotenoid present in saffron, a highly water-soluble crocin (mono and diglycosyl esters of a polyene dicarboxylic acid, called crocetin) is the main constituent responsible for its color (Alavizadeh & Hosseinzadeh, 2014; Rahaiee et al. 2015).

Black cumin (*Nigella sativa* L.) is a spice used in the preparation of pickles. Nigella oil has been shown to rich in many bioactive phytochemicals such as essential oils, showing antifungal, antibacterial and antioxidant potentials. This oil had shown complete inhibition zones against Gram-negative and Gram-positive bacteria and some fungi too. The antioxidant potential of nigella oil was even superior to that of synthetic antioxidants (Ramadan, 2015).

Green tea (*Camellia sinensis*) is an ancient beverage popular in China but now is gaining interest in Western countries mainly because of its antioxidant properties. Green tea is known to be the richest source of many bioactive polyphenolic compounds, mainly catechins (Figure 3), which may be responsible for the proposed health benefits of providing protection against CVD (Murray et al. 2015). The research data were found to be insufficient to grant a health claim to the green tea for the protection against CVD.

Fruits

Ber (Zizyphus) Fruit

Ber or jujube (*Zizyphus)* is a tropical and subtropical fruit, which grows on a spiny shrub or tree. It belongs to the genus *Zizyphus* of the family Rhamnaceae. Its tree or shrub reaches to the height of 10-40

Figure 3. Chemical structure of the major phenolic compounds in green tea
Source: Murray et al. (2015)

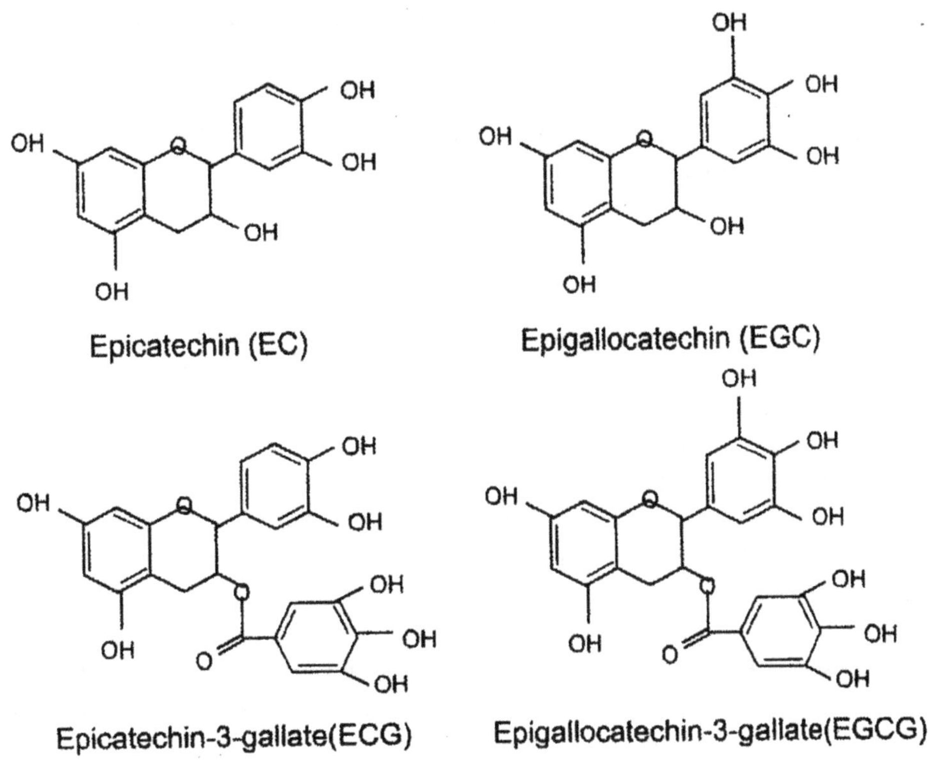

feet. *Ber* is among the ancient fruits originated in the Indo-Malaysian region of South and South Asia. Archaeological remains indicate that 7000 years ago, along with date fruits, *ber* was the main food for people in some parts of Pakistan (Ahmed, 2014), while Chinese jujube is known to be domesticated 4000 years ago (Liu, 2006). The two major dominated jujubes are however, *Zizyphus mauritiana* Lamk (Indian jujube) and *Zizyphus jujube* Mill (Chinese jujube). Although *ber* is extensively grown in India and Pakistan, it is underutilized and commercialized compared to the Chinese jujube. Chinese jujube and Indian jujube both grow in different climate such as Chinese jujube needs a temperate climate whereas Indian jujube grows in hot arid regions.

Ber fruit comes in various shapes and sizes from oval to round about 1-2.5 inch long. When fresh, its flesh is white and its skin greenish yellow that changes to red to dark maroon on ripening. The fruit is slightly juicy with sour sweet flavor and aroma. Most commonly, it is consumed raw in India and Pakistan and some as pickled and in dried form as a whole *ber* or powdered and added to other foods such as in beverages. On the other hand Chinese jujube is a highly profitable fruit with annual production of 1.4 million tons in 2001, which is 90% of the world jujube production. It is consumed mostly in fresh and dried forms and is used as an additive and flavorant to other foods. It has been used as a crude drug in traditiônal Chinese medicines palliative, analeptic and antibechic purposes for thousands of years. Chinese jujube has been studied more than any anyone else and therefore, the demand for it has increased in the last 10 years not only as a food but for pharmaceutical applications as well (Li et al., 2007).

Nutritional Characteristics

Ber is highly nutritious with abundant amount of vitamin C and a fair amount of vitamins A and B-complex. It also contains a fair amount of minerals such as iron, zinc, phosphorus and calcium. The proximate composition varies with the variety (Table 2). Ascorbic content ranges around 65-76 mg/100g whereas citric acid is 0.2-1.1 mg/100g. Other organic acids are malic and malonic acids. Pareek (2013) in their review of Jujube Fruit expressed that consumption one *ber* fruit a day fulfils the daily requirement for vitamin C of an adult as per WHO recommendations. It is known to have high vitamin P (bioflavonoid). Simple sugar content of *B*er is 22 g/100g while fiber content is 1.3 g/100g. The major simple sugars are glucose, fructose and galactose (Muchuweti et al., 2005).

Antioxidant Compounds

Antioxidants are organic compounds found in various foods that scavenge free radicals being constantly produced in the body due to oxidative stress and as a result of metabolic activities. Besides vitamins such as vitamins C, E and A, which are natural antioxidants in vegetable sources of our diet, phenolic compounds are also powerful antioxidants found in various fruits and vegetables. Increased oxidative stress in the body can cause chronic and degenerative disorders including type-2 diabetes, cardiovascular diseases and cancers (John & Shahidi, 2010). Adding a generous amount of fruits and vegetables that are a good source of antioxidants and polyphenols are recommended by health professionals.

Ber fruit is loaded with these antioxidants including vitamin C, tocopherol, vitamin A and β-carotenes as well as many phenolic compounds. The phenolic compounds found in *ber* fruit in abundance include, p-hydroxybenzoic, caffeic, ferulic and p-coumaric acids with concentrations of about 366, 31, 20 and 19 mg/kg (d. b.), respectively, whereas the least abundant is vanillic acid with a concentration of about 2.5 mg/kg (Pareek et al). Antioxidant activity and phenolic content of 12 Indian commercial cultivars of *Zizyphus mauritiana* Lamk are given in Table 3 showing a range of total phenolics from 172 to 329

Table 2. Nutrient composition of fresh Jujube fruit (units/100g)

Analysis	Nutrient (units)	Content
Proximate composition	Water (g)	77.86
	Energy (kcal)	79
	Protein (g)	1.20
	Total Lipid (g)	0.20
	Carbohydrate (g)	20.23
Minerals	Calcium, Ca (mg)	21
	Iron, Fe (mg)	0.48
	Magnesium, Mg (mg)	10
	Phosphorus, P (mg)	23
	Potassium, K (mg)	250
	Sodium, Na (mg)	3
	Zinc, Zn (mg)	0.05
Vitamins	Vitamin C (mg)	69.0
	Thiamin (mg)	0.02
	Riboflavin (mg)	0.04
	Niacin (mg)	0.9
	Vitamin B-6 (mg)	0.081
	Vitamin A, RAE (μg_RAE)	2
	Vitamin A (IU)	40

Adapted from USDA National Nutrient Database (2011)

mg GAE /100g, total flavonoids from 8 to 22 mg CAE/100g and ascorbic acid from 20 to 99 mg/100g (Koley et al. 2011). The antioxidant properties of *ber* (Z. mauritiana) fruit have been reported to decrease during irradiation but a dosage of 0.25 to 0.5 kGy was better to retain the natural antioxidants in fruit (Kavitha et al. 2015).

Similar variations in the antioxidant activities of five different Chinese jujube fruit were found. The free radical scavenging effect on the diphenyl-1-pycril-hydrazyl (DPPH) radicals reduced in the order of *Z. jujuba* cv.Jinisixiaozao > *Z. jujuba* cv. Yazao > *Z. jujuba* cv. Jianzao > *Z. jujuba* cv. Junzao > *Z. jujuba* cv. Sanbianhong. They also reported that the antioxidative activities in the extracts of these cultivars were stronger than α-tocopherol (Li et al 2005). The nutritional composition and phenolic contents are subjected to changes during growth and maturation of the fruit. For example, the ascorbic acid, sugars, carotenoids and polyphenol content of *ber* are reported to be initially low in the under ripe fruit but increase considerably when the fruit reaches a full physiological maturity (Zozio et al 2015).

Health Benefits of Ber Fruit

Consumption of foods that are high in fiber and antioxidants are promoted for various health benefits. Plant foods such as whole grains, vegetables and fruits including *ber* are known to be rich in natural antioxidants of vitamin origin as well as phenolic compounds. Health related functional characteristics and antioxidant properties of mucilage (dietary fiber) from Indian jujube fruit has been investigated by

Table 3. Total phenolics, flavonoids and ascorbic acid content of some Zizyphus genotypes

Cultivar	Total Phenolics[1]	Total Flavonoids[2]	Ascorbic Acid[3]
Chuhara	258.06 ± 37.99[cb]	8.36 ± 1.47[e]	99.49 ± 1.53[a]
Mundia	243.13 ± 41.59[dcb]	12.7 ± 1.11[edc]	93.88 ± 1.02[a]
Thornless	237.83 ± 37.09[dc]	12.38 ± 0.45[ed]	94.9 ± 2.04[a]
Jogia	241.26 ± 57.76[dc]	18.47 ± 3.03[b]	59.69 ± 0.51[d]
Gola	252.23 ± 18.29[dcb]	21.97 ± 2.09[b]	57.65 ± 4.59[d]
Kaithali	187.48 ± 34.16[ed]	13.09 ± 3.93[edc]	71.94 ± 1.53[c]
Umran	172.08 ± 31.77[e]	10.76 ± 0.85[ed]	19.54 ± 1.85[f]
Seb	203.23 ± 2.82[edc]	15.62 ± 1.92[dc]	21.95 ± 0.5[f]
ZG-3	328.65 ± 13.98[a]	14.58 ± 0.59[dc]	83.16 ± 0.51[b]
Sonaur-5	309.51 ± 46.73[ba]	11.47 ± 1.83[ed]	36.22 ± 0.51[e]
Rashmi	261.21 ± 43.68[cb]	14.71 ± 1.85[dc]	39.29 ± 3.57[e]
Elaichi	267.28 ± 18.39[cba]	16.07 ± 2.58[dc]	71.56 ± 1.15[c]

Values represent the mean of three replicates. Mean followed by the same superscripts are not significantly different ($p < 0.05$).[1]Total phenolics expressed as mg GAE/100 g.[2]Total flavonoids expressed as mg CAE/100 g. [3]Ascorbic acid expressed as mg/100 g.

Adapted from: Tammay et al. (2011)

Sangeethapriya & Siddhuraju (2014) and they suggested the crude mucilage fraction from Indian jujube fruit to have an excellent potential in nutraceutical and functional foods. Although not much scientific research is available on the health benefits of jujube fruit, but have been traditionally used for medicinal purposes in many Asian countries particularly India, Pakistan, Afghanistan, Iran, China, and Taiwan. Li et al (2005) reported its use for the treatment of simple allergies to insomnia, urinary tract infections and liver diseases in China dating back to 4000 years. In Algeria, *Zizyphus lotus* L (Desf.) is used for its medicinal effect for lowering inflammation in the body, for sedation and anti-diabetic purposes. Benammer et al (2010) analyzed the *Zizyphus lotus* L. (Desf.) the fruit pulp, seeds, leaves, stem and roots for vitamins and antioxidant content and assessed the effect of their extracts on human T-cell proliferation. Their results showed higher amount of vitamin A and C in the fruit pulp than the other parts, while the seeds were richer in vitamin C than the leaves, stem and roots. The immunosuppressive effect was exerted by extracts from all parts of the fruit however; the most dominant effect on T-cells proliferation and IL-2 mRNA expression was seen by the seed extract only.

The seeds of the Indian jujube *Zizyphus mauritiana* Lamk were also tested in hyperlipidemic rats and resulted in improved blood glucose and serum lipids levels as well as had an anti-inflammatory effect (Al-Reza et al, 2010). The antiproliferative effect on cancer cells and regulation of immune function is probably due to the presence of phenolic compounds, flavonoids, saponins that affect the protection against free radicals and cell damage against oxidative stress in biological processes (Siddiqui & Patil 2015; Dahiru & Obidoa, 2008; Kamiloglu et al. 2009; Zhang et al. 2010; Bhatia & Mishra 2010).

Jamun (*Syzygium cumini*) Fruit: The Indian Blackberry

Jamun (*Syzygium cumini* L.) belonging to Myrtaceae family, is a deep purplish blue color berry with pinkish pulp has sweet and astringent flavor. *Jamun* also known as *jamoon* or black plum in English has different names, such as, *Jambul* in Hindi, *Jamalu* in Punjabi and *Kala Jam* in Bengali. It is a summer fruit, which is available abundantly but only for short period of time. The Jamun fruit gradually changes color during ripening, starting from green color. The pigments, chlorophyll and carotenoids decrease while anthocyanins accumulate changing the original color of immature fruit from green to deep purple on full maturity. In the fully mature fruit, the total sugars increase but starch and amino acids decrease significantly (Patel & Ramana Rao 2014). *Jamun* tree is tall reaching up to a height of 30 meters, which is ever green that grows naturally in tropical and subtropical regions of Southeast Asia, such as, India, Pakistan, Bangladesh, Sri Lanka, Nepal, Myanmar, Afghanistan, Malaysia and Indonesia. The tree can live up to 100 years (Kalaivani & Chitra Devi 2013).

Health Benefits of Jamun

Jamun is known to have numerous properties and has been used as an important medicinal plant/fruit in various traditional systems of medicine for centuries. It has been shown to be effective in the treatment of type-2 diabetes, inflammation, diarrhea, and ulcers (Ayyanar et al. 2013). Swami et al (2012) have recently reviewed the food and medicinal uses of Jamun fruit. The fruit is rich in many bioactive compounds, such as, anthocyanins, glucoside, ellagic acid, isoquercetin, kaempferol and myrecetin. The seed is reported to contain alkaloid, jambosine, and glycoside jambolin, which stops diastatic activity of salivary enzyme that converts starch into sugar. The major component of its essential oil, α–pinene has significant anti-Leishmania activity (Rodrigues et al. 2015). *Jamun* fruit is reported to have antidiabetic, antiulcer, hepatoprotective, antiallergic, antiarthritic, anti-inflammatory, antihyperlipidemic, antimicrobial, antiplaque, radioprotective, antifertility, antipyretic, neuropsychopharmacological, nephroprotective, antidiarrhoeal, and antioxidant activities. These health benefits are mainly attributed to various phytochemicals, such as, tannins, steroids, flavonoids, alkaloids, fatty acids, terpenoids, phenolics, vitamins and minerals present in the fruit (Banerjee et al. 2005; Veigas et al. 2008; De Bona et al. 2011; Srivastava & Chandra 2012).

Nutritional Characteristics

The *jamun* fruit is known for its higher content of anthocyanins, plant pigments responsible for its purple color (Aqil et al. 2012). Anthocyanins have been extracted with 2% ethanol and containing 1% acetic acid and purified from *jamun* fruit using ion-exchange resin, and structural stability confirmed by HPLC-MS/MS techniques by a number of workers (Chaudhary & Mukhopadhyay 2013; Jampani et al. 2014). Prakash Maran et al (2014) have optimized the supercritical fluid extraction of anthocyanins and phenolic compounds from *jamun* fruit pulp. A pressure of 162 bar, extraction temperature of 50°C and co-solvent flow rate of 2.0g/min was suggested as optimal conditions of extraction of anthocyanins. Biochemical and histopathological effects of *jamun* juice as a source of natural antioxidants in comparison with BHT as synthetic antioxidant on rat health have been examined by El-Anany & Ali (2014). BHT produced significant changes in the liver and kidney enzymes but *jamun* juice did not cause any adverse effect on these organs.

Antioxidant Profile of Seeds and Leaves

Almost all parts of *jamun* fruit have been reported to be useful for various applications. Leaves of this tree have successfully used for the biosorption of zinc from aqueous solutions (King et al. 2008). The *jamun* seeds have been shown to possess significant anti-inflammatory activity, thus supporting the medicinal value of this plant (Kumar et al. 2008). Other applications, such as cadmium removal from aqueous solutions with *jamun* leaf powder (Srinivasa Rao et al. 2010), wound healing with seed extract (Murti et al. 2012), bio-inspired green synthesis of magnetite ($Fe3O4$) spherical magnetic nanoparticles using *jamun* seed extract (Venkateshwarlu et al., 2014), methylene blue biosorption from aqueous solutions using *jamun* leaf powder (Talathoti et al., 2014), use of *jamun* seed extract as green corrosion inhibitor in mild steel products under acidic conditions (Singh & Quraishi, 2015), use of malvidin anthocyanin in quorum quenching activity of *jamun* fruit against Klebsiella pneumoniae (Gopu et al., 2015), and use of anti-phytopathogenic activity of essential oils, hydrocarbon fractions and the other novel constituents from jamun to control fungal diseases in plants (Saroj et al., 2015), have also been reported. For antioxidant properties and the health benefits of *amla* fruit, the Indian Gooseberry (*Emblica officinalis* Gaertn or *Phyllanthus emblica* L.), the reader is referred to a chapter on super fruits by (Sidhu & Zafar, 2012).

Miscellaneous Foods

Flaxseed has attracted the attention of health professionals due to the presence of α-linolenic acid, a lignin (secoisolariciresinol diglyceride, SDG), high quality proteins, dietary fiber, phenolics, cyclic peptides, polysaccharides, alkaloids, cyanogenic glycosides, cadmium, and phytoestrogens (Shim et al, 2014; Kajla et al., 2015). Some of the diverse industrial, food and cosmetic products obtained from processing of flaxseed have been reviewed by Shim et al (2015). Flaxseed-enriched cereal-based products, such as, bread, pasta, muffins, cookies, cakes, and bars to highlight suitable processing conditions for producing healthy alternatives have been reviewed by Mercier et al (2014). The consumption of flaxseed lignan, SDG, has been suggested to prevent many diseases like cardiovascular, diabetic, lupus nephritis, bones, kidney, menopause, reproduction, mental stress, immunity, atherosclerosis, hemopoietic, liver necrosis and urinary disorders, because of its anti-inflammatory, antioxidant, antimutagenic, antimicrobial, antiobesity, antihypolipidemic and neuroprotective properties (Imran et al., 2015).

Psyllium husk is known to be an important source of water soluble dietary fiber and has been utilized to produce healthy baked products, such as, bread, buns, muffins, cake, and cookies (Ahluwalia et al., 1995; Sidhu, 2004; Bhise & Kaur, 2015). Psyllium husk has also been utilized for the production of low-fat yogurt with excellent sensory and eating qualities (Sadat-Ladjevardi et al., 2015). Okra (*Abelmoschus esculentus,* M.) is a popular health food due to its high dietary fiber, vitamin C, folate, calcium, potassium and antioxidant contents. Okra is reported to have many bioactive components (e.g., 4'-hydroxy phenethyl trans-ferulate) having anticancer properties (Ying et al., 2014). Another medicinal plant, *Aloe vera* gel has been reported to be a rich source of potent bioactive component with antioxidant (mainly phenolics) and UV absorbing activity (Ray et al., 2013). Meat and fermented meat products have been investigated as a good source of bioactive peptides having antioxidant, antihypertensive, and antimicrobial properties (Stadnik & Keska, 2015). For functional foods based on tree nuts (such as almonds, walnuts, pistachio, cashewnut and pine nuts etc.), the readers are referred to a recent publication by Kabir and Sidhu (2011).

FUTURE RESEARCH NEEDED

Since many centuries, the Asian countries have made use of many plants and animal products as medicinal foods. A number of foods have been mentioned in the folklore medicine literature. With the development of our capabilities in the analysis of food products, the role of various chemical constituents of food products is being suggested with a certain amount scientific basis. Various foods, such as, cereal grains, legumes, oilseeds, milk and milk products, herbs and condiments, exotic fruits and grain products are now being analysed for their phytochemical and other bioactive components. But still, there is a need for more research to determine complete nutritional profile of these food products to substantiate their medical and health claims for curing various human disease conditions. Obviously, more clinical studies involving human subjects are needed to elucidate the antioxidant effects on health parameters of these nutritionally important food products in order to fully appreciate their health benefits for the human population.

REFERENCES

Adom, K. K., Sorrells, M. E., & Liu, R. H. (2005). Phytochemicals and antioxidant activity of milled fractions of different wheat varieties. *Journal of Agricultural and Food Chemistry*, *53*(6), 2297–2306. doi:10.1021/jf048456d PMID:15769171

Ahluwalia, P., Kaur, A., & Sidhu, J. S. (1995). Effect of psyllium mucilloid husk as a source of fiber on baking properties of the flour and acceptability of the baked products. *Chem. Mikrobiol. Technol. Lebensm.*, *17*(3/4), 118–122.

Ahmad, A. S. (2015). Identification of potent antioxidant bioactive peptides from goat milk proteins. *Food Research International*, *74*, 80–88. doi:10.1016/j.foodres.2015.04.032

Ahmed, M. (2014). Ancient Pakistan - an archaeological history. In Harappan Civilization - The Material Culture (vol. 3). Foursome Group.

Akan, S. (2014). Health promoting properties of garlic (*Allium sativum* L.) consumption. *Akademik Gida*, *12*(2), 95–100.

Al-Hooti, S.N., Al-Saqer, J.M., Sidhu, J.S., & Al-Othman, A. (2002). Effect of raw wheat germ addition on the physical texture and objective color of a designer food (toast bread). *Nahrung/Food*, *46*(2), 68-72.

Al-Hooti, S. N., Sidhu, J. S., & Al-Saqer, J. M. (2000). Utility of CIE Tristimulus System in Measuring the Objective Crumb Color of High-fiber Toast Bread Formulations. *Journal of Food Quality*, *23*(1), 103–116. doi:10.1111/j.1745-4557.2000.tb00199.x

Al-Reza, S. M., Yoon, J. I., Kim, H. J., Kim, J. S., & Kang, S. E. (2010). Anti-inflammatory activity of seed essential oil from *Zizyphus jujube*. *Food and Chemical Toxicology*, *48*(2), 639–643. doi:10.1016/j.fct.2009.11.045 PMID:19944733

Al-Saqer, J. M., Sidhu, J. S., & Al-Hooti, S. N. (2000). Instrumental Texture and Baking Quality of High-fiber Toast Bread Formulations. *Journal of Food Processing and Preservation*, *24*(1), 1–16. doi:10.1111/j.1745-4549.2000.tb00402.x

Alavizadeh, S. H., & Hosseinzadeh, H. (2014). Bioactivity assessment and toxicity of crocin: A comprehensive review. *Food and Chemical Toxicology*, *64*, 65–80. doi:10.1016/j.fct.2013.11.016 PMID:24275090

Anderson, J. W., Randles, K. M., Kendall, C. W., & Jenkins, D. J. (2004). Carbohydrate and fiber recommendations for individuals with diabetes. A quantitative assessment and meta- analysis of the evidence. *Journal of the American College of Nutrition*, *23*(1), 5–17. doi:10.1080/07315724.2004.10719338 PMID:14963049

Anon., (2015). Functional foods and ingredients for protection against diabetes and metabolic syndrome. *Food Engg. Ingredients*, *40*(May/June), 16–18.

Aqil, F., Gupta, A., Munagala, R., Jeyabalan, J., Kausar, H., Sharma, R. J., & Gupta, R. C. et al. (2012). Antioxidant and antiproliferative activities of anthocyanin/Ellagitannin- enriched extracts from *Syzygium cumini* L. (Jamun, the Indian Blackberry). *Nutrition and Cancer*, *64*(3), 428–438. doi:10.1080/01635581.2012.657766 PMID:22420901

Ayyanar, M., Subash-Babu, P., & Ignacimuthu, S. (2013). *Syzygium cumini* L., a novel therapeutic agent for diabetes: Folk medicinal and pharmacological evidences. *Complementary Therapies in Medicine*, *21*(3), 232–243. doi:10.1016/j.ctim.2013.03.004 PMID:23642956

Bajaj, M., Kaur, A., & Sidhu, J. S. (1991). Studies on the development of nutritious cookies utilizing sunflower kernels and wheat germ. *Plant Foods for Human Nutrition (Dordrecht, Netherlands)*, *41*(4), 381–387. doi:10.1007/BF02310631 PMID:1665564

Bala, M., Kumar, S., Kumar, A., & Singh, M. (2012). Composition of antioxidant activity and bioactive compounds in leaves of selected Brassica genotypes. *Indian Journal of Agricultural Biochemistry*, *25*(2), 142–146.

Banerjee, A., Dasgupta, N., & De, B. (2005). In vitro study of antioxidant activity of *Syzygium cumini* fruit. *Food Chemistry*, *90*(4), 727–733. doi:10.1016/j.foodchem.2004.04.033

Bazzano, L. A., He, J., Ogden, L. G., Loria, C., Vipputuri, S., Myers, L., & Whelton, P. K. (2011a). Legume consumption and risk of coronary heart disease in US men and women. *Archives of Internal Medicine*, *161*(21), 2573–2578. doi:10.1001/archinte.161.21.2573 PMID:11718588

Bazzano, L. A., Thompson, A. M., Tees, M. T., Nguyen, C. H., & Winham, D. N. (2011b). Non-soy legume consumption lowers cholesterol levels: A meta-analysis of randomized controlled trials. *Nutrition, Metabolism, and Cardiovascular Diseases*, *21*(2), 94–103. doi:10.1016/j.numecd.2009.08.012 PMID:19939654

Benammar, C., Hichami, A., Yessoufou, A., Akadiri. Simonin, A.-M., Belarbi, M., Allali, H., & Khan, N. A. (2010). *Zizyphus lotus* L. (Deff.) modulates antioxidant activity and human T- cell proliferation. *BMC Complementary and Alternative Medicine*, *10*(1), 54. doi:10.1186/1472-6882-10-54 PMID:20868496

Benincasa, P., Galieni, A., Manetta, A. C., Pace, R., Guiducci, M., Pisante, M., & Stagnari, F. (2015). Phenolic compounds in grains, sprouts and wheatgrass of hulled and non-hulled wheat species. *Journal of the Science of Food and Agriculture*, *95*(9), 1795–1803. doi:10.1002/jsfa.6877 PMID:25131800

Berno, N. D., Tezotto-Uliana, J. V., Dias, C. T., & dos, . (2014). Storage temperature and type of cut affect the biochemical and physiological characteristics of fresh-cut purple onions. *Postharvest Biology and Technology*, *93*, 91–96. doi:10.1016/j.postharvbio.2014.02.012

Bhatia, A., & Mishra, T. (2010). Hypoglycemic activities of *Zizyphus mauritiana* aqueous ethanol seed extract in alloxan-induced diabetic mice. *Pharm. Biol., 48*(6), 604–610. doi:10.3109/13880200903218935 PMID:20645731

Bhise, S., & Kaur, A. (2015). Fortifying muffins with psyllium husk, oat fiber and barley fiber to improve quality and shelf life. *Carpathian Journal of Food Science and Technology., 7*(2), 5–16.

Bona, K. S. D., Belle, L. P., Bittencourt, P. E. R., Bonfanti, G., Cargnelluti, L. O., Pimentel, V. C., & Moretto, M. B. et al. (2011). Erythrocytic enzymes and antioxidant status in people with type-2 diabetes: Beneficial effect of *Syzygium cumini* leaf extract in vitro. *Diabetes Research and Clinical Practice, 94*(1), 84–90. doi:10.1016/j.diabres.2011.06.008 PMID:21737173

Bouchenak, M., & Lamri-Senhadji, M. (2013). Nutritional quality of legumes and their role in cardiometabolic risk prevention: A review. *Journal of Medicinal Food, 16*(3), 185–198. doi:10.1089/jmf.2011.0238 PMID:23398387

Brahmbhatt, M., Gundala, S. R., Asif, G., Shamsi, S. A., & Aneja, R. (2013). Ginger phytochemicals exhibit synergy to inhibit prostate cancer cell proliferation. *Nutrition and Cancer, 65*(2), 263–272. doi:10.1080/01635581.2013.749925 PMID:23441614

Brandelli, A., Dariot, D. J., & Correa, A. P. F. (2015). Whey as a source of peptides with remarkable biological activities. *Food Research International, 73*, 149–161. doi:10.1016/j.foodres.2015.01.016

Brewer, L. R., Kubola, J., Siriamornpun, S., Herald, T. J., & Shi, Y.-C. (2014). Wheat bran particle size influence on phytochemical extractability and antioxidant properties. *Food Chemistry, 152*, 483–490. doi:10.1016/j.foodchem.2013.11.128 PMID:24444965

Cais-Sokolinska, D., Pikul, J., Wojtowski, J., Dankow, R., Teichert, J., Czyzak-Runowska, G., & Bagnicka, E. (2015). Evaluation of quality of kefir from milk obtained from goats supplemented with a diet rich in bioactive compounds. *Journal of the Science of Food and Agriculture, 95*(6), 1343–1349. doi:10.1002/jsfa.6828 PMID:25042847

Camargo, A. C., Vieira, T. M. F. S., Arce, M. A. B. R., & Calori-Domingues, M. A. (2012). Gamma radiation effects on peanut skin antioxidants. *International Journal of Molecular Sciences, 13*(12), 3073–3084. doi:10.3390/ijms13033073 PMID:22489142

Charalampopoulos, D.; Wang, R.; Pandiella, S.S. & Webb, C. (2002). Application of cereals and cereal components in functional foods: a review. *International Journal of Food Microbiology, 79*(1-2), 131-141.

Chaudhary, B., & Mukhopadhyay, K. (2013). Solvent optimization for anthocyanin extraction from *Syzygium cumini* L. Skeels using response surface methodology. *International Journal of Food Sciences and Nutrition, 64*(3), 363–371. doi:10.3109/09637486.2012.738647 PMID:23121325

Chen, C. Y. N., Kamil, A., & Blumberg, J. B. (2015). Phytochemical composition and antioxidant capacity of whole wheat products. *International Journal of Food Sciences and Nutrition, 66*(1), 63–70. doi:10.3109/09637486.2014.971228 PMID:25578763

Chhabra, P., & Sidhu, J. S. (1988). Fate of phytic acid during bread making. *Die Nahrung, 32*(1), 15–19. doi:10.1002/food.19880320104

Chukwumah, Y. C., Walker, L. T., Verghese, M., Bokanga, M., Ogutu, S., & Alphonse, K. (2007). Comparison of extraction methods for the quantification of selected phytochemicals in peanuts (*Arachis hypogaea*). *Journal of Agricultural and Food Chemistry*, *55*(2), 285–290. doi:10.1021/jf062148t PMID:17227055

Dahiru, D., & Obidoa, O. (2008). Evaluation of the antioxidant effects of *Zizyphus mauritiana Lamk.* Leaf extracts against chronic ethanol-induced hepatotoxicity in rat liver. *African Journal of Traditional, Complementary, and Alternative Medicines*, *5*(1), 39–45. doi:10.4314/ajtcam.v5i1.31254 PMID:20162053

Dalton, S. M. C., Tapsell, L. C., & Probst, Y. (2012). Potential health benefits of whole wheat components. *Nutrition Today*, *47*(4), 163–174. doi:10.1097/NT.0b013e31826069d0

Darmadi-Blackberry, I., Wahlqvist, M. L., Kouris-Blazos, A., Steen, B., Lukito, W., Horie, Y., & Horie, K. (2004). Legumes: The most important dietary predictor of survival in older people of different ethnicities. *Asia Pacific Journal of Clinical Nutrition*, *13*, 217–220. PMID:15228991

Dilis, V., & Trichopoulou, A. (2009). Nutritional and health properties of pulses. *Mediterranean Journal of Nutrition and Metabolism.*, *1*(3), 149–157. doi:10.1007/s12349-008-0023-2

DiSilvestro, R. A., Joseph, E., Zhao, S., & Bomser, J. (2012). Diverse effects of a low dose supplement of lapidated curcumin in healthy middle aged people. *Nutrition Journal*, *11*(1), 79–84. doi:10.1186/1475-2891-11-79 PMID:23013352

Duenas, M., Hernandez, T., Robredo, S., Lamparski, G., Estrella, I., & Munoz, R. (2012). Bioactive phenolic compounds of soybean (Glycine max cv. Merit): Modifications by different microbiological fermentations. *Polish Journal of Food Sciences.*, *62*(4), 241–250.

Edge, M. S., Jones, J. M., & Marquart, L. (2005). A new life for whole grains. *Journal of the American Dietetic Association*, *105*(12), 1856–1860. doi:10.1016/j.jada.2005.10.022 PMID:16321586

El-Anany, A. M., & Ali, R. F. M. (2013). Biochemical and histopathological effects of administration various levels of Pomposia (*Syzygium cumini*) fruit juice as natural antioxidant on rat health. *Journal of Food Sciences and Technology.*, *50*(3), 487–495. doi:10.1007/s13197-011-0372-6 PMID:24425943

Faris, M. A. I. E., Takfufi, H. R., & Issa, A. Y. (2013). Role of lentils (*Lens culinaris* L.) in human health and nutrition: A review. *Mediterranean Journal of Nutrition And Metabolism.*, *6*(1), 3–16. doi:10.1007/s12349-012-0109-8

Garcia-Tejedor, A., Sanchez-Rivera, L., Recio, I., Salom, J. B., & Manzanares, P. (2015). Dairy *Debaryomyces hansenii* strains produce the antihypertensive casein-derived peptides LHLPLP and HLPLP. LWT-. *Food Science and Technology (Campinas.)*, *61*, 550–556.

Ghawi, S. K., Shen, Y., Niranjan, K., & Methven, L. (2014). Consumer acceptability and sensory profile of cooked broccoli with mustard seeds added to improve chemoprotective properties. *Journal of Food Science*, *79*(9), S1756–S1762. doi:10.1111/1750-3841.12556 PMID:25156799

Gopu, V., Kothandapani, S., & Shetty, P. H. (2015). Quorum quenching activity of *Syzygium cumini* L. Skeels and its anthocyanin malvidin against *Klebsiella pneumonia. Microbial Pathogenesis*, *79*, 61–69. doi:10.1016/j.micpath.2015.01.010 PMID:25637095

Guerra, E., Verardo, V., & Carboni, M. F. (2015). Determination of bioactive compounds in cream obtained as a by-product during cheese-making: Influence of cow's diet on lipid quality. *International Dairy Journal*, *42*, 16–25. doi:10.1016/j.idairyj.2014.11.004

Gundala, S. R., Mukkavilli, R., Yang, C., Yadav, P., Tandon, V., Vangala, S., & Aneja, R. et al. (2014). Enterohepatic recirculation of bioactive ginger phytochemicals is associated with enhanced tumor growth-inhibitory activity of ginger extract. *Carcinogenesis*, *35*(6), 1320–1329. doi:10.1093/carcin/bgu011 PMID:24431413

Haniadka, R., Saxena, A., Shivashankara, A. R., Fayad, R., Palatty, P. L., Nazreth, N., & Shrinath Baliga, M. et al. (2013). Ginger protects the liver against the toxic effects of xenobiotic compounds: Preclinical observations. *Journal of Nutrition and Food Sciences.*, *3*(5), 1–6.

Hermsdorff, H. H., Zulet, M. A., Abete, I., & Martinez, J. A. (2011). A legume-based hypocaloric diet reduces proinflammatory status and improves metabolic features in overweight/obese subjects. *European Journal of Nutrition*, *50*(1), 61–69. doi:10.1007/s00394-010-0115-x PMID:20499072

Hodge, A. M., English, D. R., McCredie, M. R., Severi, G., Boyle, P., Hopper, J. L., & Giles, G. G. (2004). Foods, nutrients and prostate cancer. *Cancer Causes & Control*, *15*(1), 11–20. doi:10.1023/B:CACO.0000016568.25127.10 PMID:14970730

Hosseinian, F. S., Li, W., & Beta, T. (2008). Measurement of anthocyanins and other phytochemicals in purple wheat. *Food Chemistry*, *109*(4), 916–924. doi:10.1016/j.foodchem.2007.12.083 PMID:26050008

Hyrslova, I., Chmurova, J., Krausova, G., & Curda, I. (2014). Potential of bovine colostrum for its application in fermented milk products. *Mlekarske Listy*, *25*(147S), xii–xiv.

Imran, M., Ahmad, N., Anjum, F. M., Khan, M. K., Mushtaq, Z., Nadeem, M., & Hussain, S. (2015). Potential protective properties of flax lignin secoisolariciresinol diglucoside. *Nutrition Journal*, *14*(1), 71–76. doi:10.1186/s12937-015-0059-3 PMID:26215288

Irshad, I., Kanekanian, A., Peters, A. & Masud, T. (2015). Antioxidant activity of bioactive peptides derived from bovine casein hydrolysate fractions. *Journal of Food Sciences and Technology, 52*(1), 231-239.

Isanga, J., & Zhang, G. N. (2007). Biologically active components and nutraceuticals in peanuts and related products[Review]. *Food Reviews International*, *23*(2), 123–140. doi:10.1080/87559120701224956

Isanga, J., & Zhang, G. N. (2008). Soybean bioactive components and their implications to health- a review. *Food Reviews International*, *24*(2), 252–276. doi:10.1080/87559120801926351

Jaatinen, N., Korpela, R., Poussa, T., Turpeinen, A., Mustonen, S., Merilahti, J., & Peuhkuri, K. (2014). Effects of daily intake of yogurt enriched with bioactive components on chronic stress responses: A double-blinded randomized controlled trial. *International Journal of Food Sciences and Nutrition*, *65*(4), 507–514. doi:10.3109/09637486.2014.880669 PMID:24490888

Jacobs, D. R. Jr, Pereira, M. A., Stumpf, K., Pins, J. J., & Aldercreutz, H. (2002). Whole grain food intake elevates serum enterolactone. *The British Journal of Nutrition*, *88*(2), 111–116. doi:10.1079/BJN2002601 PMID:12144714

Jager, R., Lowery, R. P., Calvanese, A. V., Joy, J. M., Purpura, M., & Wilson, J. M. (2014). Comparative absorption of curcumin formulations. *Nutrition Journal*, *13*(1), 11–18. doi:10.1186/1475-2891-13-11 PMID:24461029

Jampani, C., Naik, A., & Raghavarao, K. S. M. S. (2014). Purification of anthocyanins from *jamun* (*Syzygium cumini* L.) employing adsorption. *Separation and Purification Technology*, *125*, 170–178. doi:10.1016/j.seppur.2014.01.047

Jan, A. T., Kamli, M. R., Murtaza, I., Singh, J. B., Ali, A., & Haq, Q. M. R. (2010). Dietary flavonoid quercetin and associated health benefits- an overview. *Food Reviews International*, *26*(3), 302–317. doi:10.1080/87559129.2010.484285

John, J. A., & Shahidi, F. (2010). Phenolic compounds and antioxidant activity of Brazilian nut (*Bertholletia excelsa*). *Journal of Functional Foods*, *2*(3), 196–209. doi:10.1016/j.jff.2010.04.008

Joung, E. M., & Jung, K. H. (2014). Antioxidant activity of onion (*Allium cepa* L.) peel extracts obtained as onion by-products. *Korean Journal of Food Sciences and Technology*, *46*(3), 364–368. doi:10.9721/KJFST.2014.46.3.364

Kabagambe, E. K., Baylin, A., Ruiz-Narvarez, E., Siles, X., & Campos, H. (2005). Decreased consumption of dried mature beans is positively associated with urbanization and nonfatal acute myocardial infarction. *The Journal of Nutrition*, *135*, 17701775. PMID:15987863

Kabir, Y., & Sidhu, J. S. (2011). Antioxidative Functional Factors in Nuts. In J. Shi, C.-T. Ho, & F. Shahidi (Eds.), *Functional Foods of the East* (pp. 343–397). Taylor and Francis.

Kajla, P., Sharma, A., & Sood, D. R. (2015). Flaxseed- a potential functional food source. *Journal of Food Sciences and Technology*, *52*(4), 1857–1871. doi:10.1007/s13197-014-1293-y PMID:25829567

Kamiloglu, O., Ercisli, S., Sengul, M., Toplu, C., & Serce, S. (2009). Total phenolics and antioxidant activity of jujube (*Zizyphus jujube* Mill.) genotypes selected from Turkey. *African Journal of Biotechnology*, *8*, 303–307.

Kavaz, A., & Bakirci, I. (2009). Natural bioactive substances in milk. *Akademik Gida*, *7*(5), 44–50.

Kavitha, C., Kuna, A., Supraja, T., Blessy Sagar, S., Padmavathi, T. V. S., & Prabhakar, N. (2015). Effect of gamma irradiation on antioxidant properties of ber (*Zizyphus mauritiana*) fruit. *Journal of Food Sciences Technology.*, *52*(5), 3123–3128. doi:10.1007/s13197-014-1359-x PMID:25892819

King, P., Rakesh, N., Beena Lahiri, S., Prasanna Kumar, Y., & Prasad, V. S. R. K. (2008). Biosorption of zinc onto *Syzygium cumini* L.: Equilibrium and kinetic studies. *Chem. Engg. J.*, *144*(2), 181–187. doi:10.1016/j.cej.2008.01.019

Kisbenedek, A., Szabo, S., Polyak, E., Breitenbach, Z., Bona, A., Mark, L., & Figler, M. (2014). Analysis of trans-resveratrol in oilseeds by high-performance liquid chromatography. *Acta Alimentaria*, *43*(3), 459–464. doi:10.1556/AAlim.43.2014.3.13

Kiss, A., Naar, Z., Daroczi, L., Nemedi, E., & Kukovics, S. (2014). Development of functional sheep and goat milk products and the investigation of functionality in various packaging materials. *J. Hygienic Engg. Design*, *7*, 174–179.

Koley, T. K., Kaur, C., Nagal, S., Walia, S., & Sarika, S. (2011). *Antioxidant activity and phenolic content in genotypes of Indian jujube (Zizyphus mauritiana Lamk).* Arabian Journal of Chemistry; doi:10.1016/j.arabjc

Koliwer-Brandl, H., Siegert, N., Umnus, K., Kelm, A., Tolkach, A., Kulozik, U., & Kelm, S. et al. (2011). Lectin inhibition assays for the analysis of bioactive milk sialoglycoconjugates. *International Dairy Journal, 21*(6), 413–420. doi:10.1016/j.idairyj.2011.01.005

Kumar, A., Llavarasan, R., Jayachandran, T., Deecaraman, M., Mohan Kumar, R., Aravindan, P., & Krishan, M. R. V. et al. (2008). Anti-inflammatory activity of *Syzygium cumini* seed. *African Journal of Biotechnology, 7*(8), 941–943.

le Parc, A., Dalas, D. C., Duaut, S., Leonil, J., Martin, P., & Barile, D. (2014). Characterization of goat milk lactoferrin N-glycans and comparison with the N-Glycans of human and bovine milk. *Electrophoresis, 35*(11), 1560–1570. doi:10.1002/elps.201300619 PMID:24519758

Lee, E. J., Patil, B. S., & Yoo, K. S. (2015). Antioxidants of 15 onions with white, yellow, and red colors and their relationship with pungency, anthocyanin, and quercetin. LWT-. *Food Science and Technology (Campinas.), 63*(1), 108–114.

Levent, H., Bilgicli, N., & Ertas, N. (2015). The assessment of leavened and unleavened flat breads properties enriched with wheat germ. *Qual. Assur. Safety Crops & Foods, 7*(3), 321–326. doi:10.3920/QAS2013.0341

Li, J. W., Ding, S. D., & Ding, X. L. A. (2005). Comparison of antioxidant capacities of extracts from five cultivars of Chinese jujube. *Process Biochemistry (Barking, London, England), 40*(11), 3607–3613. doi:10.1016/j.procbio.2005.03.005

Li, J. W., Fan, L. P., Ding, S. D., & Ding, X. L. (2007). Nutritional composition of five cultivars of Chinese jujube. *Food Chemistry, 103*(2), 454–460. doi:10.1016/j.foodchem.2006.08.016

Liu, M. (2006). Chinese jujube: Botany and horticulture. *Horticultural Reviews, 32*, 229–298.

Livesey, G., Taylor, R., Hulshof, T., & Howlett, J. (2008). Glycemic response and health- A systematic review and meta-analysis: Relations between dietary glycemic properties and health outcomes. *The American Journal of Clinical Nutrition, 87*, 258S–268S. PMID:18175766

Losso, J. N., Holliday, D. L., Richard, G., Karki, N., & Finley, J. W. (2010). The health benefits of fenugreek-enriched cereal products. *Cereal Foods World, 55*(5), 236–241.

Lu, Y., Junli, L., Hao, J., Niu, Y., Whent, M., Costa, J., & Yu, L. (2015b). Genotype, environment, and their interactions on the phytochemical compositions and radical scavenging properties of soft winter wheat bran. LWT-. *Food Science and Technology (Campinas.), 60*(1), 277–283.

Lu, Y., Fuerst, E. P., Lv, J., Morris, C. F., Yu, L., Fletcher, A., & Luthria, D. et al. (2015a). Phytochemical profile and antiproliferative activity of dough and bread fractions made from refined and whole wheat flours. *Cereal Chem., 92*(3), 271–277. doi:10.1094/CCHEM-10-14-0214-R

Ma, Y., & Huang, H. (2014). Characterization and comparison of phenols, flavonoids and isoflavones of soymilk and their correlations with antioxidant activity. *International Journal of Food Science & Technology*, *49*(10), 2290–2298. doi:10.1111/ijfs.12545

Mallik, N., Bhaskar Reddy, G. V., Kiranmayi, B., Govind, V., Eswara Rao, B., & Ashalatha, P. (2013). Milk constituents as functional food components. *Indian Food Industry*, *32*(1), 17–26.

Marathe, S. A., Rajalakshmi, V., Jamdar, S. N., & Sharma, A. (2011). Comparative study on antioxidant activity of different varieties of commonly consumed legumes in India. *Food and Chemical Toxicology*, *49*(9), 2005–2012. doi:10.1016/j.fct.2011.04.039 PMID:21601612

Matysiak, M., Gawel-Beben, K., Rybczynska, K., Gminski, J., & Surma, S. (2015). Comparing selected biological properties of garlic (*Allium sativum* L.) from Poland and China. *Zywnosc*, *22*(2), 160–169.

Melnyk, J. P., Wang, S., & Marcone, M. F. (2010). Chemical and biological properties of the world's most expensive spice: Saffron. *Food Research International*, *43*(8), 1981–1989. doi:10.1016/j.foodres.2010.07.033

Mercier, S., Villeneuve, S., Moresoli, C., Mendor, M., Marcos, B., & Power, K. A. (2014). Flaxseed-enriched cereal-based products: A review of the impact of processing conditions. *Compreh. Reviews Food Sci. Food Safety*, *13*(4), 400–412. doi:10.1111/1541-4337.12075

Messina, M. J., Persky, V., Setchell, D. R., & Barnes, S. (1994). Soy intake and cancer risk: A review of the in vitro and in vivo data. *Nutrition and Cancer*, *21*(2), 113–131. doi:10.1080/01635589409514310 PMID:8058523

Mills, S., Ross, R. P., Hill, C., Fitzgerald, G. F., & Stanton, C. (2011). Mill intelligence: Mining milk for bioactive substances associated with human health. *International Dairy Journal*, *21*(6), 377–401. doi:10.1016/j.idairyj.2010.12.011

Moller, M. E., Dahl, R., & Bockman, O. C. (1998). A possible role of the dietary fiber product, wheat bran, as a nitrite scavenger. *Food and Chemical Toxicology*, *26*(10), 841–845. doi:10.1016/0278-6915(88)90024-5 PMID:2851507

Monroy, A., Lithgow, G. J., & Alavez, S. (2013). Curcumin and neurodegenerative diseases- a review. *Int. Union Biochem. Mol. Biol.*, *39*(1), 122–132.

Muchuweti, M., Zenda, G., Ndhlala, A. R., & Kasiyamhuru, A. (2005). Sugars, organic acid and phenolic compounds in *Zizyphus mauritiana* fruit. *European Journal of Food Research and Technology.*, *221*(3-4), 570–574. doi:10.1007/s00217-005-1204-6

Mukkavilli, R., Gundala, S.R., Yang, C., Donthamsetty, S., Cantuaria, G., Jadhav, G.R., Vangala, S., Reid, M.D. & Aneja, R. (2014). Modulation of cytochrome P450 metabolism and transport across intestinal epithelial barrier by ginger biophenolics. *PLOS One, 9*(9), 1-12.

Murray, M., Walchuk, C., Suh, M., & Jones, P. J. (2015). Green tea catechins and cardiovascular disease risk factors: Should a health claim be made by the United States Food and Drug Administration? *Trends in Food Science & Technology*, *41*(2), 188–197. doi:10.1016/j.tifs.2014.10.004

Murray, M., Walchuk, C., Suh, M., & Jones, P. J. (2015). Green tea catechins and cardiovascular disease risk factors: Should a health claim be made by the United States Food and Drug Administration? *Trends in Food Science & Technology*, *41*(2), 188–197. doi:10.1016/j.tifs.2014.10.004

Murti, K., & Paliwal, D. (2012). Exploration of preliminary phytochemical studies of seed of *Syzygium cumini*. *American Journal of Pharmacology and Toxicology.*, *7*(1), 12–14. doi:10.3844/ajptsp.2012.12.14

Nasir, M., & Sidhu, J. S. (2013). Chickpea, Lentil, Mung bean, Black gram, Pigeon Pea and India Vetch. In Pulses: Production, Processing and Nutritional Value. Wiley-Blackwell Publishing Co.

Nongonierma, A. B., & Fitzgerald, R. J. (2015a). The scientific evidence for the role of milk protein-derived bioactive peptides in humans: A review. *J. Functional Foods*, *17*, 640–656. doi:10.1016/j.jff.2015.06.021

Nongonierma, A. B., & Fitzgerald, R. J. (2015b). Milk proteins as a source of tryptophan- containing bioactive peptides. *Food Function*, *6*(7), 2115–2127. doi:10.1039/C5FO00407A PMID:26027501

Pareek, S. (2013). Nutritional composition of jujube fruit. *Emirates Journal of Food and Agriculture.*, *25*(6), 463–470.

Pareek, S., Kitinoja, L., Kaushik, R. A., & Paliwal, R. (2009). Postharvest physiology and storage of *ber. Stew. Posthar. Rev.*, *5*(5), 1–10. doi:10.2212/spr.2009.5.5

Pathak, L., Kanwal, A., & Agrawal, Y. (2015). Curcumin loaded self-assembled lipid-biopolymer nanoparticles for functional food applications. *J. Food Sci. Technol.*, *52*(10), 6143–6156. doi:10.1007/s13197-015-1742-2 PMID:26396362

Pekkinen, J., Rosa, N. N., Savolainen, O. I., Keski-Rahkonen, P., Mykkanen, H., Poutanen, K., & Hanihineva, K. et al. (2014). Disintegration of wheat aleurone structure has an impact on the bioavailability of phenolic compounds and other phytochemicals as evidenced by altered urinary metabolic profile of diet-induced obese mice. *Nutrition and Metabolism*, *11*(1), 1–15. doi:10.1186/1743-7075-11-1 PMID:24383425

Prakash-Maran, J., Priya, B., & Manikandan, S. (2014). Modeling and optimization of supercritical extraction of anthocyanin and phenolic compounds from *Syzygium cumini* fruit pulp. *Journal of Food Sciences and Technology.*, *51*(9), 1938–1946. doi:10.1007/s13197-013-1237-y PMID:25190849

Rahaiee, S., Moini, S., Hashemi, M., & Shojaosadati, S. A. (2015). Evaluation of antioxidant activities of bioactive compounds and various extracts obtained from saffron (*Crocus sativus* L.): A review. *Journal of Food Sciences and Technology.*, *52*(4), 1881–1888. doi:10.1007/s13197-013-1238-x PMID:25829569

Raikos, V., & Dassios, T. (2014). Health-promoting properties of bioactive peptides derived from milk proteins in infant food: A review. *Dairy Sci. Technol.*, *94*(2), 91–101. doi:10.1007/s13594-013-0152-3 PMID:24511365

Ramadan, M. F. (2015). Nutritional value and applications of Nigella sativa essential oil: A mini review. *Journal of Essential Oil Research.*, *27*(4), 271–275. doi:10.1080/10412905.2015.1045564

Ramulu, P., & Udayasekhararao, P. (2006). Total insoluble and soluble dietary fiber contents of roots, tubers, vegetables, oilseeds, spices and condiments. *Journal of Food Sciences and Technology.*, *43*(4), 399–403.

Ranich, T., Bhathena, S. J., & Velasquez, M. T. (2001). Protective effect s of dietary phytoestrogens in chronic renal disease. *Journal of Renal Nutrition*, *11*(4), 183–193. doi:10.1016/S1051-2276(01)70036-2 PMID:11679998

Ray, A., Dutta Gupta, S., & Ghosh, S. (2013). Isolation and characterization of potent bioactive fraction with antioxidant and UV absorbing activity from *Aloe vera berbadensis* Miller gel. *Journal of Plant Biochemistry and Biotechnology*, *22*(4), 483–487. doi:10.1007/s13562-012-0178-2

Ressureccion, A. V. A., Sales, J. M., Potrebko, I., Francisco, M. L. L. D., & Hitchcock, H. L. (2009). Peanuts: Bioactive food in a shell. *Food Technology*, *63*(12), 30–36.

Ricci-Cabello, I., Herrera, M. O., & Artacho, R. (2012). Possible role of milk derived bioactive peptides in the treatment and prevention of metabolic syndrome. *Nutrition Reviews*, *70*(4), 241–255. doi:10.1111/j.1753-4887.2011.00448.x PMID:22458697

Rochfort, S., & Panozzo, J. (2007). Phytochemicals for health, the role of pulses. *Journal of Agricultural and Food Chemistry*, *55*(20), 7981–7994. doi:10.1021/jf071704w PMID:17784726

Rodrigues, K. A. F., Amorim, L. V., Dias, C. N., Moraes, D. F. C., Caneiro, S. M. P., & Carvalho, F. A. A. (2015). *Syzygium cumini* L. Skeels essential oil and its major constituent α–pinene exhibit anti-Leishmania activity through immunomodulation in vitro. *Journal of Ethnopharmacology*, *160*, 32–40. doi:10.1016/j.jep.2014.11.024 PMID:25460590

Rondini, E. A., & Bannink, M. R. (2012). Microarray analysis of genes differentially expressed by diet (black beans and soy flour) during azoxymethane-induced colon carcinogenesis in rats. *Journal of Nutrition and Metabolism*, *2012*, 1–17. doi:10.1155/2012/351796 PMID:22496968

Rosa-Sibakov, N., Poutanen, K., & Micard, V. (2015). How does wheat grain, bran and aleurone structure impact their nutritional and technological properties? *Trends in Food Science & Technology*, *41*(2), 118–134. doi:10.1016/j.tifs.2014.10.003

Sadat Ladjevardi, Z., Taghi-Gharibzahedi, S. M., & Mousavi, M. (2015). Development of a stable low-fat yogurt gel using functionality of psyllium (*Plantago ovata* Forsk) husk gum. *Carbohydrate Polymers*, *125*, 272–280. doi:10.1016/j.carbpol.2015.02.051 PMID:25857984

Salgado, P. R., Lopez-Caballero, M. E., Gomez-Guillen, M. C., Mauri, A. N., & Montero, M. P. (2012). Exploration of the antioxidant and antimicrobial capacity of two sunflower protein concentrate films with naturally present phenolic compounds. *Food Hydrocolloids*, *29*(2), 374–381. doi:10.1016/j.foodhyd.2012.03.006

Sangeethapriya, M., & Sidduraja, P. (2014). Health related functional characteristics and antioxidant potential of mucilage (dietary fiber) from Zizyphus mauritiana fruits. *Food Sci. Human Wellness*, *3*(2), 79–88. doi:10.1016/j.fshw.2014.05.003

Santhosha, S. G., Prakash, J., & Prabhavathi, S. N. (2013). Bioactive components of garlic and their physiological role in health maintenance: A review. *Food Biosci.*, *3*, 59–74. doi:10.1016/j.fbio.2013.07.001

Saroj, A., Pragadheesh, V. S., Palanivelu, , Yadav, A., Singh, S. C., Samad, A., & Chanotiya, C. S. et al. (2015). Antiphytopathogenic activity of *Syzygium cumini* essential oils, hydrocarbon fractions and its novel constituents. *Industrial Crops and Products*, *74*, 327–335. doi:10.1016/j.indcrop.2015.04.065

Savolainen, O. I., Pekkinen, J., Katina, K., Poutanen, K., & Hanhineva, K. (2015). Glycosylated benzoxazinoids are degraded during fermentation of wheat bran. *Journal of Agricultural and Food Chemistry*, *65*(25), 5943–5949. doi:10.1021/acs.jafc.5b00879 PMID:26040909

Sehm, S. K., Magda, S. M., & Madiha, M. A. (2015). Effect of some plant oils and garlic on lipids of rats fed on high cholesterol diet. *International Food Research Journal*, *22*(3), 1307–1314.

Seibel, W., Sidhu, J. S., & Bruemmer, J. M. (1990). Composition of different whole wheat flours for performance in bread and *chapati*. Getreide Mehl u. *Brot.*, *44*(7), 208–210.

Shim, Y. Y., Gui, B., Arnison, P. G., Wang, Y., & Reaney, M. J. T. (2015). Flaxseed (*Linum usitatissimum* L.) bioactive compounds and peptide nomenclature: A review. *Trends in Food Science & Technology*, *38*(1), 5–20. doi:10.1016/j.tifs.2014.03.011

Shim, Y. Y., Gui, B., Wang, Y., & Reaney, M. J. T. (2015). Flaxseed (*Linum usitatissimum* L.) oil processing and selected products. *Trends in Food Science & Technology*, *43*(2), 162–177. doi:10.1016/j.tifs.2015.03.001

Shohag, M. J. I., Wei, Y., & Yang, X. (2012). Changes of folate and other potential health- promoting phytochemicals in legume seeds as affected by germination. *Journal of Agricultural and Food Chemistry*, *60*(36), 9137–9143. doi:10.1021/jf302403t PMID:22906127

Siddiqui, N. S., & Patil, M. B. (2015). Assessment of antioxidant and cytotoxic activities of extracts of some *Zizyphus* species with identification of bioactive components. *European Journal of Medicinal Plants*, *8*(4), 202–213. doi:10.9734/EJMP/2015/17351

Siddiqui, S. N., & Patil, M. B. (2015). Assessment of antioxidant and cytotoxic activities of extracts of some *Zizyphus* species with identification of bioactive components. *European Journal of Medicinal Plants*, *8*(4), 202–213. doi:10.9734/EJMP/2015/17351

Sidhu, J. S. (1995). Wheat Usage in the Indian Subcontinent. In H. Faridi & J. M. Faubion (Eds.), *Wheat End Uses Around the World* (pp. 191–213). St. Paul, MN: American Association of Cereal Chemists.

Sidhu, J. S. (2004). *Use of wheat bran and psyllium in breads and buns*. Final report, Project no. FB023C. Kuwait Institute for Scientific Research.

Sidhu, J. S., Al-Hooti, S. N., & Al-Saqer, J. M. (1999). Effect of adding wheat bran and germ fractions on the chemical composition of high-fiber toast bread. *Food Chemistry*, *67*(4), 365–371. doi:10.1016/S0308-8146(99)00123-5

Sidhu, J. S., Al-Hooti, S. N., Al-Saqer, J. M., & Al-Othman, A. (2001). Studies on the development of pan bread using raw wheat germ. *Journal of Food Quality*, *24*(3), 235–247. doi:10.1111/j.1745-4557.2001.tb00605.x

Sidhu, J. S., Kabir, Y., & Huffman, F. G. (2007). Functional foods from cereal grains. *International Journal of Food Properties*, *10*(2), 201–230. doi:10.1080/10942910601045289

Sidhu, J. S., Seibel, W., Bruemmer, J. M., & Zwingelberg, H. (1989). Effect of whole wheat flour milling procedure and bran addition on bread quality. Getreide Mehl u. *Brot.*, *43*(12), 363–365.

Sidhu, J. S., & Zafar, T. A. (2012). Super fruits: Pomegranate, Wolfberry, Aronia, Acai, Noni and Amla. In N. K. Sinha, J. S. Sidhu, J. Barta, J. S. B. Wu, & M. P. Cano (Eds.), *Handbook of Fruits and Fruit Processing* (2nd ed.; pp. 653–679). New York: John Wiley & Sons Ltd., Publishers. doi:10.1002/9781118352533.ch35

Silva, F. O., & Perrone, D. (2015). Characterization and stability of bioactive compounds from soybean meal. LWT-. *Food Science and Technology (Campinas.)*, *63*, 992–1000.

Singh, A., & Quraishi, M. A. (2015). The extract of *Jamun* (*Syzygium cumini*) seed as green corrosion inhibitor for acid media. *Res. Chem. Intermed.*, *41*(5), 2901–2914. doi:10.1007/s11164-013-1398-3

Singh, B., Bajaj, M., Kaur, A., Sharma, S., & Sidhu, J. S. (1993). Studies on the development of high protein biscuits from composite flours. *Plant Foods for Human Nutrition (Dordrecht, Netherlands)*, *43*(2), 181–189. doi:10.1007/BF01087922 PMID:8475004

Singletary, K. (2010). Ginger: An overview of health benefits. *Nutrition Today*, *45*(4), 171–183. doi:10.1097/NT.0b013e3181ed3543

Singletary, K. (2010). Turmeric: An overview of potential health benefits. *Nutrition Today*, *45*(5), 216–225. doi:10.1097/NT.0b013e3181f1d72c

Siruguri, V., & Bhat, R. V. (2015). Assessing intake of spices by pattern of spice use, frequency of consumption and portion size of spices consumed from routinely prepared dishes in southern India. *Nutrition Journal*, *14*(1), 7–15. doi:10.1186/1475-2891-14-7 PMID:25577292

Slavin, J. (2003). Why whole grains are protective: Biological mechanisms. *The Proceedings of the Nutrition Society*, *62*(1), 129–134. doi:10.1079/PNS2002221 PMID:12740067

Slavin, J. (2004). Whole grains and human health. *Nutrition Research Reviews*, *17*(01), 99–110. doi:10.1079/NRR200374 PMID:19079919

Srinivasa Rao, K., Anand, S., & Venkateswarlu, P. (2010). Cadmium removal from aqueous solution using biosorbant *Syzygium cumini* leaf powder: Kinetic and equilibrium studies. *Korean Journal of Chemical Engineering*, *27*(5), 1547–1554. doi:10.1007/s11814-010-0243-2

Srinivasan, K. (2011). Traditional Indian Functional Foods. In J. Shi, C.-T. Ho, & F. Shahidi (Eds.), *Functional foods of the East* (pp. 51–84). Boca Raton, FL: CRC Press.

Srivastava, S., & Chandra, D. (2013). Pharmacological potentials of *Syzygium cumini*: A review. *Journal of the Science of Food and Agriculture*, *93*(9), 2084–2093. doi:10.1002/jsfa.6111 PMID:23460190

Stadnik, J., & Keska, P. (2015). Meat and fermented meat products as a source of bioactive peptides. *Acta Sci. Pol. Technol. Aliment.*, *14*(3), 181–190. doi:10.17306/J.AFS.2015.3.19

Suleria, H. A. R., Butt, M. S., Anjum, F. M., Saeed, F., & Khalid, N. (2015). Onion: Nature protection against physiological threats. *Critical Reviews in Food Science and Nutrition*, *55*(1), 50–66. doi:10.1080/10408398.2011.646364 PMID:24915405

Suru, S. M., & Ugwu, C. E. (2015). Comparative assessment of onion and garlic extracts on endogenous hepatic and renal antioxidant status in rat. *Journal of Basic and Clinical Physiology and Pharmacology*, *26*(4), 347–354. doi:10.1515/jbcpp-2014-0088 PMID:25536663

Swami, S. B., Thankor, N. S. J., Patil, M. M., & Haldankar, P. M. (2013). Jamun (*Syzygium cumini* L.): A review of its food and medicinal uses. *Food Nutr. Sci.*, *3*(08), 1100–1117. doi:10.4236/fns.2012.38146

Talathoti, G. K., Satyanarayana, S. V., & King, P. (2014). Equilibrium and thermodynamic studies of methylene blue biosorption from aqueous solution using *Syzygium cumini* L. J. *Enviorn. Res. Develop.*, *8*(4), 964–973.

Tan, P. L., Peh, K. K., Gan, C. Y., & Liong, M. T. (2014). Bioactive dairy ingredients for food and non-food applications. *Acta Alimentaria*, *43*(1), 113–123. doi:10.1556/AAlim.43.2014.1.12

Taylor, J. R. N., Belton, P. S., Beta, T., & Duodu, K. G. (2014). Increasing the utilization of sorghum, millets and pseudocereals: Development in the science of their phenolic phytochemicals, biofortification and protein functionality. *Journal of Cereal Science*, *59*(3), 257–275. doi:10.1016/j.jcs.2013.10.009

Thompson, L. U. (1994). Antioxidants and hormone-mediated health benefits of whole grains. *Critical Reviews in Food Science and Nutrition*, *34*(5&6), 473–497. doi:10.1080/10408399409527676 PMID:7811379

Trio, P. Z., Sixiang, Y., He, X., He, J., Sakao, K., & Hou, D. X. (2014). Chemopreventive functions and molecular mechanisms of garlic organosulfur compounds. *Food Functions*, *5*(5), 833–844. doi:10.1039/c3fo60479a PMID:24664286

Tsen, S. Y., Siew, J., Lau, E. K. L., Afiqah bte Roslee, F., Chan, H. M., & Loke, W. M. (2014). Cow's milk as a dietary source of equol and phenolic antioxidants: Differential distribution in the milk aqueous and lipid fractions. *Dairy Sci. Technol.*, *94*(6), 625–632. doi:10.1007/s13594-014-0183-4

Tucker, L. A., & Thomas, K. S. (2009). Increasing total dietary fiber intake reduces risk of weight and fat gain in women. *The Journal of Nutrition*, *139*(3), 576–581. doi:10.3945/jn.108.096685 PMID:19158230

Vankar, P. S. (2008). Effectiveness of antioxidant properties of fresh and dry rhizomes of Curcuma longa (Long and Short varieties) with dry turmeric spice. *Int. J. Food Engg.*, *4*(8), 1–30.

Vaspreet, J., Dornez, E., Ende, W. V., Delcour, J. A., & Courtin, C. M. (2015). Cereal grain fructans: Structure, variability and potential health effects. *Trends in Food Science & Technology*, *43*(1), 32–42. doi:10.1016/j.tifs.2015.01.006

Veigas, J. M., Shrivasthava, R., & Neelwarne, B. (2008). Efficient amelioration of carbon tetrachloride induced toxicity in isolated rat hepatocytes by *Syzygium cumini* Skeels extract. *Toxicology In Vitro*, *22*(6), 1440–1446. doi:10.1016/j.tiv.2008.04.015 PMID:18538978

Velie, E. M., Schairer, C., Flood, A., He, J. P., Khattree, R., & Schatzkin, A. (2005). Empirically derived dietary patterns and risk of postmenopausal breast cancer in a large cohort study. *The American Journal of Clinical Nutrition*, *82*, 1308–1319. PMID:16332665

Venkateswarlu, S., Natesh Kumar, B., Prasad, C. H., Venkateswarlu, P., & Jyothi, N. V. V. (2014). Bio-inspired green synthesis of Fe3O4 spherical magnetic nanoparticles using *Syzygium cumini* seed extract. *Physica B, Condensed Matter*, *449*, 67–71. doi:10.1016/j.physb.2014.04.031

Vijaykumar, M. V., Pandey, V., Mishra, G. C., & Bhat, M. K. (2010). Hypolipidemic effect of fenugreek seeds is mediated through inhibition of fat accumulation and upregulation of LDL receptor. *Obesity (Silver Spring, Md.)*, *18*(4), 667–674. doi:10.1038/oby.2009.337 PMID:19851306

Vila-Donat, P., Caprioli, G., Maggi, F., Ricciutelli, M., Torregiani, E., Vittori, S., & Sagratini, G. (2015). Effective clean-up and ultra-high-performance liquid chromatography-tandem mass spectrophotometry for isoflavone determination in legumes. *Food Chemistry*, *174*, 487–494. doi:10.1016/j.foodchem.2014.11.047 PMID:25529710

Wada, Y., & Lonnerdal, B. (2014). Bioactive peptides derived from human milk proteins- mechanism of action. *The Journal of Nutritional Biochemistry*, *25*(5), 503–514. doi:10.1016/j.jnutbio.2013.10.012 PMID:24411973

Xu, B., & Chang, S. K. C. (2012). Comparative study on anti-proliferation properties and cellular antioxidant activities of commonly consumed food legumes against nine human cancer cell lines. *Food Chemistry*, *134*(3), 1287–1296. doi:10.1016/j.foodchem.2012.02.212 PMID:25005945

Xu, L., Du, B., & Xu, B. (2015). A systematic, comparative study on the beneficial health components and antioxidant activities of commercially fermented soy products marketed in China. *Food Chemistry*, *174*, 202–213. doi:10.1016/j.foodchem.2014.11.014 PMID:25529671

Ying, H., Jiang, H., Liu, H., Chen, F., & Du, Q. (2014). Ethyl acetate-n-butanol gradient solvent system for high-speed countercurrent chromatography to screen bioactive substances in okra. *J. Chromatog.*, *1359*, 117–123. doi:10.1016/j.chroma.2014.07.029 PMID:25069743

Yu, J., Ahmedna, M., & Goktepe, I. (2005). Effects of processing methods and extraction solvents on concentration and antioxidant activity of peanut skin phenolics. *Food Chemistry*, *90*(1-2), 199–206. doi:10.1016/j.foodchem.2004.03.048

Yu, S. Y., Lee, Y. J., Kim, J. D., Kang, S. N., Lee, S. K., Jang, J. Y., & Lee, O. H. et al. (2013). Phenolic composition, antioxidant activity and anti-adipogenic effect of hot water extract from safflower (*Carthamus tinctorius* L.) seed. *Nutrients*, *5*(12), 4894–4907. doi:10.3390/nu5124894 PMID:24288028

Yue, P., & Waring, S. (1998). Resistant starch in food applications. *Cereal Foods World*, *43*, 90–695.

Zhang, H., Jiang, L., Ye, S., Ye, Y., & Ren, F. (2010). Systematic evaluation of antioxidant capacities of the ethanolic extract of different tissues of jujube (*Zizyphus jujube* Mill.) from China. *Food and Chemical Toxicology*, *48*(6), 1461–1465. doi:10.1016/j.fct.2010.03.011 PMID:20230870

Zhou, K., Su, L., & Yu, L. (2004). Phytochemicals and antioxidant properties in wheat bran. *Journal of Agricultural and Food Chemistry*, *52*(20), 6108–6114. doi:10.1021/jf049214g PMID:15453674

Zhu, Y., Soroka, D., & Sang, S. (2015). Oxyphytosterols as active ingredients in wheat bran suppress human colon cancer cell growth: Identification, chemical synthesis, and biological evaluation. *Journal of Agricultural and Food Chemistry*, *63*(8), 2264–2276. doi:10.1021/jf506361r PMID:25658220

Zielinski, H. (2002). Low molecular weight antioxidants in the cereal grains- a review. *Polish J. Food Nutr. Sci.*, *11/51*(1), 3–9.

Zilic, S., Basic, Z., Sukalovic, V. H. T., Makasimovic, V., Jankovic, M., & Filipovic, M. (2014). Can the sprouting process applied to wheat improve the contents of vitamins and phenolic compounds and antioxidant capacity of the flour? *International Journal of Food Science & Technology*, *49*(4), 1040–1047. doi:10.1111/ijfs.12397

Zozio, S., Servent, A., Hiol, A., Mbeguie, D., Cosmidis, L., Lucien, J. M., & Pallet, D. (2015). Processed *Z. Mauritiana* Lamk in the formula of high nutritional value cake. *J. Food. Process. Technol.* http://dx.dio.org/10.4172/2157-7110.1000444

Chapter 17
Functional Foods in Hypertension:
Functional Foods in Cardiovascular Diseases

Anil Gupta
Eklavya Dental College and Hospital, India

ABSTRACT

Functional foods contain bioactive compounds which are endowed with remarkable biologically significant properties. These compounds have corrective and preventive potential for diseases affecting cardiovascular system, endocrine system, nervous system, alimentary canal by virtue of their capability to influence bio-macromolecules in the cells. Clinical evidence augments the anti-oxidant, anti-atherogenic, anti-ageing, cardio-protective and immune system modulatory role of the functional foods. However, additional research is necessitated to uncover concerns regarding optimal dose, duration, pharmacotherapeutics and adverse effects of active compounds in relation to the public health.

INTRODUCTION

Hypertension is a manifestation of the chronic abnormality affecting, either, vasculature, blood flow or cardiac efficiency and characterized by consistent elevation of arterial blood pressure to 140/90mmHg or above, in the body of an adult individual, as in Table1. It is expressed in systolic blood pressure and diastolic blood pressure, where, former relates to blood pressure in arteries when left ventricle contracts, whereas, latter corresponds to the relaxed state of left ventricle before the start of next contraction (Carretero & Oparil, 2000). Normotensive individuals have systolic blood pressure in the range of 100-140mmHg and diastolic blood pressure in the range of 60-90mmHg under resting condition, whereas, hypotensive persons have systolic blood pressure below 100mmHg and a decline in diastolic blood pressure below 60mmHg.

DOI: 10.4018/978-1-5225-0591-4.ch017

Hypertension is classified as primary or essential hypertension and idiopathic or secondary hypertension. In primary hypertension, a well defined etiology is unknown and this class of hypertension affects around 90% of the hypertensive population, while, secondary hypertension is ascribed to a particular cause that might be chronic renal disease, chronic diabetes mellitus, dyslipidemia, coronary artery disease and/or cushing's syndrome and further, has a marginal prevalence of around 10% out of total hypertensive patients(James et al., 2014).

In 1977, Joint National Committee (JNC-I), classified on the Detection, Evaluation, and Treatment of Hypertension, classified hypertension on the basis of diastolic blood pressure(DBP).

Later on, in 1980, (JNC-II) classified hypertension into mild (DBP 90-104 mm Hg), moderate (DBP 105-114) and severe (DBP ≥115 mm Hg). Further, in 1984, (JNC-III) report added a new term as high-normal hypertension for the patients who had DBP in the range of 85-89 mm Hg. Additionally, (JNC- III) report introduced two more terms as isolated systolic hypertension with Systolic blood pressure (SBP ≥ 160mm Hg) and borderline isolated systolic hypertension with SBP in range of (140-159mm Hg) (JNC-3, 1993).

According to the 7th report of the Joint National Committee (JNC-7) on Prevention, Detection, Evaluation, and Treatment of High Blood Pressure, the blood pressure can be classified into four categories (see Table 1) (Chobanian et al., 2003).

ETIOLOGY OF HYPERTENSION

Primary hypertension is the consequence of the interaction between diverse environmental factors and genetic factors. As such, the hypertension is attributed to various predisposing factors. Advancing age affects the elasticity of blood vessels, viscosity of blood, myocardial contractility and cardiac output, hence, negatively influences arterial blood pressure. Primary hypertension has a tendency to rise with advancing age (Kosugi et al., 2009).

Life style of an individual determines primary hypertension. Sedentary routine, coupled with minimal physical activity, habit of smoking & alcohol consumption, high fat diet, uncontrolled diabetes mellitus and emotional disturbance. Generally, personality 'Type A' individuals, who are sensitive, ambitious, status conscious, rigid in behavior & time management, have greater susceptibility to essential hypertension.

Obesity predisposes to metabolic syndrome and hypertension. Prevalence of hypertension in obese persons is higher in comparison to the normal healthy persons (Haslam & James, 2005). Insulin resistance is the cause of hyperglycemia, dyslipidemia and obesity, additionally, prompts to essential hypertension. Insulin regulates the blood glucose level in body by peripheral utilization of glucose as well as its

Table 1. Classification of hypertension

Category	Blood Pressure(mmHg)
Normotensive	SBP (90-119) & (60-79)
Pre-hypertension	SBP (120-139) or DBP (80-89)
Stage1 Hypertension	SBP (140-159) or DBP (90-99)
Stage2 Hypertension	SBP ≥160 or DBP ≥100

(DBP)- diastolic blood pressure, (SBP)- systolic blood pressure
Source: Chobanian et al. (2003)

uptake by cells. Insulin has vasodilatory effect in normotensive individuals. However, insulin resistance promotes sympathetic activity that suppresses its vasodilatory effect.

Secondary hypertension always follows a disorder in the body, hence, is associated with a particular etiology. Diseases of the kidney, namely glomerulonephritis, polycystic kidney and renal stenosis effect the renal blood circulation. There is renal hypoperfusion that stimulates rennin-angiotensin-aldosterone system. As a consequence, water & salt are retained in the body followed by development of oedema, increased cardiac output and secondary hypertension. Drugs like alcohol, non steroidal anti-inflammatory drugs, prednisolones and hormonal contraceptives are additionally responsible for hypertension. Hyperaldosteronism is a disorder of adrenal gland. In this condition, aldosterone secretion is increased, thereby, sodium reabsortion and concomitant water retention is enhanced by kidneys. So it is linked with hypertension. Another endocrine disorder, Cushing syndrome is associated with hyper secretion of cortisol. It has potent vasoconstrictive effect that causes hypertension (Dodt et al., 2009).

PATHOPHYSIOLOGY OF HYPERTENSION

Hereditary Factor

Genetic factor is of paramount importance in the pathogenesis of Primary hypertension. Monogenic and/or polygenic influences interplay with another factors towards the initiation & progression of primary hypertension. Multiple genes regulate the phenotypic expression of essential hypertension, independently & collectively.

Monogenic prerogative over the pathophysiology is responsible for a few cases of essential hypertension. Today, advancement in genetic research has led to the discovery of genes those have impact on pathophysiology of hypertension. Extensive research has been done over the Angiotensinogen gene (AGT). (Lifton, Gharavi & Geller, 2001). AGT gene expresses in multiple organs, namely liver, heart, blood vessels, brain and kidney and adipose tissues. It controls the biosynthesis of angiotensinogen, a precursor for the angiotensin protein of renin-angiotensin-aldosterone system, that is a marked regulator of blood pressure. Gene AGT exhibits polymorphism. Its variant M235T refers to the substitution of methionine by threonine at position 235(M235T) that is seriously implicated in raising the concentration of angiotensinogen in plasma, hence, involved in the instigation of exaggerated response to high salt intake and concluding greater predisposition to essential hypertension (Jeunemaitre et al., 1992).

Gene ACE is another important regulatory gene for angiotensin-converting enzyme. It has variant D and variant I. These two polymorphic forms refer to the deletion & insertion of sequence of amino acids in gene, respectively. Individuals, possessing variant D gene in their genetic constitution have embellished sensitivity to salt in comparison to those having variant I gene. In the body, RAAS system becomes hypersensitive to high salt intake, therefore, variant D gene carriers have elevated vulnerability to essential hypertension on the consumption of high salt diet (Fornage et al., 1998).

Endothelial Dysfunction

Nitric oxide is a gaseous molecule with lipophilic character. It is synthesized by vascular endothelial cells from L-arginine amino acid in the presence of endothelial nitric oxide synthase(eNO synthase) enzyme. It maintains the vascular dilator tone and regulates the adhesion & aggregation of platelets on vessel walls in blood circulation. In healthy persons, a continuous biosynthesis and release of nitric oxide(NO) preserves the elasticity of blood vessels, blood viscosity, lipid serum level and blood flow (Cai & Harrison, 2000).

Sedentary life style, smoking, alcohol consumption, dyslipidemia, anxiety trigger the start of SNS hyperactivity, renal hypoperfusion & haemodynamic changes. As a consequence, concentration of adrenaline, angiotensin II and cortisol is elevated in the blood circulation, thus, impedes the biosynthesis of nitric oxide and oxidizes the available nitric oxide in blood vessels. This endothelial dysfunction heightens the prevalence of hypertension (Fukui et al., 1997).

Renin-Angiotensin-Aldosterone System

It is a major cascading mechanism that regulates arterial blood pressure through its control over selective reabsortption of sodium ions by nephrons. Angiotensin II is the ultimate metabolite produced in this cascade of biochemical reactions. It stimulates adrenal cortex to release aldosterone which maintains reabsorption of sodium. Angiotensin II constricts blood vessels and induces the release of vassopresin from posterior pituitary gland that regulates water reabsorption. Moreover, RAAS in healthy individuals, sustains normal plasma osmolarity and total body water (Gupta, 2012).

Predisposing factors of hypertension are responsible for renal hypoperfusion and hypoxia. The decline in blood flow and ↓PO^2, accentuates the functioning of rennin-angiotensin-aldosterone system. Additionally, polymorphic variant of AGT gene in hypersensitive individuals, accountes for over production of renin in plasma. Cumulative effect is noticed by the hypersynthesis of angiotensin II. This peptide aggravates the normal physiology of sodium and water reabsorption, hence, materializes into hypertension (Mulvany, 2002).

Angiotensin II

Angiotensin II is a peptide hormone. It is a potent vasoconstrictor and important component of RAAS system. Hypersecretion of angiotensin II, stimulates the production of endothelin from the vascular endothelium through the action of endothelium converting enzyme (ECE). Angiotensin II induces oxidative stress in body. It enhances the activity of NADPH oxidase enzyme, wherein, formation of superoxide free radicals is increased. These radicals, further, react with NO and synthesizes peroxynitrites. Free radicals oxidizes arachidonic acid and produces F2-isoprostane, that amplify the vasoconstrictive effect of endothelin. Therefore, angiotensin II increases the oxidative stress in body that might pay the way for essential hypertension (Rajagopalan et al., 1996)

Hyperactivity of Sympathetic Nervous System

Predisposing factors of essential hypertension increase the activity of sympathetic nervous system, hence, secretion of catecholamines, namely adrenaline and nor-adrenaline is stimulated. These neurochemicals are potent vasoconstrictor and contribute to increased peripheral vascular resistance, increased cardiac output, raised systolic and diastolic blood pressure, moreover, potentiate the renal hypo-perfusion and hypoxia that further lead to over-activity of renin-angiotensin-aldosterone system of the body(Mark,1996).

Persistent over activity of SNS results into left ventricular hypertrophy, remodeling of blood vessels and endothelial dysfunction. It is partly due to the excess secretion of nor-adrenaline, which in turn, affects the cardiovascular system, negatively (Brook & Julius, 2000).

Vacular Remodeling

Peripheral arterioles are sensitive to catecholamines. Continuous hypersecretion of these neurochemicals induce structural changes in arterioles. They undergo stenosis and offer higher resistance to blood flow (Folkow, 1982). Indirect evidence to the above hypothesis comes from the drugs that are used to manage hypertension. These antihypertensive medication namely, calcium channel blockers, ACE inhibitors normalize the hypertension and concomitantly, relaxes the vascular smooth muscles and decreases the peripheral resistance (Schiffrin, 2001).

Metabolic Syndrome and Hypertension

Central adiposity or accumulation of visceral fat is a metabolic disturbance and it is associated with insulin resistance, dyslipidemia, diabetes mellitus, cardiovascular disease and arterial hypertension, as shown in Figure 1. These clinical conditions, collectively, constitute metabolic syndrome. Insulin resistance represents another feature associated with syndrome. Sensitivity of cells to insulin concentration is increased affecting the regulation of blood glucose level in the body. In condition of insulin resistance, cells require higher concentration of insulin for their glucose utilization. Pancrease release more insulin, hence, hyperinsulinemia stimulates liver to synthesize higher amount of fat and subsequently, results into fatty liver, haemodynamic changes and hypertension (Shulman, 2004).

Hyperinsulinemia stimulates higher lipolysis of visceral fat. Free fatty acid concentration is increased in portal and systemic circulation. Excess FFA in liver, further, aggravates insulin resistance and promotes fatty liver. Systemic FFA increases insulin resistance of skeletal muscles. Central adiposity hyper activate the SNS, which, additionally contribute to hypertension (Rahmouni et al., 2005).

Visceral fat is much less in proportion in comparison to the subcutaneous fat of the body. It is a metabolically active tissue and stimulates biosynthesis of adipokines in body, namely interleukin-6, TNF- α, macrophage chemoattractant protein. These substances accentuate insulin resistance in body tissues and liver (Lafontan, 2004).

Figure 1. Metabolic syndrome and hypertension
Source: Frayn (2000)

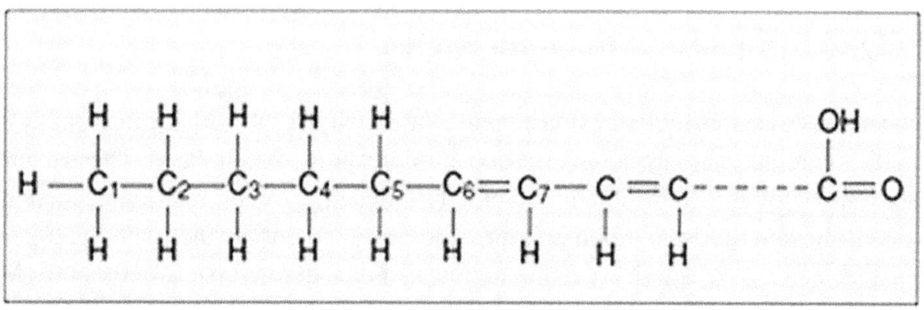

These pro-inflammatory substances worsen endothelial dysfunction and promote hyperinsulinemia, dyslipidemia and hypertension (Rupp & Maisch, 2003).

Unfortunately, concentration of Adiponectin is decreased during hyperinsulinemia and dyslipidemia. Its diminished level, further, aggravates the effect of adipokines in the body, therefore, raises the prevalence of hypertension, cardiovascular diseases and diabetes mellitus, as in Figure1.

Hyperinsulinemia, moreover, stimulates RAAS and induces hyper synthesis of angiotensin II, which has pro-atherogenic effect & it inhibits the vasodilatory effect of insulin (Shirai, 2004).

CONCEPT OF FUNCTIONAL FOODS

Hippocrates envisioned the tenet of 'Food be the medicine and medicine be the food'.

Today, health and medical professionals through the world have renewed their interest in the additional benefits rendered by the foods. Term of 'Functional foods', originated in Japan, in mid 1980. Initially, functional foods were considered as the processed foods having ingredients which can provide health benefits, apart from the nutrition function of food.

It was The Institute of Medicine's Food and Nutrition Board (IOM), 1994, that defined functional foods as "any food or food ingredient that may provide a health benefit beyond the traditional nutrients it contains." (IOM/NAS. 1994).

Another term was coined for functional foods, *Nutraceuticals*, by the United States for Innovation in medicine, 1989. It is defined as "any chemical compound which is either a food or part of a food having a medical or health benefits including prevention and treatment of diseases."

Free radicals are highly reactive species those have been implicated in the lipid peroxidation, protein denaturation and DNA damage of the tissues of the organism. A dissonance in pro-oxidant to anti-oxidant level is noticed in body manifested as oxidative stress. In this condition, either body immune system cannot scavenge free radicals or their concentration in the body exceeds the reparative capacity of body.

Oxidative stress is involved in a large number of diseases namely, coronary artery disease, hypertension, diabetes mellitus, dyslipidemia, malignancy and neurodegenerative diseases. Vitamin A, C, E and active ingredients of functional foods have anti-oxidant effect (Bjelakovic et al., 2007). Apart from nutritious role, foods can offer a prophylactic health benefit and can sustain physical & mental health through their antioxidant effect at the cellular & molecular level.

Functional foods possess pharmacologically active ingredients which provide multi organs protective effects. These foods are cardiovascular protective, hepato-protective, anti oxidant and anti ageing.

UNSATURATED FATTY ACIDS IN HYPERTENSION

Overview of LC-Unsaturated Fatty Acid Structure

Fatty acids are organic compounds having carboxylic groups and variable length of side chain that determine the fatty acids to be short chain, medium or long chain. Number of carbon atom in side chain can vary from 2C to 80C atoms. Common short chain fatty acid of biological importance is Butyric acid with (4C) present in the butter fat. Long chain fatty acids contain more than 10 carbon atoms in side chain. Further, nature of C-C bond in a fatty acid determines its structure and associated health related properties. Saturated fatty acids have a single bond present between all C-C atoms of the molecule, whereas, presence of a double bond in C-C atoms renders it unsaturated, which, either can be Mono unsaturated fatty Acid (MUFA) containing a single bond or polyunsaturated fatty acid (PUFA) having more than one double bond in the molecule.

Linoleic acid(C18:2), Figure 2, is desaturated & elongated in the presence of 6-Desaturase enzyme and Elongase enzyme and is converted into Dihomo-Gamma Linolenic acid(C20:3). It further undergoes dasturation by 5-desaturase enzyme into Arachidonic acid(C20:4). It is an essential fatty acid that is important for the biosynthesis of pharmacologically active substances namely Prostaglandins, Prostacycline, Thromboxanes in the body. Further unsaturation of Arachidonic acid produces Eicosapentaenoic acid(C20:5) and subsequent elongation and desaturation results into Docosahexaenoic acid(C22:6). All the long chain PUFA are structural constituent of the cell membrane as well as remain stored in the adipose tissues. Eicosapentaenoic acid is regulator of T-cell proliferation, platelets aggregation and vasomotor tone, hence, plays a major role in Immune response and cardiovascular dieseases. Decosahexaenoic acid is mainly concerned with dim light vision as its concentration is maxium in the rods in retina (Cunnane, Nadeau, & Likhodil, 2001).

Figure 2. Omega 6 polyunsaturated fatty acid
Source: Cicero, Ertek, and Borghi (2009)

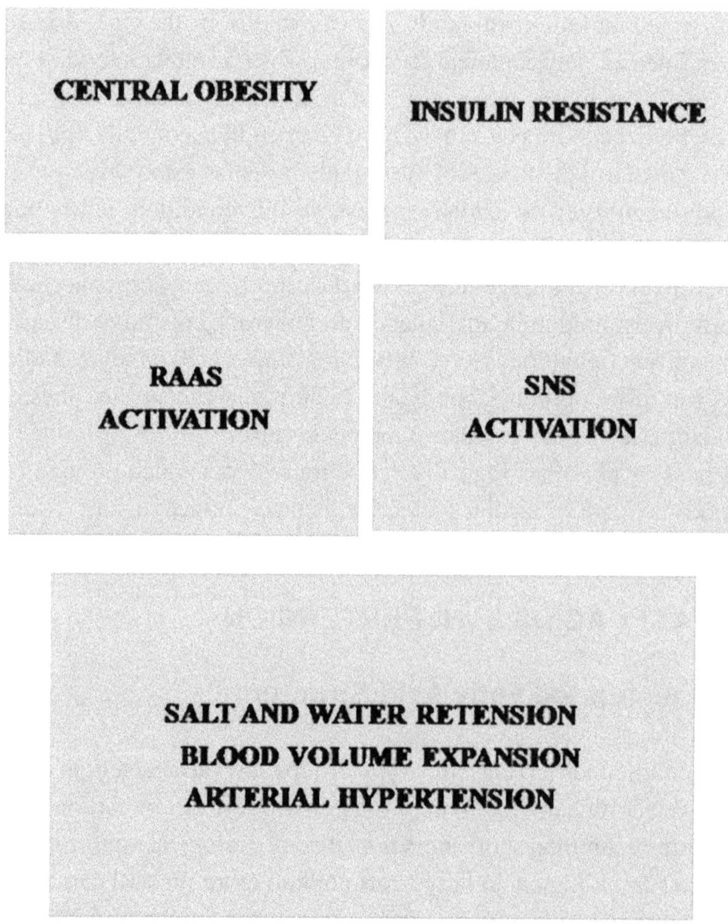

Figure 3. Omega 3 polyunsaturated fatty acid
Source: Cicero, Ertek, and Borghi (2009)

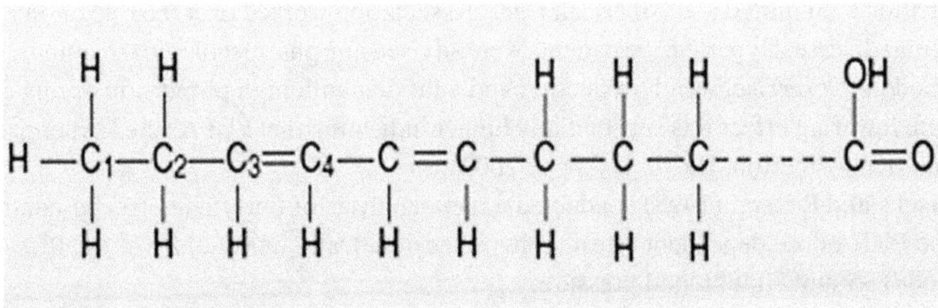

Dietary Source and Content

Table 2 clearly shows that walnut contains maximum amount of PUFA per 100gm of dietary food.

Biological Effects on Tissues

Essential blood pressure is a potential risk factor for diseases of heart and blood vessels, affecting cardiac efficiency & texture of vessels and their vasomotor tone. It is also implicated in microvascular diseases, cerebral stroke. According to WHO, hypertension is the main public health hazard and is involved in the initiation, progression and worsening of the functioning of vital organs of body namely, heart, liver, kidneys and brain (WHO, 2008). Prevalence of hypertension is higher in developing countries. Concern for its non-pharmacological management is growing all over the world utilizing yoga, acupressure, relaxation techniques. On the same approach, the use of functional foods and or dietary phytochemicals

Table 2. Content of long chain polyunsaturated fatty acid in diet

Source of lc-pufa	Contents (g/100g)
Sardine	5g
Soya bean	7g
Sea wood	11g
Olive oil	11g
Tuna	14g
Peanut butter	14.2g
Peanuts	16g
Salmon	17.3g
Seasame seeds	26g
Sunflower seeds	33g
Canola oil	34g
Walnut	47g

Source: USDA (2011)

have been in research for their efficacy in the prevention and treatment of hypertension and its associated complications.

AHA Nutrition Committed and American Heart Association worked over the role of omega 3 PUFA in cardiovascular disease. Hypertensive patients were advised non pharmacological methods, namely salt restriction, moderate exercise, weight reduction and a fat diet with high proportion of omega 3 PUFA. Blood pressure lowering effect was substantially higher indicating that PUFA acted synergistically with other methods (Kris-Etherton, Harris & Appel, 2003).

Morris, Sacks and Rosner, (1993) conducted a meta-analysis of thirty one placebo-controlled trials to find out the PUFA dose dependent effect on hypertension. Daily intake of 3g of LC PUFA showed a decline in 0.66/0.35 mm Hg of blood pressure.

In another study by Ramel et al., (2010) which focused over the effect of use of fixed dose of salmon fish (150g to be taken three time a week) and cod(150g thrice a week) providing 2.1g/day & 0.39g/day omega 3 PUFA, respectively, was compared with the consumption of capsules of fish oil yielding 1.3g/day omega 3 PUFA. Study was continued for 8 weeks involving obese patients. Study provided the daily PUFA dose related antihypertensive effect. Diastolic blood pressure in individuals having had salmon and fish oil was lower in comparison to those who had codfish.

Vascular endothelium has the pivotal role in the cardiovascular diseases due to its being the target tissues for a number of endogenous substances. Omega 3 PUFA has its anti-atherogenic and cardioprotective effect on the endothelium. Monolayer generates nitric oxide and EDHF, which are vaso-dilator. Additionally, it is the site of action of other cholesterol derived pharmacological substances namely prostaglandins, thromboxane A2, and angiotensin II and free radicals like super oxide anions, peroxynitrite and isoprostane (Abeywardena & Head, (2001).

LC-PUFA brings a modulation and normalization in the biosynthesis of vasodilators and eicosanoids derived vasoconstrictors in the body. PUFA dose dependent use increase the formation of nitric oxide and reduce the production of contracting factors (Taddei et al., 2003), hence, vasomotor tone is improved that materializes in lowering of blood pressure. There is complex network of factors that contribute to hypertension, therefore, the mechanism of action of PUFA is multi pronged.

Omega 3 fatty acid also regularize the renal sodium excretion by normalizing the hyperactivity of ACE.

Clinical Evidence for PUFA in Hypertension

Omega-3 PUFA has definite normalizing role in high blood pressure. It has been proved by studies by workers worldwide in intensive as well in observational studies. Shantakumari et al. (2014) confirmed through observational study that intake of daily supplements of 1g omega-3 PUFA for three months resulted in lowering of high blood pressure in chronic hypertensive patients.

Geleijinse et al., (2002) conducted a meta analysis of total 90 randomized clinical trials related to intake of fish oil in hypertensive amelioration and cases identified via Medline (1966-2001). Further, only 36 trials were included and 54 trials were excluded on the basis of co-administeration of drug, controls without placebo and duration (< 2 weeks). The trials included a high dose of fish oil (3.7g/day) as median value and a subsequent reduction of 2.1 mmHg of SBP & 1.6mmHg of DBP was observed. Nature of fat consumed in diet should be given the preference in comparison to the total fat intake by an individual. Moreover, the total amount of fat in diet should not exceed 30% of the total energy requirement per day. Persons who perform higher physical activities may take an additional quantity of fat that should be up to 35% of the total calories requirement (Grundy, 1999; Reddy & Katan, 2004).

Figure 4. Structure of glucosinolate
Source: Wikimedia Commons (2007)

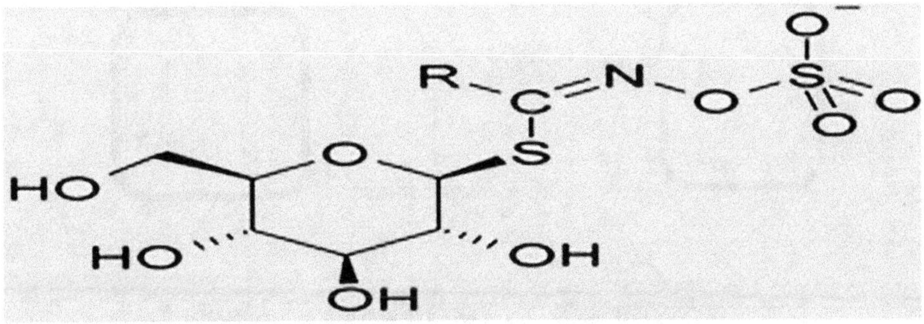

IMPACT OF GLUCOSINOLATES ON HYPERTENSION

Overview of Glucosinolate Structure

Glucosinolates are sulfur and nitrogen rich secondary metabolites in plants in family Brassicaceae which constitute important crops and vegetables namely cabbage, mustard, turnip cauliflower, radish. Glucosinolates possess a central carbon atom which is further linked to thioglucose moiety through sulfur atom on one side and its other side is attached to sulphate residue through nitrogen atom. Core carbon atom is also attached to side chain whose length is variable.

These compounds can be classified into three groups, based on the type & structure of amino acid, namely aliphatic glucosinolates derived from methionine, isoleucine, leucine and or valine. Second group of aromatic glucosinolates are derived from phenylalanine and or tyrosine and furthermore, the third group of indole glucosinolates have their origin from tryptophane amino acid. These plants additionally contain an enzyme thioglucosidase, also called as myrosinase. It can catalyze the hydrolysis of glucosinolates into bioactive phytochemicals. Generally, enzyme remains trapped within a cell wall in plants. However, cutting or chopping a plant part and chewing or cooking of a vegetable help liberate the enzyme and ensure its contact with glucosinolates in presence of water. Hydrolytic products include either isothiocyanates, oxozolidine-2-thiones, nitriles, epithionitriles or thiocyanatesand. Cooking of vegetables like cabbage, cauliflower, onions denature the myrosinase enzyme contained in plant parts. Moreover, glucosinolates are degraded by the intestinal myrosinase enzyme present in the Gut of human (Cartea & Velasco, 2008).

Dietary Source and Content of Glucosinolates

Table 3 depicts glucosinolate content of different dietary products, as mentioned in the literature of different workers. Here, name of workers have been cited against the name of dietary product and glucosinolate content.

Figure 5. Metabolites of glucosinolates after hydrolysis
Source: Ivana et al. (2004)

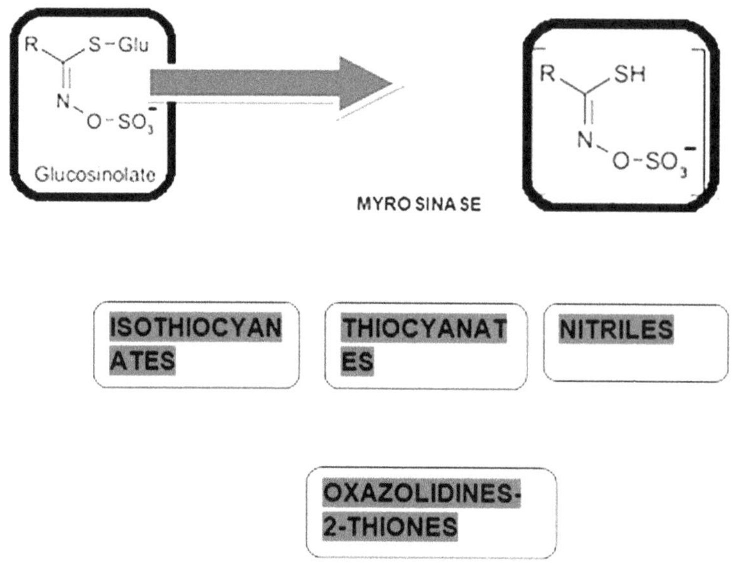

Table 3. Content of glucosinolates in diet (mg/100g)

Source of Glucosinolates	Nature	Source of Research Work	Content of Glucosinolates
Broccoli	Boiled	(Yen & Wei, 1993)	19-127mg
Brussels Sprout	Raw	(McMillan,Spinks, & Fenwick, 1986)	148mg
Cabbage Savoy	Raw	(VanEtten et al., 1980)	26.6-76.6mg
Cabbage Red	Raw	(VanEtten et al., 1980)	60-209mg
Cauliflower	Raw	(Yen & Wei, 1993)	11.7-78.7mg
Mustard Greens	Raw	(Hill et al., 1987)	118-544mg
Raddish Asian	Raw	(Carlson, Daxenbichler,& VanEtten, 1985)	138mg
Raddish European	Raw	(Carlson, Daxenbichler,& VanEtten, 1985)	44.79mg
Turnip	Raw	(Sones, Heaney, & Fenwicket, 1985)	20.4-140mg

BIOLOGICAL EFFECTS ON TISSUES AND CLINICAL EVIDENCE

Isothiocyanates can independently or synergistically with indole-3-carbinol can induce liver phase II detoxification enzymes, hence, is responsible for rapid scavenging action. Reactive oxygen species and other carcinogens are removed from body, therefore, minimizing oxidative stress. These compounds protect from cancer, cardiovascular diseases and degenerative disorders of brain. Plausible explanation is the reduction in the concentration of pro-inflammatory cytokines that is associated with reduced oxidative stress and further help improve vascular dysfunction (Jeffery & Araya, 2009).

Jeon et al., (2013) conducted a randomized placebo controlled clinical trial over obese persons to assess effect of ethanol extract of Brassica raphe. To control group, starch as placebo in dose of 2g/day and same dose of brassica ethanol extract were given for 10 weeks. Patients having had ethanol brassica extract showed improvement in high-density lipoprotein cholesterol in body and reduction of total cholesterol to HDL-C ratio along with un-esterified fatty acid and adepsin (Jeon et al., 2013).

Synthesis of ROS beyond the clearance capacity of body is a major cause for the initiation, progression of vascular injury, coronary artery diseases, neurodegenerative disorder namely ataxia, dementia. Sankhari et al., (2012) conducted a recent study on the role of anthocyanin in cabbage red over the atherogenic induced oxidative stress in rats. Anthocyanin is a red coloured pigment in red cabbage and has anti-oxidant effect. It has been proved in the study by Sankhari et al., (2012).

Another research work performed by Christiansen et al. (2010) contradicted the effect of consumption of broccoli sprouts over the improvement in endothelial dysfunction. In this study, 10g of dried broccoli sprouts were given to hypertensive individuals after randomization for 4 weeks. Daily ingestion of 10 g dried broccoli sprouts does not improve endothelial function in the presence of hypertension in human.

International study population on the macronutrients and BP, INTERMAP, led by Chan et al., (2014)researched that the intake of raw ((carrots, tomatoes, scallions) and cooked ((celery, peas, scallions, tomatoes) vegetables, definitely, lower the high blood pressure in hypertensive individuals. Daily consumption of (68 g per 1000 kcal) of of raw vegetables and (92 g per 1000 kcal) of cooked vegetable resulted in decline of (1.9 mm Hg) of systolic and (1.3 mm Hg) of diastolic blood pressure, significantly ($p<0.05$) without BMI adjustments.

EFFECT OF POLYPHENOLS ON HYPERTENSION

Overview of Polyphenol Structure

Polyphenols are the organic compounds with multiples phenol moieties. These are natural, semi-snthetic and synthetic compounds. Number and character of these phenol residues determine the properties of polyphenols. Basic structure of polyphenols has been depicted in Figure 6.

Figure 6. Favonoid skeleton
Source: Hermann (1976).

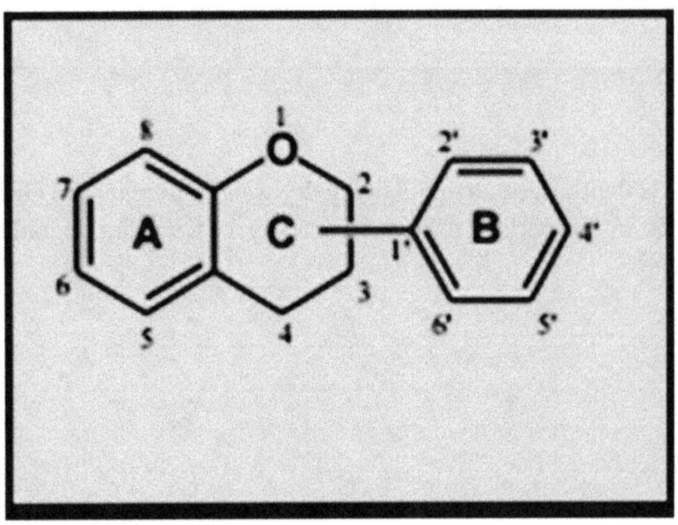

Extensive research has been undertaken to decipher and understand the antioxidant properties of dietary polyphenols affecting vascular structure & tone, cardiac functions, attenuating oxidative stress on liver, free radicals scavenger, improving functions of renal and nervous system, furthermore, exerting modulatory effect on cell receptors and enzymes, hence, affecting the endocrine glands of body. Phenolic acids have been derived from Benzoic acid and Cinnamic acid. Hydroxycinnamic acid is predominantly found in blueberries, kiwis, cherries. Hydroxybenzoic acid is present in radish, onions and red fruits.

Flavonoids

Basic structure of flavonoids have been in shown in Figure 6. The flavonols are abundant & important favonoids in foods. Good source of flavonols, namely, Quercitin and Kaempferol are the Onions, containing a 15-30mg/kg of flavonols. These are glycosylated with the addition of glucose and or rhamnose moiety. Green leafy vegetables, namely, cabbage, lettuce, cauliflower, have higher concentration of flavonols. Sun light enhance the biosynthesis of flavonols in plants, therefore, these accumulate in leaves and other aerial tissues of vegetables (Hermann, 1976). Flavones represent another sub class of flavonoids present in fruits and vegetables. The sources of flavones are Parsley and Celery that contain Leuteolin and Apigenin proteins in glycosylated forms. Isoflavones are considered the pseudohormones. These compounds have structural similarity to estrogens and the ability to bind to receptors of estrogen, hence, labeled as Phytoestrogens. Rich sources are the leguminous plants. Soyabeans has the good concentration of isoflavones in range of 580mg to 3800mg/kg of fresh weight (Cassidy, Hansley & Lamuela-Raventos, 2000).

Green tea extract and apricots contain 200mg and 250mg/kg fresh weight of catechins, Anthocyanins are the red, pink, blue or purple coloured pigmented compounds in the epidermis of flowers, stem, leaves. In diet, red wine, cereals and leafy vegetables, namely, cabbage, beans, onions, raddish, turnip and fruits like, blue berries, strawberry, green grapes have plenty of anthocyanins. Another interesting fact is that color intensity is proportional to the anthocyanins contents.

Stilbenes

Stilbenes represent a low concentration flavonoids in human diet. Resveratol is an important stillbenes having an anti cancerous activity. Its low quantity is found in Wine in range of 0.3–7 mg agycones/Liter (Vitrac et al., 2002).

Lignans

High source of lignans is the Linseed having 3.6g/kg dry weight. Cereals and Grains also have lignans but in low concentration in comparison to lignans. Intestinal microflora degrade the lignans into enterodiol and eterolactone.

BIOAVAILABILITY OF POLYPHENOLS

Intestinal absorption and metabolism

Polyphenols are polyhydroxy cyclic organic compounds with high hydrophilic character that becomes an hindrance in their intestinal mucosal absorption. Exact details about their absorption is lacking. Furthermore, a new concept of absorption has been highlighted for polyphenols. Na^+ dependent saturable transport method of absorption operates in intestinal mucosa by which Cinnamic and ferulic acid can move across the brush border epithelium of jejunum of rat (Wolfram et al., 1995). Most of the flavonoids exist in glycosylated form in foods, which resist their hydrolysis at low PH as in stomach and hence pass onto the intestine undigested. In an experiment on surgically treated rats by Gee et al. (1998), it was found that glycosides of Quercetin and Daidzein remain undigested in stomach and passed into the duodenum intact.

Agycones and glucosides are absorbed in small intestine. However, polyphenols having a rhamnose, arabinose and or xylose moiety are absorbed slowly in colon (Hollman & Ketan, 1997). Glucosidase enzyme, Lactase phlorizin hydrolase helps in hydrolysis of flavonol, isoflavone. The enzyme attached to brush border surface of intestinal epithelium. Aglycones can diffuse through the epithelium. Proanthocyanidins are unique in term of their absorption. These are high molecular weight polymers, consequently, their absorption through intestinal mucosa is largely limited and are acclaimed for their topical action in alimentary canal as antioxidants(Halliwel, Zhao & Whiteman., 2000).

Hydroxycinnamic acids after ingestion, are rapidly absorbed from the small intestine and are conjugated and, in particular, glucuronidated in the same way that flavonoids. Glucoronic acid conjugation and sulfation of polyphenols in liver render them highly hydrophilic. It has been found to enhance their anti-oxidative ability probably attributed to biosynthesis of more active metabolites from native polyphenols after conjugation in body (Kauffman et al., 1994)

Dietary Source and Content of Polyphenols

Table 4 shows the polyphenol contents of dietary products. Peppermint has highest polyphenolic content out of all the foods listed in table.

BIOLOGICAL EFFECTS OF POLYPHENOLS ON TISSUES

Koga and Meydani (2001) proved in their work that metabolites of catechin and quercitin that were formed in plasma had the modulating effect on monocyte adhesion to endothelial cells of human aorta. Daily consumption of foods, such as vegetables, fruits, cocoa, tea etc. rich in polyphenols have cardioprotective effect in man (Arts et al., 2001). Meta analysis by Di Castelnuovo et al. (2002) evaluated the effect of tea consumption in dose of three cups/day on the prevalence of coronary artery disease. Remarkable reduction of 11% in its occurrence have been found. Polyphenols can induce antioxidant enzymes to engulf reactive oxygen species from vessels and help in up-regulation of NO and lowering of blood pressure (Rein et al. 2000). In an randomized clinical trial by Taubert et al. (2007) it was found that participants who consumed 6.3g of dark chocolate (30mg of polyphenols) for 18 weeks experienced a reduction in BP.

Table 4. Contents of polyphenols in diet (mg/100g)

Source of Polyphenols	Nature	Contents of Polyphenols
Cloves	Seasoning	15188mg
peppermint	Seasoning	11960mg
Chestnut	Seed	1215mg
Rose marry dried	Seasoning	1018mg
Flaxseeds	Seed	1528mg
Spearmint	Seasoning	956mg
Black olive	Vegetable	569mg
Soya flour	Seed	466mg
Black elderberry	Fruit	1359mg
Blue berry	Fruit	836mg
Green olive	vegetable	346mg
Straw berry	Fruit	235mg
Ginger dried	Seasoning	202mg
Coffee	Beverage	214mg
Whole grain flour	Cereal	201mg
Almonds	Fruit	187mg
Apple	Fruit	136mg
Green tea	Beverage	89mg
Blood orange juice	Beverage	56mg
Potato	Vegetable	78mg
Carrot	Vegetable	14mg
Rose wine	Beverage alcoholic	10mg
Green grapes	Fruit	15mg

Source: Perez-Jimenez et al. (2015)

CLINICAL EVIDENCE IN FAVOUR OF ANTIHYPERTENSIVE EFFECT

Another study was conducted by Nagao et al. (2007) over the beneficial effects of green tea extract, wherein, a dose of 583mg and 96mg of green tea extract (catechins) was given to participants with central obesity in catechin group and control group, respectively. Reduction in body weight and blood pressure was higher in catechin group. In a placebo-controlled trial by Brown et al. (2009), after randomization, a dose of 400mg epigallocatechine was given to obese participants daily for 8 weeks. A reduction of 2.7mmHg of diastolic blood pressure was observed after eight weeks. Aviram et al. (2004) investigated the effect of pomegranate juice on the carotid artery atherosclerosis. It contains tannins and anthocyanins. In their study, 50ml/day of the juice was given to ten patients daily for one year, wherein, five out of ten continued the intake of juice for 3 years. Thickness of the middle and inner layers of carotid artery were assessed. There was an increase in thickness in control group, but the thickness of carotid artery decreased by 30% in intervention group.

LIMITATIONS

Clinical evidence based on the in vivo studies, in vitro studies on animals models and human studies involving observational & interventional clinical trials has authenticated health benefits of functional foods. However, over emphasis over the role of functional foods to alleviate diseases should be deterred.

Multiple factors, namely complex nature of bioactive chemicals in foods, their absorption & metabolism in body, nature & bioavailability of metabolites in body, ligand-receptor affinity, determination of dose & duration, potential adverse effects, interaction of phytochemicals with other xeno-substances in body and finally the nature of action of bioactive chemical, whether it is prophylactic, curative or suppressive, remain unreciprocated. Further, scientifically proved data related to pharmacodynamics and pharmacotherapeutics of phytochemicals is lacking. Another lacuna is the wide variation in experimental design regarding duration of study, optimal dose of phytochemicals, standardized source of phytochemical and participant selection has been noticed.

Intensive research is needed that must focus on these key issues and a uniformity in future clinical trials encompassing the key issues, already discussed, seem warranted.

CONCLUSION

Functional foods, as evidenced, certainly contain beneficial bioactive chemicals those can arrest and repair molecular aberrations in a cell and provide subsequent health benefits of cardiovascular, renal, nervous and other system of body. However, a conclusive research is required covering wide concerns in the context of public and clinical practice.

REFERENCES

Abeywardena, M. Y., & Head, R. J. (2001). Longchain n-3 polyunsaturated fatty acids and blood vessel function. *Cardiovascular Research*, *52*(3), 361–371. doi:10.1016/S0008-6363(01)00406-0 PMID:11738053

Arts, I. C., Jacobs, D. R. Jr, Harnack, L. J., Gross, M., & Folsom, A. R. (2001). Dietary catechins in relation to coronary heart disease death among postmenopausal women. *Epidemiology (Cambridge, Mass.)*, *12*(6), 668–675. doi:10.1097/00001648-200111000-00015 PMID:11679795

Aviram, M., Rosenblat, M., Gaitini, D., Nitecki, S., Hoffman, A., Dornfeld, L., & Hayek, T. et al. (2004). Pomegranate juice consumption for 3 years by patients with carotid artery stenosis reduces common carotid intima-media thickness, blood pressure and LDL oxidation. *Clinical Nutrition (Edinburgh, Lothian)*, *23*(3), 423–433. doi:10.1016/j.clnu.2003.10.002 PMID:15158307

Bjelakovic, G., Nikolova, D., Gluud, L. L., Simonetti, R. G., & Gluud, C. (2007). Mortality in randomized trials of antioxidant supplements for primary and secondary prevention: Systematic review and meta-analysis. *Journal of the American Medical Association*, *297*(8), 842–857. doi:10.1001/jama.297.8.842 PMID:17327526

Brook, R. D., & Julius, S. (2000). Autonomic imbalance, hypertension, and cardiovascular risk. *American Journal of Hypertension*, *13*(6), 112S–122S. doi:10.1016/S0895-7061(00)00228-4 PMID:10921530

Cai, H., & Harrison, D. G. (2000). Endothelial dysfunction in cardiovascular diseases: The role of oxidant stress. *Circulation Research*, *87*(10), 840–844. doi:10.1161/01.RES.87.10.840 PMID:11073878

Carlson, D. G., Daxenbichler, M. E., & VanEtten, C. H. (1985). Glucosinolates in radish cultivars. *Journal of the American Society for Horticultural Science*, *110*, 634–638.

Carretero, O. A., & Oparil, S. (2000). Essential Hypertension, Part -1: Definition and Etiology. *Circulation*, *101*(3), 329–335. doi:10.1161/01.CIR.101.3.329 PMID:10645931

Cartea, M. E., & Velasco, P. (2008). Glucosinolates in Brassica foods: Bioavailability in food and significance for human health. *Phytochemistry Reviews*, *7*(2), 213–229. doi:10.1007/s11101-007-9072-2

Cassidy, A., Hansley, B., & Lamuela-Raventos, R. M. (2000). Isoflavones, lignans and stilbenes—origins, metabolism and potential importance to human health. *Journal of the Science of Food and Agriculture*, *80*(7), 1044–1062. doi:10.1002/(SICI)1097-0010(20000515)80:7<1044::AID-JSFA586>3.0.CO;2-N

Chan, Q., Stamler, J., Brown, J., Daviglus, M. L., Van Horn, L., Dyer, A. R., & Elliot, P. et al. (2014). Relation of raw and cooked vegetable consumption to blood pressure: The INTERMAP Study. *Journal of Human Hypertension*, *28*(6), 353–359. doi:10.1038/jhh.2013.115 PMID:24257514

Chobanian, A. V., Bakris, G. L., Black, H. R., Cushman, W. C., Green, L. A., Izzo, J. L., & Roccella, E. et al. (2003). Joint National Committee on Prevention, Detection, Evaluation and Treatment of high blood pressure.National Heart, lung and blood Institute; National High Blood pressure Education Programme Coordination Committee. *Hypertension*, *42*(6), 1206–1252. doi:10.1161/01.HYP.0000107251.49515.c2 PMID:14656957

Christiansen, B., & Bellkosta, M. (2010). Ingestion of broccoli sprouts does not improve endothelial function in humans with hypertension. *PLoS ONE*, *5*(8), e12461. doi:10.1371/journal.pone.0012461 PMID:20805984

Cicero, A. F., Ertek, S., & Borghi, C. (2009). Omega-3 polyunsaturated fatty acids: Their potential role in blood pressure prevention and management. *Current Vascular Pharmacology*, *7*(3), 330–337. doi:10.2174/157016109788340659 PMID:19601857

Cunnane, S. C., Nadeau, C. R., & Likhodil, S. S. (2001). Alpha Linelenic acid, Figure 3, also compets for the same enzymes for the synthesis of eicosanoids and DHA. *Journal of Molecular Neuroscience*, *16*, 173–180. doi:10.1385/JMN:16:2-3:173 PMID:11478372

Dodt, C., Welhoner, J. P., Schutt, M., & Sayk, F. (2009). Glucocorticoids and Hypertension. *Der Internist*, *50*(1), 36–41. doi:10.1007/s00108-008-2197-6 PMID:19096817

Erlund, I., Koli, R., Alfthan, G., Marniemi, J., Puukka, P., Mustonen, P., & Jula, A. et al. (2008). Favorable effects of berry consumption on platelet function, blood pressure, and HDL cholesterol. *The American Journal of Clinical Nutrition*, *87*, 323–331. PMID:18258621

Folkow, B. (1982). Physiological aspects of primary hypertension. *Physiological Reviews*, *62*, 347–504. PMID:6461865

Fornage, M., Amos, C. I., Kardia, S., Sing, C. F., Turner, S. T., & Boerwinkle, E. (1998). Variation in the region of the angiotensin-converting enzyme gene influences interindividual differences in blood pressure levels in young white males. *Circulation*, *97*(18), 1773–1779. doi:10.1161/01.CIR.97.18.1773 PMID:9603530

Frayn, K. N. (2000). Visceral fat and insulin resistance--causative or correlative? *The British Journal of Nutrition*, *83*(S1Suppl 1), S71–S77. doi:10.1017/S0007114500000982 PMID:10889795

Fukui, T., Ishizaka, N., Rajagopalan, S., Laursen, J. B., Capers, Q. IV, Taylor, W. R., & Griendling, K. K. et al. (1997). p22phox mRNA expression and NADPH oxidase activity are increased in aortas from hypertensive rats. *Circulation Research*, *80*(1), 45–51. doi:10.1161/01.RES.80.1.45 PMID:8978321

Gee, J. M., Du Pont, M. S., Rhodes, M. J. C., & Johnson, I. T. (1998). Quercetin glucosides interact with the intestinal glucose transport pathway. *Free Radical Biology & Medicine*, *25*(1), 19–25. doi:10.1016/S0891-5849(98)00020-3 PMID:9655517

Geleijnse, J. M., Giltay, E. J., Grobbee, D. E., Donders, A. R., & Kok, F. J. (2002). Blood pressure response to fish oil supplementation: Metaregression analysis of randomized trials. *Journal of Hypertension*, *20*(8), 1493–1499. doi:10.1097/00004872-200208000-00010 PMID:12172309

Grundy, S. M. (1999). The optimal ratio of fat-to-carbohydrate in the diet. *Annual Review of Nutrition*, *19*(1), 325–341. doi:10.1146/annurev.nutr.19.1.325 PMID:10448527

Gupta, A. (2012). Assessing renal function in patients suffering from liver diseases. (Unpublished Doctoral Thesis). SJJT University. Retrieved from http://shodhganga.inflibnet.ac.in/handle/10603/10018

Halliwell, B., Zhao, K., & Whiteman, M. (2000). The gastrointestinal tract: A major site of antioxidant action? *Free Radical Research*, *33*(6), 819–830. doi:10.1080/10715760000301341 PMID:11237104

Haslam, D. W., & James, W. P. (2005). Obesity. *Lancet*, *366*(9492), 1197–1209. doi:10.1016/S0140-6736(05)67483-1 PMID:16198769

Herrmann, K. (1976). Flavonols and flavones in food plants: A review. *Journal of Food Technology*, *11*(5), 433–448. doi:10.1111/j.1365-2621.1976.tb00743.x

Hill, C. B., Williams, P. H., Carlson, D. G., & Tookey, H. L. (1987). Variation in glucosinolates in Oriental Brassica vegetables. *Journal of the American Society for Horticultural Science*, *112*, 309–313.

Hollman, P. C., & Katan, M. B. (1997). Absorption, metabolism and health effects of dietary flavonoids in man. *Biomedicine and Pharmacotherapy*, *51*(8), 305–310. doi:10.1016/S0753-3322(97)88045-6 PMID:9436520

Ivana, R. R., Tatjan, G., Karmela, D., & Vorkapic-Furac, J. (2004). Glucosinolates and their potential role in plant. *Periodicum Biologorum*, *110*(4), 297–309.

James, P. A., Oparil, S., Carter, B. L., Cushman, W. C., Dennison-Himmelfarb, C., Handler, J., & Ortiz, E. et al. (2014). 2014 evidence-based guideline for the management of high blood pressure in adults: Report from the panel members appointed to the Eighth Joint National Committee (JNC 8). *Journal of the American Medical Association*, *311*(5), 507–520. doi:10.1001/jama.2013.284427 PMID:24352797

Jeffery, E. H., & Araya, M. (2009). Physiological effects of broccoli consumption. *Phytochemistry Reviews*, *8*(1), 283–298. doi:10.1007/s11101-008-9106-4

Jeon, S.M., Kim, J.E., Shin, S.K.., Kwon, E.Y., Jung, U. J., Baek, N.I. (2013). Randomized double-blind placebo-controlled trial of powdered brassica rapa ethanol extract on alteration of body composition and plasma lipid and adipocytokine profiles in overweight subjects. *Journal of Medicinal Food*, *16*(2), 133-138.

Jeunemaitre, X., Soubrier, F., Kotelevtsev, Y. V., Lifton, R. P., Williams, C. S., Charru, A., & Corvol, P. et al. (1992). Molecular basis of human hypertension: Role of angiotensinogen. *Cell*, *71*(1), 169–180. doi:10.1016/0092-8674(92)90275-H PMID:1394429

Joint National Committee on the Detection, Evaluation and Treatment of High Blood Pressure (JNC-V). (1993). The fifth report of the Joint National Committee on the detection, evaluation, and treatment of high blood pressure. *Archives of Internal Medicine*, *153*(2), 154–183. doi:10.1001/archinte.1993.00410020010002 PMID:8422206

Kauffman, F. C., Zaleski, J., Thurman, R. G., & Kwei, G. Y. (1994). Biologically active conjugates of drugs and toxic chemicals. In F. C. Kauffman (Ed.), *Conjugation-deconjugation reactions in drug metabolism and toxicity* (pp. 341–366). Berlin: Springer. doi:10.1007/978-3-642-78429-3_12

Kosugi, T., Nakagawa, T., Kamath, D., & Johnson, R. J. (2009). Uric acid and Hypertension: An age-related relationship. *Journal of Human Hypertension*, *23*(2), 75–76. doi:10.1038/jhh.2008.110 PMID:18754017

Kris-Etherton, P. M., Harris, W. S., & Appel, L. J. (2003). Fatty acids and cardiovascular disease:new recommendations from the American Heart Association. AHA Nutrition Committee. and American Heart Association. *Omega-3. Arteriosclerosis, Thrombosis, and Vascular Biology*, *23*, 151–152. doi:10.1161/01.ATV.0000057393.97337.AE PMID:12588750

Lafontan, M. (2004). Fat cells: Afferent and efferent messages define new approaches to treat obesity. *Annual Review of Pharmacology and Toxicology*, *45*(1), 119–146. doi:10.1146/annurev.pharmtox.45.120403.095843 PMID:15822173

Lifton, R. P., Gharavi, A. G., & Geller, D. S. (2001). Molecular mechanisms of human hypertension. *Cell*, *104*(4), 545–556. doi:10.1016/S0092-8674(01)00241-0 PMID:11239411

Mark, A. L. (1996). The sympathetic nervous system in hypertension: A potential long term regulator of arterial pressure. *Journal of Hypertension*, *14*(S1), 59–65. PMID:9120673

McMillan, M., Spinks, E. A., & Fenwick, G. R. (1986). Preliminary observations on the effect of dietary brussels sprouts on thyroid function. *Human Toxicology*, *5*(1), 15–19. doi:10.1177/096032718600500104 PMID:2419242

Morris, M. C., Sacks, F., & Rosner, B. (1993). Does fish oil lower blood pressure? A meta-analysis of controlled trials. *Circulation*, *88*(2), 523–533. doi:10.1161/01.CIR.88.2.523 PMID:8339414

Mulvany, M. J. (2002). Small artery remodeling in hypertension. *Current Hypertension Reports*, *4*(1), 49–55. doi:10.1007/s11906-002-0053-y PMID:11790292

Nagao, T., Hase, T., & Tokimitsu, I. (2007). A green tea extract high in catechins reduces body fat and cardiovascular risks in humans. *Obesity (Silver Spring, Md.)*, *15*(6), 1473–1483. doi:10.1038/oby.2007.176 PMID:17557985

Perez-Jimenez, J., Neveu, V., Vos, F., & Scalbert, A. (2015). Identification of the 100 richest dietary sources of polyphenols: an application of the Phenol-Explorer database. *EJCN*. Retrieved from http://www.nature.com/ejcn/journal/v64/n3s/fig_tab/ejcn2010221t1.html

Rahmouni, K., Correia, M. L. G., Haynes, W. G., & Mark, A. L. (2005). Obesity-associated hypertension – new insights into mechanisms. *Hypertension*, *45*(1), 9–14. doi:10.1161/01.HYP.0000151325.83008.b4 PMID:15583075

Rajagopalan, S., Kurz, S., Munzel, T., Tarpey, M., Freeman, B. A., Griendling, K. K., & Harrison, D. G. (1996). Angiotensin II-mediated hypertension in the rat increases vascular superoxide production via membrane NADH/NADPH oxidase activation. Contribution to alterations of vasomotor tone. *The Journal of Clinical Investigation*, *97*(8), 1916–1923. doi:10.1172/JCI118623 PMID:8621776

Ramel, A., Alfredo Martinez, J., Kiely, M., Bandara, N. M., & Thorsdottir, I. (2010). Moderate consumption of fatty fish reduces diastolic blood pressure in overweight and obese European young adults during energy restriction. *Nutrition (Burbank, Los Angeles County, Calif.)*, *26*(2), 168–174. doi:10.1016/j.nut.2009.04.002 PMID:19487105

Reddy, K. S., & Katan, M. B. (2004). Diet, nutrition and the prevention of hypertension and cardiovascular diseases. *Public Health Nutrition*, *7*(1a), 167–186. doi:10.1079/PHN2003587 PMID:14972059

Rein, D., Lotito, S., Holt, R. R., Keen, C. L., Schmitz, H. H., & Fraga, C. G. (2000). Epicatechin in human plasma:In vivo determination and effect of chocolate consumption on plasma oxidation status. *The Journal of Nutrition*, *130*, 2109S–2114S. PMID:10917931

Rupp, H., & Maisch, B. (2003). Abdominal fat and sympathetic overactivity. *Herz*, *28*(8), 668–673. doi:10.1007/s00059-003-2517-5 PMID:14689100

Sankhari, J.M., Thounaojam, M.C., Jadeja, R. N., Devkar, R. V., Ramachandran, A. V. (2012). Anthocyanin-rich red cabbage (Brassica oleracea L.) extract attenuates cardiac and hepatic oxidative stress in rats fed an atherogenic diet. *Journal of Science and Food Agriculture*, *92*(8), 1688-1693.

Scalbert, A., & Williamson, G. (2000). Dietary intake and bioavailability of polyphenols. *The Journal of Nutrition*, *130*, 2073S–2085S. PMID:10917926

Schiffrin, E. L. (2001). Effects of antihypertensive drugs on vascular remodeling: Do they predict outcome in response to antihypertensive therapy? *Current Opinion in Nephrology and Hypertension*, *10*(5), 617–624. doi:10.1097/00041552-200109000-00011 PMID:11496055

Segura, J., & Ruilope, L. M. (2007). Obesity, Essential hypertension and rennin-angiotensin system. *Public Health Nutrition*, *10*(10A), 1151–1155. doi:10.1017/S136898000700064X PMID:17903324

Shantakumari, N., Eldeeb, R. A., Mabrouk Ibrahim, S. A., Sreedharan, J., & Otoum, S. (2014). Effect of PUFA on patients with hypertension: A hospital based study. *Indian Heart Journal*, *66*(4), 408–414. doi:10.1016/j.ihj.2014.05.006 PMID:25173198

Shirai, K. (2004). Obesity as the core of the metabolic syndrome and the management of coronary heart disease. *Current Medical Research and Opinion*, *20*(3), 295–304. doi:10.1185/030079903125003008 PMID:15025838

Shulman, G. I. (2004). Unraveling the cellular mechanisms of insulin resistance in humans: New insights from magnetic resonance spectroscopy. *Physiology (Bethesda, MD)*, *19*(4), 183–190. doi:10.1152/physiol.00007.2004 PMID:15304632

Sones, K., Heaney, R. K., & Fenwick, G. R. (1984a). An estimate of the mean daily intake of glucosinolates from cruciferous vegetables in the UK. *Journal of the Science of Food and Agriculture*, *35*(6), 712–719. doi:10.1002/jsfa.2740350619

Taddei, S., Ghiadoni, L., Virdis, A., Versari, D., & Salvetti, A. (2003). Mechanisms of endothelial dysfunction: Clinical significance and preventive non-pharmacological therapeutic strategies. *Current Pharmaceutical Design*, *9*(29), 2385–2402. doi:10.2174/1381612033453866 PMID:14529554

Taubert, D., Roesen, R., Lehmann, C., Jung, N., & Schoming, E. (2007). Effects of low habitual cocoa intake on blood pressure and bioactive nitric oxide: A randomized controlled trial. *JAMMA*, *298*(1), 49–60. doi:10.1001/jama.298.1.49 PMID:17609490

United States Department of Agriculture (USDA). (2011). *National Nutrient Database for standard reference release 28*. Retrieved from http://ndb.nal.usda.gov/

VanEtten, C. H., Daxenbickler, M. E., Tookey, H. L., Kwolek, W. F., Williams, P. H., & Yoder, O. C. (1980). Glucosinolates: Potential toxicants in cabbage cultivars. *Journal of the American Society for Horticultural Science*, *105*, 710–714.

Vitrac, X., Moni, J. P., Vercauteren, J., Deffieux, G., & Merillon, J. M. (2002). Direct liquid chromatography analysis of resveratrol derivatives and flavanonols in wines with absorbance and fluorescence detection. *Analytica Chimica Acta*, *458*(1), 103–110. doi:10.1016/S0003-2670(01)01498-2

Wikimedia Commons. (2007). *Chemical structure of glucosinolates*. Retrieved from https://commons.wikimedia.org/wiki/File:Glucosinolates.png

Wolfram, S., Weber, T., Grenacher, B., & Scharrer, E. (1995). A Na(+)-dependent mechanism is involved in mucosal uptake of cinnamic acid across the jejunal brush border in rats. *The Journal of Nutrition*, *125*(5), 1300–1308. PMID:7738690

World Health Organization (WHO). (2008). *The global burden of diseases: 2004 update*. Retrieved from www.who.int/healthinfo/global_burden_disease/GBD_report_2004updat

Yen, G. C., & Wei, Q. K. (1993). Myrosinase activity and total glucosinolate content of cruciferous vegetables, and some properties of cabbage myrosinase in Taiwan. *Journal of the Science of Food and Agriculture*, *61*(4), 471–475. doi:10.1002/jsfa.2740610415

Compilation of References

A 2 Z Project. (2008). *Rice fortification in developing countries: a critical review of the technical and economic feasibility*. Washington, DC: Academy for Educational Development. Retrieved from http://www.oecd.org/env/ehs/biotrack/46815658.pdf

Abd El-Salam, M. H., & El-Shibiny, S. (2013). Bioactive Peptides of Buffalo, Camel, Goat, Sheep, Mare, and Yak Milks and Milk Products. *Food Reviews International*, *29*(1), 1–23. doi:10.1080/87559129.2012.692137

Abdel Magjeed, N. (2005). Corrective effect of milk camel on some cancer biomarkers in blood of rats intoxicated with aflatoxin B1. *Journal of Saudi Chemical Society*, *9*, 253–264.

Abdel-Aal, E. M., & Rabalski, I. (2008). Bioactive compounds and their antioxidant capacity in selected primitive and modern wheat species. *The Open Agriculture Journal*, *2*(1), 7–14. doi:10.2174/1874331500802010007

Abdelgadir, W. S., Ahmed, T. K., & Dirar, H. A. (1998). The traditional fermented milk products of the Sudan. *International Journal of Food Microbiology*, *44*(1-2), 1–13. doi:10.1016/S0168-1605(98)00090-7 PMID:9849779

Abeywardena, M. Y., & Head, R. J. (2001). Longchain n-3 polyunsaturated fatty acids and blood vessel function. *Cardiovascular Research*, *52*(3), 361–371. doi:10.1016/S0008-6363(01)00406-0 PMID:11738053

Abia, W. A., Warth, B., Sulyok, M., Krska, R., Tchana, A. N., Njobeh, P. B., & Moundipa, P. F. et al. (2013). Determination of multi-mycotoxin occurrence in cereals, nuts and their products in Cameroon by liquid chromatography tandem mass spectrometry (LC-MS/MS). *Food Control*, *31*(2), 438–453. doi:10.1016/j.foodcont.2012.10.006

Abiru, Y., Ueno, T., & Uchiyama, S. (2013). Isolation and characterization of novel S-equol-producing bacteria from brines of stinky tofu, a traditional fermented soy food in Taiwan. *International Journal of Food Sciences and Nutrition*, *64*(8), 936–943. doi:10.3109/09637486.2013.816936 PMID:23869769

Abou-Soliman, N. H. (2005). *Studies on goat milk proteins: molecular and immunologicalcharacterization with respect to human health and nutrition*. (Ph.D. Thesis). Alexandria University, Egypt.

Abukutsa-Onyango, M. O. (2011). *Researching African indigenous fruits and vegetables –Why?* Retrieved July 30, 2015 from http://knowledge.cta.int/Dossiers/Commodities/Fruits/Feature-articles/Researching-African-Indigenous-Fruits-and-Vegetables-Why

Abukutsa-Onyango, M. O. (2003). Unexploited potential of indigenous African vegetables in Western Kenya. *Maseno Journal of Education. Arts and Science*, *4*(2), 103–122.

Adams, L. S., Zhang, Y., Seeram, N. P., Heber, D., & Chen, S. (2010). Pomegranate ellagitannin–derived compounds exhibit antiproliferative & antiaromatase activity in breast cancer cells in vitro. *Cancer Prevention Research (Philadelphia, Pa.)*, *3*(1), 108–113. doi:10.1158/1940-6207.CAPR-08-0225 PMID:20051378

Adebamowo, C. A., Cho, E., Sampson, L., Katan, M. B., Spiegelman, D., Willett, W. C., & Holmes, M. D. (2005). Dietary flavonols and flavonol rich foods intake and the risk of breast cancer. *International Journal of Cancer*, *114*(4), 628–633. doi:10.1002/ijc.20741 PMID:15609322

Adetunji, M., Atanda, O., Ezekiel, C. N., Sulyok, M., Warth, B., Beltrán, E., & Chilaka, C. A. et al. (2014). Fungal and bacterial metabolites of stored maize (*Zea mays,* L.) from five agro-ecological zones of Nigeria. *Mycotoxin Research*, *30*(2), 89–102. doi:10.1007/s12550-014-0194-2 PMID:24643458

Adly, A. A. M. (2010). Oxidative stress and disease: An updated review. *Research Journal of Immunology*, *3*, 129–145. doi:10.3923/rji.2010.129.145

Adom, K. K., Sorrells, M. E., & Liu, R. H. (2005). Phytochemicals and antioxidant activity of milled fractions of different wheat varieties. *Journal of Agricultural and Food Chemistry*, *53*(6), 2297–2306. doi:10.1021/jf048456d PMID:15769171

Afify, A. E. M. R., Fayed, S. A., Shalaby, E. A., & El-Shemy, H. A. (2011). *Syzygium cumini (*pomposia) active principles exhibit potent anticancer and antioxidant activities. *African Journal of Pharmacy and Pharmacology*, *5*(7), 948–956.

Agarwal, S. K., Verma, S., Singh, S. S., Tripathy, A. K., Khan, Z. K., & Kumar, S. (2000). Antifeedant and antifungal activity of chromene compounds isolated from Blepharispermum subsessile. *Journal of Ethnopharmacology*, *71*(1-2), 231–234. doi:10.1016/S0378-8741(00)00158-6 PMID:10904167

Agrahari, P., & Singh, D. K. (2014). A review on the pharmacological aspects of *Carum carvi. Journal of Biology and Earth Sciences*, *4*, M1–M13.

Agrawal, R. P., Budania, S., Sharma, P., Gupta, R., Kochar, D. K., Panwar, R. B., & Sahani, M. S. (2007). Zero prevalence of diabetes in camel milk consuming Raica community of northwest Rajasthan, India. *Diabetes Research and Clinical Practice*, *76*(2), 290–296. doi:10.1016/j.diabres.2006.09.036 PMID:17098321

Agrawal, R. P., Jain, S., Shah, S., Chopra, A., & Agarwal, V. (2011). Effect of camel milk on glycemic control and insulin requirement in patients with type 1 diabetes: 2-years randomized controlled trial. *European Journal of Clinical Nutrition*, *65*(9), 1048–1052. doi:10.1038/ejcn.2011.98 PMID:21629270

Aguiar, C. L., Baptista, A. S., Alencar, S. M., Haddad, R., & Eberlin, M. N. (2007). Analysis of isoflavonoids from leguminous plant extracts by RPHPLC/DAD and electrospray ionization mass spectrometry. *International Journal of Food Sciences and Nutrition*, *58*(2), 116–124. doi:10.1080/09637480601149350 PMID:17469767

Aguilar, A., Camacho, J. R., Chino, S., Jaquez, P., & Lopez, M. E. (1994). *Herbario Medicinal del Instituto Mexicano del Seguro Social*. Instituto Mexicano del Seguro Social Informacion Ethnobotanica. Mexico.

Ahluwalia, P., Kaur, A., & Sidhu, J. S. (1995). Effect of psyllium mucilloid husk as a source of fiber on baking properties of the flour and acceptability of the baked products. *Chem. Mikrobiol. Technol. Lebensm.*, *17*(3/4), 118–122.

Ahluwalia, V. K., & Arora, K. K. (1981). Nuclear Iso Prenylation of Poly Hydroxy Acetophenones Acid Catalyzed Condensation with Isoprene. *Tetrahedon*, *37*, 1437–1439. doi:10.1016/S0040-4020(01)92463-9

Ahmad, A. S. (2015). Identification of potent antioxidant bioactive peptides from goat milk proteins. *Food Research International*, *74*, 80–88. doi:10.1016/j.foodres.2015.04.032

Ahmed, A. H. (2013). The ability of pomegranate to ameliorate symptoms associated with Alzheimer's disease in aged transgenic mice. *Open Access Master's Theses.* Paper 146. Available at: http://digitalcommons.uri.edu/theses/146

Ahmed, M. (2014). Ancient Pakistan - an archaeological history. In Harappan Civilization - The Material Culture (vol. 3). Foursome Group.

Ahn, D. U., Olsonm, D. G., Chen, J. X., Wu, C., & Lee, J. I. (1998). Effect of muscle type packaging and irradiation on lipid oxidation volatile production, and color in raw pork patties. *Meat Science*, *47*(1), 27–39. doi:10.1016/S0309-1740(97)00101-0 PMID:22063182

Ahuja, S., Kohli, S., Krishnan, S., Dogra, D., Sharma, D., & Rani, V. (2011). Curcumin: A potential therapeutic polyphenol, prevents noradrenaline-induced hypertrophy in rat cardiac myocytes. *The Journal of Pharmacy and Pharmacology*, *63*(12), 1604–1612. doi:10.1111/j.2042-7158.2011.01363.x PMID:22060292

Aina, D. A., Jonathan, S. G., Olawuyi, O. J., & Durowoju, B. M. (2012). Antioxidant, antimicrobial and phytochemical properties of alcoholic extracts of *Cantharellus cibarius* – a Nigerian mushroom. *New York Science Journal*, *5*, 114–120.

Ajaikumar, K. B., Asheef, M., Babu, B. H., & Padikkala, J. (2005). The inhibition of gastric mucosal injury by *Punica granatum* L. (pomegranate) methanolic extract. *Journal of Ethnopharmacology*, *96*(1), 171–176. doi:10.1016/j.jep.2004.09.007 PMID:15588667

Ajay, S., Rahul, S., Sumit, G., Paras, M., Mishra, A., & Gaurav, A. (2011). Comprehensive review: *Murraya koenigii Linn. Asian Journal of Pharmacy and Life Science*, *1*(4), 417–425.

Akan, S. (2014). Health promoting properties of garlic (*Allium sativum* L.) consumption. *Akademik Gida*, *12*(2), 95–100.

Akaza, H., Miyanaga, N., Takashima, N., Naito, S., Hirao, Y., Tsukamoto, T., & Pantuck, A. J. et al. (2004). Comparisons of percent equol producers between prostate cancer patients and controls: Case-controlled studies of isoflavones in Japanese, Korean and American residents. *Japanese Journal of Clinical Oncology*, *34*(2), 86–89. doi:10.1093/jjco/hyh015 PMID:15067102

Akhtar, S., Ismail, T., Fraternale, D., & Sestili, P. (2015). Pomegranate peel and peel extracts: Chemistry and food features. *Food Chemistry*, *174*, 417–425. doi:10.1016/j.foodchem.2014.11.035 PMID:25529700

Akhtar, S., Khalid, N., Ahmed, I., Shahzad, A., & Suleria, H. A. R. (2014). Physicochemical characteristics, functional properties, and nutritional benefits of peanut oil: A review. *Critical Reviews in Food Science and Nutrition*, *54*(12), 1562–1575. doi:10.1080/10408398.2011.644353 PMID:24580558

Akomolafe, S. F., & Oboh, G. (2015). Characterization of polyphenolic constituents and radical scavenging ability of ripe tomato and red pepper fruits. *Journal of Experimental and Integrative Medicine*, *5*(1), 61–67. doi:10.5455/jeim.080215.or.123

Al Haj, O. A., & Al Kanhal, H. A. (2010). Compositional, technological and nutritional aspects of dromedary camel milk. *International Dairy Journal*, *20*, 811-821.

Alaimo, K., McDowell, M. A., & Briefel, R. R. (1994). Dietary intake of vitamins, minerals, and fiber of persons ages 2 months and over in the United States: The Third National Health and Nutrition Examination Survey, Phase 1, 1988–1991. *Advance Data*, *258*, 1–26. PMID:10138938

Alavizadeh, S. H., & Hosseinzadeh, H. (2014). Bioactivity assessment and toxicity of crocin: A comprehensive review. *Food and Chemical Toxicology*, *64*, 65–80. doi:10.1016/j.fct.2013.11.016 PMID:24275090

Al-Ayadhi, L. Y., & Elamin, N. E. (2013). Camel milk as a potential therapy as an antioxidant in autism spectrum disorder (ASD). *Evidence-Based Complementary and Alternative Medicine*, 1–8.

Albert, C. M., Gaziano, J. M., Willett, W. C., & Manson, J. E. (2002). Nut consumption and decreased risk of sudden cardiac death in the Physicians' Health Study. *Archives of Internal Medicine*, *162*(12), 1382–1387. doi:10.1001/archinte.162.12.1382 PMID:12076237

Albrecht, M., Jiang, W., Kumi-Diaka, J., Lansky, E. P., Gommersall, L. M., Patel, A., & Campbell, M. J. et al. (2004). Pomegranate extracts potently suppress proliferation, xenograft growth, & invasion of human prostate cancer cells. *Journal of Medicinal Food*, *7*(3), 274–283. doi:10.1089/jmf.2004.7.274 PMID:15383219

Alexandre, K. B., Gray, E. S., Lambson, B. E., Moore, P. L., Choge, I. A., Mlisana, K., & Morris, L. et al. (2010). Mannose-rich glycosylation patterns on HIV-1 subtype C gp120 and sensitivity to the lectins, Griffithsin, Cyanovirin-N and Scytovirin. *Virology*, *402*(1), 187–196. doi:10.1016/j.virol.2010.03.021 PMID:20392471

Alhaj, O. A. (2015). *Chromatographic determination of L- and D-amino acids in fermented camel milk*. Unpublished work, King Saud University, Kingdom of Saudi Arabia.

Alhaj, O. A., Metwalli, A. A., Ismail, E. A., Ali, H. S., Al-Khalifa, A. S., & Kanekanian, A. D. (2016). *Angiotensin Converting Enzyme - inhibitory activity and antimicrobial effect of fermented camel milk (Camelusdromedarius)*. Unpublished work, King Saud University, Kingdom of Saudi Arabia.

Alhaj, O. A., Brückner, H., & Al-Khalifa, A. S. (2012). Sequences of ACE-inhibitory precursor peptides from bacterial fermented milk of *Camelus dromedarius*. *Journal of Peptide Science*, *18*, S146–S147.

Alhaj, O. A., Kanekanian, A., & Peters, A. (2007). Investigation on whey proteins profile of commercially aviabale milk-based probiotics health drinks using fast protein liquid chromatography (FPLC). *British Food Journal*, *109*(6), 469–480. doi:10.1108/00070700710753526

Alhaj, O. A., Kanekanian, A., Peters, A., & Tatham, A. (2010). Hypocholesterolemic effect of *Bifidobacterium animalis* subsp. *Lactis* (Bb12) and trypsin casein hydrolysate. *Food Chemistry*, *123*(2), 430–435. doi:10.1016/j.foodchem.2010.04.061

Alhaj, O. A., Metwalli, A. A. M., & Ismail, E. A. (2011). Heat stability of camel milk proteins after sterilization process. *Journal of Camel Practice & Research*, *18*, 277–282.

Alhaj, O. A., Taufik, E., Handa, Y., Fukuda, K., Saito, T., & Urashima, T. (2013). Chemical characterization of oligosaccharides in commercially pasteurized dromedary camel (*camelusdromedarius*) milk. *International Dairy Journal*, *28*(2), 70–75. doi:10.1016/j.idairyj.2012.08.008

Al-Hooti, S.N., Al-Saqer, J.M., Sidhu, J.S., & Al-Othman, A. (2002). Effect of raw wheat germ addition on the physical texture and objective color of a designer food (toast bread). *Nahrung/Food, 46*(2), 68-72.

Al-Hooti, S. N., Sidhu, J. S., & Al-Saqer, J. M. (2000). Utility of CIE Tristimulus System in Measuring the Objective Crumb Color of High-fiber Toast Bread Formulations. *Journal of Food Quality*, *23*(1), 103–116. doi:10.1111/j.1745-4557.2000.tb00199.x

Alipoor, B., Haghighian, M. K., Sadat, B. E., & Asghari, M. (2012). Effect of sesame seed on lipid profile and redox status in hyperlipidemic patients. *International Journal of Food Sciences and Nutrition*, *63*(6), 674–678. doi:10.3109/09637486.2011.652077 PMID:22263599

Al-Juboori, A. J., Mohammed, M., Rashid, J., Kurian, J., & El Refaey S. (2013). Nutritional and medicinal value of camel (Camelus Dromedarius) milk. *Food & Environment II, 170*, 221-232.

Al-Khdier, A. M., Al-Saleh, A. A., Abu-Tarboush, H. M., Ismail, E. A., & Metwalli, A. A. (2014). The ability of some starter cultures to increase the conjugated linoleic acid level in cow and camel milks. *Journal of Pure and Applied Microbiology*, *8*, 363–370.

Allred, C. D., Twaddle, N. C., Allred, K. F., Goeppinger, T. S., Churchwell, M. I., Ju, Y. H., & Doerge, D. R. et al. (2005). Soy processing affects metabolism and disposition of dietary isoflavones in ovariectomized BALB/c mice. *Journal of Agricultural and Food Chemistry*, *53*(22), 8542–8550. doi:10.1021/jf051246w PMID:16248551

Al-Orf, S. M., Ahmed, M. H. M., Al-Atwai, N., Zaidi, H. A., Dehwah, A., & Dehwah, S. (2012). Review: Nutritional properties and benefits of the date fruits (*Phoenix dactylifera L.*). *Bulletin of the National Nutrition Institute of the Arab Republic of Egypt*, *39*, 98–129.

Alper, C. M., & Mattes, R. D. (2003). Peanut consumption improves indices of cardiovascular disease risk in healthy adults. *Journal of the American College of Nutrition*, *22*(2), 133–141. doi:10.1080/07315724.2003.10719286 PMID:12672709

Al-Reza, S. M., Yoon, J. I., Kim, H. J., Kim, J. S., & Kang, S. E. (2010). Anti-inflammatory activity of seed essential oil from *Zizyphus jujube*. *Food and Chemical Toxicology*, *48*(2), 639–643. doi:10.1016/j.fct.2009.11.045 PMID:19944733

Al-Saleh, A. A., Metwalli, A. A. M., Ismail, E. A., & Alhaj, O. A. (2014). Antioxidative activity of camel milk casein hydrolysates. *Journal of Camel Practice & Research*, *21*(2), 229–237. doi:10.5958/2277-8934.2014.00041.1

Al-Saqer, J. M., Sidhu, J. S., & Al-Hooti, S. N. (2000). Instrumental Texture and Baking Quality of High-fiber Toast Bread Formulations. *Journal of Food Processing and Preservation*, *24*(1), 1–16. doi:10.1111/j.1745-4549.2000.tb00402.x

Al-Sheraji, S. H., Ismail, A., Manap, M. Y., Mustafa, S., Yusof, R. M., & Hassan, F. A. (2012). Hypocholesterolemic effect of yoghurt containing Bi fidobacterium pseudocatenulatum G4 or Bi fido bacterium longum BB536. *Food Chemistry*, *135*(2), 356–361. doi:10.1016/j.foodchem.2012.04.120 PMID:22868099

Alta, M., Ramos, S., Mateos, B., Granado-Serrano, A. B., Bravo, L., & Goya, L. (2006). Quercetin Protects Human Hepatoma Hepg2 Against Oxidative Stress Induced By Tert-Butyl Hydroperoxide. *Toxicology and Applied Pharmacology*, *212*(2), 110–118. doi:10.1016/j.taap.2005.07.014 PMID:16126241

Al-Tibi, A. M., Takruri, H. R., & Ahmad, M. N. (2010). Effect of dehulling and cooking of lentils (Lens culinaris L.) on serum glucose and lipoprotein levels in streptozotocin-induced diabetic rats. *Malaysian Journalof Nutrition*, *16*(3), 409–418. PMID:22691994

Altunkaya, A., Hedegaard, R. V., Brimer, L., Gökmen, V., & Skibsted, L. H. (2013). Antioxidant capacity versus chemical safety of wheat bread enriched with pomegranate peel powder. *Food & Function*, *4*(5), 722–727. doi:10.1039/c3fo30296b PMID:23429604

Amarowicz, R. (2007). Tannins: The new natural antioxidants? *European Journal of Lipid Science and Technology*, *109*(6), 549–551. doi:10.1002/ejlt.200700145

Amarowicz, R., Karamac, M., & Weidner, S. (2001). Antioxidant activity of phenolic fraction of pea (*Pisum sativum*). *Czech Journal Food Science*, *19*, 139–142.

Amr, A. M., Takruri, H. R., Shomaf, M. S., Alhaj, O. A., & Faris, M. E. (2015). *Chemopreventive potential of probiotic fermented camel (Camelusdromedarius) and bovine (Bostaurus) milks against Azoxymethane-Induced aberrant crypt foci in Fischer 344 Rats, unpublished work*. Amman, Jordan: University of Jordan.

Andabati, A. (2014). *Nutraceutical potential of selected Ugandan traditional foods*. (Unpublished Master's Thesis). Makerere University, Uganda.

Andabati, A., & Muyonga, J. (2014). Phenolic content and antioxidant activity of selected Ugandan traditional medicinal foods. *African Journal of Food Science*, *8*(8), 427–434. doi:10.5897/AJFS2014.1136

Andersen, T., & Fogh, W. J. (2001). Weight Loss and Delayed Gastric Emptying Following a South American Herbal Preparation in Overweight Patients. *Journal of Human Nutrition and Dietetics*, *14*(3), 243–250. doi:10.1046/j.1365-277X.2001.00290.x PMID:11424516

Anderson, J. W. (1995). Dietary fibre, complex carbohydrate and coronary artery disease. *Canadian Journal Cardiology*, *11*(SG):55G – 62G.

Anderson, J. W. (2002). Dietary fiber prevents carbohydrate-induced hypertriglyceridemia. *Current Atherosclerosis Report*, 536 – 541.

Anderson, A. J., & Wynn, J. P. (2001). Microbial polyhydroxyalkanoates, polysaccharides and lipids. Cambridge University Press.

Anderson, J. W., Randles, K. M., Kendall, C. W., & Jenkins, D. J. (2004). Carbohydrate and fiber recommendations for individuals with diabetes. A quantitative assessment and meta- analysis of the evidence. *Journal of the American College of Nutrition*, *23*(1), 5–17. doi:10.1080/07315724.2004.10719338 PMID:14963049

Anesini, C., Ferraro, G., & Filip, R. (2006). Peroxidase-Like Activity of *Ilex Paraguariensis*. *Food Chemistry*, *97*(3), 459–464. doi:10.1016/j.foodchem.2005.05.025

Anon., (2015). Functional foods and ingredients for protection against diabetes and metabolic syndrome. *Food Engg. Ingredients*, *40*(May/June), 16–18.

Anonymous, . (2000). Counting the benefits of soy. *Agri-Food Res Ontario.*, *24*, 28–29.

Anonymous. (2002). The benefits of moderate beer consumption. CBMC – The Brewers of Europe.

An, S. Y., Lee, M. S., Jeon, J. Y., Ha, E. S., Kim, T. H., Ok, J. Y., & Lee, K. W. et al. (2013). Beneficial effects of fresh and fermented kimchi in prediabetic individuals. *Annals of Nutrition & Metabolism*, *63*(1-2), 111–119. doi:10.1159/000353583 PMID:23969321

Anthony, M. S., Clarkson, T. B., & Williams, J. K. (1998). Effects of soy isoflavones on ather-osclerosis: Potential mechanisms. *The American Journal of Clinical Nutrition*, *68*, 1390S–1393S. PMID:9848505

Anton, J., Meseguer, I., & Rodriguez-Valera, F. (1988). Production of an extracellular polysaccharide by Haloferax mediterranei. *Applied and Environmental Microbiology*, *54*, 23812386. PMID:16347749

Anukam, K. C., & Reid, G. (2009). African traditional fermented foods and probiotics. *Journal of Medicinal Food*, *12*(6), 1177–1184. doi:10.1089/jmf.2008.0163 PMID:20041769

Appleby, P. N., Spencer, E. A., & Key, T. J. (2004). Soy intake and blood cholesterol concentrations: A cross-sectional study of 1033 pre- and postmenopausal women in the Oxford arm of the European Prospective Investigation into Cancer and Nutrition. *The American Journal of Clinical Nutrition*, *80*, 1391–1396. PMID:15531691

Aqil, F., Gupta, A., Munagala, R., Jeyabalan, J., Kausar, H., Sharma, R. J., & Gupta, R. C. et al. (2012). Antioxidant and antiproliferative activities of anthocyanin/Ellagitannin- enriched extracts from *Syzygium cumini* L. (Jamun, the Indian Blackberry). *Nutrition and Cancer*, *64*(3), 428–438. doi:10.1080/01635581.2012.657766 PMID:22420901

Arab, L., Khan, F., & Lam, H. (2013). Epidemiologic evidence of a relationship between tea, coffee, or caffeine consumption and cognitive decline. *Advances in Nutrition*, *4*(1), 115–122. doi:10.3945/an.112.002717 PMID:23319129

Araya, H., Contreras, P., Alvina, M., Vera, G., & Pak, N. (2002). A comparison between an in vitro method to determine carbohydrate digestion rate and the glycemic response in young men. *European Journal of Clinical Nutrition*, *56*(8), 735–739. doi:10.1038/sj.ejcn.1601386 PMID:12122549

Ariga, T., Oshiba, S., & Tamada, T. (1999). Platelet aggregation inhibitor in garlic. *Lancet*, *1*, 150–151. PMID:6109819

Arlee, R., Suanphairoch, S., & Pakdeechanuan, P. (2013). Differences in chemical components and antioxidant-related substances in virgin coconut oil from coconut hybrids and their parents. *International Food Research Journal*, *20*(5), 2103–2109.

Armstrong, W. B., Kennedy, A. R., Wan, X. S., Atiba, J., McLaren, C. E., & Meyskens, F. L. (2000). Single-dose administration of Bowman-Birk inhibitor concentrate in patients with oral leukoplakia. *Cancer Epidemiology, Biomarkers & Prevention*, *9*(1), 43–47. PMID:10667462

Arnoldi, A. (2005). Functional Foods, Cardiovascular Disease and Diabetes, Woodhead Publishing Ltd, Cambridge, UK. *Carbohydrate Polymers*, *61*(4), 480–485. doi:10.1016/j.carbpol.2005.05.012

Arora, A., Nair, M. G., & Strasburg, G. M. (1998). Antioxidant activities of isoflavones and their biological metabolites in a liposomal system. *Archives of Biochemistry and Biophysics*, *356*(2), 133–141. doi:10.1006/abbi.1998.0783 PMID:9705203

Arreola, R., Quintero-Fabian, S., Lopez-Roa, R.I., Flores-Gutierrez, E.O., Reyes-Grajeda, J.P., Carrera-Quintanar, L.C., & Ortuno-Sahagun, D. (2015). Immunomodulation and Anti-Inflammatory Effects of Garlic Compounds. *Journal of Immunology Research*, 1-13.

Arsenic in your food. (2012). *Consumer Reports Magazine*.

Arthur, J. R., McKenzie, R. C., & Beckett, G. J. (2003). Selenium in the immune system. *The Journal of Nutrition*, *133*(5), 1457S–1459S. PMID:12730442

Arts, I. C., Jacobs, D. R. Jr, Harnack, L. J., Gross, M., & Folsom, A. R. (2001). Dietary catechins in relation to coronary heart disease death among postmenopausal women. *Epidemiology (Cambridge, Mass.)*, *12*(6), 668–675. doi:10.1097/00001648-200111000-00015 PMID:11679795

Asgary, S., Sahebkar, A., Afshani, M. R., Keshvari, M., Haghjooyjavanmard, S., & Rafieian-Kopaei, M. (2014). Clinical evaluation of blood pressure lowering, endothelial function improving, hypolipidemic & anti-inflammatory effects of pomegranate juice in hypertensive subjects. *Journal of Phytotherapy Research*, *28*(2), 193–199. doi:10.1002/ptr.4977 PMID:23519910

Ashenef, A. (2014). Essential and toxic metals in tea (Camellia sinensis) imported and produced in Ethiopia. *Food Additives & Contaminants: Part B*, *7*(1), 30-6. Doi:10.1080/19393210.2013.831951

Aslam, M. N., Lansky, E. P., & Varani, J. (2006). Pomegranate as a cosmeceutical source: Pomegranate fractions promote proliferation & procollagen synthesis & inhibit matrix metalloproteinase-1 production in human skin cells. *Journal of Ethnopharmacology*, *103*(3), 311–318. doi:10.1016/j.jep.2005.07.027 PMID:16221534

Aso, T., Uchiyama, S., Matsumura, Y., Taguchi, M., Nozaki, M., Takamatsu, K., Ishizuka, B., Kubota, T., Mizunuma, H., & Ohta, H. (2012). A natural S-equol supplement alleviates hot flushes and other menopausal symptoms in equol nonproducing postmenopausal Japanese women. *Journal of Womens Health (Larchmt)*, *21*, 92-100

Asseburg, H., Hagl, S., & Eckert, G. P. (2014). Nutritional approaches for healthy aging of the brain and the prevention of neurodegenerative diseases. In Pharma-Nutrition (pp. 457-479). Springer International Publishing. doi:10.1007/978-3-319-06151-1_23

Assmann, G., Buonob, P., Daniele, A., Valle, E. D., Farinaro, E., Ferns, G., & Vetrani, C. et al. (2014). Functional foods and cardiometabolic diseases: International Task Force for Prevention of Cardiometabolic Diseases. *Nutrition, Metabolism, and Cardiovascular Diseases*, *24*(12), 1272–1300. doi:10.1016/j.numecd.2014.10.010 PMID:25467217

Assmann, G., & Schulte, H. (1992). Relation of high-density lipoprotein cholesterol and triglycerides to incidence of atherosclerotic coronary artery disease (the PROCAM experience). *The American Journal of Cardiology*, *70*(7), 733–737. doi:10.1016/0002-9149(92)90550-I PMID:1519522

Association of OfficialAnalytical Chemists (AOAC). (1995). *Official methods of analysis*. AOAC International.

Assuncao, M., & Andrade, J. P. (2015). Protective action of green tea catechins in neuronal mitochondria during aging. *Frontiers in Bioscience*, *20*(2), 247–262. doi:10.2741/4307 PMID:25553449

Atale, N., Chakraborty, M., Mohanty, S., Bhattacharya, S., Nigam, D., Sharma, M., & Rani, V. (2013). Cardioprotective Role of Syzygium cumini Against Glucose- Induced Oxidative Stress in H9C2 Cardiac Myocytes. *Cardiovascular Toxicology*, *13*(3), 278–289. doi:10.1007/s12012-013-9207-1 PMID:23512199

Athayde, M. I., Coelho, G. C., & Schenkel, E. P. (2000). Caffeine and Theobromine in Epicuticular Wax of *Ilex Paraguariensis* St.Hil. *Phytochemistry*, *55*(7), 853–857. doi:10.1016/S0031-9422(00)00324-1 PMID:11190409

Atilgan, D., Parlaktas, B., Uluocak, N., Gencten, Y., Erdemir, F., Ozyurt, H., & Aslan, H. et al. (2014). Pomegranate (*Punica granatum*) juice reduces oxidative injury & improves sperm concentration in a rat model of testicular torsion-detorsion. *Journal of Experimental & Therapeutic Medicine*, *8*(2), 478–482. PMID:25009604

Atkinson, C., Berman, S., Humbert, O., & Lampe, J. W. (2004). In vitro incubation of human feces with daidzein and antibiotics suggests interindividual differences in the bacteria responsible for equol production. *The Journal of Nutrition*, *134*, 596–599. PMID:14988453

Atkinson, C., Frankenfeld, C. L., & Lampe, J. W. (2005). Gut bacterial metabolism of the soy isoflavone daidzein: Exploring the relevance to human nutrition. *Experimental Biology and Medicine*, *230*, 155–170. PMID:15734719

Aura, A.-M. (2008). Microbial metabolism of dietary phenolic compounds in the colon. *Phytochemistry Reviews*, *7*(3), 407–429. doi:10.1007/s11101-008-9095-3

Aviram, M., & Dornfeld, L. (2010). *U.S. Patent No. 7,645,469*. Washington, DC: U.S. Patent & Trademark Office.

Aviram, M., & Dornfeld, L. (2001). Pomegranate juice consumption inhibits serum angiotensin converting enzyme activity & reduces systolic blood pressure. *Atherosclerosis*, *158*(1), 195–198. doi:10.1016/S0021-9150(01)00412-9 PMID:11500191

Aviram, M., Dornfeld, L., Kaplan, M., Coleman, R., Gaitini, D., Nitecki, S., & Fuhrman, B. (2002). Pomegranate juice flavonoids inhibit low-density lipoprotein oxidation & cardiovascular diseases: Studies in atherosclerotic mice & in humans. *Drugs Under Experimental and Clinical Research*, *28*(2-3), 49–62. PMID:12224378

Aviram, M., Dornfeld, L., Rosenblat, M., Volkova, N., Kaplan, M., Coleman, R., & Fuhrman, B. et al. (2000). Pomegranate juice consumption reduces oxidative stress, atherogenic modifications to LDL, and platelet aggregation: Studies in humans and in atherosclerotic apolipoprotein E–deficient mice. *The American Journal of Clinical Nutrition*, *71*(5), 1062–1076. PMID:10799367

Aviram, M., Rosenblat, M., Gaitini, D., Nitecki, S., Hoffman, A., Dornfeld, L., & Hayek, T. et al. (2004). Pomegranate juice consumption for 3 years by patients with carotid artery stenosis reduces common carotid intima-media thickness, blood pressure and LDL oxidation. *Clinical Nutrition (Edinburgh, Lothian)*, *23*(3), 423–433. doi:10.1016/j.clnu.2003.10.002 PMID:15158307

Awika, J. M., McDonough, C. M., & Rooney, L. W. (2005). Decorticating sorghum to concentrate healthy phytochemicals. *Journal of Agricultural and Food Chemistry*, *53*(16), 6230–6234. doi:10.1021/jf0510384 PMID:16076098

Awika, J. M., & Rooney, L. W. (2004). Sorghum phytochemicals and their potential impact on human health. *Phytochemistry*, *65*(9), 1199–1221. doi:10.1016/j.phytochem.2004.04.001 PMID:15184005

Ayet, G., Burbano, C., Cuadrado, C., Pedrosa, M. M., Robredo, L. M., Muzquiz, M., & Osagie, A. et al. (1997). Effect. of Germination, under Different Environmental Conditions, on Saponins, Phytic Acid and Tannins in Lentils (Lens culinaris). *Journal of the Science of Food and Agriculture*, *74*(2), 273–279. doi:10.1002/(SICI)1097-0010(199706)74:2<273::AID-JSFA800>3.0.CO;2-L

Ayieko, M. A., & Ariaro, V. (2008). Consumption, indigeneous knowledge and cultural values of the lakefly species within the Lake Victoria region. *African Journal of Environmental Science and Technology*, *10*, 282–286.

Ayyanar, M., Subash-Babu, P., & Ignacimuthu, S. (2013). *Syzygium cumini* L., a novel therapeutic agent for diabetes: Folk medicinal and pharmacological evidences. *Complementary Therapies in Medicine*, *21*(3), 232–243. doi:10.1016/j.ctim.2013.03.004 PMID:23642956

Babich, H., Zuckerbraun, H. L., & Weinerman, S. M. (2007). In vitro cytotoxicity of (-)-catechin gallate, a minor polyphenol in green tea. *Toxicology Letters*, *171*(3), 171–180. doi:10.1016/j.toxlet.2007.05.125 PMID:17606338

Babior, B. M. (2000). Phagocytes & oxidative stress. *The American Journal of Medicine*, *109*(1), 33–44. doi:10.1016/S0002-9343(00)00481-2 PMID:10936476

Babu, A. S., Veluswami, S. K., Arena, R., Guazzi, M., & Lavie, C. J. (2014). Virgin coconut oil and its potential cardioprotective effects. *Postgraduate Medicine*, *126*(7), 76–83. doi:10.3810/pgm.2014.11.2835 PMID:25387216

Bachoual, R., Talmoudi, W., Boussetta, T., Braut, F., & El-Benna, J. (2011). An aqueous pomegranate peel extract inhibits neutrophil myeloperoxiSarmae in vitro & attenuates lung inflammation in mice. *Journal of Food & Chemical Toxicology*, *49*(6), 1224–1228. doi:10.1016/j.fct.2011.02.024 PMID:21376769

Baek, Y. H., Kwak, J. R., Kim, S. J., Han, S. S., & Song, Y. O. (2001). Effects of kimchi supplementation and/or exercise training on body composition and plasma lipids in obese middle school girls. *J. korean Soc. Food Sci. Nutr*, *30*, 906–912.

Bahkali, A.H., Hussain, M.A., & Basahy, A.Y. (1998). Protein and oil composition of sesame seeds (*Sesamum indicum*, L.) grown in the Gizan area of Saudi Arabia. *International Journal of Food Sciences and Nutrition*, *49*, 409-414.

Bai, J., Hagenmaier, R. D., & Baldwin, E. A. (2003). Coating selection for "Delicious" and other apples. *Postharvest Biology and Technology*, *28*(3), 381–390. doi:10.1016/S0925-5214(02)00201-6

Bailey, J., & Day, C. (1989). Traditional Plant Medicines as Treatments for Diabetes. *Diabetes Care*, *12*(8), 553–564. doi:10.2337/diacare.12.8.553 PMID:2673695

Bai, W., Wang, C., & Ren, C. (2013). Intakes of total and individual flavonoids by U.S. adults. *International Journal of Food Sciences and Nutrition*, *65*(1), 9–20. doi:10.3109/09637486.2013.832170 PMID:24020353

Bajaj, M., Kaur, A., & Sidhu, J. S. (1991). Studies on the development of nutritious cookies utilizing sunflower kernels and wheat germ. *Plant Foods for Human Nutrition (Dordrecht, Netherlands)*, *41*(4), 381–387. doi:10.1007/BF02310631 PMID:1665564

Baker, J. A., McCann, S. E., Reid, M. E., Nowell, S., Beehler, G. P., & Moysich, K. B. (2005). Associations between black tea and coffee consumption and risk of lung cancer among current and former smokers. *Nutrition and Cancer*, *52*(1), 15–21. doi:10.1207/s15327914nc5201_2 PMID:16090999

Bala, M., Kumar, S., Kumar, A., & Singh, M. (2012). Composition of antioxidant activity and bioactive compounds in leaves of selected Brassica genotypes. *Indian Journal of Agricultural Biochemistry*, *25*(2), 142–146.

Balasubramaniam, V., Mustar, S., Khalid, N. M., Rashed, A. A., Noh, M. F. M., Wilcox, M. D., & Pearson, J. et al. (2013). Inhibitory activities of three Malaysian edible seaweeds on lipase and α-amylase. *Journal of Applied Phycology*, *25*(5), 1405–1412. doi:10.1007/s10811-012-9964-4

Baldwin, E. A., Burns, J. K., Kazokas, W., Brecht, J. K., Hagenmaier, R. D., Bender, R. J., & Pesis, D. E. (1999). Effect of two edible coatings with different permeability characteristics on mango (*Mangifera indica* L.) ripening during storage. *Postharvest Biology and Technology*, *17*(3), 215–226. doi:10.1016/S0925-5214(99)00053-8

Bamalli, Z., Mohammed, A. S., Ghazali, H. M., & Karim, R. (2014). Baobab tree (*Adansonia digitata L*) parts: Nutrition, applications in food and uses in ethno-medicine – A Review. *Annals of Nutritional Disorders and Therapy*, *1*, 1011.

Bamdad, F., Goli, A. H., & Kadivar, M. (2006). Preparation and characterization of proteinous film from lentil (Lens culinaris): Edible film from lentil (Lens culinaris). *Food Research International*, *39*(1), 106–111. doi:10.1016/j.foodres.2005.06.006

Banerjee, A., Dasgupta, N., & De, B. (2005). In vitro study of antioxidant activity of *Syzygium cumini* fruit. *Food Chemistry*, *90*(4), 727–733. doi:10.1016/j.foodchem.2004.04.033

Banerjee, S., Maity, P., Mukherjee, S., Sil, A. K., Panda, K., Chattopadhyay, D., & Chatterjee, I. B. (2007). Black tea prevents cigarette smoke-induced apoptosis and lung damage. *Journal of Inflammation*, *4*(3). PMID:17300721

Banerjee, S., Sanjay, K. R., Chethan, S., & Malleshi, N. G. (2012). Finger millet (*Eleusine coracana*) polyphenols: Investigation of their antioxidant capacity and antimicrobial activity. *African Journal of Food Science*, *6*(13), 362–374. doi:10.5897/AJFS12.031

Bankole, S. A., & Adebanjo, A. (2003). Mycotoxins in food in West Africa: Current situation and possibilities of controlling it. *African Journal of Biotechnology*, *2*(9), 254–263. doi:10.5897/AJB2003.000-1053

Bankole, S. A., & Mabekoje, O. O. (2004). Mycoflora and occurrence of aflatoxin B1 in dried yam chips from markets in Ogun and Oyo States, Nigeria. *Mycopathologia*, *157*(1), 111–115. doi:10.1023/B:MYCO.0000012211.31618.18 PMID:15008353

Bankole, S. A., Ogunsanwo, B. M., & Mabekoje, O. O. (2004). Natural occurrence of moulds and aflatoxin B1 in melon seeds from markets in Nigeria. *Food and Chemical Toxicology*, *42*(8), 1309–1314. doi:10.1016/j.fct.2004.03.015 PMID:15207382

Baragob, A. E. A. (2015). Composition and hypoglycemic effect of camel milk in streptozotocin–induced diabetic rats. *Biochemistry and Biotechnology Research*, *3*, 38–42.

Barbana, C., & Boye, J. I. (2011). Angiotensin I-converting enzyme inhibitory properties of lentil protein hydrolysates: Determination of the kinetics of inhibition. *Food Chemistry*, *127*(1), 94–101. doi:10.1016/j.foodchem.2010.12.093

Barber, S., Camacho, J., Cerni, R., Tortosa, E., & Primo, E. (1974). Process for the stabilization of rice bran I Basic research studies. In *Proceedings of Rice byproducts utilization.*

Barber, S. (1972). Milled rice and changes during aging. In D. F. Houston (Ed.), *Rice chemistry and technology* (pp. 215–263). St Paul, MN: Am. Assoc. Cereal Chem.

Barrett-Connor, E., & Orchard, T. J. (1985). Insulin-dependent diabetes mellitus and ischemic heart disease. *Diabetes Care*, *8*(Supplement_1), S65–S70. doi:10.2337/diacare.8.1.S65 PMID:4053956

Barros, L., Duenas, M., Pinela, J., Carvalho, A. M., Buelga, C. S., & Ferreira, I. C. (2012). Characterization and quantification of phenolic compounds in four tomato (*Lycopersicon esculentum* L.) farmers' varieties in northeastern Portugal homegardens. *Plant Foods for Human Nutrition (Dordrecht, Netherlands)*, *67*(3), 229–234. doi:10.1007/s11130-012-0307-z PMID:22922837

Barros, S. G. S., Ghisolfi, E. S., Luz, L. P., Barlem, G. G., Vidal, R. M., Wolff, F. H., & Prolla, J. C. et al. (2000). Mate (Chimarrão) É Consumido Em Alta Temperature Por População Sob Risco Para O Carcinoma Epidermóide De Esófago. *Arquivos de Gastroenterologia*, *37*(1), 25–30. doi:10.1590/S0004-28032000000100006 PMID:10962624

Bart, D. & Rex, G. H. (2002). Redox control of the transsulfuration and glutathione biosynthesis pathways. *Protein and Amino Acid Metabolism*, *5*, 85-92.

Bartolmew, D. T., & Blumer, J. N. (1977). Microbial interactions in country-style hams. *Journal of Food Science*, *42*(2), 498–502. doi:10.1111/j.1365-2621.1977.tb01531.x

Bassa, S., Mestre, C., Hell, K., Vervia, P., & Cardwell, K. (2001). First report of aflatoxin in dried yam chips in Benin. *Plant Disease*, *85*(9), 1032. doi:10.1094/PDIS.2001.85.9.1032A

Bastos, D. H. M., Moura de Oliveira, D., Texeira Matsumoto, R. L., Oliveira Carvalho, D., & Lima Ribeiro, M. (2007). *Yerba mate*: Pharmacological Properties, Research and Biotechnology. *Med. Arom. Plant Sci. Biotech.*, *1*(1), 37–46.

Bastos, D. M. H., Fornari, A. C., Queiroz, Y. S., Soares, R. A. M., & Torres, E. A. F. S. (2005). The Chlorogenic Acid and Caffeine Content of Yerba Mate (*Ilex Paraguariensis*) Beverages. *Acta Farm. Bonaer.*, *24*, 91–95.

Bastos, D. M. H., & Torres, E. A. F. S. (2003). Bebidas à Base de Erva-Mate (*Ilex Paraguariensis*) e Saúde Pública. *Nutrire: Rev. Soc. Bras. Aliment. Nutri.*, *26*, 77–89.

Bates, M. N., Hopenhayn, C., Rey, O. A., & Moore, L. E. (2007). Bladder Cancer and Mate Consumption in Argentina: A Case-Control Study. *Cancer Letters*, *246*(1-2), 268–273. doi:10.1016/j.canlet.2006.03.005 PMID:16616809

Battu, G., Male, C. K. V. L. S. N. A., Haripriya, T., Malleswari, V. N., & Reeshma, S. (2011). A phytopharmacological review on vigna species. *Pharmanest*, *2*, 62–67.

Bauman, D. E., Mather, I. H., Wall, R. J., & Lock, A. L. (2006). Major advances associated with the biosynthesis of milk. *Journal of Dairy Science*, *89*(4), 1235–1243. doi:10.3168/jds.S0022-0302(06)72192-0 PMID:16537956

Baurenfiend, J. C., & DeRitter, E. (1991). Foods considered for nutrient addition: cereal grain products. In *Nutrient Additions to Food*. Academic Press.

Bayan, L., Koulivand, P. H., & Gorji, A. (2013). Garlic: A review of potential therapeutic effects. *The American Journal of Physiology*, *4*, 1–14. PMID:25050296

Bazzano, L. A., He, J., Ogden, L. G., Loria, C. M., Vupputuri, S., Myers, L., & Whelton, P. K. (2002). Fruit and vegetable intake and risk of cardiovascular disease in us adults: The first national health and nutrition examination survey epidemiologic follow-up study. *The American Journal of Clinical Nutrition*, *76*, 93–99. PMID:12081821

Bazzano, L. A., Thompson, A. M., Tees, M. T., Nguyen, C. H., & Winham, D. M. (2011). Non-soy legume consumption lowers cholesterol levels: A meta-analysis of randomized controlled trials. *Nutrition, Metabolism, and Cardiovascular Diseases*, *21*(2), 94–103. doi:10.1016/j.numecd.2009.08.012 PMID:19939654

Bazzano, L., He, J., Ogden, L. G., Loria, C., Vuputuri, S., & Myers, L. et al.. (2001). Legume consumption and risk of coronary heart disease in US men and women. *Archives of Internal Medicine*, *161*(21), 2573–2578. doi:10.1001/archinte.161.21.2573 PMID:11718588

Bechtel, D. B., & Pomeranz, Y. (1978). Ultrastructure of the mature ungerminated rice (Oryza sativa) caryopsis. The starchy endosperm. *American Journal of Botany*, *65*, 684–691.

Bednar, G. E., Patil, A. R., Murray, S. M., Grieshop, C. M., Merchen, N. R., & Fahey, G. C. (2001). Starch and fiber fractions in selected food and feed ingredients affect their small intestinal digestibility and fermentability and their large bowel fermentability in vitro in a canine model. *The Journal of Nutrition*, *131*(2), 276–286. PMID:11160546

Benammar, C., Hichami, A., Yessoufou, A., Akadiri. Simonin, A.-M., Belarbi, M., Allali, H., & Khan, N. A. (2010). *Zizyphus lotus* L. (Deff.) modulates antioxidant activity and human T- cell proliferation. *BMC Complementary and Alternative Medicine*, *10*(1), 54. doi:10.1186/1472-6882-10-54 PMID:20868496

Bendini, A., Cerretani, L., Carrasco-Pancorbo, A., Gomez-Caravaca, A. M., Segura-Carretero, A., Fernandez-Gutierrez, A., & Lercker, G. (2007). Phenolic molecules in virgin olive oils: A survey of their sensory properties, health effects, antioxidant activity and analytical methods. An overview of the last decade. *Molecules (Basel, Switzerland)*, *12*(8), 1679–1719. doi:10.3390/12081679 PMID:17960082

Benincasa, P., Galieni, A., Manetta, A. C., Pace, R., Guiducci, M., Pisante, M., & Stagnari, F. (2015). Phenolic compounds in grains, sprouts and wheatgrass of hulled and non-hulled wheat species. *Journal of the Science of Food and Agriculture*, *95*(9), 1795–1803. doi:10.1002/jsfa.6877 PMID:25131800

Benkerroum, N., Mekkaoui, M., Bennani, N., & Kamal, H. (2004). Antimicrobial activity of camel's milk against pathogenic strains of Escherichia coli and Listeria monocytogene. *International Journal of Dairy Technology*, *57*(1), 39–43. doi:10.1111/j.1471-0307.2004.00127.x

Berno, N. D., Tezotto-Uliana, J. V., Dias, C. T., & dos, . (2014). Storage temperature and type of cut affect the biochemical and physiological characteristics of fresh-cut purple onions. *Postharvest Biology and Technology*, *93*, 91–96. doi:10.1016/j.postharvbio.2014.02.012

Bhadoriya, S. S., Ganeshpurkar, A., Narwaria, J., Rai, G., & Jain, A. P. (2011). *Tamarindus indica*: Extent of explored potential. *Pharmacognosy Review*, *5*(9), 73–81. doi:10.4103/0973-7847.79102 PMID:22096321

Bhagwat, S., Haytowitz, D. B., & Holden, J. M. (2011). USDA database for the flavonoid content of selected foods Release 3. U.S. Department of Agriculture. Retrieved from http://www.ars.usda.gov/nutrientdata

Bhathena, S. J., & Velasquez, M. T. (2002). Beneficial role of dietary phytoestrogens in obesity and diabetes. *The American Journal of Clinical Nutrition*, *76*, 1191–1201. PMID:12450882

Bhatia, A., & Mishra, T. (2010). Hypoglycemic activities of *Zizyphus mauritiana* aqueous ethanol seed extract in alloxan-induced diabetic mice. *Pharm. Biol.*, *48*(6), 604–610. doi:10.3109/13880200903218935 PMID:20645731

Bhattacharya, S., Narasimha, H. V., & Bhattacharya, S. (2005). The moisture dependent physical and mechanical properties of whole lentil pulse and split cotyledon. *International Journal of Food Science & Technology*, *40*(2), 213–221. doi:10.1111/j.1365-2621.2004.00933.x

Bhatty, R., & Christison, G. (1984). Composition and nutritional quality of pea (*Pisumsativum* L.), faba bean (*Vicia faba* L. spp. minor) and lentil (*Lens culinaris* Medik.) meals, protein concentrates and isolates. *Plant Foods for Human Nutrition (Dordrecht, Netherlands)*, *34*(1), 41–51. doi:10.1007/BF01095071

Bhise, S., & Kaur, A. (2015). Fortifying muffins with psyllium husk, oat fiber and barley fiber to improve quality and shelf life. *Carpathian Journal of Food Science and Technology.*, *7*(2), 5–16.

Bialonska, D., Kasimsetty, S. G., Khan, S. I., & Ferreira, D. (2009). Urolithins, intestinal microbial metabolites of pomegranate ellagitannins, exhibit potent antioxidant activity in a cell-based assay. *Journal of Agricultural and Food Chemistry*, *57*(21), 10181–10186. doi:10.1021/jf9025794 PMID:19824638

Biesalski, H. K. (2005). Meat as a component of a healthy diet—Are there any risks or benefits if meat is avoided in the diet? *Meat Science*, *70*(3), 509–524. doi:10.1016/j.meatsci.2004.07.017 PMID:22063749

Bilal, I., Chowdhury, A., Davidson, J., & Whitehead, S. (2014). Phytoestrogens and prevention of breast cancer: The contentious debate. *World Journal of Clinical Oncology*, *5*(4), 705–712. doi:10.5306/wjco.v5.i4.705 PMID:25302172

Bingham, S. A., Day, N. E., Luben, R., Ferrari, P., Slimani, N., Norat, T., & Riboli, E. et al. (2003). Dietary fiber in food & protection against colorectal cancer in the European Prospective Investigation into Cancer & Nutrition (EPIC): An observational study. *Lancet*, *361*, 1496–1501. doi:10.1016/S0140-6736(03)13174-1 PMID:12737858

Biswas, T. K., & Mukherjee, B. (2003). Plant medicines of Indian origin for wound healing activity: A review. *The International Journal of Lower Extremity Wounds*, *2*(1), 25–39. doi:10.1177/1534734603002001006 PMID:15866825

Bjelakovic, G., Nikolova, D., Gluud, L. L., Simonetti, R. G., & Gluud, C. (2007). Mortality in randomized trials of antioxidant supplements for primary and secondary prevention: Systematic review and meta-analysis. *Journal of the American Medical Association*, *297*(8), 842–857. doi:10.1001/jama.297.8.842 PMID:17327526

Block, G., Patterson, B., & Subar, A. (1992). Fruit, vegetables, and cancer prevention: A review of the epidemiological evidence. *Nutrition and Cancer*, *18*(1), 1–29. doi:10.1080/01635589209514201 PMID:1408943

Bloedon, L. T., & Szapary, P. O. (2004). Flaxseed and Cardiovascular Risk. *Nutrition Reviews*, *62*(1), 18–27. doi:10.1111/j.1753-4887.2004.tb00002.x PMID:14995053

Boehm, G., & Stahl, B. (2003). Oligosaccharides. In Functional Dairy Products (pp. 203-243). Cambridge, UK: Woodhead Publishers.

Boehm, G., & Stahl, B. (2007). Oligosaccharides from Milk. *The Journal of Nutrition*, *137*, 847S–849S. PMID:17311985

Boker, L. K., Van der Schouw, Y. T., De Kleijn, M. J., Jacques, P. F., Grobbee, D. E., & Peeters, P. H. (2002). Intake of dietary phytoestrogens by Dutch women. *The Journal of Nutrition*, *132*, 1319–1328. PMID:12042453

Bolaños, R., Del Castillo, A., & Francia, J. (2010). Soy isoflavones versus placebo in the treatment of climacteric vasomotor symptoms: Systematic review and meta-analysis. *Menopause (New York, N.Y.)*, *17*, 660–666. PMID:20464785

Bolca, S., Possemiers, S., Herregat, A., Huybrechts, I., Heyerick, A., De Vriese, S., & Van de Wiele, T. et al. (2007). Microbial and dietary factors are associated with the equol producer phenotype in healthy postmenopausal women. *The Journal of Nutrition*, *137*, 2242–2246. PMID:17885005

Boles, J. A., Shand, P. J., Patience, J. F., McCurdy, A. R., & Schaefer, A. L. (1993). Acid base status of stress susceptible pigs affects sensory quality of loin roasts. *Journal of Food Science*, *58*(6), 1254–1257. doi:10.1111/j.1365-2621.1993.tb06159.x

Bona, K. S. D., Belle, L. P., Bittencourt, P. E. R., Bonfanti, G., Cargnelluti, L. O., Pimentel, V. C., & Moretto, M. B. et al. (2011). Erythrocytic enzymes and antioxidant status in people with type-2 diabetes: Beneficial effect of *Syzygium cumini* leaf extract in vitro. *Diabetes Research and Clinical Practice*, *94*(1), 84–90. doi:10.1016/j.diabres.2011.06.008 PMID:21737173

Bonithon-Kopp, C., Coudray, C., Berr, C., Touboul, P. J., Feve, J. M., Favier, A., & Ducimetiere, P. (1997). Combined effects of lipid peroxidation and antioxidant status on carotid atherosclerosis in a population aged 59–71 year. The EVA study. Etude sur le Vieillisement Arteriel. *The American Journal of Clinical Nutrition*, *65*, 121–127. PMID:8988923

Bookheimer, S. Y., Renner, B. A., Ekstrom, A., Li, Z., Henning, S. M., Brown, J. A., & Small, G. W. et al. (2013). Pomegranate juice augments memory & FMRI activity in middle-aged & older adults with mild memory complaints. *Evidence-Based Complementary & Alternative Medicine. Article ID*, *946298*. doi:10.1155/2013/946298

Bordoni, A., Hrelia, S., Angeloni, C., Giordano, E., Guarnieri, C., Caldarera, C. M., & Biagi, P. L. (2002). Green tea protection of hypoxia/reoxygenation injury in cultured cardiac cells. *The Journal of Nutritional Biochemistry*, *13*(2), 103–111. doi:10.1016/S0955-2863(01)00203-0 PMID:11834226

Borghi, C., & Cicero, A. (2006). Recent evidence of the role of omega-3 polyunsaturated fatty acids on blood pressure control and hypertension-related complications. *Future Lipidology*, *1*(5), 569–577. doi:10.2217/17460875.1.5.569

Borneo, R., & Leon, A.E. (2012). Whole grain cereals: functional components and health benefits. *Food and Function*, *3*, 110-119.

Borras-Linares, I., Stojanovic, Z., Quirantes-Pine, R., Arraez-Roman, D., Svarc-Gajic, J., Fernandez-Gutierrez, A., & Segura-Carretero, A. (2014). *Rosmarinus officinalis* leaves as a natural source of bioactive compounds. *International Journal of Molecular Sciences*, *15*(11), 20585–20606. doi:10.3390/ijms151120585 PMID:25391044

Borrelli, F., & Ernst, E. (2010). Alternative and complementary therapies for the menopause. *Maturitas*, *66*(4), 333–343. doi:10.1016/j.maturitas.2010.05.010 PMID:20580501

Bouayed, J., & Bohn, T. (2010). Exogenous antioxidants— double-edged swords in cellular redox state. *Oxidative Medicine and Cellular Longevity*, *3*(4), 228–237. doi:10.4161/oxim.3.4.12858 PMID:20972369

Bouchenak, M., & Lamri-Senhadji, M. (2013). Nutritional quality of legumes and their role in cardiometabolic risk prevention: A review. *Journal of Medicinal Food*, *16*(3), 185–198. doi:10.1089/jmf.2011.0238 PMID:23398387

Boullata, J. I., & Nace, A. M. (2000). Safety issues with herbal medicine. *Pharmacotherapy*, *20*(3), 257–356. doi:10.1592/phco.20.4.257.34886 PMID:10730682

Bouzid, K., Benali, F. T., Chadli, R., Bouzouina, M., Bouzid, A., Benchohra, A., & Bouzid, S. et al. (2015). Extraction, identification and quantitative HPLC analysis of flavonoids from fruit extracts of *Arbutus unedo* L. from Tiaret area (Western Algeria). *Basic Research Journal of Agricultural Science and Review*, *4*(1), 24–30.

Boye, J. I., Roufik, S., Pesta, N., & Barbana, C. (2010). Angiotensin I-converting enzyme inhibitory properties and SDS-PAGE of red lentil protein hydrolysates. *LWT-Food Science and Technology*, *43*(6), 987–991. doi:10.1016/j.lwt.2010.01.014

Boyer, J., & Liu, R. H. (2004). Apple phytochemicals and their health benefits. *Nutrition Journal*, *3*(1), 5. doi:10.1186/1475-2891-3-5 PMID:15140261

Brahmbhatt, M., Gundala, S. R., Asif, G., Shamsi, S. A., & Aneja, R. (2013). Ginger phytochemicals exhibit synergy to inhibit prostate cancer cell proliferation. *Nutrition and Cancer*, *65*(2), 263–272. doi:10.1080/01635581.2013.749925 PMID:23441614

Brandelli, A., Dariot, D. J., & Correa, A. P. F. (2015). Whey as a source of peptides with remarkable biological activities. *Food Research International*, *73*, 149–161. doi:10.1016/j.foodres.2015.01.016

Bravo, I., Goya, L., & Lecumberri, E. (2007). LC/MS Characterization of Phenolic Constituents of Mate (*Ilex paraguariensis* St Hil.) and Its Antioxidant Activity Compared to Commonly Consumed Beverages. *Food Research International*, *11*, 401–407.

Breitling, L. (2002). Insulin and anti diabetic activity of camel milk. *Journal of Camel Practice and Research*, *9*, 43–45.

Brewer, L. R., Kubola, J., Siriamornpun, S., Herald, T. J., & Shi, Y.-C. (2014). Wheat bran particle size influence on phytochemical extractability and antioxidant properties. *Food Chemistry*, *152*, 483–490. doi:10.1016/j.foodchem.2013.11.128 PMID:24444965

Brewer, M. S., Ikins, W. G., & Harbers, C. A. Z. (1992). TBA values, sensory characteristics, and volatiles in ground pork during long term frozen storage: Effects of packaging. *Journal of Food Science*, *57*(3), 558–580. doi:10.1111/j.1365-2621.1992.tb08042.x

Brigelius-flohe, R., & Traber, M. G. (1999). Vitamin E: Function and metabolism. *The FASEB Journal*, *13*, 1145–1155. PMID:10385606

Brodie, A., Sabnis, G., & Jelovac, D. (2006). Aromatase & breast cancer. *The Journal of Steroid Biochemistry and Molecular Biology*, *102*(1), 97–102. doi:10.1016/j.jsbmb.2006.09.002 PMID:17113978

Brook, R. D., & Julius, S. (2000). Autonomic imbalance, hypertension, and cardiovascular risk. *American Journal of Hypertension*, *13*(6), 112S–122S. doi:10.1016/S0895-7061(00)00228-4 PMID:10921530

Brouns, E. (2002). Soya isoflavones: A new and promising ingredient for the health foods sector. *Food Research International*, *35*(2-3), 187–193. doi:10.1016/S0963-9969(01)00182-X

Brown, N. M., Galandi, S. L., Summer, S. S., Zhao, X., Heubi, J. E., King, E. C., & Setchell, K. D. (2014). S-(-)equol production is developmentally regulated and related to early diet composition. *Nutrition Research (New York, N.Y.)*, *34*(5), 401–409. doi:10.1016/j.nutres.2014.03.005 PMID:24916553

Bruce, W. R., Giacca, A., & Medline, A. (2000). Possible mechanisms relating diet and risk of colon cancer. *Cancer Epidemiology, Biomarkers & Prevention*, *9*(12), 1271–1279. PMID:11142411

Brückner, H., & Fujii, N. (2010). *D-Amino Acids in Chemistry, Life Sciences and Biotechnology*. Weinheim, Germany: Verlag Helvetica ChimicaActa, Zürich, Switzerland and Wiley-VCH.

Brueckner, H., & Hausch, M. (1990). D-amino acids in dairy products: Detection, origin and nutritional aspects. I. Milk, fermented milk, fresh cheese and acid crude cheese. *Milchwissenschaft. Milk Science International*, *45*, 357–360.

Bubols, G. B., Viann, D. R., Medina-Remónd, A., Poser, G., Lamuela-Raventos, R. M., Eifler-Lim, V. L., & Garcia, S. C. (2013). The antioxidant activity of coumarins and flavonoids. *Mini Reviews in Medicinal Chemistry*, *13*, 1–17. PMID:22876957

Buffa, C. W. (1976). Rice bran wax, a new wax for cosmetics, drugs & toiletries. *Cosmet Toiletries*, *91*, 14–16.

Bulotta, S., Celano, M., Lepore, S. M., Montalcini, T., Pujia, A., & Russo, D. (2014). Beneficial effects of the olive oil phenolic components oleuropein and hydroxytyrosol: Focus on protection against cardiovascular and metabolic diseases. *Journal of Translational Medicine*, *12*(1), 219. doi:10.1186/s12967-014-0219-9 PMID:25086598

Burri, B. J. (1997). Beta-carotene and human health: A review of current research. *Nunition Research*, *1*(17), 547–580. doi:10.1016/S0271-5317(97)00011-0

Burris, K. P., Harte, F. M., Michael Davidson, P., Neal Stewart, C. Jr, & Zivanovic, S. (2012). Composition and Bioactive Properties of Yerba Mate (*Ilex paraguariensis* A. St.-Hil.): A review. *Chilean J. Agric. Res.*, *72*(2), 268–274. doi:10.4067/S0718-58392012000200016

Burt, S. (2004). Essential oils: Their antibacterial properties and potential applications in foods—A review. *International Journal of Food Microbiology*, *94*(3), 223–253. doi:10.1016/j.ijfoodmicro.2004.03.022 PMID:15246235

Busambwa, K., Miller-Cebert, R., Aboagye, L., Dalrymple, L., Boateng, J., Shackelford, L., & Verghese, M. et al. (2014). Inhibitory effect of lentils, green split and yellow peas (sprouted and non-sprouted) on azoxymethane-induced aberrant crypt foci in Fisher 344 male rats. *International Journal of Cancer Research*, *10*(1), 27–36. doi:10.3923/ijcr.2014.27.36

Businco, L., Bruno, G., Giampietro, P. G., & Cantoni, A. (1992). Allergenicity and nutritional adequacy of soy protein formulas. *The Journal of Pediatrics*, *121*(5), S21–S28. doi:10.1016/S0022-3476(05)81402-7 PMID:1447630

Butt, M. S., & Sultan, M. T. (2011). Ginger and its health claims: Molecular aspects. *Critical Reviews in Food Science and Nutrition*, *51*(5), 383–393. doi:10.1080/10408391003624848 PMID:21491265

Cabrera, C., Artacho, R., & Gimeanez, R. (2006). Beneficial effects of green tea - A review. *Journal of the American College of Nutrition*, *25*(2), 79–99. doi:10.1080/07315724.2006.10719518 PMID:16582024

Cabrera, C., Gimeanez, R., & Loapez, M. C. (2003). Determination of tea components with antioxidant activity. *Journal of Agricultural and Food Chemistry*, *51*(15), 4427–4435. doi:10.1021/jf0300801 PMID:12848521

Cagri, A., Ustunol, Z., & Ryser, E. T. (2004). Antimicrobial edible films and coatings. *Journal of Food Protection*, *67*(4), 833–848. PMID:15083740

Cai, H., & Harrison, D. G. (2000). Endothelial dysfunction in cardiovascular diseases: The role of oxidant stress. *Circulation Research*, *87*(10), 840–844. doi:10.1161/01.RES.87.10.840 PMID:11073878

Cais-Sokolinska, D., Pikul, J., Wojtowski, J., Dankow, R., Teichert, J., Czyzak-Runowska, G., & Bagnicka, E. (2015). Evaluation of quality of kefir from milk obtained from goats supplemented with a diet rich in bioactive compounds. *Journal of the Science of Food and Agriculture*, *95*(6), 1343–1349. doi:10.1002/jsfa.6828 PMID:25042847

Calabrese, V., Cornelius, C., Dinkova-Kostova, A. T., Iavicoli, I., Di Paola, R., Koverech, A., & Calabrese, E. J. (1822). (2012) Cellular stress responses, hormetic phytochemicals and vitagenes in aging and longevity. *Biochimica et Biophysica Acta*, 753–783.

Caldwell, C. R., Britz, S. J., & Mirecki, R. M. (2005). Effect of temperature, elevated carbon dioxide, and drought during seed development on the isoflavone content of dwarf soybean [*Glycine max* (L.) Merrill] grown in controlled environments. *Journal of Agricultural and Food Chemistry*, *53*(4), 1125–1129. doi:10.1021/jf0355351 PMID:15713029

Calnek, B. W., Luginbuhl, R. E., & Helmboldt, C. F. (1977). Disease of Poultry. Iowa State University.

Calvino, A. (2005). Note: Caffeine Content and Dynamical Bitterness of Yerba Mate *Ilex paraguariensis* Infusions. *Food Science & Technology International*, *11*(6), 401–407. doi:10.1177/1082013205060624

Camara, C. R. S., Urrea, C. A., & Schlegel, V. (2013). Pinto beans (*Phaseolus vulgaris* L.) as a functional food: Implications on human health. *Agriculture*, *3*(1), 90–111. doi:10.3390/agriculture3010090

Camargo, A. C., Vieira, T. M. F. S., Arce, M. A. B. R., & Calori-Domingues, M. A. (2012). Gamma radiation effects on peanut skin antioxidants. *International Journal of Molecular Sciences*, *13*(12), 3073–3084. doi:10.3390/ijms13033073 PMID:22489142

Campos-Vega, R., Loarca-Piña, G., & Oomah, B. D. (2010). Minor components of pulses and their potential impact on human health. *Food Research International*, *43*(2), 461–482. doi:10.1016/j.foodres.2009.09.004

Canani, R. B., Costanzo, M., Leone, L., Pedata, M., Meli, R., & Calignano, A. (2011). Potential beneficial effects of butyrate in intestinal and extra intestinal diseases. *World Journal of Gastroenterology*, *17*(12), 1519–1528. doi:10.3748/wjg.v17.i12.1519 PMID:21472114

Cao, Y., Calafat, A. M., Doerge, D. R., Umbach, D. M., Bernbaum, J. C., Twaddle, N. C., & Rogan, W. J. et al. (2009). Isoflavones in urine, saliva, and blood of infants: Data from a pilot study on the estrogenic activity of soy formula. *Journal of Exposure Science & Environmental Epidemiology*, *19*(2), 223–234. doi:10.1038/jes.2008.44 PMID:18665197

Caplice, E., & Fitzgerald, G. F. (1999). Food fermentations: Role of microorganisms in food production and preservation. *International Journal of Food Microbiology*, *50*(1-2), 131–149. doi:10.1016/S0168-1605(99)00082-3 PMID:10488849

Cardak, A. D., Yetismeyen, A., & Bruckner, H. (2003). Quantitative comparison of free fatty acids in camel, goat and cow milk. *Milchwissenschaft. Milk Science International*, *58*, 127–130.

Carini, M., Facino, R. M., Aldini, G., Calloni, M., & Colombo, L. (1998). Characterization of Phenolic Antioxidants from Mate (*Ilex paraguariensis*) by Liquid Chromatography Mass Spectrometry and Liquid Chromatography Tandem Mass Spectrometry. *Rapid Communications in Mass Spectrometry*, *12*(22), 1813–1819. doi:10.1002/(SICI)1097-0231(19981130)12:22<1813::AID-RCM379>3.0.CO;2-#

Carlsen, M. H., Halvorsen, B. L., Holte, K., Bøhn, S. K., Dragland, S., Sampson, L., & Blomhoff, R. et al. (2010). The total antioxidant content of more than 3100 foods, beverages, spices, herbs and supplements used worldwide. *Nutrition Journal*, *9*(1), 3. doi:10.1186/1475-2891-9-3 PMID:20096093

Carlson, D. G., Daxenbichler, M. E., & VanEtten, C. H. (1985). Glucosinolates in radish cultivars. *Journal of the American Society for Horticultural Science*, *110*, 634–638.

Carr, A., & Frei, B. (1999). Does vitamin C act as a pro-oxidant under physiological conditions? *The FASEB Journal*, *13*, 1007–1024. PMID:10336883

Carretero, O. A., & Oparil, S. (2000). Essential Hypertension, Part -1: Definition and Etiology. *Circulation*, *101*(3), 329–335. doi:10.1161/01.CIR.101.3.329 PMID:10645931

Cartea, M. E., Francisco, M., Soengas, P., & Velasco, P. (2011). Phenolic compounds in *Brassica* vegetables. *Molecules (Basel, Switzerland)*, *16*(1), 251–280. doi:10.3390/molecules16010251 PMID:21193847

Cartea, M. E., & Velasco, P. (2008). Glucosinolates in Brassica foods: Bioavailability in food and significance for human health. *Phytochemistry Reviews*, *7*(2), 213–229. doi:10.1007/s11101-007-9072-2

Cassidy, A., Albertazzi, P., Lise Nielsen, I., Hall, W., Williamson, G., Tetens, I., & Branca, F. et al. (2006). Critical review of health effects of soyabean phyto-oestrogens in post-menopausal women. *The Proceedings of the Nutrition Society*, *65*(01), 76–92. doi:10.1079/PNS2005476 PMID:16441947

Cassidy, A., Hansley, B., & Lamuela-Raventos, R. M. (2000). Isoflavones, lignans and stilbenes—origins, metabolism and potential importance to human health. *Journal of the Science of Food and Agriculture*, *80*(7), 1044–1062. doi:10.1002/(SICI)1097-0010(20000515)80:7<1044::AID-JSFA586>3.0.CO;2-N

Cassidy, A., Mukamal, K. J., Liu, L., Franz, M., Eliassen, A. H., & Rimm, E. B. (2013). High anthocyanin intake is associated with a reduced risk of myocardial infarction in young and middle-aged women. *Circulation*, *127*(2), 188–196. doi:10.1161/CIRCULATIONAHA.112.122408 PMID:23319811

Castaner, O., Covas, M. I., Khymenets, O., Nyyssonen, K., Konstantinidou, V., Zunft, H. F., & Fito, M. et al. (2012). Protection of LDL from oxidation by olive oil polyphenols is associated with a downregulation of CD40-ligand expression and its downstream products in vivo in humans. *The American Journal of Clinical Nutrition*, *95*(5), 1238–1244. doi:10.3945/ajcn.111.029207 PMID:22440854

Castelnuovo, A. D. (2012). Consumption of cocoa, tea and coffee and risk of cardiovascular disease. *European Journal of Internal Medicine*, *23*(1), 15–25. doi:10.1016/j.ejim.2011.07.014 PMID:22153525

Caulifield, L. E., & Black, R. E. (2004). Zinc Deficiency. In Comparative quantification of health risks: Global and regional burden of disease attributable to selected major risk factors (vol. 1, pp. 257-279). Geneva, Switzerland: World Health Organisation.

Chagas, V.T., Franca, L.M., Malik, S., & Paes, A.M.D. (2015). Syzygium cumini (L.) skeels: a prominent source of bioactive molecule against cardiometabolic disease. *Frontiers in Pharmacology, 6*(259), 1-8.

Challier, B., Perarnau, J. M., & Viel, J. F. (1998). Garlic, onion and cereal fiber as protective factors for breast cancer: French case-control study. *European Journal of Epidemiology, 14*(8), 737–747. doi:10.1023/A:1007512825851 PMID:9928867

Champagne, C. P., Tompkins, T. A., Buckley, N. D., & Green-Johnson, J. M. (2010). Effect of fermentation by pure and mixed cultures of *Streptococcus thermophilus* and *Lactobacillus helveticus* on isoflavone and B-vitamin content of a fermented soy beverage. *Food Microbiology, 27*(7), 968–972. doi:10.1016/j.fm.2010.06.003 PMID:20688240

Champ, M. M.-J. (2002). Non-nutrient bioactive substances of pulses. *The British Journal of Nutrition, 88*(S3), 307–319. doi:10.1079/BJN2002721 PMID:12498631

Chan, E. W. C., Soh, E. Y., Tie, P. P., & Law, Y. P. (2011). Antioxidant and antibacterial properties of green, black and herbal teas of Camellia sinensis. *Pharmacognosy Research, 3*(4), 266-72.

Chandrashekar, P., Kumar, P. K. P., Ramesh, H. P., Lokesh, B. R., & Krishna, A. G. G. (2014). Hypolipidemic effect of oryzanol concentrate and low temperature extracted crude rice bran oil in experimental male wistar rats. *Journal of Food Science and Technology, 51*(7), 1278–1285. doi:10.1007/s13197-012-0628-9 PMID:24966420

Chanes, & Arias, P. (Eds.). (2008). *Food Engineering: Integrated Approaches*. New York: Springer.

Chang, U. J., Kim, D. G., Kim, J. M., Suh, H. J., & Oh, S. H. (2003). Weight reduction effect of extract of fermented red pepper on female college students. *J. Korean Soc. Food Sci. Nutr, 32*(3), 479–484. doi:10.3746/jkfn.2003.32.3.479

Chan, J. Y., Yuen, A. C., Chan, R. Y., & Chan, S. W. (2013). A review of the cardiovascular benefits and antioxidant properties of allicin. *Phytotherapy Research, 27*(5), 637–646. doi:10.1002/ptr.4796 PMID:22888009

Chan, Q., Stamler, J., Brown, J., Daviglus, M. L., Van Horn, L., Dyer, A. R., & Elliot, P. et al. (2014). Relation of raw and cooked vegetable consumption to blood pressure: The INTERMAP Study. *Journal of Human Hypertension, 28*(6), 353–359. doi:10.1038/jhh.2013.115 PMID:24257514

Chan, Y., Demonty, I., Pelled, D., & Jones, P. J. (2007). Olive oil containing olive oil fatty acid esters of plant sterols and dietary diacylglycerol reduces low-density lipoprotein cholesterol and decreases the tendency for peroxidation in hypercholesterolaemic subjects. *The British Journal of Nutrition, 98*(03), 563–570. doi:10.1017/S0007114507730775 PMID:17559697

Charalampopoulos, D.; Wang, R.; Pandiella, S.S. & Webb, C. (2002). Application of cereals and cereal components in functional foods: a review. *International Journal of Food Microbiology, 79*(1-2), 131-141.

Charles, C., Yuskavage, J., Carlson, O., John, M., Tagalicud, A. S., Maggio, M., & Basaria, S. et al. (2009). Effects of high-dose isoflavones on metabolic and inflammatory markers in healthy postmenopausal women. *Menopause (New York, N.Y.), 16*(2), 395–400. doi:10.1097/gme.0b013e3181857979 PMID:18981951

Cha, S. D., Yu, J. W., Kim, T. W., Cho, H. S., & Lee, D. H. (2012). Effects of Lactobacillus plantarum CIB 001 on lipid metabolism of hypercholesterolemic rats. *Korean J. Food Sci. Technol, 44*(3), 324–330. doi:10.9721/KJFST.2012.44.3.324

Chaudhary, B., & Mukhopadhyay, K. (2013). Solvent optimization for anthocyanin extraction from *Syzygium cumini* L. Skeels using response surface methodology. *International Journal of Food Sciences and Nutrition, 64*(3), 363–371. doi:10.3109/09637486.2012.738647 PMID:23121325

Cheigh, H. S., Park, K. Y., & Lee, C. Y. (1994). Biochemical, microbiological, and nutritional aspects of kimchi (Korean fermented vegetable products). *Critical Reviews in Food Science and Nutrition, 34*(2), 175–203. doi:10.1080/10408399409527656 PMID:8011144

Cheigh, H. S., Song, E. S., & Jeon, Y. S. (1999). Changes of chemical and antioxidative characteristics of cholorophylls in the model system of mustard leaf kimchi during ferementation. *J. Korean Soc. Food Sci Nutr*, *28*(3), 520–525.

Chelule, P. K., Mbongwa, H. P., Carries, S., & Gqaleni, N. (2010b). Lactic acid fermentation improves the quality of amahewu, a traditional South African maize-based porridge. *Food Chemistry*, *122*(3), 656–661. doi:10.1016/j.foodchem.2010.03.026

Chelule, P. K., Mokoena, M. P., & Gqaleni, N. (2010a). Advantages of traditional lactic acid bacteria fermentation of food in Africa. In A. Méndez-Vilas (Ed.), *Current Research, Technology and Education Topics in Applied Microbiology and Microbial Biotechnology* (pp. 1160–1167). Badajoz: Formatex Research Center.

Chemfaces. (2015). *Theaflavin-3'-gallate:Number, C. A. S.28543-07-9*. Retrieved November 9, 2015 from http://www.chemfaces.com/natural/Theaflavin-3-gallate-CFN98599.html

Chen, C. L., Chiou, H. Y., Hsu, L. I., Hsueh, Y. M., Wu, M. M., Wang, Y. H., & Chen, C. J. (2010). Arsenic in drinking water and risk of urinary tract cancer: A follow-up study from northeastern Taiwan. *Cancer Epidemiology, Biomarkers & Prevention*, *19*(1), 101–110. doi:10.1158/1055-9965.EPI-09-0333 PMID:20056628

Chen, C. Y. N., Kamil, A., & Blumberg, J. B. (2015). Phytochemical composition and antioxidant capacity of whole wheat products. *International Journal of Food Sciences and Nutrition*, *66*(1), 63–70. doi:10.3109/09637486.2014.971228 PMID:25578763

Chen, C., & Kong, A.-N. T. (2005). Dietary cancer-chemopreventive compounds: From signaling and gene expression to pharmacological effects. *Trends in Pharmacological Sciences*, *26*(6), 318–326. doi:10.1016/j.tips.2005.04.004 PMID:15925707

Chen, H., Siebenmorgen, T., & Griffin, K. (1998). Quality characteristics of long-grain rice milled in two commercial systems. *Cereal Chemistry.*, *75*(4), 560–565. doi:10.1094/CCHEM.1998.75.4.560

Chen, P., Kuo, W., Chiang, C., Chiou, H., Hsieh, Y., & Chu, S. (2006). Black rice anthocyanins inhibit cancer cells invasion via repressions of MMPs and uPA expression. *Chemico-Biological Interactions*, *163*(3), 218–229. doi:10.1016/j.cbi.2006.08.003 PMID:16970933

Chen, W. C., Hsieh, S. R., Chiu, C. H., Hsu, B. D., & Liou, Y. M. (2014). Molecular identification for epigallocatechin-3-gallate-mediated antioxidant intervention on the H2O2-induced oxidative stress in H9c2 rat cardiomyoblasts. *Journal of Biomedical Science*, *21*, 56. PMID:24913014

Chen, Y., Graziano, J. H., Parvez, F., Liu, M., Slavkovich, V., Kalra, T., & Ahsan, H. et al. (2011). Arsenic exposure from drinking water and mortality from cardiovascular disease in Bangladesh: Prospective cohort study. *BMJ (Clinical Research Ed.)*, *342*(may05 2), d2431. doi:10.1136/bmj.d2431 PMID:21546419

Cheung, A. H., & Ng, T. B. (2007). Isolation and characterization of a trypsin-chymotrypsin inhibitor from the seeds of green lentil (*Lens culinaris*). *Protein and Peptide Letters*, *14*(9), 859–864. doi:10.2174/092986607782110310 PMID:18045226

Chevion, M. (1988). A site-specific mechanism for free radical induced biological damage: The essential role of redox-active transition metals. *Free Radical Biology & Medicine*, *5*(1), 27–37. doi:10.1016/0891-5849(88)90059-7 PMID:3075945

Chhabra, P., & Sidhu, J. S. (1988). Fate of phytic acid during bread making. *Die Nahrung*, *32*(1), 15–19. doi:10.1002/food.19880320104

Chiang, A., Wu, H., Yeh, H., Chu, C., Lin, H., & Lee, W. (2006). Antioxidant effects of black rice extract through the induction of superoxide dismutase and catalase activities. *Lipids*, *41*(8), 797–803. doi:10.1007/s11745-006-5033-6 PMID:17120934

Chidambara Murthy, K. N., Reddy, V. K., Veigas, J. M., & Murthy, U. D. (2004). Study on wound healing activity of Punica granatum peel. *Journal of Medicinal Food*, *7*(2), 256–259. doi:10.1089/1096620041224111 PMID:15298776

Chilaka, C. A., De Kock, S., Phoku, J. Z., Mwanza, M., Egbuta, M. A., & Dutton, M. F. (2012). Fungal and mycotoxin contamination of South African comercial maize. *Journal of Food Agriculture and Environment*, *10*, 296–303.

Chiou, A., Karathanos, V. T., Mylona, A., Salta, F. N., Preventi, F., & Andrikopoulos, N. K. (2007). Currants (*Vitis vinifera* L.) content of simple phenolics and antioxidant activity. *Food Chemistry*, *102*(2), 516–522. doi:10.1016/j.foodchem.2006.06.009

Chipley, J. (2005). Sodium benzoate and benzoic acid. In P. M. Davidson, J. N. Sofos, & A. L. Branen (Eds.), *Antimicrobials in Food* (pp. 11–48). Boca Raton, FL: CRC Press.

Chobanian, A. V., Bakris, G. L., Black, H. R., Cushman, W. C., Green, L. A., Izzo, J. L., & Roccella, E. et al. (2003). Joint National Committee on Prevention, Detection, Evaluation and Treatment of high blood pressure.National Heart, lung and blood Institute; National High Blood pressure Education Programme Coordination Committee. *Hypertension*, *42*(6), 1206–1252. doi:10.1161/01.HYP.0000107251.49515.c2 PMID:14656957

Cho, H. S., Kim, S., Lee, S. Y., Park, J. A., Kim, S. J., & Chun, H. S. (2008). Protective effect of the green tea component, L-theanine on environmental toxins-induced neuronal cell death. *Neurotoxicology*, *29*(4), 656–662. doi:10.1016/j.neuro.2008.03.004 PMID:18452993

Cho, H. S., Park, W. J., Hong, G. E., Kim, J. H., Ju, M. G., & Lee, C. H. (2015). Antioxidant activity of Allium hookeri root extract and its effect on lipid stability of sulfur-fed pork patties. *Korean J. Food Sci. An.*, *35*(1), 32–40. PMID:26761799

Choi, K. H. (2014). *Antiviral effects of Lactobacillus plantarum YML009 isolated from Kimchi on influenza virus H1N1*. (MS Thesis). Youngnam University, Daegu, Korea.

Choi, S. M. (2001). *Antiobesity and anticancer effects of red pepper powder and kimchi*. (Ph.D Thesis). Pusan National University, Busan, Korea.

Choi, E. J., & Kim, G. H. (2014). The antioxidant activity of daidzein metabolites, *O*-desmethylangolensin and equol, in HepG2 cells. *Molecular Medicine Reports*, *9*, 328–332. PMID:24154619

Choi, H. J., Kim, J., & Jhon, M. S. (1999). Viscoelastic characterization of biodegradable poly (3-hydroxy butyrate-co-3-hydroxy valerate). *Polymer*, *40*, 4135–4138. doi:10.1016/S0032-3861(98)00627-2

Choi, I. H., Noh, J. S., Han, J. S., Kim, H. J., Han, E. S., & Song, Y. O. (2013). Kimchi, a fermented vegetable, improves serum lipid profiles in healthy young adults: Randomized clinical trial. *Journal of Medicinal Food*, *16*(3), 223–229. doi:10.1089/jmf.2012.2563 PMID:23444963

Choi, J. H., & Han, I. K. (1974). Effects of substitution of sodium on sodium sulphate for methionine on performance and nutrient metabolism of broiler chickens. *Korean Journal of Animal Sciences*, *16*, 20–36.

Choi, M. W., Kim, K. H., & Park, K. Y. (1997). Effects of kimchi extracts on the growth of sarcoma-180 cells and phagocytic activity of mice. *J. Korean Soc. Food Sci Nutr*, *26*, 254–260.

Choi, S. H., Kim, H. J., Kwon, M. J., Baek, Y. H., & Song, Y. O. (2001). The effect of kimchi pill supplementation on plasma lipid concentration in healthy people. *J. Korean Soc. Food Sci. Nutr.*, *30*, 913–920.

Choi, Y., Jeong, H. S., & Lee, J. (2007). Antioxidant activity of methanolic extracts from some grains consumed in Korea. *Food Chemistry*, *103*(1), 130–138. doi:10.1016/j.foodchem.2006.08.004

Cho, J. H., Min, B. J., Kwon, O. S., Shon, K. S., Jin, Y. G., Kim, H. J., & Kim, I. H. (2005). Effect of MSM (Methyl Sulfonyl Methane) supplementation on growth performance and digestibility of CA and N in pigs. *Journal of Korean Soc. Food Sci. Nutr.*, *34*(3), 361–365. doi:10.3746/jkfn.2005.34.3.361

Choudhury, N. H., & Juliano, B. O. (1980). Effect of' amylose content on the lipids of mature rice grain. *Phytochemistry*, *19*(7), 1385–1389. doi:10.1016/0031-9422(80)80179-8

Cho, W. M., Yang, S. H., Lee, S. M., Jang, S. S., Kim, H. C., Hong, S. K., & Kim, H. S. (2012). Effects of different additives on the growth performance and carcass characteristics of Holstein steers. *Journal of Life Science*, *22*(22), 61–166.

Christiansen, B., & Bellkosta, M. (2010). Ingestion of broccoli sprouts does not improve endothelial function in humans with hypertension. *PLoS ONE*, *5*(8), e12461. doi:10.1371/journal.pone.0012461 PMID:20805984

Chukwumah, Y. C., Walker, L. T., Verghese, M., Bokanga, M., Ogutu, S., & Alphonse, K. (2007). Comparison of extraction methods for the quantification of selected phytochemicals in peanuts (*Arachis hypogaea*). *Journal of Agricultural and Food Chemistry*, *55*(2), 285–290. doi:10.1021/jf062148t PMID:17227055

Chung, H. (2009). *Characterization of antioxidant activities of soybeans and assessment of their bioaccessibility after in vitro digestion. Ph.D thesis*. Virginia Polytechnic Institute and State University. Retrieved from http://vtechworks.lib.vt.edu/handle/10919/29638?show=full

Chung, H.-J., Liu, Q., Pauls, K. P., Fan, M. Z., & Yada, R. (2008). In vitro starch digestibility, expected glycemic index and some physicochemical properties of starch and flour from common bean (*Phaseolus vulgaris* L.) varieties grown in Canada. *Food Research International*, *41*(9), 869–875. doi:10.1016/j.foodres.2008.03.013

Chung, J. Y., Huang, C., Meng, X., Dong, Z., & Yang, C. S. (1999). Inhibition of activator protein 1 activity and cell growth by purified green tea and black tea polyphenols in H-ras-transformed cells: Structure-activity relationship and mechanisms involved. *Cancer Research*, *59*(18), 4610–4617. PMID:10493515

Chung, M. J., Walker, P. A., & Hogstrand, C. (2006). Dietary phenolic antioxidants, caffeic acid and Trolox, protect rainbow trout gill cells from nitric oxide-induced apoptosis. *Aquatic Toxicology (Amsterdam, Netherlands)*, *80*(4), 321–328. doi:10.1016/j.aquatox.2006.09.009 PMID:17113165

Chung, T. K., & Baker, D. H. (1992). Efficiency of dietary methionine utilization by young pigs. *The Journal of Nutrition*, *122*, 1862–1869. PMID:1512636

Cicero, A. F., Ertek, S., & Borghi, C. (2009). Omega-3 polyunsaturated fatty acids: Their potential role in blood pressure prevention and management. *Current Vascular Pharmacology*, *7*(3), 330–337. doi:10.2174/157016109788340659 PMID:19601857

Cisneros-Zevallos, L., & Krochta, J. M. (2003). Dependence of coating thickness on viscosity of coating solution applied to fruits and vegetables by dipping method. *Journal of Food Science*, *68*(2), 503–510. doi:10.1111/j.1365-2621.2003.tb05702.x

Claeys, W. L., Verraes, C., Cardoen, S., De Block, J., Huyghebaert, A., Raes, K., & Herman, L. et al. (2014). Consumption of raw or heated milk from different species: An evaluation of the nutritional and potential health benefits. *Food Control*, *42*, 188–201. doi:10.1016/j.foodcont.2014.01.045

Clavel, T., Charrier, C., Braune, A., Wenning, M., Blaut, M., & Haller, D. (2009). Isolation of bacteria from the ileal mucosa of TNFdeltaARE mice and description of *Enterorhabdus mucosicola* gen. nov., sp. nov. *International Journal of Systematic and Evolutionary Microbiology*, *59*(7), 1805–1812. doi:10.1099/ijs.0.003087-0 PMID:19542111

Clavel, T., Fallani, M., Lepage, P., Levenez, F., Mathey, J., Rochet, V., & Coxam, V. et al. (2005). Isoflavones and functional foods alter the dominant intestinal microbiota in postmenopausal women. *The Journal of Nutrition, 135*, 2786–2792. PMID:16317121

Clavel, T., Lepage, P., & Charrier, C. (2014). The family *Coriobacteriaceae*. In E. Rosenberg, E. F. DeLong, S. Lory, E. Stackebrandt, & F. Thompson (Eds.), *The Prokaryotes-Actinobacteria* (pp. 201–238). Berlin: Springer-Verlag.

Clavel, T., & Mapesa, J. O. (2013). Phenolics in human nutrition: importance of the intestinal microbiome for isoflavone and lignin bioavailability. In K. G. Ramawat & J. M. Merillon (Eds.), *Handbook of Natural Products*. Berlin: Springer-Verlag. doi:10.1007/978-3-642-22144-6_94

Coates, A. M., & Howe, P. R. (2007). Edible nuts and metabolic health. *Current Opinion in Lipidology, 18*(1), 25–30. doi:10.1097/MOL.0b013e3280123a47 PMID:17218828

Collaborative group of the primary prevention project (PPP). (2001). Low-dose aspirin and vitamin E in people at cardiovascular risk: a randomized trial in general practice. *Lancet, 357*, 89-95.

Conner, E. M., & Grisham, M. B. (1996). Inflammation, free radicals, & antioxidants. *The Journal of Nutrition, 12*(4), 274–277. doi:10.1016/S0899-9007(96)00000-8 PMID:8862535

Connor, W. E. (1994). n-3 Fatty acids and heart disease. In: Kritchevsky D, Carroll KK, editors. Nutrition and disease update: heart disease. Champaign, IL: American Oil Chemists' Society.

Connor, W. E. (2000). Importance of n-3 fatty acids in health and disease. *The American Journal of Clinical Nutrition, 71*, 171S–175S. PMID:10617967

Conway, V., Couture, P., Richard, C., Gauthier, S. F., Pouliot, Y., & Lamarche, B. (2013). Impact of buttermilk consumption on plasma lipids and surrogate markers of cholesterol homeostasis in men and women. *Nutrition, Metabolism, and Cardiovascular Diseases, 23*(12), 1255–1262. doi:10.1016/j.numecd.2013.03.003 PMID:23786821

Cooper, R., Morre, D. J., & Morre, D. M. (2005). Medicinal benefits of green tea: Part I. Review of noncancer health benefits. *Journal of Alternative and Complementary Medicine (New York, N.Y.), 11*(3), 521–528. doi:10.1089/acm.2005.11.521 PMID:15992239

Cornelio Favarin, D., Martins Teixeira, M., Lemos de Andrade, E., de Freitas Alves, C., Lazo Chica, J. E., Artério Sorgi, C., & Paula Rogerio, A. et al. (2013). Anti-inflammatory effects of ellagic acid on acute lung injury induced by acid in mice. *Mediators of Inflammation. Article ID, 164202*. doi:10.1155/2013/164202

Cornwell, T., Cohick, W., & Raskin, I. (2004). Dietary phytoestrogens and health. *Phytochemistry, 65*(8), 995–1016. doi:10.1016/j.phytochem.2004.03.005 PMID:15110680

Corpet, D. E., & Taché, S. (2002). Most effective colon cancer chemopreventive agents in rats: A systematic review of aberrant crypt foci and tumor data, ranked by potency. *Nutrition and Cancer, 43*(1), 1–21. doi:10.1207/S15327914NC431_1 PMID:12467130

Corrao, G., Rubbiati, L., Bagnardi, V., Zambon, A., & Poikolainen, K. (2000). Alcohol and coronary heart disease: A meta-analysis. *Addiction (Abingdon, England), 95*(10), 1505–1523. doi:10.1046/j.1360-0443.2000.951015056.x PMID:11070527

Correa, P. (1981). Epidemiological correlations between diet and cancer frequency. *Cancer Research, 41*(9 Part 2), 3685–3689. PMID:6266659

Corrigan, C. J., & Kay, A. B. (1992). T cells and eosinophils in the pathogenesis of asthma. *Immunology Today, 13*(12), 501–507. doi:10.1016/0167-5699(92)90026-4 PMID:1361126

Corti, R., Flammer, A. J., Hollenberg, N. K., & Luscher, T. F. (2009). Cocoa and Cardiovascular Health. *Circulation, 119*(10), 1433–1441. doi:10.1161/CIRCULATIONAHA.108.827022 PMID:19289648

Costa, R. L., & Summa, M. A. (2000). Soy protein in the management of hyperlipidemia. *Annales Pharmaceutiques, 34*, 931–935. doi:10.1345/aph.19371 PMID:10928406

Craig, W. J. (1999). Health-promoting properties of common herbs. *The American Journal of Clinical Nutrition, 70*, 491s–499s. PMID:10479221

Craig, W., & Beck, L. (1999). Phytochemicals: Health protective effects. *Canadian Journal of Dietetic Practice and Researc, 60*, 78–84. PMID:11551345

Crawford, S. L., Jackson, E. A., Churchill, L., Lampe, J. W., Leung, K., & Ockene, J. K. (2013). Impact of dose, frequency of administration, and equol production on efficacy of isoflavones for menopausal hot flashes: A pilot randomized trial. *Menopause (New York, N.Y.), 20*(9), 936–945. doi:10.1097/GME.0b013e3182829413 PMID:23511704

Crouse, J. R. III, Morgan, T., Terry, J. G., Ellis, J., Vitolins, M., & Burke, G. L. (1999). A ran-domized trial comparing the effect of casein with that of soy protein contain-ing varying amounts of isoflavones on plasma concentrations of lipids and lipoproteins. *Archives of Internal Medicine, 159*(17), 2070–2076. doi:10.1001/archinte.159.17.2070 PMID:10510993

Crozier, A., Jaganath, I. B., & Clifford, M. N. (2009). Dietary phenolics: Chemistry, bioavailability and effects on health. *Natural Product Reports, 26*(8), 1001–1043. doi:10.1039/b802662a PMID:19636448

Cruz, M. J. S., Garitta, L. V., & Hough, G. (2003). Note: Relationships of consumer acceptability and sensory attributes of Yerba Mate (*Ilex paraguariensis* St. Hil.) using preference mapping. *Food Science & Technology International, 9*(5), 347–362. doi:10.1177/1082013203038376

Cui, H., Kong, Y., & Zhang, H. (2012). Oxidative stress, mitochondrial dysfunction, and aging. *Journal of Signal Transduction*, 646354. PMID:21977319

Cunnane, S. C., Nadeau, C. R., & Likhodil, S. S. (2001). Alpha Linelenic acid, Figure 3, also compets for the same enzymes for the synthesis of eicosanoids and DHA. *Journal of Molecular Neuroscience, 16*, 173–180. doi:10.1385/JMN:16:2-3:173 PMID:11478372

D'Aniello, G., Grieco, N., Filippo, M. A., Capiello, F., Topo, E., D'Aniello, E., & Ronsini, S. (2007). Reproductive implicatin of D-aspartic acid in human pre-ovulatory follicular fluid. *Human Reproduction (Oxford, England), 22*(12), 3178–3183. doi:10.1093/humrep/dem328 PMID:17951582

Dabai, F. D., Walker, A. F., Sambrook, I. E., Welch, V. A., Owen, R. W., & Abeyasekera, S. (1996). Comparative effects on blood lipids and faecal steroids of five legume species incorporated into a semi-purified, hypercholesterolaemic rat diet. *The British Journal of Nutrition, 75*(04), 557–571. doi:10.1079/BJN19960159 PMID:8672408

Dagher, S. M. (1991). *Traditional Foods in the Near East*. FAO.

Dahiru, D., & Obidoa, O. (2008). Evaluation of the antioxidant effects of *Zizyphus mauritiana Lamk.* Leaf extracts against chronic ethanol-induced hepatotoxicity in rat liver. *African Journal of Traditional, Complementary, and Alternative Medicines, 5*(1), 39–45. doi:10.4314/ajtcam.v5i1.31254 PMID:20162053

Dalié, D. K. D., Deschamps, A. M., & Richard-Forget, F. (2010). Lactic acid bacteria - Potential for control of mould growth and mycotoxins: A review. *Food Control, 21*(4), 370–380. doi:10.1016/j.foodcont.2009.07.011

Dalton, S. M. C., Tapsell, L. C., & Probst, Y. (2012). Potential health benefits of whole wheat components. *Nutrition Today, 47*(4), 163–174. doi:10.1097/NT.0b013e31826069d0

Dana, N., & Rafiee, L. (2015). Antiangiogenic & antiproliferative effects of black pomegranate peel extract on melanoma cell line. *Research in Pharmaceutical Sciences*, *10*(2), 117–124. PMID:26487888

Danesi, F., Di Nunzio, M., Boschetti, E., & Bordoni, A. (2009). Green tea extract selectively activates peroxisome proliferator-activated receptor beta/delta in cultured cardiomyocytes. *The British Journal of Nutrition*, *101*(12), 1736–1739. doi:10.1017/S0007114508145871 PMID:19055854

Daniel, M., Denni, M., & Chauhan, D. (2012). Polyphenols, phospholipids and fixed oil composition of pearl millet. *International Journal of Pharmacy & Life Sciences*, *3*(11), 2098–2102.

Daniel, M., & Tollefsbol, T. O. (2015). Epigenetic linkage of aging, cancer and nutrition. *The Journal of Experimental Biology*, *218*(Pt 1), 59–70. doi:10.1242/jeb.107110 PMID:25568452

Darmadi-Blackberry, I., Wahlqvist, M. L., Kouris-Blazos, A., Steen, B., Lukito, W., Horie, Y., & Horie, K. (2004). Legumes: The most important dietary predictor of survival in older people of different ethnicities. *Asia Pacific Journal of Clinical Nutrition*, *13*, 217–220. PMID:15228991

Dasaroju, S., & Gottumukkala, K. M. (2014). Current trends in the research of *emblica officinalis (amla):* A pharmacological perspective. *International Journal of Pharmaceutical Sciences Review and Research*, *24*(2), 150–159.

Dasgupta, A., & Klein, K. (2014). *Tea, Coffee, and Chocolate: Rich Sources of Antioxidants*. Antioxidants in Food, Vitamins and Supplements Prevention and Treatment of Disease. doi:10.1016/B978-0-12-405872-9.00013-6

Das, S., Santani, D. D., & Dhalla, N. S. (2007). Experimental evidence for the cardioprotective effects of red wine. *Experiments in Clinical Cardiology*, *12*(1), 5–10. PMID:18650973

Das, S., & Sarma, P. H. U. L. E. N. (2014). A study on the anticonvulsant and antianxiety activity of ethanolic extract of punica granatum linn. *International Journal of Pharmacy and Pharmaceutical Sciences*, *6*(2), 389–392.

Dauchet, L., Amouyel, P., Hercberg, S., & Dallongeville, J. (2006). Fruit and vegetable consump-tion and risk of coronary heart disease: A meta-analysis of cohort studies. *The Journal of Nutrition*, *136*(10), 2588–2593. PMID:16988131

Dauqan, E. M. A., Abdullah, A., & Sani, H. A. (2011). Natural antioxidants, lipid profile, lipid peroxidation, antioxidant enzymes of different vegetable oils. *Advance Journal of Food Science and Technology*, *3*(4), 308–316.

Davidson, M. H., Maki, K. C., Dicklin, M. R., Feinstein, S. B., Witchger, M. S., Bell, M., & Aviram, M. et al. (2009). Effects of consumption of pomegranate juice on carotid intima–media thickness in men & women at moderate risk for coronary heart disease. *The American Journal of Cardiology*, *104*(7), 936–942. doi:10.1016/j.amjcard.2009.05.037 PMID:19766760

Davidson, P. M. (2005). Parabens. In P. M. Davidson, J. N. Sofos, & A. L. Branen (Eds.), *Antimicrobials in Foods* (pp. 291–303). Boca Raton, FL: CRC Press.

Davis, M. A., Mackenzie, T. A., Cottingham, K. L., Gilbert-Diamond, D., Punshon, T., & Karagas, M. R. (2012). Rice consumption and urinary arsenic concentrations in U.S. children. *Environmental Health Perspectives*, *120*(10), 1418–1424. doi:10.1289/ehp.1205014 PMID:23008276

de Almeida Costa, G. E., da Silva Queiroz-Monici, K., Reis, S. M. P. M., & de Oliveira, A. C. (2006). Chemical composition, dietary fibre and resistant starch contents of raw and cooked pea, common bean, chickpea and lentil legumes. *Food Chemistry*, *94*(3), 327–330. doi:10.1016/j.foodchem.2004.11.020

de Cremoux, P., This, P., Leclercq, G., & Jacquot, Y. (2010). Controversies concerning the use of phytoestrogens in menopause management: Bioavailability and metabolism. *Maturitas*, *65*(4), 334–339. doi:10.1016/j.maturitas.2009.12.019 PMID:20080366

De Datta, S. K. (1981). *Principles and Practices of Rice Production*. New York, NY: John Wiley and Sons, Inc.

De Deckere, E. A. M., & Korver, O. (1996). Minor constituents of rice brain oil as functional foods. *Nutrition Reviews*, *54*(11), S120–S126. doi:10.1111/j.1753-4887.1996.tb03831.x PMID:9110588

De Filippo, C., Cavalieri, D., Di Paola, M., Ramazzotti, M., Poullet, J. B., Massart, S., & Lionetti, P. et al. (2010). Impact of diet in shaping gut microbiota revealed by a comparative study in children from Europe and rural Africa. *Proceedings of the National Academy of Sciences of the United States of America*, *107*(33), 14691–14696. doi:10.1073/pnas.1005963107 PMID:20679230

De Mejía, E. G., & Prisecaru, V. I. (2005). Lectins as bioactive plant proteins: A potential in cancer treatment. *Critical Reviews in Food Science and Nutrition*, *45*(6), 425–445. doi:10.1080/10408390591034445 PMID:16183566

de Oliveira, J. F., Garreto, D. V., da Silva, M. C., Fortes, T. S., de Oliveira, R. B., Nascimento, F. R., & Nicolete, R. et al. (2013). Therapeutic potential of biodegradable microparticles containing Punica granatum L.(pomegranate) in murine model of asthma. *Inflammation Research*, *62*(11), 971–980. doi:10.1007/s00011-013-0659-3 PMID:23979691

de Pascual-Teresa, S., Moreno, D. A., & Garcia-Viguera, C. (2010). Flavanols and Anthocyanins in Cardiovascular Health: A Review of Current Evidence. *International Journal of Molecular Sciences*, *11*(4), 1679–1703. doi:10.3390/ijms11041679 PMID:20480037

de Pascual-Teresa, S., & Sanchez-Ballesta, M. T. (2008). Anthocyanins: From plant to health. *Phytochemistry Reviews*, *7*(2), 281–299. doi:10.1007/s11101-007-9074-0

De, B. K., & Bhattacharyya, D. K. (1998). Physical refiningof rice bran oil in relation to degumming & dewaxing. *Journal of the American Oil Chemists' Society*, *75*(11), 1683–1686. doi:10.1007/s11746-998-0112-x

Debeufort, F., Quezada-Gallo, J. A., & Voilley, A. (1998). Edible films and coatings: Tomorrow's packaging: A review. *Critical Reviews in Food Science and Nutrition*, *38*(4), 299–313. doi:10.1080/10408699891274219 PMID:9626488

Decroos, K., Eeckhaut, E., Possemiers, S., & Verstraete, W. (2006). Administration of equol-producing bacteria alters the equol production status in the Simulator of the Gastrointestinal Microbial Ecosystem (SHIME). *The Journal of Nutrition*, *136*, 946–952. PMID:16549455

Decroos, K., Vanhemmens, S., Cattoir, S., Boon, N., & Verstraete, W. (2005). Isolation and characterisation of an equol-producing mixed microbial culture from a human faecal sample and its activity under gastrointestinal conditions. *Archives of Microbiology*, *183*(1), 45–55. doi:10.1007/s00203-004-0747-4 PMID:15578160

del Rio, D., Rodriguez-Mateos, A., Spencer, J. P., Tognolini, M., Borges, G., & Crozier, A. (2013). Dietary (poly)phenolics in human health: Structures, bioavailability, and evidence of protective effects against chronic diseases. *Antioxidants & Redox Signalling*, *18*(14), 1818–1892. doi:10.1089/ars.2012.4581 PMID:22794138

del Rosario, A. R., Briones, V. P., Vidal, A. J., & Juliano, B. O. (1968). Composition and endosperm structure of developing and mature rice kernel. *Cereal Chemistry*, *45*, 225–235.

Delzenne, N. M., Daubioul, C., Neyrinck, A., Lasa, M., & Taper, H. S. (2002). Inulin and oligofructose modulate lipid metabolism in animals: Review of biochemical events and future prospects. *The British Journal of Nutrition*, *87*(S2), S255–S259. doi:10.1079/BJN/2002545 PMID:12088526

Demirbas, A. (2005). β-Glucan and mineral nutrient contents of cereals grown in Turkey. *Food Chemistry*, *90*(4), 773–777. doi:10.1016/j.foodchem.2004.06.003

Deokate, U. A., & Khadabadi, S. S. (2012). Pharmacology and phytochemistry of *Coccinia indica*. *Pharmacophore*, *3*, 179–185.

Department of Health and Human Services (HHS). (1997). *New dietary ingredients: Brickellia cavanillesii*. Retrieved November 14, 2015 from: http://www.fda.gov/OHRMS/DOCKETS/95s0316/rpt0010_.pdf

Desilets, D. J., Davis, K. E., Nair, P. P., Salata, K. F., Maydonovitch, C. L., Howard, R. S., & Wong, R. K. et al. (1999). Lectin. binding to human colonocytes is predictive of colonic neoplasia. *The American Journal of Gastroenterology*, *94*(3), 744–750. doi:10.1111/j.1572-0241.1999.00946.x PMID:10086661

Deu John Mahandi Cruz. (2006). *Lactic acid bacteria isolated from kimchi and shrimp (Palaeomon macrodactylus) inhibit the infection of porcine epidemic diarrhea virus in vitro*. (Master Thesis). Chungnam National University, Gwangju, Korea.

Devlieghere, F., Vermeulen, A., & Debevere, J. (2004). Chitosan: Antimicrobial activity, interactions with food components and applicability as a coating on fruit and vegetables. *Food Microbiology*, *21*(6), 703–714. doi:10.1016/j.fm.2004.02.008

Dexter, P. B. (1998). *Rice fortification for developing countries*. Fayetteville, AR: OMNI/USAID. Retrieved from http://www.mostproject.org/PDF/rice4.pdf

Dharmananda, S. (2005). *Neuroprotective herbs and active constituents approaches to preventing degenerative diseases*. Retreated from: http://www.itmonline.org/arts/neuro.htm

Dickel, M. I., Rates, S. M., & Ritter, M. R. (2007). Plants Popularly Used for Losing Weight Purposes in Porto Alegre, South Brazil. *Journal of Ethnopharmacology*, *109*(1), 60–71. doi:10.1016/j.jep.2006.07.003 PMID:16963210

Diedhiou, P. M., Bandyopadhyay, R., Atehnkeng, J., & Ojiambo, P. S. (2011). Aspergillus colonization and aflatoxin contamination of maize and sesame kernels in two agroecological zones in Senegal. *Journal of Phytopathology*, *159*(4), 268–275. doi:10.1111/j.1439-0434.2010.01761.x

Dilis, V., & Trichopoulou, A. (2009). Nutritional and health properties of pulses. *Mediterranean Journal of Nutrition and Metabolism.*, *1*(3), 149–157. doi:10.1007/s12349-008-0023-2

Ding, E. L., Hutfless, S. M., Ding, X., & Girotra, S. (2006). Chocolate and prevention of cardiovascular disease: A systematic review. *Nutrition & Metabolism*, *3*(1), 2. doi:10.1186/1743-7075-3-2 PMID:16390538

Ding, W. K., & Shah, N. P. (2010). Enhancing the biotransformation of isoflavones in soymilk supplemented with lactose using probiotic bacteria during extended fermentation. *Journal of Food Science*, *75*(3), M140–M149. doi:10.1111/j.1750-3841.2010.01526.x PMID:20492303

DiSilvestro, R. A., DiSilvestro, D. J., & DiSilvestro, D. J. (2009). Pomegranate extract mouth rinsing effects on saliva measures relevant to gingivitis risk. *Journal of Phytotherapy Research*, *23*(8), 1123–1127. doi:10.1002/ptr.2759 PMID:19170139

DiSilvestro, R. A., Joseph, E., Zhao, S., & Bomser, J. (2012). Diverse effects of a low dose supplement of lapidated curcumin in healthy middle aged people. *Nutrition Journal*, *11*(1), 79–84. doi:10.1186/1475-2891-11-79 PMID:23013352

Dkhil, M. A. (2013). Anti-coccidial, anthelmintic & antioxidant activities of pomegranate (Punica granatum) peel extract. *Journal of Parasitology Research*, *112*(7), 2639–2646. doi:10.1007/s00436-013-3430-3 PMID:23609599

Dodt, C., Welhoner, J. P., Schutt, M., & Sayk, F. (2009). Glucocorticoids and Hypertension. *Der Internist*, *50*(1), 36–41. doi:10.1007/s00108-008-2197-6 PMID:19096817

Donkor, O. N., Henriksson, A., Singh, T. K., Vasiljevic, T., & Shah, N. P. (2007). ACE-inhibitory activity of probiotic yoghurt. *International Dairy Journal*, *17*(11), 1321–1331. doi:10.1016/j.idairyj.2007.02.009

Doores, S. (1993). Organic acids. In Antimicrobials in Food (pp. 95–136). Marcel Dekker, Inc.

Dorchies, O. M., Wagner, S., Buetler, T. M., & Ruegg, U. T. (2009). Protection of dystrophic muscle cells with polyphenols from green tea correlates with improved glutathione balance and increased expression of 67LR, a receptor for (-)-epigallocatechin gallate. *BioFactors (Oxford, England)*, *35*(3), 279–294. doi:10.1002/biof.34 PMID:19322813

Dreosti, I. E. (2000). Antioxidant polyphenols in tea, cocoa, and wine. *Nutrition (Burbank, Los Angeles County, Calif.)*, *16*(7/8), 692–694. doi:10.1016/S0899-9007(00)00304-X PMID:10906600

Drewnoski, M. E., Pogge, D. J., & Hanse, S. L. (2014). *Journal of Animal Science.* American Society of Animal Science. Retrieved from http://www.journalofanimalscience.org/content/early/2014/06/30/jas.2013-7242

Drewnowski, A., & Gomez-Carneros, C. (2000). Bitter taste, phytonutrients and the consumer: A review. *Amarican journal of Clinical. Nutrition (Burbank, Los Angeles County, Calif.)*, *72*, 1424–1435.

Drinkine, J., Lopes, P., Kennedy, J. A., Teissedre, P. L., & Saucier, C. (2007). Ethylidene-Bridged Flavan-3-ols in Red Wine and Correlation With Wine Age. *Journal of Agricultural and Food Chemistry*, *55*(15), 6292–6299. doi:10.1021/jf070038w PMID:17602645

Duane, W. (1997). Effects of legume consumption on serum cholesterol, biliary lipids, and sterol metabolism in humans. *Journal of Lipid Research*, *38*(6), 1120–1128. PMID:9215540

Duan, L. P., Wang, H. H., & Wang, D. Q. H. (2004). Cholesterol absorption is mainly regulated by the jejunal and ileal ATP-binding cassette sterol efflux transporters Abcg5 and Abcg8 in mice. *Journal of Lipid Research*, *45*(7), 1312–233. doi:10.1194/jlr.M400030-JLR200 PMID:15102882

Dubey, P., & Cheema, S. K. (2006). Molecular mechanisms involved in the regulation of lipid and lipoprotein metabolism by fish oil. *Future Lipidology*, *1*(5), 559–568. doi:10.2217/17460875.1.5.559

Dueñas, M., Hernández, T., & Estrella, I. (2002). Phenolic composition of the cotyledon and the seed coat of lentils (*Lens culinaris* L.). *European Food Research and Technology*, *215*(6), 478–483. doi:10.1007/s00217-002-0603-1

Duenas, M., Hernandez, T., & Estrella, I. (2006). Assessment of in vitro antioxidant capacity of the seed coat and the cotyledon of legumes in relation to their phenolic contents. *Food Chemistry*, *98*(1), 95–103. doi:10.1016/j.foodchem.2005.05.052

Duenas, M., Hernandez, T., Robredo, S., Lamparski, G., Estrella, I., & Munoz, R. (2012). Bioactive phenolic compounds of soybean (Glycine max cv. Merit): Modifications by different microbiological fermentations. *Polish Journal of Food Sciences.*, *62*(4), 241–250.

Dueñas, M., Sun, B., Hernández, T., Estrella, I., & Spranger, M. I. (2003). Proanthocyanidin composition in the seed coat of lentils (*Lens culinaris* L.). *Journal of Agricultural and Food Chemistry*, *51*(27), 7999–8004. doi:10.1021/jf0303215 PMID:14690386

Duffy, R., Wiseman, H., & File, S. E. (2003). Improved cognitive function in postmenopausal women after 12 weeks of consumption of a soya extract containing isoflavones. *Pharmacology, Biochemistry, and Behavior*, *75*(3), 721–729. doi:10.1016/S0091-3057(03)00116-3 PMID:12895690

Du, Q., Xu, Y., Li, L., Zhao, Y., Jerz, G., & Winterhalter, P. (2011). Antioxidant constituents in the fruits of *Luffa cylindrica* (L.) Roem. *Food Chemistry*, *127*, 609–614. PMID:23140707

Duranti, M. (2006). Grain legume proteins and nutraceutical properties. *Fitoterapia*, *77*(2), 67–82. doi:10.1016/j.fitote.2005.11.008 PMID:16406359

Duriez, P., & Fruchart, J.-C. (1993). Vitamine E et athérosclerose. *Méd Nutr.*, *29*, 17–19.

Du, Y., & Lou, H. (2008). Catechin and proanthocyanidin B4 from grape seeds prevent doxorubicin induced toxicity in cardiomyocytes. *European Journal of Pharmacology*, *591*(1-3), 96–101. doi:10.1016/j.ejphar.2008.06.068 PMID:18611398

Dweck, A. C., & Data, D. (2015). *A review of Guava (*Psidium guajava*)*. Retreated from: www.dweckdata.co.uk/Published_papers/Psidium_guajava.pdf

Dwivedi, S., Sahrawat, K., Puppala, N., & Ortiz, R. (2014). Plant prebiotics and human health: Biotechnology to breed prebiotic-rich nutritious food crops. *Electronic Journal of Biotechnology*, *17*(5), 238–245. doi:10.1016/j.ejbt.2014.07.004

Dykes, L. & Roonwy, L.W. (2007). *Phenolic compounds in cereals grains and their health benefit.* Cereal Foods World, AACC International Inc. doi:10.1094/CFW-52-3-0105

Dykes, L., & Rooney, L. W. (2006). Sorghum and millet phenols and antioxidants. *Journal of Cereal Science*, *44*(3), 236–251. doi:10.1016/j.jcs.2006.06.007

Edeoga, H. O., Okwu, D. E., & Mbaebie, B. O. (2005). Phytochemical constituents of some Nigerian medicinal plants. *African Journal of Biotechnology*, *4*(7), 685–688. doi:10.5897/AJB2005.000-3127

Edge, M. S., Jones, J. M., & Marquart, L. (2005). A new life for whole grains. *Journal of the American Dietetic Association*, *105*(12), 1856–1860. doi:10.1016/j.jada.2005.10.022 PMID:16321586

Egert, S., Bosy-Westphal, A., Seiberl, J., Kurbitz, C., Settler, U., Plachta-Danielzik, S., & Muller, M. J. et al. (2009). Quercetin reduces systolic blood pressure and plasma oxidised low-density lipoprotein concentrations in overweight subjects with a high-cardiovascular disease risk phenotype: A double-blinded, placebo-controlled cross-over study. *The British Journal of Nutrition*, *102*(7), 1065–1074. PMID:19402938

Eidi, A., & Eidi, M. (2009). Antidiabetic effects of sage (*Salvia officinalis* L.) leaves in normal and streptozotocin-induced diabetic rats. *Diabetes & Metabolic Syndrome: Clinical Research & Reviews*, *3*(1), 40–44. doi:10.1016/j.dsx.2008.10.007

Eisenberg, D. M., Davis, R. B., Erner, S. L., Appel, S., Wilkey, S., Van Rompay, M., & Kessler, R. C. (1998). Trends in alternative medicine use in the United States, 1990-1997: Results of a follow-up national survey. *Journal of the American Medical Association*, *280*(18), 1569–1575. doi:10.1001/jama.280.18.1569 PMID:9820257

Eisenberg, D. M., Kessler, R. C., Foster, C., Norlock, F. E., Calkins, D. R., & Delbanco, T. L. (1993). Unconventional medicine in the United States: Prevalence, costs, and patterns of use. *The New England Journal of Medicine*, *328*(4), 246–252. doi:10.1056/NEJM199301283280406 PMID:8418405

Ekor, M. (2014). The growing use of herbal medicines: issues relating to adverse reactions and challenges in monitoring safety. *Frontiers in Pharmacology, 4*(177), 1-10. Doi: 10.3389/fphar.2013.00177

El Hag, I. M. N., Ahmed, I. A. M., Ahmed, S. O., Eltayeb, M. M., & Babiker, E. E. (2013). Effect of processing methods on antinutritional factors, protein digestibility and minerals extractability of winter sorghum cultivars. *Australian Journal of Basic and Applied Sciences*, *7*(12), 229–237.

El-Adawy, T., Rahma, E., El-Bedawey, A., & El-Beltagy, A. (2003). Nutritional potential and functional properties of germinated mung bean, pea and lentil seeds. *Plant Foods for Human Nutrition (Dordrecht, Netherlands)*, *58*(3), 1–13. doi:10.1023/B:QUAL.0000040339.48521.75 PMID:12859008

El-Agamy, E. I. (2000). Effect of heat treatment on camel milk proteins with respectto antimicrobial factors: A comparison with cows' and buffalo milk proteins. *Food Chemistry*, *68*(2), 227–232. doi:10.1016/S0308-8146(99)00199-5

El-Agamy, E. I. (2007). The challenge of cow milk protein allergy. *Small Ruminant Research*, *68*(1-2), 64–72. doi:10.1016/j.smallrumres.2006.09.016

El-Agamy, E. I., Nawar, M., Shamsia, S. M., Awad, S., & Haenlein, G. F. W. (2009). Are camel milk proteins convenient to the nutrition of cow milk allergic children? *Small Ruminant Research*, *82*(1), 1–6. doi:10.1016/j.smallrumres.2008.12.016

El-Agamy, E. I., Ruppanner, R., Ismail, A., Champagne, C. P., & Assaf, R. (1992). Antibacterial and antiviral activity of camel milk protective proteins. *The Journal of Dairy Research*, *59*(02), 169–175. doi:10.1017/S0022029900030417 PMID:1319434

El-Anany, A. M., & Ali, R. F. M. (2013). Biochemical and histopathological effects of administration various levels of Pomposia (*Syzygium cumini*) fruit juice as natural antioxidant on rat health. *Journal of Food Sciences and Technology.*, *50*(3), 487–495. doi:10.1007/s13197-011-0372-6 PMID:24425943

El-Baky, H. H. (2009). Enhancing antioxidant availability in grains of wheat plants grown under seawater-stress in response to microalgae extracts treatments. *African Journal of Biochemistry Research*, *3*(4), 77–83.

Elekofehinti, O. O. (2015). Saponins: Anti-diabetic principles from medicinal plants–A review. *Pathophysiology*, *22*(2), 95–103. doi:10.1016/j.pathophys.2015.02.001 PMID:25753168

Elvevoll, E. O., Barstad, H., Breimo, E. S., Brox, J., Eilertsen, K. E., Lund, T., & Osterud, B. et al. (2006). Enhanced incorporation of n-3 fatty acids from fish compared with fish oils. *Lipids*, *41*(12), 1109–1114. doi:10.1007/s11745-006-5060-3 PMID:17269556

Emery, R. S., Smith, C. K., & Huffman, C. F. (1957). Utilization of inorganic sulfate by rumen microorganisms. I. incorporation of inorganic sulfate into amino acids. APP. *Microbiol*, *5*, 360–363. PMID:13488436

Engel, R. R., & Smith, A. H. (1994). Arsenic in drinking water and mortality from vascular disease: An ecologic analysis in 30 counties in the United States. *Archives of Environmental & Occupational Health*, *49*(5), 418–427. doi:10.1080/00039896.1994.9954996 PMID:7944575

Erkkila, A., & Lichtenstein, A. (2006). Fiber and cardiovascular disease risk: How strong is the evidence? *The Journal of Cardiovascular Nursing*, *21*(1), 3–8. doi:10.1097/00005082-200601000-00003 PMID:16407729

Erlund, I., Koli, R., Alfthan, G., Marniemi, J., Puukka, P., Mustonen, P., & Jula, A. et al. (2008). Favorable effects of berry consumption on platelet function, blood pressure, and HDL cholesterol. *The American Journal of Clinical Nutrition*, *87*, 323–331. PMID:18258621

Escandón-Rivera, S., González-Andrade, M., Bye, R., Linares, E., Navarrete, A., & Mata, R. (2012). α-glucosidase inhibitors from Brickellia cavanillesii. *Journal of Natural Products*, *75*(5), 968–974. doi:10.1021/np300204p PMID:22587572

Escudero, F. E., Munoz, A. M., Alvarado-Ortiz, C., Alvarado, A., & Yanez, J. A. (2012). Purple corn (*Zea mays* L.). Phenolic compounds profile and its assessment as an agent against oxidative stress in isolated mouse organs. *Journal of Medicinal Food*, *15*(2), 206–215. doi:10.1089/jmf.2010.0342 PMID:22082063

Eshak, E. S., Iso, H., Date, C., Yamagishi, K., Kikuchi, S., Watanabe, Y., & Tamakoshi, A. et al. (2011). JACC Study Group. Rice intake is associated with reduced risk of mortality from cardiovascular disease in Japanese men but not women. *The Journal of Nutrition*, *141*(4), 595–602. doi:10.3945/jn.110.132167 PMID:21346103

Eshak, E. S., Iso, H., Yamagishi, K., Kokubo, Y., Saito, I., Yatsuya, H., & Tsugane, S. et al. (2014). Rice consumption is not associated with risk of cardiovascular disease morbidity or mortality in Japanese men and women: A large population-based, prospective cohort study. *The American Journal of Clinical Nutrition*, *141*(1), 199–207. doi:10.3945/ajcn.113.079038 PMID:24740204

Eshiet, E. R. (2010). *Chemical characterization of diabetic herbal tea and in vitro evaluation of glucose transport and metabolism gene expression profile.* (Unpublished Doctoral Dissertation). Texas Tech University, Lubbock, TX.

Eshiet, E. R., Zhu, J., Anderson, T. A., & Smith, E. E. (2014a). Chemical characterization of Brickellia cavanillesii (Asteraceae) using gas chromatographic methods. *Food Sci Nutr*, *2*(2), 105–113. doi:10.1002/fsn3.52 PMID:24804069

Eshiet, E. R., Zhu, J., & Smith, E. E. (2014b). Lyophilized tea extracts of Brickellia cavanillesii (Asteraceae): In vitro characterization of biological activity. *Journal of Food Science*, *79*(7), T1454–T1461. doi:10.1111/1750-3841.12519 PMID:24962327

Eshiet, E. R., Zhu, J., & Smith, E. E. (2015). The biologic potential of lyophilized extracts of Brickellia cavanillesii (Asteraceae): Apoptosis and glut 2 gene expression. *Journal of Food Processing & Technology*, *7*(1). doi:10.4172/2157-7110.1000541

Euromonitor, I. (2010). *Cardiovascular health: A key area of functional food and drinks development*. London: Euromonitor International. Retrieved July 10, 2015, from http://www.euromonitor.com/cardiovascular-health-a-key-area-of-functional-food-and-drinks-development/report

European Food Science Authority. (2012). Scientific Opinion on the substantiation of health claims related to soy isoflavones and maintenance of bone mineral density (ID 1655) and reduction of vasomotor symptoms associated with menopause (ID 1654, 1704, 2140, 3093, 3154, 3590) (further assessment) pursuant to Article 13(1) of Regulation (EC) No 1924/2006. *EFSA Journal*, *10*, 2847.

Everitt, A. V., Hilmer, S. N., Brand-Miller, J. C., Jamieson, H. A., Truswell, A. S., Sharma, A. P., & Le Couteur, D. G. et al. (2006). Dietary Approaches that Delay Age-Related Diseases. *Journal of Clinical Interventions in Aging*, *1*(1), 11–31. doi:10.2147/ciia.2006.1.1.11 PMID:18047254

Ezekiel, C. N., Abia, W. A., Ogara, I. M., Sulyok, M., Warth, B., & Krska, R. (2015). Fate of mycotoxins in two popular traditional cereal-based beverages (*kunu-zaki and pito*) from rural Nigeria. *LWT -. Food Science and Technology (Campinas.)*, *60*, 137–141.

Ezekiel, C. N., Sulyok, M., Babalola, D. A., Warth, A., Ezekiel, V. C., & Krska, R. (2013). Incidence and consumer awareness of toxigenic *Aspergillus* section Flavi and aflatoxin B1 in peanut cake from Nigeria. *Food Control*, *30*(2), 596–601. doi:10.1016/j.foodcont.2012.07.048

Ezekiel, C. N., Sulyok, M., Warth, B., Odebode, A. C., & Krska, R. (2012). Natural occurrence of mycotoxins in peanut cake from Nigeria. *Food Control*, *27*(2), 338–342. doi:10.1016/j.foodcont.2012.04.010

Ezekiel, R., Singh, N., Sharma, S., & Kaur, A. (2013). Beneficial phytochemicals in potato — a review. *Food Research International*, *50*(2), 487–496. doi:10.1016/j.foodres.2011.04.025

Fabec, B., Hellstrom, T., Henrysdotter, G., Hjulmand-Lassen, M., Nilsson, J., Rudinger, L., . . . Tuomala, V. (2000). *Active and intelligent food Packaging. A Nordic report on the legislative aspects*. Retrieved from www.norden.org/ pub/ebook/2000-584.pdf

Fagundes, R. B., Abnet, C. C., Strickland, P. T., Kamangar, F., Roth, M. J., Taylor, P. R., & Dawsey, S. M. (2006). Higher Urine 1-Hydroxy Pyrene Glucuronide (1-OHPG) is Associated with Tobacco Smoke Exposure and Drinking Mate in Healthy Subjects from Rio Grande do Sul, Brazil. *BMC Cancer*, *6*(1), 139–145. doi:10.1186/1471-2407-6-139 PMID:16729889

Falanga, V. (2005). Wound healing & its impairment in the diabetic foot. *Lancet*, *366*(9498), 1736–1743. doi:10.1016/S0140-6736(05)67700-8 PMID:16291068

Fandohan, P., Zoumenou, D., Hounhouigan, D. J., Marasas, W. F. O., Wingfield, M. J., & Hell, K. (2005). Fate of aflatoxins and fumonisins during the processing of maize into food products in Benin. *International Journal of Food Microbiology*, *98*(3), 249–259. doi:10.1016/j.ijfoodmicro.2004.07.007 PMID:15698686

FAO (Food and Agriculture Organization of the United Nations). (2004). Rice is life.*Proceedings of the FAO Rice Conference*. Food and Agriculture Organization of the United Nations.

FAO, IFAD, & WFP. (2014). *The State of Food Insecurity in the World 2014. Strengthening the enabling environment for food security and nutrition*. Rome: FAO.

FAO. (1954). *Rice and rice diets – a nutritional survey* (rev. ed.). Rome: FAO.

FAO. (1995). *Sorghum and millets in human nutrition*. Retrieved April 20, 2015, from http://www.fao.org/docrep/t0818e/t0818e00.htm

FAO. (2008). *Camels and camel milk*. Retrieved June 5, 2015, from http://www.fao.org/docrep/003/x6528e/X6528E04.htm

FAO. (2010). *Composition of selected foods from West Africa*. Rome: Food and Agriculture Organisation.

FAO. (2013). *Edible insects: Future prospects for food and feed security*. Rome: Food and Agriculture Organisation.

FAO. (2015). *A resource book for teachers of agriculture*. Retrieved March 25, 2015 from http://www.fao.org/docrep/w0078e/w0078e06.htm

FAOSTAT (The Statistics Division of the Food and Agriculture Organization of the United Nations). (2012). *Database of Food and Agricultural Organization*. Available from: http://faostat3.fao.org/

FAOSTAT. (2013). *Camel milk*. Retrieved May 15, 2015 from http://faostat3.fao.org/home/E

FAOSTAT. (2013). Retrieved March 25, 2015 from http://faostat.fao.org/site/567/DesktopDefault.aspx?PageID=567#ancor

Farahani, M. (2012). Assessment of antiherpetic effect of Camellia sinensis against herpes simplex virus type 1. *Journal of Isfahan Medical School, 30*(207).

Farah, Z. (1996). *Camel milk properties and products*. St. Gallen, Switzerland: SKAT, Swiss Centre for Developments Cooperation in Technology and Management.

Farbstein, D., Kozak-Blickstein, A., & Levy, A. P. (2010). Antioxidant vitamins and their use in preventing cardiovascular disease. *Molecules (Basel, Switzerland), 15*(11), 8098–8110. doi:10.3390/molecules15118098 PMID:21063272

Faria, A. F., Marques, M. C., & Mercadante, A. Z. (2011). Identification of bioactive compounds from jambolao (*Syzygium cumini*) and antioxidant capacity evaluation in different pH conditions. *Food Chemistry, 126*(4), 1571–1578. doi:10.1016/j.foodchem.2010.12.007 PMID:25213929

Faris, M. A. I. E., & Takruri, H. R. (2003). Study of the effect of using different levels of tahinah (sesame butter) on the protein digestibility-corrected amino acid score (PDCAAS) of chickpea dip. *Journal of the Science of Food and Agriculture, 83*(1), 7–12. doi:10.1002/jsfa.1273

Faris, M. A. I. E., Takruri, H. R., & Issa, A. Y. (2013). Role of lentils (*Lens culinaris* L.) in human health and nutrition: A review. *Mediterranean Journal of Nutrition and Metabolism, 6*(1), 3–16. doi:10.1007/s12349-012-0109-8

Faris, M. A. I. E., Takruri, H. R., Shomaf, M. S., & Bustanji, Y. K. (2009). Chemopreventive effect of raw and cooked lentils (*Lens culinaris* L) and soybeans (Glycine max) against azoxymethane-induced aberrant crypt foci. *Nutrition Research (New York, N.Y.), 29*(5), 355–362. doi:10.1016/j.nutres.2009.05.005 PMID:19555818

Fawzy, A. G., Abdallah, H. M., Marzonk, M. S. A., Soliman, F. M., & Sleem, A. (2008). Antidiabetic and antioxidant activities of major flavonoids of Cynanchum acutum L. (Asclepiadaceae) growing in Egypt. Z. *Naturforsch., 63c*, 658–662. PMID:19040103

Fellman, J. K., Rudell, D. R., Mattinson, D. S., & Mattheis, J. P. (2003). Relationship of harvest maturity to Flavor regeneratin after CA storage of 'Delicious' apples. *Postharvest Biology and Technology*, *27*(1), 39–51. doi:10.1016/S0925-5214(02)00193-X

Ferlay, J., Shin, H. R., Bray, F., Forman, D., Mathers, C., & Parkin, D. M. (2010). Estimates of worldwide burden of cancer in 2008: GLOBOCAN 2008. *International Journal of Cancer*, *127*(12), 2893–2917. doi:10.1002/ijc.25516 PMID:21351269

Fernandez-Orozco, R., Zieliński, H., & Piskuła, M. K. (2003). Contribution of low-molecular weight antioxidants to the antioxidant capacity of raw and processed lentil seeds. *Food/Nahrung*, *47*(5), 291-299.

Ferrari, C. K. B. (1998). Oxidação lipídica em alimentos e sistemas biológicos: Mecanismos gerais e conseqüências nutricionais e patológicas. *Rev Nutr*, *11*(1), 3–14. doi:10.1590/S1415-52731998000100001

Ferrari, C. K. B., & Torres, E. A. F. S. (2003). Biochemical pharmacology of functional foods and prevention of chronic diseases of aging. *Biomedicine and Pharmacotherapy*, *57*(5-6), 251–260. doi:10.1016/S0753-3322(03)00032-5 PMID:12888262

Ferreira, F., Vázquez, A., Güntner, C., & Moyna, P. (1997). Inhibition of the Passive Diffusion of Chol. Acid by the *Ilex Paraguariensis* St. Hil. saponins. *Phytotherapy Research*, *11*(1), 79–81. doi:10.1002/(SICI)1099-1573(199702)11:1<79::AID-PTR34>3.0.CO;2-R

Ferreira, J. F. S., & Jannick, J. (Eds.). (1996). *Progress in new crops*. Arlington, VA: ASHS press.

Fiedor, J., & Burda, K. (2014). Potential role of carotenoids as antioxidants in human health and disease. *Nutrients*, *6*(2), 466–488. doi:10.3390/nu6020466 PMID:24473231

Fielding, J. M., Rowley, K. G., Cooper, P., & O'Dea, K. (2005). Increases in plasma lycopene concentration after consumption of tomatoes cooked with olive oil. *Asia Pacific Journal of Clinical Nutrition*, *14*, 131–136. PMID:15927929

Filip, R., Lotito, S. B., Ferraro, G., & Praga, C. G. (2000). Antioxidant Activity of *Ilex paraguariensis* and Related Species. *Nutrition Research (New York, N.Y.)*, *20*(10), 1437–1446. doi:10.1016/S0271-5317(00)80024-X

Finke, B. (2000). *Isolierung und charakterisierung von oligosaccharide naushumanen und tierischenmilchen*. (Ph.D. thesis). University of Giessen, Shaker Verlag, Aachen, Germany.

Finkina, E. I., Shramova, E. I., Tagaev, A. A., & Ovchinnikova, T. V. (2008). A novel defensin from the lentil Lens culinaris seeds. *Biochemical and Biophysical Research Communications*, *371*(4), 860–865. doi:10.1016/j.bbrc.2008.04.161 PMID:18468512

Finucane, M.M., Stevens, G.A., Cowan, M.J., Danaei, G., Lin, J.K., Paciorek, C.J., … Ezzati, M. (2011). Global Burden of Metabolic Risk Factors of Chronic Diseases Collaborating Group (Body Mass Index). National, regional, and global trends in body-mass index since 1980: systematic analysis of health examination surveys and epidemiological studies with 960 country-years and 9·1 million participants. *Lancet*, *377*(9765), 557-67.

Fiordaliso, M., Kok, N., Desager, J. P., Goethals, F., Deboyser, D., Roberfroid, M., & Delzenne, N. (1995). Dietary oligofructose lowers triglycerides, phospholipids and cholesterol in serum and very low density lipoproteins of rats. *Lipids*, *30*(2), 163–167. doi:10.1007/BF02538270 PMID:7769973

Firestone, D. (1997) Officialmethods & recommended practices of the AOCS (5th ed.). AOCS Press.

Fischer, U. A., Carle, R., & Kammerer, D. R. (2011). Identification and quantification of phenolic compounds from pomegranate (*Punica granatum* L.) peel, mesocarp, aril and differently produced juices by HPLC-DAD–ESI/MS^n. *Food Chemistry*, *127*(2), 807–821. doi:10.1016/j.foodchem.2010.12.156 PMID:23140740

Flight, I., & Clifton, P. (2006). Cereal grains and legumes in the prevention of coronary heart disease and stroke: A review of the literature. *European Journal of Clinical Nutrition*, *60*(10), 1145–1159. doi:10.1038/sj.ejcn.1602435 PMID:16670693

Folch, J., Lees, M., & Sloane-Stanley, G. H. (1957). A simple method for the isolation and purification of total lipids from animal tissue. *The Journal of Biological Chemistry*, *226*, 497. PMID:13428781

Folkow, B. (1982). Physiological aspects of primary hypertension. *Physiological Reviews*, *62*, 347–504. PMID:6461865

Food and Agricultural Organisation. (2013). *FAOSTAT Database*. Rome: Food and Agricultural Organization.

Food and Agriculture Organization (FAO). (1988). *Traditional Food Plants*. Rome: FAO.

Food and Agriculture Organization (FAO). (2011). *Economic and Social Department: The Statistical Division*. Retrieved from http://faostat.fao.org/site/567/DesktopDefault.aspx?PageID=567#ancor

Food and Agriculture Organization. (2006). *Rice International commodity profile*. Rome: Food and Agricultural Organization. Retrieved from http://www.fao.org/fileadmin/templates/est/COMM_MARKETS_MONITORI G/Rice/Documents/Rice_Profile_Dec-06.pdf

Food and Agriculture Organization/World Health Organization. (2013). Dietary protein quality evaluation in human nutrition. Report of an FAO expert consultation. Food and Agriculture Organization. *Food and Nutrition Paper, 92.*

Food and Drug Administration. (1999). Food labeling, health claims, soy protein, and coronary heart disease. *Federal Register*, *57*, 699–733.

Food and Drug Administration. (1999). Food labeling: Health claims; soy protein and coronary heart disease. Food and Drug Administration, HHS. Final rule. *Federal Register*, *64*, 57700–57733. PMID:11010706

Food and Drug Administration. (2003). *Qualified Health Claims: Letter of Enforcement Discretion – Nuts and Coronary Heart Disease. docket no. 02P-0505*. Washington, DC: FDA.

Food and Nutrition Press. (2013). *FAORiceMarket Monitor*. Accessed June 29, (2013). http://www.fao.org/economic/est/publications/rice-ublications/rice%20marketmonitor-FoodandAgricultureOrganization

Fooks, L. J., Fuller, R., & Gibson, G. R. (1999). Prebiotics, probiotics and human gut microbiology. *International Dairy Journal*, *9*(1), 53–61. doi:10.1016/S0958-6946(99)00044-8

Fornage, M., Amos, C. I., Kardia, S., Sing, C. F., Turner, S. T., & Boerwinkle, E. (1998). Variation in the region of the angiotensin-converting enzyme gene influences interindividual differences in blood pressure levels in young white males. *Circulation*, *97*(18), 1773–1779. doi:10.1161/01.CIR.97.18.1773 PMID:9603530

Foster-Powell, K., Holt, S. H., & Brand-Miller, J. C. (2002). International table of glycemic index and glycemic load values. *The American Journal of Clinical Nutrition*, *76*(1), 5–56. PMID:12081815

Foster-Powell, K., Holt, S. H., & Brand-Miller, J. C. (2002). International table of glycemic index and glycemic load values: 2002. *The American Journal of Clinical Nutrition*, *76*(1), 5–56. PMID:12081815

Fouchier, R. A., Munster, V., Wallensten, A., Bestebroer, T. M., Herfst, S., Smith, D., & Osterhaus, A. D. et al. (2005). Characterization of a novel influenza A virus hemagglutinin subtype (H16) obtained from black-headed gulls. *Journal of Virology*, *79*(5), 2814–2822. doi:10.1128/JVI.79.5.2814-2822.2005 PMID:15709000

Fournier, L. R., Ryan Borchers, T. A., Robison, L. M., Wiediger, M., Park, J. S., Chew, B. P., & Beerman, K. A. et al. (2007). The effects of soy milk and isoflavone supplements on cognitive performance in healthy, postmenopausal women. *The Journal of Nutrition, Health & Aging*, *11*, 155–164. PMID:17435957

Fox, C., & Eberl, M. (2002). Phytic acid (IP6), novel broad spectrum anti-neoplastic agent: A systematic review. *Complementary Therapies in Medicine*, *10*(4), 229–234. doi:10.1016/S0965-2299(02)00092-4 PMID:12594974

Fox, P. F., & McSweeney, P. L. H. (1998). Lactose chapter. In *Dairy Chemistry and Biochemistry* (pp. 21–66). Thomson Science.

Francini, A., & Sebastiani, L. (2013). phenolic compounds in apple (Malus X domestica Borkh.): Compounds characterization and stability during postharvest and after processing. *Antioxidants*, *2*(3), 181–193. doi:10.3390/antiox2030181 PMID:26784345

Franke, A. A., Lai, J. F., & Halm, B. M. (2014). Absortion, distribution, metabolism, and excretion of isoflavonoids after soy intake. *Archives of Biochemistry and Biophysics*, *59*, 24–28. doi:10.1016/j.abb.2014.06.007 PMID:24946051

Franke, A. A., Lai, J. F., Halm, B. M., Pagano, I., Kono, N., Mack, W. J., & Hodis, H. N. (2012). Equol production changes over time in postmenopausal women. *The Journal of Nutritional Biochemistry*, *23*(6), 573–579. doi:10.1016/j.jnutbio.2011.03.002 PMID:21775122

Frankenfeld, C. L. (2011). *O*-desmethylangolensin: The importance of equol's lesser known cousin to human health. *Advances in Nutrition*, *2*(4), 317–324. doi:10.3945/an.111.000539 PMID:22332073

Franssen, L. R., & Krochta, J. M. (2003). Edible Coatings containing natural antimicrobials for processed foods. In S. Roller (Ed.), Naturals antimicrobials for the minimal processing of foods (pp. 120-132). Boca Raton, FL: CRC Press. doi:10.1533/9781855737037.250

Franz, C. M. A. P., Hucha, M., Mathara, J. M., Abriouel, H., Benomar, N., Reid, G., & Holzapfel, W. H. et al. (2014). African fermented foods and probiotics. *International Journal of Food Microbiology*, *190*, 84–96. doi:10.1016/j.ijfoodmicro.2014.08.033 PMID:25203619

Fraser, G. E., Lindsted, K. D., & Beeson, W. L. (1995). Effect of risk factor values on lifetime risk of and age at that first coronary event. The Adventist Health Study. *American Journal of Epidemiology*, *142*, 746–758. PMID:7572946

Fraser, G. E., Sabate, J., Beeson, W. L., & Strahan, T. M. (1992). A possible protective effect of nut consumption on risk of coronary heart disease. The Adventist Health Study. *Archives of Internal Medicine*, *152*(7), 1416–1424. doi:10.1001/archinte.1992.00400190054010 PMID:1627021

Fratianni, F., Cardinale, F., Cozzolino, A., Granese, T., Albanese, D., Di Matteo, M., & Nazzaro, F. et al. (2014). Polyphenol composition and antioxidant activity of different grass pea (*Lathyrussativus*), lentils (*Lens culinaris*), and chickpea (*Cicer arietinum*) ecotypes of the Campania region (Southern Italy). *Journal of Functional Foods*, *7*, 551–557.

Frayn, K. N. (2000). Visceral fat and insulin resistance--causative or correlative? *The British Journal of Nutrition*, *83*(S1Suppl 1), S71–S77. doi:10.1017/S0007114500000982 PMID:10889795

Freier, T. C., & Rüdiger, H. E. (1990). Lectin-binding proteins from lentil seeds as mitogens for murine B lymphocytes. *Phytochemistry*, *29*(5), 1459–1461. doi:10.1016/0031-9422(90)80100-U

Fritz, H., Seely, D., Flower, G., Skidmore, B., Fernandes, R., Vadeboncoeur, S., & Fergusson, D. et al. (2013). Soy, red clover, and isoflavones and breast cancer: A systematic review. *PLoS ONE*, *8*(11), e81968. doi:10.1371/journal.pone.0081968 PMID:24312387

Fritz, H., Seely, D., Kennedy, D. A., Fernandes, R., Cooley, K., & Fergusson, D. (2013). Green tea and lung cancer: A systematic review. *Integrative Cancer Therapies*, *12*(1), 7–24. doi:10.1177/1534735412442378 PMID:22532034

Frohlich, R. H., Kunze, M., & Kiefer, I. (1997). Cancer preventive value of natural, non-nutritive food constituents. *Acta Medica Austriaca*, *23*, 108–113. PMID:9312973

Fry, A. C., Bonner, E., Lewis, D. L., Johnson, R. L., Stone, M. H., & Kraemer, W. J. (1997). The effects of gamma-oryzanol supplementation during resistance exercise training. *International Journal of Sport Nutrition*, *7*, 318–329. PMID:9407258

Fu, C., Wang, T., Wang, Y., Chen, X., Jiao, J., Ma, F., & Bi, K. et al. (2011). Metabonomics study of the protective effects of green tea polyphenols on aging rats induced by d-galactose. *Journal of Pharmaceutical and Biomedical Analysis*, *55*(5), 1067–1074. doi:10.1016/j.jpba.2011.03.011 PMID:21444175

Fuhrman, B., & Aviram, M. (2005).Pomegranate & cardiovascular diseases: pomegranate juice polyphenolic antioxidants protect against oxidative stress & atherosclerosis development.*International Symposium on Human Health Effects of Fruits & Vegetables*, *744*, 205-216.

Fujiki, H., Imai, K., Nakachi, K., Shimizu, M., Moriwaki, H., & Suganuma, M. (2012). Challenging the effectiveness of green tea in primary and tertiary cancer prevention. *Journal of Cancer Research and Clinical Oncology*, *138*(8), 1259–1270. doi:10.1007/s00432-012-1250-y PMID:22699930

Fujiki, H., Suganuma, M., Okabe, S., Sueoka, E., Suga, K., Imai, K., & Nakachi, K. (2000). A new concept of tumor promotion by tumor necrosis factor-alpha, and cancer preventive agents (-)-epigallocatechin gallate and green tea--a review. *Cancer Detection and Prevention*, *24*(1), 91–99. PMID:10757128

Fukuda, K., Yamamoto, A., Ganzorig, K., Khuukhenbaatar, J., Senda, A., Saito, T., & Urashima, T. (2010). Chemical characterization of the oligosaccharides in Bactrian camel (*Camelusbactrianus*) milk and colostrums. *Journal of Dairy Science*, *93*(12), 5572–5587. doi:10.3168/jds.2010-3151 PMID:21094729

Fukui, T., Ishizaka, N., Rajagopalan, S., Laursen, J. B., Capers, Q. IV, Taylor, W. R., & Griendling, K. K. et al. (1997). p22phox mRNA expression and NADPH oxidase activity are increased in aortas from hypertensive rats. *Circulation Research*, *80*(1), 45–51. doi:10.1161/01.RES.80.1.45 PMID:8978321

Fukushi, J. (1966). Antioxidant effects of oryzanol. In Edible rice bran oil part – III. Hokkaido-Ritsu Eisei Kenkyushoho.

Fung, W. (2009). *Early childhood malnutrition and adult obesity: Evidence from the 1959-61 China famine.* Retrieved March 25, 2015 from http://www.cpc.unc.edu/projects/china/ publications/1219

Fung, T. T., Hu, F. B., Pereira, M. A., Liu, S., Stampfer, M. J., Coldtz, G. A., & Willet, W. C. (2002). Whole-grain intake and the risk of type 2 diabetes: A prospective study in men. *The American Journal of Clinical Nutrition*, *76*, 535–540. PMID:12197996

Gale, C. R., Ashurst, H. E., Powers, H. J., & Martyn, C. N. (2001). Antioxidant vitamin status and carotid atherosclerosis in the elderly. *The American Journal of Clinical Nutrition*, *74*, 402–408. PMID:11522566

Galgani, J. E., Ryan, D. H., & Ravussin, E. (2010). Effect of capsinoids on energy metabolism in human subjects. *The British Journal of Nutrition*, *103*(01), 38–42. doi:10.1017/S0007114509991358 PMID:19671203

Gamel, T., & Abdel-Aal, E.-S. (2012). Phenolic acid and antioxidant properties of barley wholegrain and pearling fractions. *Agricultural and Food Science*, *21*, 118–131.

Garber, K. (2012). At loose ends: Telomere theories of aging and cancer begin to converge. *Journal of the National Cancer Institute*, *104*(11), 803–806. doi:10.1093/jnci/djs271 PMID:22673587

García-Alonso, A., Goñi, I., & Saura-Calixto, F. (1998). Resistant starch and potential glycaemic index of raw and cooked legumes (lentils, chickpeas and beans). *ZeitschriftfürLebensmitteluntersuchung und-Forschung A*, *206*(4), 284-287.

Garcia, E., & Barret, D. M. (2002). Preservative treatments for fresh cut fruits and vegetables. In O. Lamikanra (Ed.), *Fresh-Cut Fruits and Vegetables* (pp. 267–304). Boca Raton, FL: CRC Press.

Garcia-Mora, P., Peñas, E., Frias, J., & Martínez-Villaluenga, C. (2014). Savinase, the most suitable enzyme for releasing peptides from lentil (*Lens culinaris* var. Castellana) protein concentrates with multifunctional properties. *Journal of Agricultural and Food Chemistry*, *62*(18), 4166–4174. doi:10.1021/jf500849u PMID:24738747

Garcia-Tejedor, A., Sanchez-Rivera, L., Recio, I., Salom, J. B., & Manzanares, P. (2015). Dairy *Debaryomyces hansenii* strains produce the antihypertensive casein-derived peptides LHLPLP and HLPLP. LWT-. *Food Science and Technology (Campinas.)*, *61*, 550–556.

Gardana, C., Canzi, E., & Simonetti, P. (2014). R(-)-*O*-desmethylangolensin is the main enantiomeric form of daidzein metabolite produced by human in vitro and in vivo. *Journal of Chromatography. B, Analytical Technologies in the Biomedical and Life Sciences*, *953-954*, 30–37. doi:10.1016/j.jchromb.2014.01.048 PMID:24561352

Gareau, M. G., Sherman, P. M., & Walker, W. A. (2010). Probiotics and the gut microbiota in intestinal health and disease. *Nature Reviews in Gastroenterology and Hepatology*, *7*(9), 503–514. doi:10.1038/nrgastro.2010.117 PMID:20664519

Gautam, R. U. P. E. S. H., & Sharma, S. (2012). Antiulcer activity of *Punica granatum* Linn. in diabetic rats. *International Journal of Pharmacy & Pharmaceutical Sciences*, *4*, 459–461.

Gawlik-Dziki, U. (2008). Effect of hydrothermal treatment on the antioxidant properties of broccoli (*Brassica oleracea* var. botrytis italica) florets. *Food Chemistry*, *109*(2), 393–401. doi:10.1016/j.foodchem.2007.12.058 PMID:26003363

Gebremariam, M. M., Zarnkow, M., & Becker, T. (2012). Teff (*Eragrostis tef*) as a raw material for malting, brewing and manufacturing of gluten-free foods and beverages: a review. *Journal of Food Science & Technology*. DOI 10.1007/s13197-012-0745-5

Gee, J. M., Du Pont, M. S., Rhodes, M. J. C., & Johnson, I. T. (1998). Quercetin glucosides interact with the intestinal glucose transport pathway. *Free Radical Biology & Medicine*, *25*(1), 19–25. doi:10.1016/S0891-5849(98)00020-3 PMID:9655517

Geleijnse, J. M., Giltay, E. J., Grobbee, D. E., Donders, A. R., & Kok, F. J. (2002). Blood pressure response to fish oil supplementation: Metaregression analysis of randomized trials. *Journal of Hypertension*, *20*(8), 1493–1499. doi:10.1097/00004872-200208000-00010 PMID:12172309

Germaine, K. A., Samman, S., Fryirs, C. G., Griffiths, P. J., Johnson, S. K., & Quail, K. J. (2008). Comparison of in vitro starch digestibility methods for predicting the glycaemic index of grain foods. *Journal of the Science of Food and Agriculture*, *88*(4), 652–658. doi:10.1002/jsfa.3130

Ghawi, S. K., Shen, Y., Niranjan, K., & Methven, L. (2014). Consumer acceptability and sensory profile of cooked broccoli with mustard seeds added to improve chemoprotective properties. *Journal of Food Science*, *79*(9), S1756–S1762. doi:10.1111/1750-3841.12556 PMID:25156799

Ghosh, A. K., Banerjee, S., Mullick, H. I., & Banerjee, J. (2011). Zingiber officinale: A natural gold. *International Journal of Pharma and Bio Sciences*, *2*, 283–294.

Ghosh, D. (2009). Future perspectives of nutrigeonomics foods: Benefits vs risks. *Indian Journal of Biochemistry & Biophysics*, *46*, 31–36. PMID:19374251

Ghosh, D. (2015). Tannins from foods to combat diseases. *International Journal of Pharma Research & Review*, *4*(5), 40–44.

Giada, M. L. R. (2013). Food phenolic compounds: Main classes, sources and their antioxidant power, oxidative stress and chronic degenerative diseases - a role for antioxidants. In Oxidative stress and chronic degenerative diseases - A role for antioxidants (pp. 87-112). IntTech Publisher.

Gianetti, J., Pedrinelli, R., Petrucci, R., Lazzerini, G., De Caterina, M., Bel-lomo, G., & De Catarina, R. (2002). Inverse association between carotid intima-media thickness and the antioxidant lycopene in atherosclerosis. *American Heart Journal*, *143*(3), 467–474. doi:10.1067/mhj.2002.120776 PMID:11868053

Gibaldi, M. (2001). Are phytoestrogens a "natural alternative" to estrogen replacement therapy? *The Western Journal of Medicine*, *173*(4), 273. doi:10.1136/ewjm.173.4.273 PMID:11017999

Giday, M., Teklehaymanot, T., Animut, A., & Mekonnen, Y. (2007). Medicinal plants of the Shinasha, Agew-awi and Amhara peoples in northwest Ethiopia. *Journal of Ethnopharmacology*, *110*(3), 516–525. doi:10.1016/j.jep.2006.10.011 PMID:17101251

Gilani, G. S., Nimal Ratnayke, W. M., Mueller, R., & Mazza, G. (2009). Effects of source of protein and supplementary extracted isoflavones and anthocyanins on longevity of Stroke-prone Spontaneously Hypertensive (SHRSP) rats. *The Journal of Toxicological Sciences*, *34*(3), 335–341. doi:10.2131/jts.34.335 PMID:19483387

Gilbert-Diamond, D., Cottingham, K. L., Gruber, J. F., Punshon, T., Sayarath, V., Gandolfi, A. J., & Karagas, M. (2011). Rice consumption contributes to arsenic exposure in US women. *Proceedings of the National Academy of Sciences of the United States of America*, *108*(51), 20656–20660. doi:10.1073/pnas.1109127108 PMID:22143778

Gilchrest, B. A. (1984). *Skin and Aging Process*. Boca Raton, FL: CRC Press. Inc.

Gill, C., & Rowland, I. (2003). Cancer. In Functional Dairy Products (pp. 19-53). Cambridge, UK: Woodhead Publishers.

Girish, T. K., Pratape, V. M., & Rao, U. J. S. P. (2012). Nutrient distribution, phenolic acid composition, antioxidant and alphaglucosidase inhibitory potentials of black gram (*Vigna mungo* L.) and its milled byproducts. *Food Research International*, *46*(1), 370–377. doi:10.1016/j.foodres.2011.12.026

Gnädig, S., Xue, Y., Berdeaux, O., Chardigny, J. M., & Sebedio, J. L. (2003). Conjugated linoleic acid (CLA) as a functional ingredient. In Functional Dairy Products (pp. 263-298). CRC Press.

Gobbetti, M., Minervini, F., & Rizzello, C. G. (2004). Angiotensin I-converting enzyme-inhibitory and antimicrobial bioactive peptides. *International Journal of Dairy Society*, *57*(2-3), 173–188. doi:10.1111/j.1471-0307.2004.00139.x

Goenka, P., Sarawgi, A., Karun, V., Nigan, A., Dutta, S., & Marwah, N. (2013). Camellia sinensis (tea): implications and role in preventing dental decay. *Pharmacognosy Reviews*, *7*(14), 152-6.

Goffman, F. D., & Bergman, C. J. (2004). Rice kernel phenolic content and its relationship with antiradical efficiency. *Journal of the Science of Food and Agriculture*, *84*(10), 1235–1240. doi:10.1002/jsfa.1780

Gohari, A. R., Saeidnia, S., & Mahmoodabadi, M. K. (2013). An overview on saffron, phytochemicals, and medicinal properties. *Pharmacognocy Reviews*, *7*(13), 61–66. doi:10.4103/0973-7847.112850 PMID:23922458

Golden, E. B., Lam, P. Y., Kardosh, A., Gaffney, K. J., Cadenas, E., Louie, S. G., & Schönthal, A. H. et al. (2009). Green tea polyphenols block the anticancer effects of bortezomib and other boronic acid-based proteasome inhibitors. *Blood*, *113*(23), 5927–5937. doi:10.1182/blood-2008-07-171389 PMID:19190249

González-Granillo, M., Steffensen, K. R., Granados, O., Torres, N., Korach-André, M., Ortiz, V., & Tovar, A. R. et al. (2012). Soy protein isoflavones differentially regulate liver X receptor isoforms to modulate lipid metabolism and cholesterol transport in the liver and intestine in mice. *Diabetologia*, *55*, 2469–2478. PMID:22739758

González-Sarrías, A., Giménez-Bastida, J. A., García-Conesa, M. T., Gómez-Sánchez, M. B., García-Talavera, N. V., Gil-Izquierdo, A., & Espín, J. C. et al. (2010). Occurrence of urolithins, gut microbiota ellagic acid metabolites & proliferation markers expression response in the human prostate gland upon consumption of walnuts & pomegranate juice. *Journal of Molecular Nutrition & Food Research*, *54*(3), 311–322. doi:10.1002/mnfr.200900152 PMID:19885850

Gopala Krishna, A. G., Khatoon, S., Sheila, P. M., Sarmandal, C. V., & Indira, T. N. (2001). Effect of refining crude rice bran oil on the retention of oryzanol in the refined oil. *Journal of the American Oil Chemists' Society*, *78*(2), 127–131. doi:10.1007/s11746-001-0232-0

Gopala Krishna, A. G., Prabhakar, J. V., & Sen, D. P. (1984). Effect of degree of milling on tocopherol content of rice bran. *Journal of Food Science and Technology*, *21*, 222–224.

Gopu, V., Kothandapani, S., & Shetty, P. H. (2015). Quorum quenching activity of *Syzygium cumini* L. Skeels and its anthocyanin malvidin against *Klebsiella pneumonia. Microbial Pathogenesis*, *79*, 61–69. doi:10.1016/j.micpath.2015.01.010 PMID:25637095

Gorgen, M., Turatti, K., Medeiros, A. R., Buffon, A., Bonan, C. D., Sarkis, J. J., & Pereira, G. S. (2005). Aqueous Extract of *Ilex paraguariensis* Decreases Nucleotide Hydrolysis in Rat Blood Serum. *Journal of Ethnopharmacology*, *97*(1), 73–77. doi:10.1016/j.jep.2004.10.015 PMID:15652278

Gorinstein, S., Cvikrov, M., Machackova, I., Haruenkit, R., Park, Y., Junge, S., & Trakhtenberg, S. et al. (2004). Characterization of antioxidant compounds in Jaffa sweeties and white grapefruits. *Food Chemistry*, *84*(4), 503–510. doi:10.1016/S0308-8146(03)00127-4

Gorzalczany, S., Filip, R., Alonso, M. R., Mino, J., Ferraro, G. E., & Acevedo, C. (2001). Choleretic Effect and Intestinal Propulsion of 'Mate' (*Ilex paraguariensis*) and its Substitutes or Adulterants. *Journal of Ethnopharmacology*, *75*(2-3), 291–294. doi:10.1016/S0378-8741(01)00179-9 PMID:11297866

Gosmann, G., Guillaume, D., Taketa, A. T., & Schenkel, E. P. (1995). Triterpenoid Saponins from *Ilex paraguariensis. Journal of Natural Products*, *58*(3), 438–441. doi:10.1021/np50117a015 PMID:7775986

Gossé, F., Guyot, S., Roussi, S., Lobstein, A., Fischer, B., Seiler, N., & Raul, F. (2005). Chemopreventive properties of apple procyanidins on human colon cancer-derived metastatic SW620 cells and in a rat model of colon carcinogenesis. *Carcinogenesis*, *26*(7), 1291–1295. doi:10.1093/carcin/bgi074 PMID:15790589

Gotto, A. M. Jr. (2003). Antioxidants, statins, and atherosclerosis. *Journal of the American College of Cardiology*, *41*(7), 1205–1210. doi:10.1016/S0735-1097(03)00082-2 PMID:12679223

Goufo, P., & Trindade, H. (2014). Rice antioxidants: Phenolic acids, flavonoids, anthocyanins, proanthocyanidins, tocopherols, tocotrienols, γ-oryzanol, and phytic acid. *Food Science Nutrition*, *2*(2), 75–104. doi:10.1002/fsn3.86 PMID:24804068

Gou, Z., Jiang, S., Zheng, C., Tian, Z., & Lin, X. (2015). Equol inhibits LPS-induced oxidative stress and enhances the immune response in chicken HD11 macrophages. *Cellular Physiology and Biochemistry*, *36*(2), 611–621. doi:10.1159/000430124 PMID:25997976

Graf, D., Di Cagno, R., Fåk, F., Flint, H. J., Nyman, M., Saarela, M., & Watzl, B. (2015). Contribution of diet to the composition of the human gut microbiota. *Microbial Ecology in Health and Disease*, *26*, 26164. PMID:25656825

Graf, E., & Eaton, J. W. (1990). Antioxidant functions of phytic acid. *Free Radical Biology & Medicine*, *8*(1), 61–69. doi:10.1016/0891-5849(90)90146-A PMID:2182395

Graham, H. W. (1992). Green tea composition, consumption, and polyphenol chemistry. *Preventive Medicine*, *21*(3), 334–350. doi:10.1016/0091-7435(92)90041-F PMID:1614995

Granito, M., Champ, M., David, A., Bonnet, C., & Guerra, M. (2001). Identification of gas-producing components in different varieties of *Phaseolus vulgaris* by in vitro fermentation. *Journal of the Science of Food and Agriculture*, *81*(6), 543–550. doi:10.1002/jsfa.839

Grassi, D., Necozione, S., Lippi, C., Croce, G., Valeri, L., Pasqualetti, P., & Ferri, C. et al. (2005). Cocoa reduces blood pressure and insulin resistance and improves endothelium-dependent vasodilation in hypertensives. *Hypertension*, *46*(2), 398–405. doi:10.1161/01.HYP.0000174990.46027.70 PMID:16027246

Greenwald, P., Clifford, C., & Milner, J. (2001). Diet and cancer prevention. *European Journal of Cancer*, *37*(8), 948–965. doi:10.1016/S0959-8049(01)00070-3 PMID:11334719

Grundy, S. M. (1999). The optimal ratio of fat-to-carbohydrate in the diet. *Annual Review of Nutrition*, *19*(1), 325–341. doi:10.1146/annurev.nutr.19.1.325 PMID:10448527

Grzeskowiak, L., Collado, M. C., Mangani, C., Maleta, K., Laitinen, K., Ashorn, P., & Salminen, S. et al. (2012). Distinct gut microbiota in southeastern African and northern European infants. *Journal of Pediatric Gastroenterology and Nutrition*, *54*(6), 812–816. doi:10.1097/MPG.0b013e318249039c PMID:22228076

Guadamuro, L., Delgado, S., Redruello, B., Flórez, A. B., Suárez, A., Martínez-Camblor, P., & Mayo, B. (2015). Equol status and changes in faecal microbiota in menopausal women receiving long-term treatment for menopause symptoms with a soy-isoflavone concentrate. *Frontiers in Microbiology*, *6*, 777. doi:10.3389/fmicb.2015.00777 PMID:26300856

Guan, L., Huang, Y., & Chen, Z. Y. (2008). Developmental and reproductive toxicity of soybean isoflavones to immature SD rats. *Biomedical and Environmental Sciences*, *21*(3), 197–204. doi:10.1016/S0895-3988(08)60029-X PMID:18714816

Güçlü-Üstündağ, Ö., & Mazza, G. (2007). Saponins: Properties, applications and processing. *Critical Reviews in Food Science and Nutrition*, *47*(3), 231–258. doi:10.1080/10408390600698197 PMID:17453922

Guerra, E., Verardo, V., & Carboni, M. F. (2015). Determination of bioactive compounds in cream obtained as a by-product during cheese-making: Influence of cow's diet on lipid quality. *International Dairy Journal*, *42*, 16–25. doi:10.1016/j.idairyj.2014.11.004

Guilbert, S. (1986). Technology and application of edible protective films. In M. Mathlouthi (Ed.), *Food packaging and preservation: Theory and practice* (pp. 371–393). London: Elsevier Applied Science Publishing Co.

Guillamon, E., Pedrosa, M. M., Burbano, C., Cuadrado, C., de Cortes Sánchez, M., & Muzquiz, M. (2008). The trypsin inhibitors present in seed of different grain legume species and cultivar. *Food Chemistry*, *107*(1), 68–74. doi:10.1016/j.foodchem.2007.07.029

Gundala, S. R., Mukkavilli, R., Yang, C., Yadav, P., Tandon, V., Vangala, S., & Aneja, R. et al. (2014). Enterohepatic recirculation of bioactive ginger phytochemicals is associated with enhanced tumor growth-inhibitory activity of ginger extract. *Carcinogenesis*, *35*(6), 1320–1329. doi:10.1093/carcin/bgu011 PMID:24431413

Gupta, A. (2012). Assessing renal function in patients suffering from liver diseases. (Unpublished Doctoral Thesis). SJJT University. Retrieved from http://shodhganga.inflibnet.ac.in/handle/10603/10018

Gupta, M., Sharma, S., Gautam, A. K., & Bhadauria, R. (2011). *Momordica charantia* Linn. (karela): Nature's silent healer. *International Journal of Pharmaceutical Sciences Review and Research*, *11*, 32–37.

Gupta, R. K., Patel, A. K., Shah, N., Choudhary, A. K., Jha, U. K., Yadav, U. C., & Pakuwal, U. et al. (2014). Oxidative stress and antioxidants in disease and cancer: A review. *Asian Pacific Journal of Cancer Prevention*, *15*(11), 4405–4409. doi:10.7314/APJCP.2014.15.11.4405 PMID:24969860

Gurfinkel, D., & Rao, A. (2003). Soyasaponins: The relationship between chemical structure and colon anticarcinogenic activity. *Nutrition and Cancer*, *47*(1), 24–33. doi:10.1207/s15327914nc4701_3 PMID:14769534

Gutteridge, J. M. (1995). Lipid peroxidation and antioxidants as biomarkers of tissue damage. *Clinical Chemistry*, *41*, 1819–1828. PMID:7497639

Habauzit, V., & Morand, C. (2012). Evidence for a protective effect of polyphenols-containing foods on cardiovascular health: An update for clinicians. *Therapeutic Advances in Chronic Diseases*, *3*(2), 87–106. doi:10.1177/2040622311430006 PMID:23251771

Hagenmaier, R. D., & Shaw, P. E. (1990). Moisture permeability of edible films made with fatty acid and (hydroxypropyl) methylcellulose. *Journal of Agricultural and Food Chemistry*, *38*(9), 1799–1803. doi:10.1021/jf00099a004

Haggblade, S., Duodu, G., Kabasa, J. D., Minnaar, A., Ojijo, N., & Taylor, J. R. N. (2014). *Bending the curve in Africa's nutrition transition*. Retrieved July 20, 2015 from http://www.ifama.org/files/conf/2014%20Conference/T1Bending%281%29.pdf

Hahn, Y.S., & Oh, J.Y., & Song, J.E. (2002). The study on amylolytic enzyme and protease activities of kimchi. *Korean J. Food Sci. Technol.*, *34*, 269–273.

Hak, A. E., Stampfer, M. J., Campos, H., Sesso, H. D., Gaziano, J. M., Willett, W., & Ma, J. (2003). Plasma carotenoids and tocopherols and risk of myocardial infarction in a low-risk population of US male physicians. *Circulation*, *108*(7), 802–807. doi:10.1161/01.CIR.0000084546.82738.89 PMID:12900344

Halliwell, B., & Chirico, S. (1993). Lipid peroxidation: Its mechanism, measure-ment, and significance. *The American Journal of Clinical Nutrition*, *57*(Suppl), 715–725. PMID:8475889

Halliwell, B., & Gutteridge, J. M. C. (1999). *Free radicals in biology and medicine* (2nd ed.). Oxford, UK: Clarendon Press.

Halliwell, B., Zhao, K., & Whiteman, M. (2000). The gastrointestinal tract: A major site of antioxidant action? *Free Radical Research*, *33*(6), 819–830. doi:10.1080/10715760000301341 PMID:11237104

Hall, M. C., O'Brien, B., & McCormack, T. (2007). Equol producer status, salivary estradiol profile and urinary excretion of isoflavones in Irish Caucasian women, following ingestion of soymilk. *Steroids*, *72*(1), 64–70. doi:10.1016/j.steroids.2006.10.010 PMID:17157887

Halton, T. L., Willett, W. C., Liu, S., Manson, J. E., Albert, C. M., Rexrode, K., & Hu, F. B. (2006). Low carbohydrate-diet score and the risk of coronary heart disease in women. *The New England Journal of Medicine*, *355*(19), 1991–2002. doi:10.1056/NEJMoa055317 PMID:17093250

Hamden, K., Jaouadi, B., Carreau, S., Aouidet, A., & Elfeki, A. (2011). Therapeutic effects of soy isoflavones on α-amylase activity, insulin deficiency, liver-kidney function and metabolic disorders in diabetic rats. *Natural Product Research*, *25*(3), 244–255. doi:10.1080/14786411003683117 PMID:21108110

Hammond N (1994). Functional & nutritional characteristics of rice bran extracts. *Cereal Foods World, 39*, 752-754.

Hamzah, R. U., Jagam, A. A., Makun, H. A., & Engwin, E. C. (2013). *Antioxidant properties of selected African vegetables, fruits and mushrooms: A review.* Retrieved March 25, 2015 from

Hamzah, R. U., Jigam, A. A., Makun, H. A., & Egwim, E. C. (2014). Phytochemical screening and invitro antioxidant activity of methanolic extract of selected Nigerian vegetables. *Asian Journal of Basis and Applied Sciences*, *1*(1), 1–14.

Han, C., Zhao, Y., Leonard, S. W., & Traber, M. G. (2004). Edible coatings to improve storability and enhance nutritional value of fresh and frozen strawberries *Fragaria ananassa*) and raspberries (*Rubus ideaus*). *Postharvest Biology and Technology*, *33*(1), 67–78. doi:10.1016/j.postharvbio.2004.01.008

Han, I. H. (2005). *Oligosaccharide reduction, protein digestibility improvement, antioxidant activity determination and phenolic compounds identification in legumes*. Washington State University.

Haniadka, R., Saxena, A., Shivashankara, A. R., Fayad, R., Palatty, P. L., Nazreth, N., & Shrinath Baliga, M. et al. (2013). Ginger protects the liver against the toxic effects of xenobiotic compounds: Preclinical observations. *Journal of Nutrition and Food Sciences.*, *3*(5), 1–6.

Han, J. S., Lee, S. H., Lee, K. I., & Park, K. Y. (1995). Standardizations of traditional special kimchi in Kyungsang province. *The East Asian Society of Dietary Life*, *5*(2), 27–38.

Han, K., Bose, S., Wang, J. H., Kim, B. S., Kim, M. J., Kim, E. J., & Kim, H. (2015). Contrasting effects of fresh and fermented kimchi consumption on gut microbiota composition and gene expression related to metabolic syndrome in obese Korean women. *Molecular Nutrition & Food Research*, *59*(5), 1004–1008. doi:10.1002/mnfr.201400780 PMID:25688926

Hanmoungjai, P., Pyle, D. L., & Niranjan, K. (2001). Enzymatic process for extracting oil & protein from rice bran. *Journal of the American Oil Chemists' Society*, *78*(8), 817–821. doi:10.1007/s11746-001-0348-2

Hanson, M. G., Zahradka, P., & Taylor, C. G. (2014). Lentil-based diets attenuate hypertension and large-artery remodelling in spontaneously hypertensive rats. *The British Journal of Nutrition*, *111*(04), 690–698. doi:10.1017/S0007114513002997 PMID:24063808

Han, X., Shen, T., & Lou, H. (2007). Dietary polyphenols and their biological significance. *International Journal of Molecular Sciences*, *8*(9), 950–988. doi:10.3390/i8090950

Harland, J., & Haffner, T. (2008). Systematic review, meta-analysis and regression of randomised controlled trials reporting an association between an intake of circa 25 g soya protein per day and blood cholesterol. *Atherosclerosis*, *200*(1), 13–27. doi:10.1016/j.atherosclerosis.2008.04.006 PMID:18534601

Harrison, R. (2006). Milk xanthine oxidase: Properties and physiological roles. *International Dairy Journal*, *16*(6), 546–554. doi:10.1016/j.idairyj.2005.08.016

Haslam, D. W., & James, W. P. (2005). Obesity. *Lancet*, *366*(9492), 1197–1209. doi:10.1016/S0140-6736(05)67483-1 PMID:16198769

Hassan, M. A. M., & Youssef, A. M. K. (2012). Effect of toasting and microwaving on gross chemical composition, total phenolics, antioxidant activity and phenolic acids fractionation of white beans flour (*Phaseolus vulgaris* L.). *World Applied Sciences Journal*, *18*, 731–736.

Hayouni, E. A., Miled, K., Boubaker, S., Bellasfar, Z., Abedrabba, M., Iwaski, H., & Hamdi, M. et al. (2011). Hydroalcoholic extract based-ointment from *Punica granatum* L. peels with enhanced in vivo healing potential on dermal wounds. *Phytomedicine*, *18*(11), 976–984. doi:10.1016/j.phymed.2011.02.011 PMID:21466954

Heber, D., Seeram, N. P., Wyatt, H., Henning, S. M., Zhang, Y., Ogden, L. G., & Hill, J. O. et al. (2007). Safety and antioxidant activity of a pomegranate ellagitannin-enriched polyphenol dietary supplement in overweight individuals with increased waist size. *Journal of Agricultural and Food Chemistry*, *55*(24), 10050–10054. doi:10.1021/jf071689v PMID:17966977

Heck, C. I., & De Mejia, E. G. (2007). Yerba Mate Tea (*Ilex paraguariensis*): A Comprehensive Review on Chemistry, Health Implications and Technological Considerations. *Journal of Food Science*, *72*(9), 138–151. doi:10.1111/j.1750-3841.2007.00535.x PMID:18034743

Hedlund, T. E., Johannes, W. U., & Miller, G. J. (2003). Soy isoflavonoid equol modulates the growth of benign and malignant prostatic epithelial cells *in vitro*. *The Prostate*, *54*(1), 68–78. doi:10.1002/pros.10137 PMID:12481257

He, F. J., & Chen, J. Q. (2013). Consumption of soybean, soy foods, soy isoflavones and breast cancer incidence: Differences between Chinese women and women in Western countries and possible mechanisms. *Food Science and Human Wellness*, *2*(3-4), 146–161. doi:10.1016/j.fshw.2013.08.002

Hefni, M., Öhrvik, V., Tabekha, M., & Witthöft, C. (2010). Folate content in foods commonly consumed in Egypt. *Food Chemistry*, *121*(2), 540–545. doi:10.1016/j.foodchem.2009.12.044

Hegde, A. M., Rai, K., & Padmanabhan, V. (2009). Total antioxidant capacity of saliva and its relation with early childhood caries and rampant caries. *The Journal of Clinical Pediatric Dentistry*, *33*(3), 231–234. doi:10.17796/jcpd.33.3.c730518021m56077 PMID:19476096

Hegsted, M., & Windhauser, M. M. (1993). Reducing human heart disease risk with rice bran. *Louisiana Agriculture*, *36*, 22–23.

Heim, K. E., Tagliaferro, A. R., & Bobilya, D. J. (2002). Flavonoid antioxidants: Chemistry, metabolism and structure-activity relationships. *The Journal of Nutritional Biochemistry*, *13*(10), 527–584. doi:10.1016/S0955-2863(02)00208-5 PMID:12550068

Heinonen, S., Hoikkala, A., Wähälä, K., & Adlerreutz, H. (2003). Metabolism of the soy isoflavones daidzein, genistein and glycitein in human subjects. Identification of new metabolites having an intact isoflavonoid skeleton. *The Journal of Steroid Biochemistry and Molecular Biology*, *87*(4-5), 285–299. doi:10.1016/j.jsbmb.2003.09.003 PMID:14698210

Heiss, M. L., & Heiss, R. J. (2007). *The story of tea: a cultural history and drinking guide*. New York: Ten Speed Press.

Helen, S. (2010). *Tea, a global history*. Reaktion Books Ltd.

Hemavathy, J., & Prabhakar, J. V. (1987). Lipid composition of rice (*Oryza sativa* L.) bran. J. *Journal of the American Oil Chemists' Society*, *64*(7), 1016–1019. doi:10.1007/BF02542441

Hemmati, A. A., Rezaie, A., & Darabpour, P. (2013). Preventive effects of pomegranate seed extract on bleomycin-induced pulmonary fibrosis in rat. *Jundishapur Journal of Natural Pharmaceutical Products*, *8*(2), 76–80. doi:10.17795/jjnpp-8821 PMID:24624192

Henon, G., Recseg, K., & Kovari, K. (2001). Wax analysis of vegetable oils using liquid chromatography on a double adsorbent layer of silica gel & silver nitrate impregnated silica gel. *Journal of the American Oil Chemists' Society*, *78*(4), 401–410. doi:10.1007/s11746-001-0275-2

Herb Palace. (2004). *History of Herbal Medicine.* Retrieved November 9, 2015 from, http://www.herbpalace.com/alternative-medicine/herbal-medicine.html

Hermenegildo, C., Oviedo, P. J., García-Pérez, M. A., Tarín, J. J., & Cano, A. (2005). Effects of phytoestrogens genistein and daidzein on prostacyclin production by human endothelial cells. *The Journal of Pharmacology and Experimental Therapeutics*, *315*(2), 722–728. doi:10.1124/jpet.105.090456 PMID:16046614

Hermsdorff, H. H., Zulet, M. A., Abete, I., & Martinez, J. A. (2011). A legume-based hypocaloric diet reduces proinflammatory status and improves metabolic features in overweight/obese subjects. *European Journal of Nutrition*, *50*(1), 61–69. doi:10.1007/s00394-010-0115-x PMID:20499072

Hernandez-Munoz, P., Almenar, E., Ocio, M. J., & Gavara, R. (2006). Effect of calcium dips and chitosan coatings on postharvest life of strawberries (Fragaria × Ananassa). *Postharvest Biology and Technology*, *39*(3), 247–253. doi:10.1016/j.postharvbio.2005.11.006

Hernández-Salazar, M., Osorio-Diaz, P., Loarca-Piña, G., Reynoso-Camacho, R., Tovar, J., & Bello-Pérez, L. A. (2010). *In vitro* fermentability and antioxidant capacity of the indigestible fraction of cooked black beans (*Phaseolus vulgaris* L.), lentils (*Lens culinaris* L.) and chickpeas (*Cicer arietinum* L.). *Journal of the Science of Food and Agriculture*, *90*(9), 1417–1422. doi:10.1002/jsfa.3954 PMID:20549791

Herrmann, K. (1976). Flavonols and flavones in food plants: A review. *Journal of Food Technology*, *11*(5), 433–448. doi:10.1111/j.1365-2621.1976.tb00743.x

Hertog, M. G. L., Kromhout, D., Aravanis, C., Blackburn, H., Buzina, R., Fidanza, F., & Nedeljkovic, S. et al. (1995). Flavonoid intake and long-term risk of coronary heart disease and cancer in the Seven Countries Country. *Archives of Internal Medicine*, *155*(4), 381–386. doi:10.1001/archinte.1995.00430040053006 PMID:7848021

Hertog, M. G., Feskens, E. J., Hollman, P. C., Katan, M. B., & Kromhout, D. (1993). Dietary antioxidant flavonoids and risk of coronary heart disease: The Zutphen Elderly study. *Lancet*, *342*(8878), 1007–1011. doi:10.1016/0140-6736(93)92876-U PMID:8105262

Hibino, K., Kidzu, T., Masumura, T., Ohtsuki, K., Tanaka, K., Kawabata, K., & Fujii, S. (1989). Amino acid composition of rice prolamin polypeptides. *Agricultural and Biological Chemistry*, *53*, 513–518.

Higdon, J. (2002). *Tea*. Linus Pauling Institute. Retrieved November 2, 2015 from http://lpi.oregonstate.edu/book/export/html/435

Higdon, J. V., & Frei, B. (2006). Coffee and health: A review of recent human research. *Critical Reviews in Food Science and Nutrition*, *46*(2), 101–123. doi:10.1080/10408390500400009 PMID:16507475

Hill, C. B., Williams, P. H., Carlson, D. G., & Tookey, H. L. (1987). Variation in glucosinolates in Oriental Brassica vegetables. *Journal of the American Society for Horticultural Science*, *112*, 309–313.

Hilliam, M. (2003). Future for dairy products ingredients in the functional foods market. *Australian Journal of Dairy Technology*, *58*, 98–103.

Hinton, J. J. C., & Shaw, B. (1954). The distribution of nicotinic acid in the rice grain. *The British Journal of Nutrition*, *8*(01), 65–71. doi:10.1079/BJN19540010 PMID:13140830

Hodge, A. M., English, D. R., McCredie, M. R., Severi, G., Boyle, P., Hopper, J. L., & Giles, G. G. (2004). Foods, nutrients and prostate cancer. *Cancer Causes & Control*, *15*(1), 11–20. doi:10.1023/B:CACO.0000016568.25127.10 PMID:14970730

Hodge, A. M., English, D. R., O'Dea, K., & Giles, G. G. (2004). Glycemic index and dietary fiber and the risk of type 2 diabetes. *Diabetes Care*, *27*(11), 2701–2706. doi:10.2337/diacare.27.11.2701 PMID:15505008

Holden, J. M., Bhagwat, S. A., Haytowitz, D. B., Gebhardt, S. E., Dwyen, J. T., Peterson, J., & Balentine, D. et al. (2005). Development of a database of critically evaluated flavonoids data: Application of USDA's data quality evaluation system. *Journal of Food Composition and Analysis*, *18*(8), 829–844. doi:10.1016/j.jfca.2004.07.002

Hollman, P. C. H., & Katan, M. B. (1999, September). (199) Dietary flavonoids: Intake, health effects and bioavailability. *Food and Chemical Toxicology*, *37*(9-10), 937–942. doi:10.1016/S0278-6915(99)00079-4 PMID:10541448

Hollman, P. C., & Katan, M. B. (1997). Absorption, metabolism and health effects of dietary flavonoids in man. *Biomedicine and Pharmacotherapy*, *51*(8), 305–310. doi:10.1016/S0753-3322(97)88045-6 PMID:9436520

Holse, M., Husted, S., & Hansen, A. (2010). Chemical composition of Marama beans (*Tylosema esculentum*): A wild African bean with unexploited potential. *Journal of Food Composition and Analysis*, *23*(6), 648–657. doi:10.1016/j.jfca.2010.03.006

Hong, H. J., Kim, E., Cho, D., & Kim, T. S. (2010). Differential suppression of heat-killed lactobacilli isolated from kimchi, a Korean traditional food, on airway hyperresponsiveness in mice. *Journal of Clinical Immunology*, *30*(3), 449–458. doi:10.1007/s10875-010-9375-8 PMID:20204477

Hong, S. J., Kim, S. I., Kwon, S. M., Lee, J. R., & Chung, B. C. (2002). Comparative study of concentration of isoflavones and lignans in plasma and prostatic tissues of normal control and benign prostatic hyperplasia. *Yonsei Medical Journal*, *43*(2), 236–241. doi:10.3349/ymj.2002.43.2.236 PMID:11971218

Hong, Y. J., Tomas-Barberan, F. A., Kader, A. A., & Mitchell, A. E. (2006). The flavonoid glycosides and procyanidin composition of deglet noor dates (*Phoenix dactylifera*). *Journal of Agricultural and Food Chemistry*, *54*(6), 2405–2411. doi:10.1021/jf0581776 PMID:16536626

Hooper, L., Kroon, P. A., Rimm, E. B., Cohn, J. S., Harvey, I., Le Cornu, K. A., & Cassidy, A. et al. (2008). Flavonoids, flavonoid-rich foods, and cardiovascular risk: A meta-analysis of randomized controlled trials. *The American Journal of Clinical Nutrition*, *88*, 38–50. PMID:18614722

Hoover, R., Hughes, T., Chung, H., & Liu, Q. (2010). Composition, molecular structure, properties, and modification of pulse starches: A review. *Food Research International*, *43*(2), 399–413. doi:10.1016/j.foodres.2009.09.001

Hoover, R., & Ratnayake, W. (2002). Starch characteristics of black bean, chick pea, lentil, navy bean and pinto bean cultivars grown in Canada. *Food Chemistry*, *78*(4), 489–498. doi:10.1016/S0308-8146(02)00163-2

Hoque, M. M., Bari, I. M. L., Inatsu, Y., & Kawamoto, S. (2006). Antibacterial activity of some Asian Spices and Herbs against Selected Potent Food Borne Pathogens and Spoilage Bacteria. In *Proceeding of the Japan-Bangladesh Joint International Conference on Microbiology Education and the Prospect of Japanese Collaboration in Education and Research* (*vol. 2*, pp. 22-30). Academic Press.

Hoque, M. M., Bari, I. M. L., Vijay, Y. K. J., & Kawampto, S. (2008). Antibacterial activity of cloves and cinnamon extracts against food borne pathogens and spoilage bacteria and inactivation of *Listeria monocytogenes* in ground chicken meat with their essential oils. *Rep. Natural Food Researh*, *72*, 9–21.

Hornych, A., Girault, F., Oravec, S., Forette, B., & Horrobin, D. (2001). Effect of gamma-linolenic acid on plasma and membrane lipids and renal prostaglandins in old subjects. *Klin Biochem Metab*, *9*, 28–34.

Ho, S. C., Chan, S. G., Yip, Y. B., Chan, C. S., Woo, J. L., & Sham, A. (2008). Change in bone mineral density and its determinants in pre- and perimenopausal Chinese women: The Hong Kong Perimenopausal Women Osteoporosis Study. *Osteoporosis International*, *19*(12), 1785–1796. doi:10.1007/s00198-008-0614-2 PMID:18437272

Hosoda, K., Furuta, T., & Ishii, K. (2011). Metabolism and disposition of isoflavone conjugated metabolites in humans after ingestion of kinako. *Drug Metabolism and Disposition: the Biological Fate of Chemicals*, *39*(9), 1762–1767. doi:10.1124/dmd.111.038281 PMID:21622628

Hossain, M. (1997). Rice supply and demand in Asia: a socioeconomic and biophysical analysis. In *Proceedings of the Second International Symposium on Systems Approaches for Agricultural Development*. doi:10.1007/978-94-011-5416-1_20

Hosseinian, F. S., Li, W., & Beta, T. (2008). Measurement of anthocyanins and other phytochemicals in purple wheat. *Food Chemistry*, *109*(4), 916–924. doi:10.1016/j.foodchem.2007.12.083 PMID:26050008

Hou, I. C., Amarnani, S., Chong, M. T., & Bishayee, A. (2013). Green tea and the risk of gastric cancer: Epidemiological evidence. *World Journal of Gastroenterology*, *19*(24), 3713–3722. doi:10.3748/wjg.v19.i24.3713 PMID:23840110

Houston, M. C. (2005). Nutraceuticals, vitamins, antioxidants, and minerals in the prevention and treatment of hypertension. *Progress in Cardiovascular Diseases*, *47*(6), 396–449. doi:10.1016/j.pcad.2005.01.004 PMID:16115519

Hsieh, Y. L., Pai, P., Ho, T. J., Chung, L. C., Cheng, Y. C., Wu, C. H., & Huang, C. Y. et al. (2014). Effects of Garlic Oil on Interleukin-6 Mediated Cardiac Hypertrophy in Hypercholesterol-Fed Hamsters. *The Chinese Journal of Physiology*, *57*(6), 320–328. doi:10.4077/CJP.2014.BAC261 PMID:25575520

Hsu, E. (2006). Reflections on the discovery of the antimalarial qinghao. *British Journal of Clinical Pharmacology*, *61*(6), 666–670. doi:10.1111/j.1365-2125.2006.02673.x PMID:16722826

Hsu, S. P., Wu, M. S., Yang, C. C., Huang, K. C., Liou, S. Y., Hsu, S. M., & Chien, C. T. (2007). Chronic green tea extract supplementation reduces hemodialysis-enhanced production of hydrogen peroxide and hypochlorous acid, atherosclerotic factors, and proinflammatory cytokines. *The American Journal of Clinical Nutrition*, *86*, 539–547. PMID:17991670

Huang, T., Duan, K., Huang, S., & Chen, C. W. (2006). Production of polyhydroxyalkanoates from inexpensive extruded rice bran & starch by Haloferax mediterranei. *Journal of Industrial Microbiology & Biotechnology*, *33*(8), 701–706. doi:10.1007/s10295-006-0098-z PMID:16491353

Hu, C., Zawistowski, J., Ling, W., & Kitts, D. D. (2003). Black rice (*Oryza sativa* L. *indica*) pigmented fraction suppresses both reactive oxygen species and nitric oxide in chemical and biological model systems. *Journal of Agricultural and Food Chemistry*, *51*(18), 5271–5277. doi:10.1021/jf034466n PMID:12926869

Hudson, E. A., Dinh, P. A., Kokubun, T., Simmonds, M. S. J., & Gescher, A. (2000). Characterization of potentially chemopreventive phenols in extracts of brown rice that inhibit the growth of human breast and colon cancer cells. *Cancer Epidemiology, Biomarkers & Prevention*, *9*, 1163–1170. PMID:11097223

Hu, E., Pan, A., Malik, V., & Sun, Q. (2012). White rice consumption and risk of type 2 diabetes: Meta-analysis and systematic review. *BMJ (Clinical Research Ed.)*, *344*(mar15 3), e1454. doi:10.1136/bmj.e1454 PMID:22422870

Huebner, F. R., Bietz, J. A., Webb, B. D., & Juliano, B. O. (1990). Rice cultivar identification by high-performance liquid chromatography of endosperm proteins. *Cereal Chemistry*, *67*, 129–135.

Hu, F. B., Stampfer, M. J., Manson, J. E., Rimm, E. B., Colditz, G. A., Ros-ner, B. A., & Willet, W. et al. (1998). Frequent nut consumption and risk of coronary heart disease in women: Prospective cohort study. *British Medical Journal*, *317*(7169), 1341–1345. doi:10.1136/bmj.317.7169.1341 PMID:9812929

Hu, J., La, V. C., Negri, E., Chatenoud, L., Bosetti, C., Jia, X., & Wang, C. et al. (1999). Diet and brain cancer in adults: A case-control study in northeast China. *International Journal of Cancer*, *81*(1), 20–23. doi:10.1002/(SICI)1097-0215(19990331)81:1<20::AID-IJC4>3.0.CO;2-2 PMID:10077146

Hummelova, J., Rondevaldova, J., Balastikova, A., Lapcik, O., & Kokoska, L. (2015). The relationship between structure and *in vitro* antibacterial activity of selected isoflavones and their metabolites with special focus on anti-staphylococcal effect of demethyltexasin. *Letters in Applied Microbiology*, *60*(3), 242–247. doi:10.1111/lam.12361 PMID:25421722

Hu, N., Yu, J., Tan, L., Wang, Y., Sun, Y., Sun, L., & Tan, L. (2013). Nutrition and the risk of Alzheimer's disease. *Biomed Research International*, *2013*, 1–12. PMID:23865055

Hunt, J. V., Smith, C. C., & Wolff, S. P. (1990). Autoxidative glycosylation & possible involvement of peroxides & free radicals in LDL modification by glucose. *Journal of Diabetes*, *39*(11), 1420–1424. doi:10.2337/diab.39.11.1420 PMID:2227114

Huxley, R. R., & Neil, H. A. (2003). The relation between dietary flavonol intake and coronary heart disease mortality: A meta-analysis of prospective cohort studies. *European Journal of Clinical Nutrition*, *57*(8), 904–908. doi:10.1038/sj.ejcn.1601624 PMID:12879084

Hwang, E. Y., Ryu, H. S., Chun, S. S., Park, K. Y., & Rhee, S. H. (1995). Effect of Godulbaegi (Korean Lettuce, *lxeris sonchifolia* H.) Kimchi on the in vitro digestibility of proteins. *J. Korean Soc. Food Nutr.*, *24*, 1010–1015.

Hyrslova, I., Chmurova, J., Krausova, G., & Curda, I. (2014). Potential of bovine colostrum for its application in fermented milk products. *Mlekarske Listy*, *25*(147S), xii–xiv.

Hyun, J. W., & Chung, H. S. (2004). Cyanidin and malvidin from *Oryza sativa* cv. Heugjinjubyeo mediate cytotoxicity against human monocytic leukemia cells by arrest of G2/M phase and induction of apoptosis. *Journal of Agricultural and Food Chemistry*, *52*(8), 2213–2217. doi:10.1021/jf030370h PMID:15080622

ICRAF. (2004). *Agroforestry Database, a tree species reference and selection guide*. Nairobi: ICRAF.

IFIC. (2011). *Functional foods*. International Food Information Council Foundation. Retrieved July 12, 2015, from http://www.foodinsight.org

IFIC. (2013). *Functional Foods, consumer survey*. International Food Information Council Foundation. Retrieved July 17, 2015 from http://www.foodinsight.org

IFIC. (2015). *Food & health survey*. International Food Information Council Foundation. Retrieved July 20, 2015 from http://www.foodinsight.org

Iinuma, M., Roberts, M. F., Matlin, S. A., Stacey, V. E., Timmermann, B. N., Mabryd, T. J., & Browne, R. (1985). Synthesis and revised structure of the flavone Brickellin. *Phytochemistry*, *24*(6), 1367–1368. doi:10.1016/S0031-9422(00)81135-8

ILSI. (1999). Scientific concepts of functional foods in Europe: Consensus document. *The British Journal of Nutrition*, *81*(04), s1–s27. doi:10.1017/S0007114599000471 PMID:10999022

Imai, K., Suga, K., & Nakachi, K. (1997). Cancer-preventive effects of drinking green tea among a Japanese population. *Preventive Medicine*, *26*(6), 769–775. doi:10.1006/pmed.1997.0242 PMID:9388788

Imran, M., Ahmad, N., Anjum, F. M., Khan, M. K., Mushtaq, Z., Nadeem, M., & Hussain, S. (2015). Potential protective properties of flax lignin secoisolariciresinol diglucoside. *Nutrition Journal*, *14*(1), 71–76. doi:10.1186/s12937-015-0059-3 PMID:26215288

Inoue, T., Nagatomi, Y., Uyama, A., & Mochizuki, N. (2013). Fate of mycotoxins during beer brewing and fermentation. *Bioscience, Biotechnology, and Biochemistry*, *77*(7), 1410–1415. doi:10.1271/bbb.130027 PMID:23832360

International Agency for Research on Cancer (IARC) Monograph. (n.d.). *Chemical composition of tea*. Retrieved July 27, 2015 from http://monographs.iarc.fr/ENG/Monographs/vol51/mono51-8B.pdf

International Fund for Agricultural Development, World Food Programme, Food and Agricultural Organization. (2012). *The State of Food Insecurity in the World (2012). Economic growth is necessary but not sufficient to accelerate reduction of hunger and malnutrition*. Rome: Food and Agricultural Organization. Accessed June 29, 2013. http://www.fao.org/publications/sofi/(2012)/en/

International Organization for Standardization. Geneva, Switzerland (ISO) 13299 Sensory Analysis Methodology. (1998). General guidance for establishing a sensory profile. ISO.

International Rice Research Institute. (2013). *Rice knowledge bank*. Los Ba˜nos, the Philippines: Author. Retrieved from http://www.knowledgebank.irri.org/rkb/rice-milling.html

International Rice Research Institute. (2013). *World Rice Statistics (2013)*. Los Ba˜nos, the Philippines: IRRI. Retrieved from http://irri.org/index.php?option=com_k2&view=item&id=9081&Itemid=100481&lang=en

Iqbal, S., Bhanger, M. I., & Anwar, F. (2005). Antioxidant properties and components of some commercially available varieties of rice bran in Pakistan. *Food Chemistry*, *93*(2), 265–272. doi:10.1016/j.foodchem.2004.09.024

Iqbal, S., Haleem, S., Akhtar, M., Zia-Ul-Haq, M., & Akbar, J. (2008). Efficiency of pomegranate peel extracts in stabilization of sunflower oil under accelerated conditions. *Food Research International*, *41*(2), 194–200. doi:10.1016/j.foodres.2007.11.005

IRRI. (1990). *(199lb). Program report for*. Manila: IRRI.

Irshad, I., Kanekanian, A., Peters, A. & Masud, T. (2015). Antioxidant activity of bioactive peptides derived from bovine casein hydrolysate fractions. *Journal of Food Sciences and Technology, 52*(1), 231-239.

Irvine, S. L., Hummelen, R., & Hekmat, S. (2011). Probiotic yogurt consumption may improve gastrointestinal symptoms,productivity, and nutritional intake of people living with humanimmunodeficiency virus in Mwanza, Tanzania. *Nutrition Research (New York, N.Y.)*, *31*(12), 875–881. doi:10.1016/j.nutres.2011.10.005 PMID:22153512

Isanga, J., & Zhang, G. N. (2007). Biologically active components and nutraceuticals in peanuts and related products[Review]. *Food Reviews International*, *23*(2), 123–140. doi:10.1080/87559120701224956

Isanga, J., & Zhang, G. N. (2008). Soybean bioactive components and their implications to health- a review. *Food Reviews International*, *24*(2), 252–276. doi:10.1080/87559120801926351

Isao, M., Fumiaki, I., Manson, J. E., Frank, H. B., Walter, W. C., & Rob, D. M. et al.. (2013). Fruit consumption and risk of type 2 diabetes: Results from three prospective longitudinal cohort studies. *British Medical Journal*, *347*(1), f5001. doi:10.1136/bmj.f5001 PMID:23990623

Ishikawa, A., Kuriyama, S., Tsubono, Y., Fukao, A., Takahashi, H., Tachiya, H., & Tsuji, I. (2006). Smoking, alcohol drinking, green tea consumption and the risk of esophageal cancer in Japanese men. *Journal of Epidemiology*, *16*(5), 185–192. doi:10.2188/jea.16.185 PMID:16951537

Islam, M. A., Punt, A., Spenkelink, B., Murk, A. J., Rolaf van Leeuwen, F. X., & Rietjens, I. M. (2014). Conversion of major soy isoflavone glucosides and aglycones *in vitro* intestinal models. *Molecular Nutrition & Food Research*, *58*(3), 503–515. doi:10.1002/mnfr.201300390 PMID:24668774

Islam, M. S., & Choi, H. (2009). Antidiabetic effect of Korean traditional Baechu (Chinese cabbage) kimchi in a type 2 diabetes model of rats. *Journal of Medicinal Food*, *12*(2), 292–297. doi:10.1089/jmf.2008.0181 PMID:19459728

Ismail, T., Akhtar, S., Riaz, M., & Ismail, A. (2014). Effect of pomegranate peel supplementation on nutritional, organoleptic & stability properties of cookies. *International Journal of Food Sciences and Nutrition*, *65*(6), 661–666. doi:10.3109/09637486.2014.908170 PMID:24725173

Isolabella, S., Cogoi, L., Lopes, P., Anesini, C., Ferraro, G., & Filip, R. (2010). Study of the Bioactive Compounds Variation During Yerba Mate (*Ilex paraguariensis*) Processing. *Food Chemistry*, *122*(3), 695–699. doi:10.1016/j.foodchem.2010.03.039

Isolauri, E., Juntunen, M., Rautanen, T., Sillanaukee, P., & Koivula, T. (1991). A human *Lactobacillus*strain (*Lactobacillus casei*sp. strain GG) promotes recovery from acute diarrhea in children. *Pediatrics*, *88*, 90–97. PMID:1905394

Issa, A. Y., Volate, S. R., & Wargovich, M. J. (2006). The role of phytochemicals in inhibition of cancer and inflammation: New directions and perspectives. *Journal of Food Composition and Analysis*, *19*(5), 405–419. doi:10.1016/j.jfca.2006.02.009

Itani, T., Tatemoto, H., Okamoto, M., Fujii, K., & Muto, N. (2002). A comparative study on antioxidative activity and polyphenol content of colored kernel rice. *Journal of Japanese Society of Nutrition and Food Science*, *49*(8), 540–543. doi:10.3136/nskkk.49.540

Ito, E., Crozier, A., & Ashihara, H. (1997). Theophylline Metabolism in Higher Plants. *Biochimica et Biophysica Acta*, *1336*(2), 323–330. doi:10.1016/S0304-4165(97)00045-7 PMID:9305805

Ito, M. (2003). Characterization of natural waxes & their application to cosmetic foundations. *Fragrance Journal*, *31*, 38–46.

Ivana, R. R., Tatjan, G., Karmela, D., & Vorkapic-Furac, J. (2004). Glucosinolates and their potential role in plant. *Periodicum Biologorum*, *110*(4), 297–309.

Iwama, F., & Maruta, S. (1969). Composition of hard portion of crude rice bran wax. *Kogyo Kagaku Zassh*, *722*, 605–2608.

Iwuoha, C. I., & Eke, O. S. (1996). Nigerian Indigenous Fermented foods: Their traditional process operations, inherent problems, improvements and current status. *Food Research International*, *29*(5-6), 527–540. doi:10.1016/0963-9969(95)00045-3

Iwuoha, G. N., Ubeng, G. G., & Onwuachu, U. I. (2013). Detoxification effect of fermentation on cyanide content of cassava tuber. *Journal of Applied Sciences and Environmental Management*, *17*(4), 567–570.

Iyidogan, N. F., & Bayindirli, A. (2004). Effect of L-cysteine, kojic acid and 4- hexylresorcinol combination on inhibition of enzymatic browning in Amasya apple juice. *Journal of Food Engineering*, *62*(3), 299–304. doi:10.1016/S0260-8774(03)00243-7

Jaatinen, N., Korpela, R., Poussa, T., Turpeinen, A., Mustonen, S., Merilahti, J., & Peuhkuri, K. (2014). Effects of daily intake of yogurt enriched with bioactive components on chronic stress responses: A double-blinded randomized controlled trial. *International Journal of Food Sciences and Nutrition*, *65*(4), 507–514. doi:10.3109/09637486.2014.880669 PMID:24490888

Jackson, K. G., & Lovegrove, J. A. (2002). Functional foods, blood lipids and coronary heart disease. *Fd Sci Tech Bull.*, 1-11.

Jackson, R. L., Greiwe, J. S., & Schwen, R. J. (2011). Emerging evidence of the health benefits of S-equol, an estrogen receptor β agonist. *Nutrition Reviews*, *69*(8), 432–448. doi:10.1111/j.1753-4887.2011.00400.x PMID:21790611

Jacobs, A., Wegewitz, U., Sommerfeld, C., Grossklaus, R., & Lampen, A. (2009). Efficacy of isoflavones in relieving vasomotor menopausal symptoms. A systematic review. *Molecular Nutrition & Food Research*, *53*(9), 1084–1097. doi:10.1002/mnfr.200800552 PMID:19653225

Jacobs, D. R. Jr, & Gallaher, D. D. (2004). Whole grain intake and cardiovascular disease, a review. *Current Atherosclerosis Reports*, *6*(6), 414–423. doi:10.1007/s11883-004-0081-y PMID:15485586

Jacobs, D. R. Jr, Marquart, L., Slavin, J., & Kushi, L. H. (1998). Whole-grain intake andcancer: An expanded review and meta-analysis. *Nutrition and Cancer*, *30*(2), 85–96. doi:10.1080/01635589809514647 PMID:9589426

Jacobs, D. R. Jr, Pereira, M. A., Stumpf, K., Pins, J. J., & Aldercreutz, H. (2002). Whole grain food intake elevates serum enterolactone. *The British Journal of Nutrition*, *88*(2), 111–116. doi:10.1079/BJN2002601 PMID:12144714

Jacques, R. A., dos Santos Freitas, I., Perez, V. F., Dariva, C., de Oliveira, A. P., de Oliveira, J. V., & Caramao, E. B. (2007). The Use of Ultrasound in the Extraction of *Ilex paraguariensis* Leaves: A Comparison with Maceration. *Ultrasonics Sonochemistry*, *14*(1), 6–12. doi:10.1016/j.ultsonch.2005.11.007 PMID:16439181

Jager, R., Lowery, R. P., Calvanese, A. V., Joy, J. M., Purpura, M., & Wilson, J. M. (2014). Comparative absorption of curcumin formulations. *Nutrition Journal*, *13*(1), 11–18. doi:10.1186/1475-2891-13-11 PMID:24461029

Jain, S. K., McVie, R., Jaramillo, J. J., Palmer, M., Smith, T., Mea-chum, Z. D., & Little, R. L. (1996). The effect of modest vitamin E supplementation on lipid peroxidation products and other cardiovascular risk factors in diabetic patients. *Lipids*, *31*(1Suppl), 87–90. doi:10.1007/BF02637057 PMID:8729100

Jaiswal, P. K. (1983). Specification of rice bran oil and extractions. In *Rice bran oil: status and prospects. Proceedings of a seminar*. Oil Technologists' Association of India.

Jameel, M., Ali, A., & Ali, M. (2015a). Isolation of antioxidant phytoconstituents from the seeds of *Lens culinaris* Medik. *Food Chemistry*, *175*, 358–365. doi:10.1016/j.foodchem.2014.11.130 PMID:25577092

Jameel, M., Ali, A., & Ali, M. (2015b). New fatty acid and glycosides from the seeds of *Lens culinaris* Medik. *International Journal of Advances in Pharmacy Medicine and Bioallied Sciences*, *3*, 50–54.

James, P. A., Oparil, S., Carter, B. L., Cushman, W. C., Dennison-Himmelfarb, C., Handler, J., & Ortiz, E. et al. (2014). 2014 evidence-based guideline for the management of high blood pressure in adults: Report from the panel members appointed to the Eighth Joint National Committee (JNC 8). *Journal of the American Medical Association*, *311*(5), 507–520. doi:10.1001/jama.2013.284427 PMID:24352797

Jamil, S. S., Nizami, Q., & Salam, M. (2007). *Centella asiatica* (Linn.) urban oA review. *Natural Product Radiance*, *6*, 158–170.

Jampani, C., Naik, A., & Raghavarao, K. S. M. S. (2014). Purification of anthocyanins from *jamun* (*Syzygium cumini* L.) employing adsorption. *Separation and Purification Technology*, *125*, 170–178. doi:10.1016/j.seppur.2014.01.047

Jan, A. T., Kamli, M. R., Murtaza, I., Singh, J. B., Ali, A., & Haq, Q. M. R. (2010). Dietary flavonoid quercetin and associated health benefits- an overview. *Food Reviews International*, *26*(3), 302–317. doi:10.1080/87559129.2010.484285

Jane, P. (2004). The discovery of Tea. In *Afternoon tea* (p. 10). The Jarrold Group.

Jang, A., & Lee, M. (2005). Purification and identification of angiotensin converting enzyme inhibitory peptides from beef hydrolysates. *Meat Science*, *69*(4), 653–661. doi:10.1016/j.meatsci.2004.10.014 PMID:22063143

Jang, H. D., Yoo, J. S., Chae, S. J., Park, S. I., Jung, J. C., & Kim, H. J. Kim & Seok, H. B. (2006). Effect of dietary methyl sulfonyl methane on growth performance and meat quality characteristics in growing finishing pigs. *Korean Journal of International Agriculture*, *18*, 116–120.

Jang, K. S., Kim, M. J., Oh, Y. A., Kang, M. S., & Kim, S. D. (1991). Changes in carotene content of Chinese cabbage kimchi containing various submaterials and lactic acid bacteria during fermention. *J. Food Sci. Nutr.*, *20*(1), 5–12.

Jang, Y. R., Kim, Y. K., Kwon, I. B., & Lee, H. Y. (1998). Screening and identification of the fibrinolytic bacterial strain from Jeot-gal, salt-fermented fish. *Korean J. Food Sci. Technol.*, *30*, 655–650.

Jansen van Rensburg, W. S., Venter, S. L., Netshiluuhi, T. R., Van der Heever, E., Vorster, H. J., & De Rorde, J. A. (2004). Role of indigenous leafy vegetables in combating hunger and malnutrition. *South African Journal of Botany*, *70*(1), 116–123. doi:10.1016/S0254-6299(15)30268-4

Jeffery, E. H., & Araya, M. (2009). Physiological effects of broccoli consumption. *Phytochemistry Reviews*, *8*(1), 283–298. doi:10.1007/s11101-008-9106-4

Jenkins, D. J., Kendall, C. W., Marchie, A., Faulkner, D. A., Wong, J. M., de Souza, R., & Connelly, P. W. et al. (2005). Direct comparison of a dietary portfolio of cholesterol-lowering foods with a statin in hypercholesterolemic participants. *The American Journal of Clinical Nutrition*, *81*, 380–387. PMID:15699225

Jenkins, D., Wolever, T., Taylor, R. H., Barker, H., Fielden, H., Baldwin, J. M., & Goff, D. V. et al. (1981). Glycemi.c index of foods: A physiological basis for carbohydrate exchange Am*erica.n. The Journal of Clinical Nutrition*, *34*(3), 362–366.

Jenkins, D., Wong, G. S., Patten, R., Bird, J., Hall, M., Buckley, G. C., & Little, J. A. et al. (1983). Legumin.ous seeds in the dietary management of hyperlipidemia. *The American Journal of Clinical Nutrition*, *38*(4), 567–573. PMID:6624698

Jenks, B. H., Iwashita, S., Nakagawa, Y., Ragland, K., Lee, J., Carson, W. H., & Uchiyama, S. et al. (2012). A pilot study on the effects of S-equol compared to soy isoflavones on menopausal hot flash frequency. *Journal of Women's Health*, *21*(6), 674–782. doi:10.1089/jwh.2011.3153 PMID:22409590

Jeon, S.M., Kim, J.E., Shin, S.K.., Kwon, E.Y., Jung, U. J., Baek, N.I. (2013). Randomized double-blind placebo-controlled trial of powdered brassica rapa ethanol extract on alteration of body composition and plasma lipid and adipocytokine profiles in overweight subjects. *Journal of Medicinal Food*, *16*(2), 133-138.

Jepson, R. G. I., & Craig, J. C. (2008). Cranberries for preventing urinary tract infections. *Cochrane Database Syst Rev*, *23*(1). 10.1002/14651858.CD001321.pub4

Jeune, M. L., Kumi-Diaka, J., & Brown, J. (2005). Anticancer activities of pomegranate extracts & genistein in human breast cancer cells. *Journal of Medicinal Food*, *8*(4), 469–475. doi:10.1089/jmf.2005.8.469 PMID:16379557

Jeunemaitre, X., Soubrier, F., Kotelevtsev, Y. V., Lifton, R. P., Williams, C. S., Charru, A., & Corvol, P. et al. (1992). Molecular basis of human hypertension: Role of angiotensinogen. *Cell*, *71*(1), 169–180. doi:10.1016/0092-8674(92)90275-H PMID:1394429

Jiang, F., Zhang, Y., & Dusting, G. J. (2011). NADPH oxidase-mediated redox signaling: Roles in cellular stress response, stress tolerance, and tissue repair. *Pharmacological Reviews*, *63*(1), 218–242. doi:10.1124/pr.110.002980 PMID:21228261

Jiang, G., Lin, S., Wen, L., Jiang, Y., Zhao, M., Chen, F., & Yang, B. et al. (2013). Identification of a novel phenolic compound in litchi (Litchi chinensis Sonn.) pericarp and bioactivity evaluation. *Food Chemistry*, *136*(2), 563–568. doi:10.1016/j.foodchem.2012.08.089 PMID:23122098

Jiang, Z. Y., Parini, P., Eggertsem, G., Davis, M. A., Hu, H., Suo, G. J., & Einarsson, C. et al. (2008). Increased expression of LXR alpha, ABCG5, ABCG8, and SR-BI in the liver from normolipidemic, nonobese Chinese gallstone patients. *Journal of Lipid Research*, *49*(2), 464–472. doi:10.1194/jlr.M700295-JLR200 PMID:18007013

Jing, Z., & Wei-Jie, Y. (2015). Effects of soy protein containing isoflavones in patients with chronic kidney disease: A systematic review and meta-analysis. *Clinical Nutrition (Edinburgh, Lothian)*. doi:10.1016/j.clnu.2015.03.012 PMID:25882339

Jin, J. S., Kitahara, M., Sakamoto, M., Hattori, M., & Benno, Y. (2010). *Slackia equolifaciens* sp. nov., a human intestinal bacterium capable of producing equol. *International Journal of Systematic and Evolutionary Microbiology*, *60*(8), 1721–1724. doi:10.1099/ijs.0.016774-0 PMID:19734283

JNC-7 Guidelines. (2004). The seventh report of the joint national committee on prevention, detection, evaluation, & treatment of high blood pressure. National Heart, Lung, and Blood Institute (US). Report. No. 04-5230.

John Hopkins Medicine. (2015). *Herbal medicine*. Retrieved November 14, 2015 from: http://www.hopkinsmedicine.org/healthlibrary/conditions/complementary_and_alternative_medicine/herbal_medicine_85,P00181/

John, J. A., & Shahidi, F. (2010). Phenolic compounds and antioxidant activity of Brazilian nut (*Bertholletia excelsa*). *Journal of Functional Foods*, *2*(3), 196–209. doi:10.1016/j.jff.2010.04.008

Johnson, C. R., Combs, G. F., & Thavarajah, P. (2013). Lentil (*Lens culinaris* L.): A prebiotic-rich whole food legume. *Food Research International*, *51*(1), 107–113. doi:10.1016/j.foodres.2012.11.025

Johnson, E. A., & Larson, A. E. (2005). Lysozyme. In M. P. Davidson, J. N. Sofos, & A. L. Branen (Eds.), *Antimicrobials in Food* (pp. 361–387). Boca Raton, FL: CRC Press.

Johnson, L. A., & Lusas, E. W. (1983). Comparison of alternative solvents for oil extraction. *Journal of the American Oil Chemists' Society*, *60*(2), 229–242. doi:10.1007/BF02543490

Johns, T., & Sthapit, B. (2004). Biocultural diversity in the sustainability of developing country food systems. *Food and Nutrition Bulletin*, *25*(2), 143–155. doi:10.1177/156482650402500207 PMID:15214260

Johri, R. K. (2011). *Cuminum cyminum* and *Carum carvi*: An update. *Pharmacognosy Review*, *5*(9), 63–72. doi:10.4103/0973-7847.79101 PMID:22096320

Joint National Committee on the Detection, Evaluation and Treatment of High Blood Pressure (JNC-V). (1993). The fifth report of the Joint National Committee on the detection, evaluation, and treatment of high blood pressure. *Archives of Internal Medicine*, *153*(2), 154–183. doi:10.1001/archinte.1993.00410020010002 PMID:8422206

Jolly, C. I., Narayanan, S., & Prabhu, S. K. (2000). Antihypertensive activity of flowers of *Punica granatum* Linn. (Variety-Gulnar). *Indian Journal of Natural Products*, *16*(1), 3–7.

Jomova, K., Jenisova, Z., Feszterova, M., Baros, S., Liska, J., Hudecova, D., & Valko, M. et al. (2011). Arsenic: Toxicity, oxidative stress and human disease. *Journal of Applied Toxicology*, *31*, 95–107. PMID:21321970

Jones, P. J. (2002). Clinical nutrition: 7. Functional foods — more than just nutrition. *Canadian Medical Association Journal*, *166*(12), 1555–1563. PMID:12074125

Jones, P. J. H., & Raeini-Sarjaz, M. (2001). Plant sterols and their derivatives; the current spread of results. *Nutrition Reviews*, *59*(1), 21–24. doi:10.1111/j.1753-4887.2001.tb01901.x PMID:11281249

Jones, P. J., Raeini-Sarjaz, M., Ntanios, F. V., Vanstone, C. A., Feng, J. Y., & Parsons, W. E. (2000). Modulation of plasma lipid levels and cholesterol kinetics by phytosterol versus phytostanol esters. *Journal of Lipid Research*, *41*(5), 697–705. PMID:10787430

Joung, E. M., & Jung, K. H. (2014). Antioxidant activity of onion (*Allium cepa* L.) peel extracts obtained as onion by-products. *Korean Journal of Food Sciences and Technology*, *46*(3), 364–368. doi:10.9721/KJFST.2014.46.3.364

Joy, S., Siow, R. C., Rowlands, D. J., Becker, M., Wyatt, A. W., Aaronson, P. I., & Mann, G. E. et al. (2006). The isoflavone equol mediates rapid vascular relaxation: Ca2+-independent activation of endothelial nitric-oxide synthase/Hsp90 involving ERK1/2 and Akt phosphorylation in human endothelial cells. *The Journal of Biological Chemistry*, *281*(37), 27335–27345. doi:10.1074/jbc.M602803200 PMID:16840783

Jrad, Z., Girardet, J.-M., Adt, I., Oulahal, N., Degraeve, P., Khorchani, T., & El Hatmi, H. (2014). Antioxidant activity of camel milk casein. *Mljekarstvo*, *64*, 287–294. doi:10.15567/mljekarstvo.2014.0408

Jukanti, A. K., Gaur, P. M., Gowda, C. L. L., & Chibbar, R. N. (2012). Nutritional quality and health benefits of chickpea (*Cicer arietinum* L.): A review. *The British Journal of Nutrition*, *108*(S1), S11–S26. doi:10.1017/S0007114512000797 PMID:22916806

Juliano, B. O. (1972). The rice caryopsis and its composition. In D. F. Houston (Ed.), *Rice chemistry and technology* (pp. 16–74). St Paul, MN: American Association of Cereal Chemistry.

Juliano, B. O. (1979). The chemical basis of rice grain quality. In *Proceedings, Workshop on Chemical Aspects of Rice Grain Quality*. Los Baños, Laguna, the Philippines: IRRI.

Juliano, B. O. (1993). *Rice in Human Nutrition*. Rome: Food and Agriculture Organization of the United Nations.

Juliano, B. O. (Ed.). (1985b). *Rice: chemistry and technology* (2nd ed.). St Paul, MN: American Association of Cereal Chemistry.

Juliano, B. O., & Bechtel, D. B. (1985). The rice grain and its gross compo sition. In B. O. Juliano (Ed.), *Rice chemistry and technology* (2nd ed.; pp. 17–57). St Paul, MN: American Association of Cereal Chemistry.

Juliano, B. O., & Goddard, M. S. (1986). Cause of varietal difference in insulin and glucose responses to ingested rice. *Qualitas Plantarum Plant Foods for Human Nutrition*, *36*(1), 35–41. doi:10.1007/BF01091751

Jumah, R. Y., Shaker, R. R., & Abu-Jadayil, B. (2001). Effect of milk source on therheological properties of yoghurt during the gelation process. *International Journal of Dairy Technology*, *54*(3), 89–93. doi:10.1046/j.1364-727x.2001.00012.x

Jumpertz, R., Le, D. S., Turnbaugh, P. J., Trinidad, C., Bogardus, C., Gordon, J. I., & Krakoff, J. (2011). Energy-balance studies reveal associations between gut microbes, caloric load, and nutrient absorption in humans. *The American Journal of Clinical Nutrition*, *94*(1), 58–65. doi:10.3945/ajcn.110.010132 PMID:21543530

Jung, D. H., & Jung, S. H. (2005). *Garlic Science, World science, Israel Goldberg, Functional Foods*. New York: Chapman & Hall.

Jung, H. A., Su, B. N., Keller, W. J., Mehta, R. G., & Kinghorn, A. D. (2006). Antioxidant xanthones from the pericarp of *Garcinia mangostana* (Mangosteen). *Journal of Agricultural and Food Chemistry*, *54*(6), 2077–2082. doi:10.1021/jf052649z PMID:16536578

Jung, K. H. (2004). *Effect of the processed sulfur on the growth performance, antivirus and meat quality in pigs*. Chonnam University.

Jung, K. O., Lee, K. I., Suh, K. J., & Park, K. Y. (1999). Antimutagenic and anticancer effects of Buchu Kimchi. *J. Food Sci. Nutr.*, *4*, 33–37.

Jung, Y. K., Yang, Y. S., Kang, J. O., Kong, Y. S., & Kim, J. O. (1995). Fibrinolysis of fermented kimchi. *Korean Society of Life Science*, *5*(4), 203–210.

Jurenka, J. (2008). Therapeutic application of pomegranate (*Punica granatum*): *A Review. Alternative Medicine Review*, *13*, 128–144. PMID:18590349

Kabagambe, E. K., Baylin, A., Ruiz-Narvarez, E., Siles, X., & Campos, H. (2005). Decreased consumption of dried mature beans is positively associated with urbanization and nonfatal acute myocardial infarction. *The Journal of Nutrition*, *135*, 17701775. PMID:15987863

Kabir, Y., & Sidhu, J. S. (2011). Antioxidative Functional Factors in Nuts. In J. Shi, C.-T. Ho, & F. Shahidi (Eds.), *Functional Foods of the East* (pp. 343–397). Taylor and Francis.

Kader, A. A. (1986). Biochemical and physiological basis for effects of controlled and modified atmospheres on fruits and vegetables. *Food Technology*, *40*(5), 99–104.

Kaefer, C. M., & Milner, J. A. (2008). The role of herbs and spices in cancer prevention. *The Journal of Nutritional Biochemistry*, *19*(6), 347–361. doi:10.1016/j.jnutbio.2007.11.003 PMID:18499033

Kagawa, H., Hirano, H., & Kikuchi, E. (1988). Variation in glutelin seed storage protein in rice (*Oryza sativa* L.). *Japanese Journal of Breeding, 38*, 327-332.

Kajla, P., Sharma, A., & Sood, D. R. (2015). Flaxseed- a potential functional food source. *Journal of Food Sciences and Technology*, *52*(4), 1857–1871. doi:10.1007/s13197-014-1293-y PMID:25829567

Kakuda, T. (2002). Neuroprotective effects of the green tea components theanine and catechins. *Biological & Pharmaceutical Bulletin*, *25*(12), 1513–1518. doi:10.1248/bpb.25.1513 PMID:12499631

Kakuda, T., Nozawa, A., Sugimoto, A., & Niino, H. (2002). Inhibition by theanine of binding of [3H]AMPA, [3H]kainate, and [3H]MDL 105,519 to glutamate receptors. *Bioscience, Biotechnology, and Biochemistry*, *66*(12), 2683–2686. doi:10.1271/bbb.66.2683 PMID:12596867

Kaliora, A. C., & Dedoussis, G. V. Z. (2007). Natural antioxidant compounds in risk factors for CVD. *Pharmacological Research*, *56*(2), 99–109. doi:10.1016/j.phrs.2007.04.018 PMID:17572098

Kalogeropoulos, N., Chiou, A., Ioannou, M., Karathanos, V. T., Hassapidou, M., & Andrikopoulos, N. K. (2010). Nutritional evaluation and bioactive microconstituents (phytosterols, tocopherols, polyphenols, triterpenic acids) in cooked dry legumes usually consumed in the Mediterranean countries. *Food Chemistry*, *121*(3), 682–690. doi:10.1016/j.foodchem.2010.01.005

Kamga, R. T., Kouame, C., Atangana, A. R., Chagomoka, T., & Ndango, R. (2013). Nutritional Evaluation of Five African Indigenous Vegetables. *Journal of Horticultural Research*, *21*(1), 99–106. doi:10.2478/johr-2013-0014

Kamiloglu, O., Ercisli, S., Sengul, M., Toplu, C., & Serce, S. (2009). Total phenolics and antioxidant activity of jujube (*Zizyphus jujube* Mill.) genotypes selected from Turkey. *African Journal of Biotechnology*, *8*, 303–307.

Kamiyama, M., Kishimoto, Y., Tani, M., Utsunomiya, K., & Kondo, K. (2009). Effects of equol on oxidized low-density lipoprotein-induced apoptosis in endothelial cells. *Journal of Atherosclerosis and Thrombosis*, *16*(3), 239–249. doi:10.5551/jat.1057 PMID:19638716

Kanavos, P. (2006). The rising burden of cancer in the developing world. *Annals of Oncology, 17*(suppl 8), 15-23.

Kang, J. H. (2009). *Studies on the biofunctional properties of capsaicin in modulating obesity-induced inflammation and metabolic diseases*. (Ph.D Thesis). Ulsan University, Ulsan, Korea.

Kang, J., Badger, T. M., Ronis, M. J., & Wu, X. (2010). Non-isoflavone phytochemicals in soy and their health effects. *Journal of Agricultural and Food Chemistry*, *58*(14), 8119–8133. doi:10.1021/jf100901b PMID:20578706

Kankolongo, M. A., Hell, K., & Nawa, I. N. (2009). Assessment for fungal, mycotoxin and insect spoilage in maize stored for human consumption in Zambia. *Journal of the Science of Food and Agriculture*, *89*(8), 1366–1375. doi:10.1002/jsfa.3596

Kanu, P. J., Bahsoon, J. Z., Kanu, J. B., & Kandeh, J. B. A. (2010). Nutraceutical Importance of Sesame Seed and Oil: A Review of the Contribution of their Lignans. Sierra Leone. *Journal of Biomedical Research*, *2*, 4–16.

Kapoor, S. (2015). Bioactives and therapeutic potential of legumes: A review. *International Journal of Pharmacy and Biological Sciences*, *5*, 65–74.

Kappeler, S. (1998). *Compositional and structural analysis of camel milk proteins with emphasis on protective proteins*. (Ph.D. Thesis). Swiss Federal Institute of Technology, Zürich, Switzerland.

Kappeler, S., Farah, Z., & Puhan, Z. (1999). Alternative splitting of lactophorin mRNA from lactating mammary gland of the camel (*Camelus dromedarius*). *Journal of Dairy Science*, *82*(10), 2084–2093. doi:10.3168/jds.S0022-0302(99)75450-0 PMID:10531593

Kappeler, S., Farah, Z., & Puhan, Z. (2003). 5'-Flanking regions of camel milk genesare highly similar to homologue regions of other species and can be divided into two distinct groups. *Journal of Dairy Science*, *86*(2), 498–508. doi:10.3168/jds.S0022-0302(03)73628-5 PMID:12647956

Karlsen, A., Retterstol, L., Laake, P., Paur, I., Kjolsrud-Bohn, S., Sandvik, L., & Blomhoff, R. (2007). Anthocyanins inhibit nuclear factor-kB activation in monocytes and reduce plasma concentrations of pro-inflammatory mediators in healthy adults. *The Journal of Nutrition*, *137*, 1951–1954. PMID:17634269

Karunamoorthi, K., Kim, H., Jegajeevanram, K., Xavier, J., & Vijayalakshmi, J. (2014). Papaya: Agifted nutraceutical plant -acritical review of recent human health research. *TANG*, *4*, 1–17.

Karvaj, M., Beno, P., & Fedor-Freybergh, P. G. (2007). Positive effect of flavonoids to cardiovascular and central nervous system. *Neuroendocrinology Letters*, *28*, 1–3. PMID:18030258

Kasimsetty, S. G., Bialonska, D., Reddy, M. K., Ma, G., Khan, S. I., & Ferreira, D. (2010). Colon cancer chemopreventive activities of pomegranate ellagitannins and urolithins. *Journal of Agricultural and Food Chemistry*, *58*(4), 2180–2187. doi:10.1021/jf903762h PMID:20112993

Katan, M. B., & de Roos, N. M. (2004). Promises and problems of functional foods. *Critical Reviews in Food Science and Nutrition*, *44*(5), 369–377. doi:10.1080/10408690490509609 PMID:15540650

Katan, M. B., Grundy, S. M., Jones, P., Law, M., Miettinen, T., & Paoletti, R. (2003). Efficacy and safety of plant stanols and sterols in the management of blood cholesterol levels. *Mayo Clinic Proceedings*, *78*(8), 965–978. doi:10.1016/S0025-6196(11)63144-3 PMID:12911045

Kauffman, F. C., Zaleski, J., Thurman, R. G., & Kwei, G. Y. (1994). Biologically active conjugates of drugs and toxic chemicals. In F. C. Kauffman (Ed.), *Conjugation-deconjugation reactions in drug metabolism and toxicity* (pp. 341–366). Berlin: Springer. doi:10.1007/978-3-642-78429-3_12

Kaufman, D. W., Kelly, J. P., Rosemberg, L., Anderson, T. E., & Mitchell, A. A. (2002). Recent patterns of medication use in the ambulatory adult population of the United States. *Journal of the American Medical Association*, *287*(3), 337–344. doi:10.1001/jama.287.3.337 PMID:11790213

Kaufman, P. B., Duke, J. A., Brielmann, H., Boik, J., & Hoyt, J. E. (1997). A comparative survey of leguminous plants as sources of the isoflavones, genistein and daidzein: Implications for human nutrition and health. *Journal of Alternative and Complementary Medicine (New York, N.Y.)*, *3*(1), 7–12. doi:10.1089/acm.1997.3.7 PMID:9395689

Kavaz, A., & Bakirci, I. (2009). Natural bioactive substances in milk. *Akademik Gida*, *7*(5), 44–50.

Kavitha, C., Kuna, A., Supraja, T., Blessy Sagar, S., Padmavathi, T. V. S., & Prabhakar, N. (2015). Effect of gamma irradiation on antioxidant properties of ber (*Zizyphus mauritiana*) fruit. *Journal of Food Sciences Technology.*, *52*(5), 3123–3128. doi:10.1007/s13197-014-1359-x PMID:25892819

Kawada, T., Watanabe, T., Takaishi, T., Tanaka, T., & Iwai, K. (1986). Capsaicin induced b-adrenergic action on energy metabolism in rats: Influence of capsaicin on oxygen consumption, the respiratory quotient and substrate utilization. *Proceedings of the Society for Experimental Biology and Medicine*, *183*, 350–256. PMID:2876434

Kawakami, M., & Kobayashi, A. (1991). Volatile Constituents of Green Mate and Roasted Mate. *Journal of Agricultural and Food Chemistry*, *39*(7), 1275–1279. doi:10.1021/jf00007a016

Kawarazuka, N. (2010). *The contribution of fish intake, aquaculture, and small-scale fisheries to improving nutrition: A literature review*. The World Fish Center Working Paper No.2106. The World Fish Center.

Kawarazuka, N., & Be'ne´, C. (2010). The potential role of small fish species in improving micronutrient deficiencies in developing countries: Building evidence. *Public Health Nutrition*, *14*(11), 1927–1938. doi:10.1017/S1368980011000814 PMID:21729489

Kayode, A.A., & Kayode, O.T. (2010). Some medicinal values of *Telfairia occidentalis:* A review. *American Journal of Biochemistry and Molecular Biology*, *1*(1), 30-38.

Kays, S. J., & Paull, R. E. (2004). Stress in harvested products. In Postharvest Biology (pp. 355-414). Athens, GA: Exon Press.

Kays, S. J. (1999). Preharvest factors affecting appearance. *Postharvest Biology and Technology*, *15*(3), 233–247. doi:10.1016/S0925-5214(98)00088-X

Kemperman, R. A., Bolca, S., Loger, L. C., & Vaughan, E. E. (2010). Novel approaches for analyzing gut microbes and dietary polyphenols: Challenges and opportunities. *Microbiology*, *156*(11), 3224–3231. doi:10.1099/mic.0.042127-0 PMID:20724384

Kennedy, A. R. (1998). The Bowman-Birk inhibitor from soybeans as an anticarcinogenic agent. *The American Journal of Clinical Nutrition*, *68*(6), 1406S–1412S. PMID:9848508

Kerr, B. J., Weber, T. E., Ziemer, C. J., Spence, C., Cotta, M. A., & Whitehead, T. R. (2011). Effect of dietary inorganic sulfur level on growth performance, fecal composition, and measures of inflammation and sulfate-reducing bacteria in the intestine of growing pigs. *Journal of Animal Science*, *89*(2), 426–437. doi:10.2527/jas.2010-3228 PMID:20952529

Key, T. J. (2011). Fruit and vegetables and cancer risk. *British Journal of Cancer*, *104*(1), 6–11. doi:10.1038/sj.bjc.6606032 PMID:21119663

Khan, A. A., Alzohiary, M. A., & Mohieldein, A. H. (2012). Antidiabetic effects of camel milk in streptozotocin (STZ)-induced diabetic rats. *American Journal of Biochemistry and Molecular Biology*. DOI:10.3923/ajbmb.2012

Khan, A., Sankhyan, P., & Kumar, S. (2013). Biochemical characterization of mustard oil (*Brassica campestris* L.) with special reference to its fatty acid composition. *Asian Journal of Advances in Basic Sciences*, *1*, 1–9.

Khandelwal, S., Demonty, I., Jeemon, P., Lakshmy, R., Mukherjee, R., Gupta, R., & Reddy, K. S. et al. (2009). Independent and interactive effects of plant sterols & fish oil n-3 long chain polyunsaturated fatty acids on the plasma lipid profile of mildly hyperlipidemic Indian adults. *The British Journal of Nutrition*, *102*(5), 722–732. doi:10.1017/S0007114509297170 PMID:19296875

Khan, G. N., Gorin, M. A., Rosenthal, D., Pan, Q., Bao, L. W., Wu, Z. F., & Merajver, S. D. et al. (2009). Pomegranate fruit extract impairs invasion & motility in human breast cancer. *Integrative Cancer Therapies*, *8*(3), 242–253. doi:10.1177/1534735409341405 PMID:19815594

Khan, S., Choudhary, S., Pandey, A., Khan, M. K., & Thomas, G. (2015). Sunflower oil: Efficient oil source for human consumption. *Emer Life Science Research*, *1*, 1–3.

Khaskheli, M., Arain, M. A., Chaudhry, S., Soomro, A. H., & Qureshi, T. A. (2005). Physico-chemical quality of camel milk. *Journal of Agriculture and Social Sciences*, *2*, 164–166.

Khatiwada, J., Verghese, M., Walker, L., Shackelford, L., Chawan, C., & Sunkara, R. (2006). Combination of green tea, phytic acid, and inositol reduced the incidence of azoxymethane-induced colon tumors in Fisher 344 male rats. *LWT-Food Science and Technology*, *39*(10), 1080–1086. doi:10.1016/j.lwt.2005.07.018

Khush, G. (2004). *Harnessing science and technology for sustainable rice based production systems*. Presented at the FAO Rice Conference, Rome, Italy.

Khush, G. (1997). Origin, dispersal, cultivation and variation of rice. *Plant Molecular Biology*, *35*(1/2), 25–34. doi:10.1023/A:1005810616885 PMID:9291957

Kim, H. (2012). *Selection of Lactobacillus strains for cholesterol reduction study and the mechanism through regulating ABCG5/8*. (Master Thesis). Handong Global University, Pohang, Korea.

Kim, B. K., Park, K. Y., Kim, H. Y., Ahn, S. C., & Cho, E. J. (2011). Anti-aging effects and mechanisms of kimchi during fermentation under stress-induced premature senescence cellular system. *Food Science and Biotechnology*, *20*(3), 643–649. doi:10.1007/s10068-011-0091-9

Kim, E. K., An, S. Y., Lee, M. S., Kim, T. H., Lee, H. K., Hwang, W. S., & Lee, K. W. et al. (2011). Fermented kimchi reduces body weight and improves metabolic parameters in overweight and obese patients. *Nutrition Research (New York, N.Y.)*, *31*(6), 436–443. doi:10.1016/j.nutres.2011.05.011 PMID:21745625

Kim, G. S., Jung, Y. R., Lee, N. J., Hong, S. H., Yu, J. H., Jeong, J. H., & Kang, J. K. (2006). The composition of the toxicity of processed sulfur with non processed sulfur in Sprague-Dawley rats. *J. Vet. Med. Biotechnol.*, *7*, 183–190.

Kim, H. J., Lee, J. S., Chung, H. Y., Song, S. H., Suh, H., Noh, J. S., & Song, Y. O. (2007). 3-(4′-hydroxyl-3′, 5′-dimethoxyphenyl) propionic acid, an active principle of kimchi, inhibits development of atherosclerosis in rabbits. *Journal of Agricultural and Food Chemistry*, *55*(25), 10486–10492. doi:10.1021/jf072454m PMID:18004805

Kim, H. J., Sung, Y. B., Song, Y. O., Kang, M. R., Kim, T. W., Park, S. H., & Jang, J. Y. (2012). Kimchi suppresses 7-ketocholesterol-induced endoplasmic reticulum stress in macrophages. *Food Science and Biotechnology*, *21*(5), 1293–1299. doi:10.1007/s10068-012-0170-6

Kim, H., Oh, S. Y., Kang, M. H., Kim, K. N., Kim, Y., & Chang, N. (2014). Association between kimchi intake and asthma in Korean adults: The fourth and fifth Korea National Health and Nutrition Examination Survey (2007-2011). *Journal of Medicinal Food*, *17*(1), 172–178. doi:10.1089/jmf.2013.3013 PMID:24456368

Kim, J. H., Lee, H. R., Pyun, C. W., Hong, G. H., Kim, S. K., & Lee, C. H. (2015). Changes in physiochemical, microbiological and sensory properties of dry-cured ham in processed sulfur-fed pigs. *Journal of Food Processing and Preservation*, *39*(6), 829–839. doi:10.1111/jfpp.12293

Kim, J. H., Pyun, C. W., Hong, G. H., Kim, S. K., Yang, C. Y., & Lee, C. H. (2014). Changes in physiochemical and microbiological properties of isoflavone-treated dry-cured sausage from sulfur-fed pork during storage. *Journal of Animal Sciences and Technology*, *56*(1), 21. doi:10.1186/2055-0391-56-21 PMID:26290710

Kim, J. H., Ryu, J. D., Lee, H. G., Park, J. H., Moon, G. S., Cheigh, H. S., & Song, Y. O. (2002a). The effect of kimchi on production of free radicals and anti-oxidative enzyme activities in the brain of SAM. *Journal of the Korean Society of Food Science and Nutrition*, *31*(1), 117–123. doi:10.3746/jkfn.2002.31.1.117

Kim, J. H., Ryu, J. D., & Song, Y. O. (2002b). The effect of kimchi intake on free radical production and the inhibition of oxidation in young adults and the elderly people. *Korean Journal of Community Nutrition*, *7*, 257–265.

Kim, K. H., Kim, S. H., & Park, K. Y. (2001). Effects of kimchi extracts on production of nitric oxide by activated macrophages, transforming growth factor β1 of tumor cells and interleukin-6 in splenocytes. *J. Food Sci. Nutr.*, *6*, 126–132.

Kim, K. H., Kim, S. H., Rhee, S. H., & Park, K. Y. (1998). Effects of kimchi extracts on interleukin-2 production and natural killer cell activity in mice. *J. Food Sci. Nutr.*, *3*, 282–286.

Kim, M. J., Song, Y. S., & Song, Y. O. (1998). The Fibrinolytic activity of kimchi and its ingredients in *vivo* and in *vitro. J. Korean Soc. Food Sci. Nutr.*, *27*(4), 633–638.

Kim, M., Kim, S. I., Han, J., Wang, X. L., Song, D. G., & Kim, S. U. (2009). Stereospecific biotransformation of dihydrodaidzein into (3S)-equol by the human intestinal bacterium *Eggerthella* strain Julong 732. *Applied and Environmental Microbiology*, *75*(10), 3062–3068. doi:10.1128/AEM.02058-08 PMID:19304836

Kim, N. D., Mehta, R., Yu, W., Neeman, I., Livney, T., Amichay, A., & Lansky, E. et al. (2002). Chemopreventive & adjuvant therapeutic potential of pomegranate (*Punica granatum*) for human breast cancer. *Breast Cancer Research and Treatment*, *71*(3), 203–217. doi:10.1023/A:1014405730585 PMID:12002340

Kingman, S. M., Walker, A. F., Low, A., Sambrook, I., Owen, R., & Cole, T. (1993). Comparative effects of four legume species on plasma lipids and faecal steroid excretion in hypercholesterolaemic pigs. *The British Journal of Nutrition*, *69*(02), 409–421. doi:10.1079/BJN19930043 PMID:8489997

King, P., Rakesh, N., Beena Lahiri, S., Prasanna Kumar, Y., & Prasad, V. S. R. K. (2008). Biosorption of zinc onto *Syzygium cumini* L.: Equilibrium and kinetic studies. *Chem. Engg. J.*, *144*(2), 181–187. doi:10.1016/j.cej.2008.01.019

Kinsella, J. E., Frankel, E., German, B., & Kanner, J. (1993). Possible mechanisms for the protective role of antioxidants in wine and plant foods. *Food Technology*, *47*(4), 85–89.

Kinyuru, J. N., Kenji, G. M., Muhoho, S. N., & Ayieko, M. (2010). Nutritional potential of longhorn grasshopper (*Ruspolia differens*) consumed in Siaya District. *Journal of Agriculture, Science and Technology*, *12*, 32–47.

Kinyuru, J. N., Konyole, S. O., Roos, N., Onyango, C. A., Owino, V. O., Owuor, B. O., & Kenji, G. M. et al. (2013). Nutrient composition of four species of winged termites consumed in western Kenya. *Journal of Food Composition and Analysis*, *30*(2), 120–124. doi:10.1016/j.jfca.2013.02.008

Kirjanvainen, P. V. (2003). Probiotic and the management of food allergy. In Functional Dairy Products (pp. 108-131). Cambridge, UK: Woodhead Publishers.

Kirsner, R. S., & Eaglstein, W. H. (1993). The wound healing process. *Journal of Dermatologic Clinics*, *11*(4), 629–640. PMID:8222347

Kisbenedek, A., Szabo, S., Polyak, E., Breitenbach, Z., Bona, A., Mark, L., & Figler, M. (2014). Analysis of trans-resveratrol in oilseeds by high-performance liquid chromatography. *Acta Alimentaria*, *43*(3), 459–464. doi:10.1556/AAlim.43.2014.3.13

Kiss, A., Naar, Z., Daroczi, L., Nemedi, E., & Kukovics, S. (2014). Development of functional sheep and goat milk products and the investigation of functionality in various packaging materials. *J. Hygienic Engg. Design*, *7*, 174–179.

Kitts, D., & Weiler, K. (2003). Bioactive proteins and peptides from food sources. Applications of bioprocesses used in isolation and recovery. *Current Pharmaceutical Design*, *9*(16), 1309–1323. doi:10.2174/1381612033454883 PMID:12769739

Klaenhammer, T., Altermann, E., Arigoni, F., Bolotin, A., Breidt, F., Broadbent, J., & Siezen, R. J. et al. (2002). Discovering lactic acid bacteria by genomics. *Antonie van Leeuwenhoek*, *82*(1/4), 29–58. doi:10.1023/A:1020638309912 PMID:12369195

Klayman, D. L., Lin, A. J., Acton, N., Scovill, J. P., Hotch, J. M., Millous, W. K., & Dobek, A. S. et al. (1984). Isolation of artemisinin (qinghaosu) from Artemisia annua growing in the United States. *Journal of Natural Products*, *47*(4), 715–717. doi:10.1021/np50034a027 PMID:6387056

Kleijnen, J., Knipschild, P., & ter Riet, G. T. (1989). Garlic, onions and cardiovascular risk factors. A review of the evidence from human experiments with emphasis on commercially available preparations. *British Journal of Clinical Pharmacology*, *28*(5), 535–544. doi:10.1111/j.1365-2125.1989.tb03539.x PMID:2686739

Klein & Mordechai. (n.d.). *Pomegranate-derived Products for the Treatment of Skin Sores & Lesions.* U.S. Patent Application, 12, 676-957.

Kochhar, S. P. (2000). Stable and healthful frying oil for the 21st century. *Inform (Silver Spring, Md.)*, *11*, 642–647.

Kohli, S., Chhabra, A., Jaiswal, A., Rustagi, Y., Sharma, M., & Rani, V. (2013). Curcumin Suppresses Gelatinase B Mediated Norepinephrine Induced Stress in H9c2 Cardiomyocytes. *PLoS ONE*, *8*(10), e76519. doi:10.1371/journal.pone.0076519 PMID:24116115

Kohlmeier, L., Kark, J. D., Gomez-Gracia, E., Martin, B. C., Steck, S. E., Kardinaal, A. F., & Kok, F. J. et al. (1997). Lycopene and myocardial infarction risk in the EURAMIC study. *American Journal of Epidemiology*, *146*(8), 618–626. doi:10.1093/oxfordjournals.aje.a009327 PMID:9345115

Koji, I. (2009). Present condition and problems of rice industry under socio-economic transformation in Cambodia. PhD dissertation. Japan: Graduate School of International Development,Nagoya University. Retrieved from http://www2.gsid.nagoya-u.ac.jp/blog/anda/files/2009/06/21_ishikawa.pdf

Koley, T. K., Kaur, C., Nagal, S., Walia, S., & Sarika, S. (2011). *Antioxidant activity and phenolic content in genotypes of Indian jujube (Zizyphus mauritiana Lamk).* Arabian Journal of Chemistry; doi:10.1016/j.arabjc

Koliwer-Brandl, H., Siegert, N., Umnus, K., Kelm, A., Tolkach, A., Kulozik, U., & Kelm, S. et al. (2011). Lectin inhibition assays for the analysis of bioactive milk sialoglycoconjugates. *International Dairy Journal*, *21*(6), 413–420. doi:10.1016/j.idairyj.2011.01.005

Konuspayeva, G., Faye, B., & Loiseau, G. (2009). The composition of camel milk: A meta-analysis of the literature data. *Journal of Food Composition and Analysis*, *22*(2), 95–101. doi:10.1016/j.jfca.2008.09.008

Korashy, H. M., Maayah, Z. H., Abd-Allah, A. R., El-Kadi, A. O. S., & Alhaider, A. A. (2012). Camel Milk Triggers Apoptotic Signaling Pathways in Human Hepatoma HepG2 and Breast CancerMCF7 Cell Lines through Transcriptional Mechanism. *Journal of Biomedicine & Biotechnology*, 1–9. doi:10.1155/2012/593195

Korea Food Research Institute. (1997). *Development of technology on production of commercial kimchi products with constant quality.* Research Report 389.

Korhonen, H., & Pihlanto, A. (2003). Food-derived bioactive peptides - opportunities for designing future foods. *Current Pharmaceutical Design*, *9*(16), 1297–1308. doi:10.2174/1381612033454892 PMID:12769738

Ko, S., Janes, M. E., Hettiarachchy, N. S., & Johnson, M. G. (2001). Physical and chemical properties of edible films containing nisin and their action against Listeria monocytogenes. *Journal of Food Science*, *66*(7), 1006–1011. doi:10.1111/j.1365-2621.2001.tb08226.x

Kostova, I., Bhatia, S., Grigorov, P., Balkansky, S., Parmar, V. S., Prasad, A. K., & Saso, L. (2011). Coumarins as antioxidants. *Current Medicinal Chemistry*, *18*, 3929–3951. doi:10.2174/092986711803414395 PMID:21824098

Kosugi, T., Nakagawa, T., Kamath, D., & Johnson, R. J. (2009). Uric acid and Hypertension: An age-related relationship. *Journal of Human Hypertension*, *23*(2), 75–76. doi:10.1038/jhh.2008.110 PMID:18754017

Koyama, S., Cobb, L. J., Mehta, H. H., Seeram, N. P., Heber, D., Pantuck, A. J., & Cohen, P. (2010). Pomegranate extract induces apoptosis in human prostate cancer cells by modulation of the IGF–IGFBP axis. *Growth Hormone & IGF Research*, *20*(1), 55–62. doi:10.1016/j.ghir.2009.09.003 PMID:19853487

Kreijkamp-Kaspers, S., Kok, L., Grobbee, D. E., de Haan, E. H., Aleman, A., & van der Schouw, Y. T. (2007). Dietary phytoestrogen intake and cognitive function in older women. *The Journals of Gerontology. Series A, Biological Sciences and Medical Sciences*, *62*(5), 556–562. doi:10.1093/gerona/62.5.556 PMID:17522362

Krinsky, N. I., & Johnson, E. J. (2005). Carotenoid actions and their relation to health and disease. *Molecular Aspects of Medicine*, *26*(6), 459–516. doi:10.1016/j.mam.2005.10.001 PMID:16309738

Kris-Etherton, P. M., Etherton, T. D., Carlson, J., & Gardner, C. (2002). Recent discoveries in inclusive food-based approaches and dietary patterns for reduction in risk for cardiovascular disease. *Current Opinion in Lipidology*, *13*(4), 397–407. doi:10.1097/00041433-200208000-00007 PMID:12151855

Kris-Etherton, P. M., Harris, W. S., & Appel, L. J. (2003). Fatty acids and cardiovascular disease:new recommendations from the American Heart Association. AHA Nutrition Committee. and American Heart Association. *Omega-3. Arteriosclerosis, Thrombosis, and Vascular Biology*, *23*, 151–152. doi:10.1161/01.ATV.0000057393.97337.AE PMID:12588750

Kris-Etherton, P. M., Hecker, K. D., Bonanome, A., Coval, S. M., Binkoski, A. E., Hilpert, K. F., & Etherton, T. D. et al. (2002). Bioactive compounds in foods: Their role in the prevention of cardiovascular disease and cancer. *The American Journal of Medicine*, *113*(9), 71–88. doi:10.1016/S0002-9343(01)00995-0 PMID:12566142

Kris-Etherton, P. M., Hu, F. B., Ros, E., & Sabaté, J. (2008). The role of tree nuts and peanuts in the prevention of coronary heart disease: Multiple potential mechanisms. *The Journal of Nutrition*, *138*(9), 1746S–1751S. PMID:18716180

Kris-Etherton, P. M., Zhao, G., Binkoski, A. E., Coval, S. M., & Etherton, T. D. (2001). The effects of nuts on coronary heart disease risk. *Nutrition Reviews*, *59*(4), 103–111. doi:10.1111/j.1753-4887.2001.tb06996.x PMID:11368503

Krishna, K. L., Paridhavi, M., & Patel, J. A. (2008). Review on nutritional, medicinal and pharmacological properties of papaya (*Carica papaya* Linn.). *Natural Product Radiance*, *7*, 364–373.

Krishnaswamy, K. (2006). *Turmeric-The salt of the orient is the spice of life*. New Delhi, India: Allied Publishers Pvt. Ltd.

Kritchevsky, S. B., Shimakawa, T., Tell, G. S., Dennis, B., Carpenter, M., Eck-feldt, J. H., & Heiss, G. et al. (1995). Dietary antioxidants and carotid artery wall thickness. The ARIC study. Atherosclerosis Risk in Communities study. *Circulation*, *92*(8), 2142–2150. doi:10.1161/01.CIR.92.8.2142 PMID:7554194

Krochta, J. M., & Mulder-Johnston, C. D. (1997). Edible and biodegradable polymer films: Challenges and opportunities. *Food Technology*, *51*, 61–74.

Kubo, K., Saito, M., Tadokoro, T., & Mackawa, A. (1997). Changes in Susceptibility of Tissues to Lipid Peroxidation after Ingestion of Various Levels of Docosahexanoic Acid and Vitamin E. *The British Journal of Nutrition*, *78*(04), 655–669. doi:10.1079/BJN19970181 PMID:9389890

Kulig, M., Bergmann, R., Klettke, U., Wahn, V., Tacke, U., & Wahn, U. (1999). Natural course of sensitization to food and inhalant allergens during the first 6 years of life. *The Journal of Allergy and Clinical Immunology*, *103*(6), 1173–1179. doi:10.1016/S0091-6749(99)70195-8 PMID:10359902

Kulkarni, M., Nagasampagi, B. A., Deshpande, S. G., & Sharma, R. N. (1987). Five chromenes from Blepharispermum subsessile. *Phytochemistry*, *26*(11), 2969–2971. doi:10.1016/S0031-9422(00)84573-2

Kumar, A., Llavarasan, R., Jayachandran, T., Deecaraman, M., Mohan Kumar, R., Aravindan, P., & Krishan, M. R. V. et al. (2008). Anti-inflammatory activity of *Syzygium cumini* seed. *African Journal of Biotechnology*, *7*(8), 941–943.

Kumari, A., Dora, J., Kumar, A., & Kumar, A. (2012). Pomegranate (*Punica granatum*)-Overview. *International Journal of Pharmaceutical and Chemical Sciences*, *1*(4), 1218–1222.

Kumar, S., & Pandey, A. K. (2013). Chemistry and biological activities of flavonoids: An overview. *TheScientificWorld-Journal*, *2013*, 1–16. PMID:24470791

Kumar, S., Prasad, A. K., Iyer, S. V., & Vaidya, S. K. (2013). Systematic pharmacognostical, phytochemical and pharmacological review on an ethno medicinal plant, *Basella alba* L. *Journal of Pharmacognosy and Phytotherapy*, *5*, 53–58.

Kundhal, K., & Lok, C. (2005). Clinical epidemiology of cardiovascular disease in chronic kidney disease. *Nephron. Clinical Practice*, *101*(2), 47–c52. doi:10.1159/000086221 PMID:15942250

Kunwar, A., & Priyadarsini, K. I. (2011). Free radicals, oxidative stress and importance of antioxidants in human health. *Journal of Medical & Allide Science*, *1*(2), 53–60.

Kunyanga, C. N., Imungi, J. K., & Vellingiri, V. (2013). Nutritional evaluation of indigenous foods with potential food-based solution to alleviate hunger and malnutrition in Kenya. *Journal of Applied Biosciences*, *67*(0), 5277–5288. doi:10.4314/jab.v67i0.95049

Kunz, C., & Rudloff, S. (2006). Health promoting aspects of milk oligosaccharides. *International Dairy Journal*, *16*(11), 1341–1346. doi:10.1016/j.idairyj.2006.06.020

Kuriyama, S., Shimazu, T., Ohmori, K., Kikuchi, N., Nakaya, N., Nishino, Y., & Tsuji, I. et al. (2006). Green tea consumption and mortality due to cardiovascular disease, cancer, and all causes in Japan: The Ohsaki study. *Journal of the American Medical Association*, *296*(10), 1255–1265. doi:10.1001/jama.296.10.1255 PMID:16968850

Kurosawa, T., Itoh, F., Nozaki, A., Nakano, Y., Katsuda, S., Osakabe, N., & Itakura, H. et al. (2005). Suppressive effect of cocoa powder on atherosclerosis in Kurosawa and Kusanagi-hypercholesterolemic rabbits. *Journal of Atherosclerosis and Thrombosis*, *12*(1), 20–28. doi:10.5551/jat.12.20 PMID:15725692

Kushi, L. H., Meyer, K. A., & Jacobs, D. R. Jr. (1999). Cereals, legumes, and chronic disease risk reduction: Evidence from epidemiologic studies. *The American Journal of Clinical Nutrition*, *70*, 451S–458S. PMID:10479217

Kuwabara, Y., Nagai, S., Yoshimitsu, N., Nakagawa, I., Watanabe, Y., & Tamai, Y. (1995). Antihypertensive effect of the milk fermented by culturing with various lactic acid bacteria and yeast. *Journal of Fermentation and Bioengineering*, *80*(3), 294–295. doi:10.1016/0922-338X(95)90834-M

Kwak, J. S., Kim, J. Y., Paek, J. E., Lee, Y. J., Kim, H. R., Park, D. S., & Kwon, O. (2014). Garlic powder intake and cardiovascular risk factors: A meta-analysis of randomized controlled clinical trials. *Nutrition Research and Practice*, *8*(6), 644–654. doi:10.4162/nrp.2014.8.6.644 PMID:25489404

Kwenin, W. K. J., Wolli, M., & Dzomeku, B. M. (2011). Assessing the nutritional value of some African indigenous green Leafy Vegetables in Ghana. *Journal of Animal & Plant Sciences*, *10*, 1300–1305.

Kwon, M. J., Chun, J. H., Song, Y. S., & Song, Y. O. (1999). Daily kimchi consumption and its hypolipidemic effect in middle-aged men. *J. Korean Soc. Food Sci. Nutr.*, *28*, 1144–1150.

Kwon, M. J., Song, Y. S., Choi, M. S., Park, S. J., Jeong, K. S., & Song, Y. O. (2003a). Cholesteryl ester transfer protein activity and atherogenic parameters in rabbit supplemented with cholesterol and garlic powder. *Life Sciences*, *72*(26), 2953–2964. doi:10.1016/S0024-3205(03)00234-0 PMID:12706483

Kwon, M. J., Song, Y. S., Choi, M. S., & Song, Y. O. (2003b). Red pepper attenuates cholesteryl ester transfer protein activity and atherosclerosis in cholesterol-fed rabbits. *Clinica Chimica Acta*, *332*(1-2), 37–44. doi:10.1016/S0009-8981(03)00118-9 PMID:12763278

Kwon, M. J., Song, Y. S., & Song, Y. O. (1997). Effects of Kimchi on tissue and fecal lipid composition and apolipoprotein and thyroxine levels in rats. *J. Korean Food Sci. Nutr.*, *26*(3), 507–513.

Kwon, M. J., Song, Y. S., & Song, Y. O. (1998a). Antioxidative effect of kimchi ingredients on rabbits fed cholesterol diet. *Journal of the Korean Society of Food Science and Nutrition*, *27*, 1189–1196.

Kwon, Y., & Magnuson, B. A. (2007). Effect of azoxymethane and curcumin on transcriptional levels of cyclooxygenase-1 and-2 during initiation of colon carcinogenesis. *Scandinavian Journal of Gastroenterology*, *42*(1), 72–80. doi:10.1080/00365520600825216 PMID:17190766

Kwon, Y., Malik, M., & Magnuson, B. A. (2004). Inhibition of colonic aberrant crypt foci by curcumin in rats is affected by age. *Nutrition and Cancer*, *48*(1), 37–43. doi:10.1207/s15327914nc4801_6 PMID:15203376

Lafontan, M. (2004). Fat cells: Afferent and efferent messages define new approaches to treat obesity. *Annual Review of Pharmacology and Toxicology*, *45*(1), 119–146. doi:10.1146/annurev.pharmtox.45.120403.095843 PMID:15822173

Lai, H. T. M., Threapleton, D. E., Day, A. J., Williamson, G., Cade, J. E., & Burley, V. J. (2015). Fruit intake and cardiovascular disease mortality in the UK Women's Cohort Study. *European Journal of Epidemiology*, *30*(9), 1035–1048. doi:10.1007/s10654-015-0050-5 PMID:26076918

Lai, P. K., & Roy, J. (2004). Antimicrobial and chemopreventive properties of herbs and spices. *Current Medicinal Chemistry*, *11*(11), 1451–1460. doi:10.2174/0929867043365107 PMID:15180577

Lai, S., Zhou, Q., Zhang, Y., & Shang, J. Yu. T. (2009). Effects of pomegranate tannins onexperimental gastric damages. *Zhongguo Zhong Yao Za Zhi*, *34*(10), 1290–1294. PMID:19673398

Lajolo, F. M., & Genovese, M. I. (2002). Nutritional significance of lectins and enzyme inhibitors from legumes. *Journal of Agricultural and Food Chemistry*, *50*(22), 6592–6598. doi:10.1021/jf020191k PMID:12381157

Lala, G., Malik, M., Zhao, C., He, J., Kwon, Y., Giusti, M. M., & Magnuson, B. A. (2006). Anthocyanin-rich extracts inhibit multiple biomarkers of colon cancer in rats. *Nutrition and Cancer*, *54*(1), 84–93. doi:10.1207/s15327914nc5401_10 PMID:16800776

Lambert, J. D., & Elias, R. J. (2010). The antioxidant and pro-oxidant activities of green tea polyphenols: A role in cancer prevention. *Archives of Biochemistry and Biophysics*, *501*(1), 65–72. doi:10.1016/j.abb.2010.06.013 PMID:20558130

Lampe, J. W. (1999). Health effects of vegetables and fruit: Assessing mecha-nisms of action in human experimental studies. *The American Journal of Clinical Nutrition*, *70*(Suppl), 475–490. PMID:10479220

Lamuela-Raventos, R. M., Gimeno, E., Fito, M., Castellote, A. I., Covas, M., de la Torre-Boronat, M. C., & Lopez-Sabater, M. C. (2004). Interaction of olive oil phenol antioxidant components with low-density lipo protein. *Biological Research*, *37*(2), 247–252. doi:10.4067/S0716-97602004000200011 PMID:15455654

Lamy, S., Akla, N., Ouanouki, A., Lord-Dufour, S., & Beliveau, R. (2012). Diet-derived polyphenols inhibit angiogenesis by modu-lating the interleukin-6/STAT3 pathway. *Experimental Cell Research*, *318*(13), 1568–1596. doi:10.1016/j.yexcr.2012.04.004 PMID:22522122

Landete, J. M. (2012). Updated knowledge about polyphenols: Functions, bioavailability, metabolism, and health. *Critical Reviews in Food Science and Nutrition*, *52*(10), 936–948. doi:10.1080/10408398.2010.513779 PMID:22747081

Landete, J. M., Arqués, J., Medina, M., Gaya, P., De La Rivas, B., & Muñoz, R. (2015). Bioactivation of Phytoestrogens: Intestinal Bacteria and Health. *Critical Reviews in Food Science and Nutrition*, 00. doi:10.1080/10408398.2013.789823 PMID:25848676

Lansky, E. P., Harrison, G., Froom, P., & Jiang, W. G. (2005). Pomegranate (Punica granatum) pure chemicals show possible synergistic inhibition of human PC-3 prostate cancer cell invasion across Matrigel™. *Investigational New Drugs*, *23*(2), 121–122. doi:10.1007/s10637-005-5856-7 PMID:15744587

Lansky, E., Shubert, S., & Neeman, I. (2004). Pharmacological and therapeutic properties of pomegranate. *Israel. CIHEAM-Options Mediterraneennes*, *42*, 231–235.

Lardos, A. (2006). The botanical materiamedica of the Iatrosophikon-a collection of prescriptions from a monastery in Cyprus. *Journal of Ethnopharmacology*, *104*(3), 387–406. doi:10.1016/j.jep.2005.12.035 PMID:16459038

Larrosa, M., González-Sarrías, A., Yáñez-Gascón, M. J., Selma, M. V., Azorín-Ortuño, M., Toti, S., & Espín, J. C. (2010). Anti-inflammatory properties of a pomegranate extract & its metabolite urolithin-A in a colitis rat model & the effect of colon inflammation on phenolic metabolism. *The Journal of Nutritional Biochemistry*, *21*(8), 717–725. doi:10.1016/j.jnutbio.2009.04.012 PMID:19616930

Latha, G., Sindhu, P. G., Suja, S. R., Geetha, B. S., Pushpangadan, P., & Rajasekharan, S. (2005). Pharmacology and chemistry of Myristica fragrans Houtt. A review. *Journal of Spices and Aromatic Crops*, *14*(2), 94–101.

Laura, M. (2007). *Tea: The Drink that Changed the World*. Tuttle Publishing.

Laurie, S. A., Miller, V. A., Grant, S. C., Kris, M. G., & Ng, K. K. (2005). Phase I study of green tea extract in patients with advanced lung cancer. *Cancer Chemotherapy and Pharmacology*, *55*(1), 33–38. doi:10.1007/s00280-004-0859-1 PMID:15309507

Law, M. (2000). Plant sterol and stanol margarines and health. *British Medical Journal*, *320*(7238), 861–864. doi:10.1136/bmj.320.7238.861 PMID:10731187

Law, M. R., Wald, N. J., & Thompson, S. G. (1994). By how much and how quickly does reduction in serum cholesterol concentration lower risk of ischaemic heart disease? *BMJ (Clinical Research Ed.)*, *308*(6925), 367–372. doi:10.1136/bmj.308.6925.367 PMID:8043072

le Parc, A., Dalas, D. C., Duaut, S., Leonil, J., Martin, P., & Barile, D. (2014). Characterization of goat milk lactoferrin N-glycans and comparison with the N-Glycans of human and bovine milk. *Electrophoresis*, *35*(11), 1560–1570. doi:10.1002/elps.201300619 PMID:24519758

Lebesi, D. M., & Tzia, C. (2009). Effect of the addition of dietary fiber& edible cereal bran sources on the baking & sensory characteristics of cupcakes. *Food and Bioprocess Technology*, *4*(5), 710–722. doi:10.1007/s11947-009-0181-3

LeClair, K. (2000). Breaking the sensory barrier for functional foods. *Food Product Design*, *7*, 59–63.

Lecumberri, E., Dupertuis, Y. M., Miralbell, R., & Pichard, C. (2013). Green tea polyphenol epigallocatechin-3-gallate (EGCG) as adjuvant in cancer therapy. *Clinical Nutrition (Edinburgh, Lothian)*, *32*(6), 894–903. doi:10.1016/j.clnu.2013.03.008 PMID:23582951

Lee, P. Y., Taha, A. B. A., Lin, K., Ghazali, S. R., & Almashoor, S. H. S. A. (2007). Usage of complimentary and alternative medicine among primary care clinic attendees, Kuching, Sarawak, Malaysia, January – April, 2004. *Asia Pacific Journal of Family Medicine, 6*(1).

Lee, S. Y. (2001). *Anti-aging effects of kimchi diet in senescence accelerated mice (SAM P-8)*. (M. S. Thesis). Pusan National Univ, Korea.

Lee, W. J. (2003). *Effect of capsaicin on uncoupling protein-2 expression in 3T3-L1 cell line*. (M.S. Thesis). Inje University, Gimhae, Korea.

Lee, C. J., Chen, L. G., Liang, W. L., & Wang, C. C. (2010). Anti-inflammatory effects of Punica granatum Linne invitro & in vivo. *Journal of Food Chemistry*, *118*(2), 315–322. doi:10.1016/j.foodchem.2009.04.123

Lee, E. J., Patil, B. S., & Yoo, K. S. (2015). Antioxidants of 15 onions with white, yellow, and red colors and their relationship with pungency, anthocyanin, and quercetin. LWT-. *Food Science and Technology (Campinas.)*, *63*(1), 108–114.

Lee, G. R., Shin, M. K., Yoon, D. J., Kim, A. R., Yu, R., Park, N. H., & Han, I. S. (2013). Topical application of capsaicin reduces visceral adipose fat by affecting adipokine levels in high-fat diet-induced obese mice. *Obesity (Silver Spring, Md.)*, *21*(1), 115–122. doi:10.1002/oby.20246 PMID:23505175

Lee, J. I., Min, H. K., Lee, J. W., Jeong, J. D., Ha, Y. J., Kwack, S. C., & Park, J. S. (2009). Changes in the quality of loin from pigs supplemented with dietary methyl sulfonyl methane during cold storage. *Korean J. Food Sci*, *2*(2), 229–237. doi:10.5851/kosfa.2009.29.2.229

Lee, J. J., Lee, Y. M., Kim, A. R., Chang, H. C., & Lee, M. Y. (2008). Effect of Leuconostoc kimchi GJ2 isolated from kimchi (fermented Korean Cabbage) on lipid metabolism in high cholesterol-fed rats. *Korean J. Food Preserv*, *15*, 760–768.

Lee, J. S., Kwon, J. K., Han, S. H., An, I. J., Kim, S. J., Lee, S. H., & Jung, J. Y. et al. (2010). Toxicity study of detoxification sulfur at 3 months post-treatment in rats. *J F Hyg Safety*, *25*, 263–268.

Lee, J., Koo, N., & Min, D. B. (2004). Reactive oxygen species, aging, and antioxidative nutraceuticals. *Comprehensive Reviews in Food Science and Food Safety*, *3*(1), 21–33. doi:10.1111/j.1541-4337.2004.tb00058.x

Lee, J., Lee, H. J., Park, J. D., Lee, S. K., Lee, S. I., Lim, H. D., & Kim, E. C. et al. (2008). Anti-cancer activity of highly purified sulfur in immortalized and malignant human oral keratinocytes. *Toxicology In Vitro*, *22*(1), 87–95. doi:10.1016/j.tiv.2007.08.016 PMID:17920232

Lee, K. E., Choi, U. H., & Ji, G. E. (1996). Effect of kimchi intake on the composition of human large intestinal bacteria. *Korean J. Food Science and Technology (Campinas.)*, *28*, 981.

Lee, K. E., Choi, U. H., & Ji, G. E. (1996). Effect of kimchi intake on the composition of human large intestinal bacteria. *J. Korean Soc. Food Sci Tecbnol*, *28*, 981–986.

Lee, K. G., & Shibamoto, T. (2000). Antioxidant properties of aroma compounds isolated from soybeans and mung beans. *Journal of Agricultural and Food Chemistry*, *48*(9), 4290–4293. doi:10.1021/jf000442u PMID:10995351

Lee, K. O., Kim, S. N., & Kim, Y. C. (2014). Anti-wrinkle Effects of Water Extracts of Teas in Hairless Mouse. *Toxicological Reviews*, *30*(4), 283–289. doi:10.5487/TR.2014.30.4.283 PMID:25584148

Lee, S. H., & Kim, S. D. (1988). Effect of various ingredients of kimchi on the kimchi fermentation. *J. Food Sci. Nutr.*, *17*(3), 249–254.

Lee, Y. M., Kwon, M. J., Kim, J. K., Suh, H. S., Chio, J. S., & Song, Y. O. (2004). Isolation and identification of active principle in Chinese cabbage kimchi responsible for antioxidant activity. *Korean Journal of Food Science and Technology*, *36*, 129–133.

Lehmann, L., Esch, H. L., Wagner, J., Rohnstock, L., & Metzler, M. (2005). Estrogenic and genotoxic potential of equol and two hydroxylated metabolites of Daidzein in cultured human Ishikawa cells. *Toxicology Letters*, *158*(1), 72–86. doi:10.1016/j.toxlet.2005.02.011 PMID:15993745

Lei, V., & Jakobsen, M. (2004). Microbiological characterization and probiotic potentialof *koko* and *kokosourwater*, African spontaneously fermented millet porridge and drink. *Journal of Applied Microbiology*, *96*(2), 384–397. doi:10.1046/j.1365-2672.2004.02162.x PMID:14723700

Lentils. (2003). InGrant, G. D. M., & Alonso, R. (Eds.), *Encyclopedia of Food Science and Nutrition*. London: Elsevier Science Ltd.

Leong, H., Mathur, P. S., & Greene, G. L. (2008). Green tea catechins inhibit angiogenesis through suppression of STAT3 activation. *Breast Cancer Research and Treatment*, *117*(3), 505–515. doi:10.1007/s10549-008-0196-x PMID:18821062

Léonil, J., Gagnaire, V., Mollé, D., Pezennec, S., & Bouhallab, S. (2000). Application of chromatography and mass spectrometry to the characterization of food proteins and derived peptides. *Journal of Chromatography. A*, *881*(1-2), 1–21. doi:10.1016/S0021-9673(00)00071-6 PMID:10905689

Leopoldini, M., Russo, N., & Toscano, M. (2011). The molecular basis of working mechanism of natural polyphenolic antioxidants. *Food Chemistry*, *125*(2), 288–306. doi:10.1016/j.foodchem.2010.08.012

Lephart, E. D., West, T. W., Weber, K. S., Rhees, R. W., Setchell, K. D., Adlercreutz, H., & Lund, T. D. (2002). Neurobehavioral effects of dietary soy phytoestrogens. *Neurotoxicology and Teratology*, *24*(1), 5–16. doi:10.1016/S0892-0362(01)00197-0 PMID:11836067

Lethavy, A., Marjoribanks, J., Kronenberg, F., Roberts, H., Eden, J., & Brown, J. (2013). Phytoestrogens for menopausal vasomotor symptoms[Review]. *Cochrane Database of Systematic Reviews*, *12*(no. CD001395). doi:10.1002/14651858.CD001395.pub4 PMID:24323914

Levent, H., Bilgicli, N., & Ertas, N. (2015). The assessment of leavened and unleavened flat breads properties enriched with wheat germ. *Qual. Assur. Safety Crops & Foods*, *7*(3), 321–326. doi:10.3920/QAS2013.0341

Levi, F., Pasche, C., La Vecchia, C., Lucchini, F., & Franceschi, S. (1999). Food groups and colorectal cancer risk. *British Journal of Cancer*, *79*(7/8), 1283–1287. doi:10.1038/sj.bjc.6690206 PMID:10098773

Lewis, M. W. (2012). Hot, caffeinated, and expanding: the global geography of coffee, tea, and yerba mate. *GeoCurrents*. Retrieved October 26, 2015 from http://www.geocurrents.info/economic-geography/hot-caffeinated-and-expanding-the-global-geography-of-coffee-tea-and-yerba-mate

Lewis, D. R., Southwick, J. W., Ouellet-Hellstrom, R., Rench, J., & Calderon, R. L. (1999). Drinking water arsenic in Utah: A cohort mortality study. *Environmental Health Perspectives*, *107*(5), 359–365. doi:10.1289/ehp.99107359 PMID:10210691

Ley, J. P., Blings, M., Paetz, S., Krammer, G. B., & Bertram, H. J. (2006). New bitter-masking compounds: Hydroxylated benzoic acid amides of aromatic amines as structural analogues of homoeriodictyol. *Journal of Agricultural and Food Chemistry*, *54*(22), 8574–8579. doi:10.1021/jf0617061 PMID:17061836

Liang, Y. C., Chen, Y. C., Lin, Y. L., Lin-Shiau, S. Y., Ho, C. T., & Lin, J. K. (1999). Suppression of extracellular signals and cell proliferation by the black tea polyphenol, theaflavin-3,3'-digallate. *Carcinogenesis*, *20*(4), 733–736. doi:10.1093/carcin/20.4.733 PMID:10223207

Liao, Y. T., Chen, C. J., Li, W. F., Hsu, L. I., Tsai, L. Y., Huang, Y. L., & Wang, S. L. et al. (2012). Elevated lactate dehydrogenase activity and increased cardiovascular mortality in the arsenic-endemic areas of southwestern Taiwan. *Toxicology and Applied Pharmacology*, *262*(3), 232–237. doi:10.1016/j.taap.2012.04.028 PMID:22569360

Lichtenstein, A. H., Ausman, L. M., Carrasco, W., Gualtieri, L. J., Jenner, J. L., Ordovas, J. M., & Schaefer, E. J. et al. (1994). Rice br.an oil consumption & plasma lipid levels in moderately hypercholesterolemic humans Ar*terio.sclerosis. Thrombosis, and Vascular Biology*, *14*, 549–556. doi:10.1161/01.ATV.14.4.549

Lifton, R. P., Gharavi, A. G., & Geller, D. S. (2001). Molecular mechanisms of human hypertension. *Cell*, *104*(4), 545–556. doi:10.1016/S0092-8674(01)00241-0 PMID:11239411

Li, G. H., Le, G. W., Shi, Y. H., & Shrestha, S. (2004). Angiotensin I-converting enzyme inhibitory peptides derived from food proteins and their physiological and pharmacological effects. *Nutrition Research (New York, N.Y.), 24*(7), 469–486. doi:10.1016/S0271-5317(04)00058-2

Li, J. W., Ding, S. D., & Ding, X. L. A. (2005). Comparison of antioxidant capacities of extracts from five cultivars of Chinese jujube. *Process Biochemistry (Barking, London, England), 40*(11), 3607–3613. doi:10.1016/j.procbio.2005.03.005

Li, J. W., Fan, L. P., Ding, S. D., & Ding, X. L. (2007). Nutritional composition of five cultivars of Chinese jujube. *Food Chemistry, 103*(2), 454–460. doi:10.1016/j.foodchem.2006.08.016

Lilley, D. M., & Stillwell, R. H. (1965). Probiotics promoting factors produced by microorganisms. *Science, 147*(3659), 747–748. doi:10.1126/science.147.3659.747 PMID:14242024

Li, N., Han, C., & Chen, J. (1999). Tea preparations protect against DMBA-induced oral carcinogenesis in hamsters. *Nutrition and Cancer, 35*(1), 73–79. doi:10.1207/S1532791473-79 PMID:10624709

Lin, L., Allemekinders, H., Dansby, A., Campbell, L., Durance-Tod, S., Berger, A., & Jones, P. J. (2013). Evidence of health benefits of canola oil. *Nutrition Reviews, 71*(6), 370–385. doi:10.1111/nure.12033 PMID:23731447

Liolios, C. C., Gortzi, O., Lalas, S., Tsaknis, J., & Chinou, I. (2009). Liposomal incorporation of carvacrol and thymol isolated from the essential oil of *Origanum dictamnus* L. and in vitro antimicrobial activity. *Food Chemistry, 112*(1), 77–83. doi:10.1016/j.foodchem.2008.05.060

Li, S., Chen, G., Zhang, C., Wu, M., Wu, S., & Liu, Q. (2014). Research progress of natural antioxidants in foods for thetreatment of diseases. *Food Science and Human Wellness, 3*, 110–116.

Lisabeth, L. D., Ahn, H. J., Chen, J. J., Sealy-Jefferson, S., Burke, J. F., & Meliker, J. R. (2010). Arsenic in drinking water and stroke hospitalizations in Michigan. *Stroke, 41*(11), 2499–2504. doi:10.1161/STROKEAHA.110.585281 PMID:20947858

Liu, L., Guo, X. E., Zhou, Y. Q., & Xia, J. L. (2003). Prevalence of dementia in China. *Dementia and Geriatric Cognitive Disorders, 15*(4), 226–230. doi:10.1159/000068784 PMID:12626856

Liu, M. (2006). Chinese jujube: Botany and horticulture. *Horticultural Reviews, 32*, 229–298.

Liu, R. H. (2007). Whole grain phytochemicals and health. *Journal of Cereal Science, 46*(3), 207–219. doi:10.1016/j.jcs.2007.06.010

Liu, S., Manson, J. E., Lee, I.-M., Cole, S. R., Hennekens, C. H., Willet, W. C., & Buring, J. E. (2000). Fruit and vegetable intake and risk of cardiovascular disease: The Women's Health Study. *The American Journal of Clinical Nutrition, 72*, 922–928. PMID:11010932

Liu, Z. M., Ho, S. C., Woo, J., Chen, Y. M., & Wong, C. (2014). Randomized controlled trial of whole soy and isoflavone daidzein on menopausal symptoms in equol-producing Chinese postmenopausal women. *Menopause (New York, N.Y.), 21*(6), 653–660. doi:10.1097/GME.0000000000000102 PMID:24149925

Livesey, G., Taylor, R., Hulshof, T., & Howlett, J. (2008). Glycemic response and health- A systematic review and meta-analysis: Relations between dietary glycemic properties and health outcomes. *The American Journal of Clinical Nutrition, 87*, 258S–268S. PMID:18175766

Li, W., Liang, H., Zhang, M., Zhang, R., Deng, Y., Wei, Z., & Tang, X. et al. (2012). Phenolic profiles and antioxidant activity of litchi (*Litchi chinensis* Sonn.) fruit pericarp from different commercially available cultivars. *Molecules (Basel, Switzerland), 17*(12), 14954–14967. doi:10.3390/molecules171214954 PMID:23247368

Li, Y. W., Zhang, Y., Zhang, L., Li, X., Yu, J. B., Zhang, H. T., & Liu, H. G. et al. (2014). Protective effect of tea polyphenols on renal ischemia/reperfusion injury via suppressing the activation of TLR4/NF-κB p65 signal pathway. *Gene*, *542*(1), 46–51. doi:10.1016/j.gene.2014.03.021 PMID:24630969

Li, Y., Guo, C., Yang, J., Wei, J., Xu, J., & Cheng, S. (2006). Evaluation of antioxidant properties of pomegranate peel extract in comparison with pomegranate pulp extract. *Food Chemistry*, *96*(2), 254–260. doi:10.1016/j.foodchem.2005.02.033

Li, Y., Liu, L., Andrews, L. G., & Tollefsbol, T. O. (2009). Genistein depletes telomerase activity through cross-talk between genetic and epigenetic mechanisms. *International Journal of Cancer*, *125*(2), 286–296. doi:10.1002/ijc.24398 PMID:19358274

Li, Y., Zhao, S., Zhang, W., Zhao, P., He, B., Wu, N., & Han, P. (2011). Epigallocatechin-3-O-gallate (EGCG) attenuates FFAs-induced peripheral insulin resistance through AMPK pathway and insulin signaling pathway in vivo. *Diabetes Research and Clinical Practice*, *93*(2), 205–214. doi:10.1016/j.diabres.2011.03.036 PMID:21514684

Llaneza, P., González, C., Fernández-Iñarrea, J., Alonso, A., Díaz, F., Arnott, I., & Ferrer-Barriendos, J. (2010). Soy isoflavones, diet and physical exercise modify serum cytokines in healthy obese postmenopausal women. *Phytomedicine*, *18*(4), 245–250. doi:10.1016/j.phymed.2010.07.011 PMID:20732799

Lock, A. L., Destaillats, F., Kraft, J., & German, J. B. (2008). Introduction to the proceedings of the symposium 'Scientific update on dairy fats and cardiovascular disease'. *Journal of the American College of Nutrition*, *27*(6), 720S–722S. doi:10.1080/07315724.2008.10719749 PMID:19155431

Loganathan, R., Selvaduray, K. R., Radhakrishnan, A., & Nesaretnam, K. (2010). Palm oil: Risch in health promoting phytonutrients. *Palm Oil Developments*, *50*, 16–25.

Lombardi-Boccia, G., Ruggeri, S., Aguzzi, A., & Cappelloni, M. (2003). Globulins enhance in vitro iron but not zinc dialysability: A study on six legume species. *Journal of Trace Elements in Medicine and Biology*, *17*(1), 1–5. doi:10.1016/S0946-672X(03)80037-8 PMID:12755494

López-Fandiño, R., Otte, J., & Van Camp, J. (2006). Review: Physiological, chemicaland technological aspects of milk-protein-derived peptides with antihypertensiveand ACE-inhibitory activity. *International Dairy Journal*, *16*(11), 1277–1293. doi:10.1016/j.idairyj.2006.06.004

Lopriore, C., & Muehlhoff, E. (2003). *Food security and nutrition trends in West Africa - Challenges and the way forward.* Retrieved April 15, 2015 from ftp://ftp.fao.org/es/esn/nutrition/ouagafinal.pdf

Losso, J. N. (2008). The biochemical and functional food properties of the Bowman-Birk inhibitor. *Critical Reviews in Food Science and Nutrition*, *48*(1), 94–118. doi:10.1080/10408390601177589 PMID:18274967

Losso, J. N., Holliday, D. L., Richard, G., Karki, N., & Finley, J. W. (2010). The health benefits of fenugreek-enriched cereal products. *Cereal Foods World*, *55*(5), 236–241.

Loughmiller, J. A., Nelssen, J. L., Goodband, R. D., Tokach, M. D., Titgemeyer, E. C., & Kim, I. H. (1998). Influence of dietary total sulfur amino acids and methionine on growth performance and carcass characteristics of finishing gilts. *Journal of Animal Science*, *76*(8), 2129–2137. PMID:9734863

Loughmiller, J. A., Tokach, M. D., Goodband, R. D., Nelssen, J. L., Titgemeyer, E. C., Kim, I. H., & Dritz, S. (1996). Dietary total sulfur amino acid requirement for optimal growth performance and carcass characteristics in finishing gilts. In *Kansas State University Swine Day. Report of Progress* (pp. 133–135). Kansas State University.

Lovegrove, J. A., & Jackson, K. G. (2011). Functional foods and coronary heart disease (CHD). In Functional Foods - Concept to Product (2nd ed.). Woodhead Publishing Series in Food Science, Technology and Nutrition.

Low, Y. L., Dunning, A. M., Dowsett, M., Luben, R. N., Khaw, K. T., Wareham, N. J., & Bingham, S. A. (2006). Implications of gene-environment interaction in studies of gene variants in breast cancer: An example of dietary isoflavones and the D356N polymorphism in the sex hormone-binding globulin gene. *Cancer Research*, *66*(18), 8980–8983. doi:10.1158/0008-5472.CAN-06-2432 PMID:16982738

Lukmanji, Z., Hertzmark, E., Mlingi, N., Assey, V., & Ndossi, G. et al.. (2008). *Tanzania food composition Tables. MUHAS-TFNC*. Dar es Salaam, Tanzania: HSPH.

Lu, L. J. W., Anderson, K. E., Graddy, J. J., & Nagamani, M. (1996). Effects of soya consumption for one month on steroid hormones in premenopausal women: Implications for breast cancer risk reduction. *Cancer Epidemiology, Biomarkers & Prevention*, *5*, 63–70. PMID:8770469

Lunceford, N., & Gugliucci, A. (2005). *Ilex paraguariensis* extracts inhibit AGE formation more efficiently than green tea. *Fitoterapia*, *76*(5), 419–427. doi:10.1016/j.fitote.2005.03.021 PMID:15894431

Lund, T. D., Munson, D. J., Haldy, M. E., Setchell, K. D., Lephart, E. D., & Handa, R. J. (2004). Equol is a novel antiandrogen that inhibits prostate growth and hormone feedback. *Biology of Reproduction*, *70*(4), 1188–1195. doi:10.1095/biolreprod.103.023713 PMID:14681200

Luthria, A., Singh, K., & D'souza, M. (2014). *In vitro* antioxidant activity of black gram, cowpea, desi chickpea and yellow mustard as affected by sprouting. *Journal of Global Biosciences*, *3*(1), 385–389.

Lu, Y., Junli, L., Hao, J., Niu, Y., Whent, M., Costa, J., & Yu, L. (2015b). Genotype, environment, and their interactions on the phytochemical compositions and radical scavenging properties of soft winter wheat bran. LWT-. *Food Science and Technology (Campinas.)*, *60*(1), 277–283.

Lu, Y., Fuerst, E. P., Lv, J., Morris, C. F., Yu, L., Fletcher, A., & Luthria, D. et al. (2015a). Phytochemical profile and antiproliferative activity of dough and bread fractions made from refined and whole wheat flours. *Cereal Chem.*, *92*(3), 271–277. doi:10.1094/CCHEM-10-14-0214-R

MacCalla, A. F. (1994). *Agriculture and Food Need to 2025, Why we should be concerned*. Washington, DC: CGIAR.

Macfarlane, A., & Macfarlane, I. (2004). The empire of tea. The Overlook Press.

Maclean, J. L., Dawe, D. C., Hardy, B., & Hettel, G. P. (Eds.). (2002). Rice Almanac. CABI Publishing.

Maclure, M. (1993). Demonstration of deductive meta-analysis: Ethanol intake and risk of myocardial infarction. *Epidemiologic Reviews*, *15*(2), 328–351. PMID:8174661

MacRae, W. D., & Towers, G. H. N. (1984). Biological activities of lignans. *Phytochemistry*, *23*(6), 1207–1220. doi:10.1016/S0031-9422(00)80428-8

Maenthaisong, R., Chaiyakunapruk, N., Niruntrapom, S., & Kongkaew, C. (2007). The efficacy of Aloe vera used for burn wound healing: A systematic review. *Burns*, *33*(6), 713–718. doi:10.1016/j.burns.2006.10.384 PMID:17499928

Magala-Nyago, C. M., Kikafunda, J.K., Mwasaru, M.A., Kenji, G.M., & Connely, R.K. (2005). Evaluation of nutritional value of malted and extruded finger millet based complementary foods. In *Proceedings of African Crop Science Conference* (*vol. 7*, pp 677-686). Kampala, Uganda: ACSJ.

Mahmood, A. A., Sidik, K., Salmah, I., Suzainur, K. A. R., & Yusoff, K. M. (2004). Cytoprotective effects of honey and methanol extracts from *P. granatum* L. fruit peel and *N. sativa* L seeds on ethanol-induced gastric damage in rats. *Journal of Food Technology*, *2*(3), 136–141.

Mahmoud, A. M., Yang, W., & Bosland, M. C. (2014). Soy isoflavones and prostate cancer: A review of molecular mechanisms. *The Journal of Steroid Biochemistry and Molecular Biology*, *140*, 116–132. doi:10.1016/j.jsbmb.2013.12.010 PMID:24373791

Maldonado, J., Gil, A., Narbona, E., & Molina, J. A. (1998). Special formulas in infant nutrition: A review. *Early Human Development*, *53*, S23–S32. doi:10.1016/S0378-3782(98)00062-0 PMID:10102652

Malhomme, H., Seagrove, S., Mehta, A., Divekar, P., Campbell, S., & Curnow, A. (2010). Using natural dietary sources of antioxidants to protect against ultraviolet and visible radiation-induced DNA damage: an investigation of human green tea ingestion. *Journal of Photochemistry and Photobiology B*, *101*(2), 169-173.

Malik, A., Afaq, F., Sarfaraz, S., Adhami, V. M., Syed, D. N., & Mukhtar, H. (2005). Pomegranate fruit juice for chemoprevention & chemotherapy of prostate cancer. *Proceedings of the National Academy of Sciences of the United States of America*, *102*(41), 14813–14818. doi:10.1073/pnas.0505870102 PMID:16192356

Maliro, M. F. A. (2001). The role and potential of traditional tuber crops in Malawi. In D. Pasternak & A. Schlissel (Eds.), *Combating Desertification with Plants* (pp. 55–64). Kluwer Academic Press. doi:10.1007/978-1-4615-1327-8_5

Mallik, N., Bhaskar Reddy, G. V., Kiranmayi, B., Govind, V., Eswara Rao, B., & Ashalatha, P. (2013). Milk constituents as functional food components. *Indian Food Industry*, *32*(1), 17–26.

Mandel, S. A., Amit, T., Weinreb, O., & Youdim, M. B. (2011). Understanding the broad-spectrum neuroprotective action profile of green tea polyphenols in aging and neurodegenerative diseases. *Journal of Alzheimer's Disease*, *25*(2), 187–208. PMID:21368374

Manful, J. T., Swetman, A. A., Coker, R. D., & Drunis, A. (2007). Changes in the thiamine and riboflavin contents of rice during artisanal parboiling in Ghana. *Tropical Science*, *47*(4), 211–217. doi:10.1002/ts.215

Manjula, K., Hell, K., Fandohan, P., Abass, A., & Bandyopadhyay, R. (2009). Aflatoxin and fumonisin contamination of cassava products and maize grain from markets in Tanzania and Republic of Congo. *Toxin Reviews*, *28*(2-3), 63–69. doi:10.1080/15569540802462214

Mantovani, D., Cardozo Filho, L., Santos, L. C., de Souza, V. L., & Watanabe, C. S. (2009). Chromatographic quantification of isoflavone content from soy derivates using HPLC technique. *Journal of Chromatographic Science*, *47*(9), 766–769. doi:10.1093/chromsci/47.9.766 PMID:19835685

Marathe, S. A., Rajalakshmi, V., Jamdar, S. N., & Sharma, A. (2011). Comparative study on antioxidant activity of different varieties of commonly consumed legumes in India. *Food and Chemical Toxicology*, *49*(9), 2005–2012. doi:10.1016/j.fct.2011.04.039 PMID:21601612

Marchione, M. (2009). Two billion, five hundred million dollars spent, no alternative cures. *Phys.org*. Retrieved November 13, 2015 from http://phys.org/news/2009-06-25b-spent-alternative-med.html

Marcinkiewicz, J. (2010). Taurine bromamine (TauBr) - its role in immunity and new perspectives for clinical use. *Journal of Biomedical Science*, *17*(Suppl 1), S3. doi:10.1186/1423-0127-17-S1-S3 PMID:20804605

Margetts, B.M., Thompson, R., & Duffy, S. (1994). *A Review of the Epidemiological Literature Linking Fruit and Vegetable Consumption to Risk of Cancer*. Nutritional Epidemiology Working Group on Diet and Cancer.

Marina, A. M., Man, Y. B., Nazimah, S. A., & Amin, I. (2009). Antioxidant capacity and phenolic acids of virgin coconut oil. *International Journal of Food Sciences and Nutrition*, *60*(sup2Suppl 2), 114–123. doi:10.1080/09637480802549127 PMID:19115123

Marinangeli, C. P., & Jones, P. J. (2012). Pulse grain consumption and obesity: Effects on energy expenditure, substrate oxidation, body composition, fat deposition and satiety. *The British Journal of Nutrition*, *108*(S1), S46–S51. doi:10.1017/S0007114512000773 PMID:22916815

Mark, A. L. (1996). The sympathetic nervous system in hypertension: A potential long term regulator of arterial pressure. *Journal of Hypertension*, *14*(S1), 59–65. PMID:9120673

Marks, G., Aydos, R. D., Fagundes, D. J., Pontes, E. R. J. C., Takita, L. C., Amaral, E. G. A. S., & Ynouye, C. M. et al. (2006). Modulation of transforming growth factor beta2 (TGF-beta2) by inositol hexaphosphate in colon carcinogenesis in rats. *Acta Cirurgica Brasileira*, *21*, 51–56. doi:10.1590/S0102-86502006001000012 PMID:17293967

Marles, R. J., & Farnsworth, N. R. (1994). Plants as Sources of Antidiabetic Agents. *Economic and Medicinal Plant Research*, *6*, 149–187.

Marrian, G. F., & Haslewood, G. A. (1932). Equol, a new inactive phenol isolated from the ketohydroxyoestrin fraction of mares' urine. *The Biochemical Journal*, *26*(4), 1227–1232. doi:10.1042/bj0261227 PMID:16744928

Martin, L. C. (2007). Tea: the drink that changed the world. Turtle Publishing.

Martinez, M. (1954). Plantas utiles de la flora Mexico. Mexico. *Ediciones Botas, 400.*

Martinez, I., Kim, J., Duffy, P. R., Schlegel, V. L., & Walter, J. (2010). Resistant starches types 2 and 4 have differential effects on the composition of the fecal microbiota in human subjects. *PLoS ONE*, *5*(11), e15046. doi:10.1371/journal.pone.0015046 PMID:21151493

Martin, M. J., Martin-Sosa, S., Garcia-Pardo, L. A., & Hueso, P. (2001). Distribution of bovine sialoglycoconjugates during lactation. *Journal of Dairy Science*, *84*(5), 995–1000. doi:10.3168/jds.S0022-0302(01)74558-4 PMID:11384055

Martino, H. S. D. M., Cardoso, L. M., Ribeiro, S. M. R., Dantas, M. I. S., Piovesan, N. D., & Mejia, E. D. (2011). Nutritional and bioactive compounds of soybean: benefits on human health, soybean and health. InTech Publisher.

Martins, J. M., Riottot, M., de Abreu, M. C., Lança, M. J., Viegas-Crespo, A. M., Almeida, J. A., & Bento, O. P. et al. (2004). Dietary raw peas (*Pisum sativum* L.) reduce plasma total and LDL cholesterol and hepatic esterified cholesterol in intact and ileorectal anastomosed pigs fed cholesterol-rich diets. *The Journal of Nutrition*, *134*(12), 3305–3312. PMID:15570030

Martins, J. M., Riottot, M., de Abreu, M. C., Viegas-Crespo, A. M., Lança, M. J., Almeida, J. A., & Bento, O. P. et al. (2005). Cholesterol-lowering effects of dietary blue lupin (Lupinus angustifolius L.) in intact and ileorectal anastomosed pigs. *Journal of Lipid Research*, *46*(7), 1539–1547. doi:10.1194/jlr.M500129-JLR200 PMID:15834122

Maruo, T., Sakamoto, M., Ito, C., Toda, T., & Benno, Y. (2008). *Adlercreutzia equolifaciens* gen. nov., sp. nov., an equol-producing bacterium isolated from human faeces, and emended description of the genus *Eggerthella*. *International Journal of Systematic and Evolutionary Microbiology*, *58*(5), 1221–1227. doi:10.1099/ijs.0.65404-0 PMID:18450717

Masibo, M., & He, Q. (2008). Major mango polyphenols and their potential significance to human health. *Comprehensive Reviews in Food Science and Food Safety*, *7*(4), 309–319. doi:10.1111/j.1541-4337.2008.00047.x

Mastan, S. K., Chaitanya, G., Latha, T. B., Srikanth, A., Sumalatha, G., & Kumar, K. E. (2009). Cardioprotective effect of methanolic extract of Syzygium cumini seeds on isoproterenol-induced myocardial infarction in rats. *Der Pharmacia Lettre*, *1*(1), 143–149.

Masuda, M., Suzui, M., Lim, J. T., & Weinstein, I. B. (2003). Epigallocatechin-3-gallate inhibits activation of HER-2/neu and downstream signaling pathways in human head and neck and breast carcinoma cells. *Clinical Cancer Research*, *9*(9), 3486–3491. PMID:12960141

Mata, R., & Escandón, S. (2012). Calein C, an Alpha-Glucosidase Inhibitor from Brickellia cavanillesii. *Planta Medica*, *78*(05), 96. doi:10.1055/s-0032-1307604

Mathanghi, S. K., & Sudha, K. (2012). Functional properties of finger millet (*Eleusine coracana L.*) for health. *International Journal of Pharmaceutical. Chemical and Biological Sciences*, *2*(4), 431–438.

Mathangi, S. K. (2012). Nutraceutical properties of great millet – *Sorghum vulgare. International Journal of Food. Agriculture and Veterinary Sciences*, *2*, 40–45.

Mathangi, S. K., & Sudha, K. (2012). Functional and phytochemical properties of finger millet (*Eleusine coracana* L.) for health. *International Journal of Pharmaceutical Chemical and Biological Sciences*, *2*, 431–438.

Mathé, G. (1999). Red wine, green tea and vitamins: Do their antioxidants play a role in immunologic protection against cancer or even AIDS? *Biomedicine and Pharmacotherapy*, *53*(4), 165–167. doi:10.1016/S0753-3322(99)80084-5 PMID:10392288

Mathieu, G., & Meissa, D. (2007). Traditional leafy vegetables in Senegal: Diversity and Medicinal Uses. *African Journal of Traditional, Complementary, and Alternative Medicines*, *4*(4), 469–475. doi:10.4314/ajtcam.v4i4.31239 PMID:20161914

Matthies, A., Blaut, M., & Braune, A. (2009). Isolation of a human intestinal bacterium capable of daidzein and genistein conversion. *Applied and Environmental Microbiology*, *75*(6), 1740–1744. doi:10.1128/AEM.01795-08 PMID:19139227

Matthies, A., Clavel, T., Gütschow, M., Engst, W., Haller, D., Blaut, M., & Braune, A. (2008). Conversion of daidzein and genistein by an anaerobic bacterium newly isolated from the mouse intestine. *Applied and Environmental Microbiology*, *74*(15), 4847–4852. doi:10.1128/AEM.00555-08 PMID:18539813

Matthies, A., Loh, G., Blaut, M., & Braune, A. (2012). Daidzein and genistein are converted to equol and 5-hydroxy-equol by human intestinal *Slackia isoflavoniconvertens* in gnotobiotic rats. *The Journal of Nutrition*, *142*(1), 40–66. doi:10.3945/jn.111.148247 PMID:22113864

Matumba, L., Monjerezi, M., Khonga, E. B., & Lakudzala, D. D. (2011). Aflatoxins in sorghum, sorghum malt and traditional opaque beer in southern Malawi. *Food Control*, *22*(2), 266–268. doi:10.1016/j.foodcont.2010.07.008

Matumba, L., Van Poucke, C., Biswick, T., Monjerezi, M., Mwatseteza, J., & De Saeger, S. (2014). A limited survey of mycotoxins in traditional maize based opaque beers in Malawi. *Food Control*, *36*(1), 253–256. doi:10.1016/j.foodcont.2013.08.032

Matysiak, M., Gawel-Beben, K., Rybczynska, K., Gminski, J., & Surma, S. (2015). Comparing selected biological properties of garlic (*Allium sativum* L.) from Poland and China. *Zywnosc*, *22*(2), 160–169.

Maubach, J., Bracke, M. E., Heyerick, A., Depypere, H. T., Serreyn, R. F., Mareel, M. M., & De Keukeleire, D. (2003). Quantitation of soy-derived phytoestrogens in human breast tissue and biological fluids by high-performance liquid chromatography. *Journal of Chromatography. B, Analytical Technologies in the Biomedical and Life Sciences*, *784*(1), 137–144. doi:10.1016/S1570-0232(02)00789-4 PMID:12504192

Maurya, P. K., & Rizvi, S. I. (2009). Protective role of tea catechins on erythrocytes subjected to oxidative stress during human aging. *Natural Product Research*, *23*(12), 1072–1079. doi:10.1080/14786410802267643 PMID:18846469

Ma, W. W., Heinstein, P. P., & McLaughlin, J. L. (1989). Additional Toxic, Bitter Saponins from the Seeds of *Chenopodium quinoa. Journal of Natural Products*, *52*(5), 1132–1135. doi:10.1021/np50065a035 PMID:2607350

Ma, Y., & Huang, H. (2014). Characterization and comparison of phenols, flavonoids and isoflavones of soymilk and their correlations with antioxidant activity. *International Journal of Food Science & Technology*, *49*(10), 2290–2298. doi:10.1111/ijfs.12545

Mazur, W. M., Duke, J. A., Wähälä, K., Rasku, S., & Adlercreutz, H. (1998). Isoflavonoids and lignans in legumes: Nutritional and health aspects in humans. *The Journal of Nutritional Biochemistry*, *9*(4), 193–200. doi:10.1016/S0955-2863(97)00184-8

Mbatia, B., Awuor, O. L., Kirwa, M. E., & Kackim, M. F. (2014). Antioxidative and functional properties of *Rastrineobola argentea* (dagaa) fish protein hydrolysate. *Discourse Journal of Agriculture and Food Sciences*, *2*, 180–189.

McCrory, M. A., Hamaker, B. R., Lovejoy, J. C., & Eichelsdoerfer, P. E. (2010). Pulse consumption, satiety, and weight management. *Advances in Nutrition: An International Review Journal*, *1*(1), 17–30. doi:10.3945/an.110.1006 PMID:22043448

McInnes, G. T. (2004). How important is optimal blood pressure control? *Clinical Therapeutics*, *26*, 3–11. doi:10.1016/S0149-2918(04)90140-3 PMID:15291374

McKay, D. L., & Blumberg, J. B. (2002). The role of tea in human health: An update. *Journal of the American College of Nutrition*, *21*(1), 1–13. doi:10.1080/07315724.2002.10719187 PMID:11838881

McMillan, M., Spinks, E. A., & Fenwick, G. R. (1986). Preliminary observations on the effect of dietary brussels sprouts on thyroid function. *Human Toxicology*, *5*(1), 15–19. doi:10.1177/096032718600500104 PMID:2419242

Medrano, M. A., Boix, R., Pastor-Barriuso, R., Palau, M., Damián, J., Ramis, R., & Navas-Acien, A. et al. (2010). Arsenic in public water supplies and cardiovascular mortality in Spain. *Environmental Research*, *110*(5), 448–454. doi:10.1016/j.envres.2009.10.002 PMID:19880104

Mehra, R., & Kelly, P. (2006). Milk oligosaccharides: Structural and technological aspects[Review]. *International Dairy Journal*, *16*(11), 1334–1340. doi:10.1016/j.idairyj.2006.06.008

Mehta, R., & Lansky, E. P. (2004). Breast cancer chemopreventive properties of pomegranate (Punica granatum) fruit extracts in a mouse mammary organ culture. *European Journal of Cancer Prevention*, *13*(4), 345–348. doi:10.1097/01.cej.0000136571.70998.5a PMID:15554563

Meisel, H. (2004). Multifunctional peptides encrypted in milk proteins. *BioFactors (Oxford, England)*, *21*(1-4), 55–61. doi:10.1002/biof.552210111 PMID:15630170

Meisel, H., & Bockelmann, W. (1999). Bioactive peptides encrypted in milk proteins: Proteolytic activation and thropho-functional properties. *Antonie van Leeuwenhoek*, *76*(1/4), 207–215. doi:10.1023/A:1002063805780 PMID:10532380

Meisel, H., Walsh, D. J., Murray, B., & FitzGerald, R. J. (2006). ACE inhibitory peptides. In Y. Mine & F. Shahidi (Eds.), *Nutraceutical Proteins and Peptides in Health and Disease* (Vol. 4, pp. 269–315). Taylor & Francis Group Publisher.

Mekky, R. H., Contreras, M. M., El-Gindi, M. R., Abdel-Monem, A. R., Abdel-Sattar, E., & Segura-Carretero, A. (2015). Profiling of phenolic and other compounds from Egyptian cultivars of chickpea (*Cicer arietinum* L.) and antioxidant activity: A comparative study. *RSC Advances*, *5*(23), 17751–17767. doi:10.1039/C4RA13155J

Meliker, J. R., Wahl, R. L., Cameron, L. L., & Nriagu, J. O. (2007). Arsenic in drinking water and cerebrovascular disease, diabetes mellitus, and kidney disease in Michigan: A standardized mortality ratio analysis. *Environmental Health*, *6*(1), 4. doi:10.1186/1476-069X-6-4 PMID:17274811

Melnyk, J. P., Wang, S., & Marcone, M. F. (2010). Chemical and biological properties of the world's most expensive spice: Saffron. *Food Research International*, *43*(8), 1981–1989. doi:10.1016/j.foodres.2010.07.033

Meng, Q., Velalar, C. N., & Ruan, R. (2008). Regulating the age-related oxidative damage, mitochondrial integrity, and antioxidative enzyme activity in Fischer 344 rats by supplementation of the antioxidant epigallocatechin-3-gallate. *Rejuvenation Research*, *11*(3), 649–660. doi:10.1089/rej.2007.0645 PMID:18593283

Mensah, J. K., Okoli, R. I., Ohaju-Obodo, J. O., & Eifediyi, K. (2008). Phytochemical, nutritional and medical properties of some leafy vegetables consumed by Edo people of Nigeria. *African Journal of Biotechnology*, *7*, 2305–2309.

Mensah, P. (1997). Fermentation - the key to food safety assurance in Africa? *Food Control*, *8*(5-6), 271–278. doi:10.1016/S0956-7135(97)00020-0

Mercanligil, S. M., Arslan, P., Alasalvar, C., Okut, E., Akgul, E., Pinar, A., & Shahidi, F. et al. (2007). Effects of hazelnut-enriched diet on plasma cholesterol and lipoprotein profiles in hypercholesterolemic adult men. *European Journal of Clinical Nutrition*, *61*(2), 212–220. doi:10.1038/sj.ejcn.1602518 PMID:16969381

Mercier, S., Villeneuve, S., Moresoli, C., Mendor, M., Marcos, B., & Power, K. A. (2014). Flaxseed-enriched cereal-based products: A review of the impact of processing conditions. *Compreh. Reviews Food Sci. Food Safety*, *13*(4), 400–412. doi:10.1111/1541-4337.12075

Messina, M. (2000). Soyfoods and shoybean phyto-oestrogens (isoflavones) as possible alternatives to hormone replacement therapy. *European Journal of Cancer*, *36*, S71–S77. doi:10.1016/S0959-8049(00)00233-1 PMID:11056326

Messina, M. (2010). A brief historical overview of the past two decades of soy and isoflavone research. *The Journal of Nutrition*, *140*(7), 1350S–1354S. doi:10.3945/jn.109.118315 PMID:20484551

Messina, M. J., Persky, V., Setchell, D. R., & Barnes, S. (1994). Soy intake and cancer risk: A review of the in vitro and in vivo data. *Nutrition and Cancer*, *21*(2), 113–131. doi:10.1080/01635589409514310 PMID:8058523

Messina, M., Nagata, C., & Wu, A. H. (2006). Estimated Asian adult soy protein and isoflavone intakes. *Nutrition and Cancer*, *55*(1), 1–12. doi:10.1207/s15327914nc5501_1 PMID:16965235

Mestres, C., Bassa, S., Fagbohoun, E., Nogo, M., Hell, K., Vernier, P., & Cardwell, K. F. et al. (2004). Yam chip food subsector: Hazardous practices and presence of aflatoxins in Benin. *Journal of Stored Products Research*, *40*(5), 575–585. doi:10.1016/j.jspr.2003.11.003

Meydani, M., Lipman, R. D., Han, S. N., Wu, D., Beharka, A., Mar-tin, K., & Meydani, S. N. et al. (1998). The effect of long-term dietary supplementation with antioxidants. *Annals of the New York Academy of Sciences*, *854*(1), 352–360. doi:10.1111/j.1749-6632.1998.tb09915.x PMID:9928443

Micallef, M. A., & Garg, M. L. (2008). The lipid-lowering effects of phytosterols and (n-3) polyunsaturated fatty acids are synergistic and complementary in hyperlipidemic men and women. *The Journal of Nutrition*, *138*, 1086–1090. PMID:18492838

Michaud, D. S., Spiegelman, D., Clinton, S. K., Rimm, S. K., Willett, W. C., & Giovannucci, E. L. (1999). Fruit and vegetable intake and incidence of bladder cancer in a male prospective cohort. *Journal of the National Cancer Institute*, *7*(7), 605–613. doi:10.1093/jnci/91.7.605 PMID:10203279

Miettinen, T. A., Vuoristo, M., Nissinen, M., Jarvinen, H. J., & Gylling, H. (2000). Serum, biliary, and fecal cholesterol and plant sterols in cholectomized patients before and during consumption of stanol ester margarine. *The American Journal of Clinical Nutrition*, *71*(5), 1095–1102. PMID:10799370

Mikami, M., Sekikawa, M., & Shimada, K. I. (2007). Non-heated meat products (Dry cured ham). *FFI Journal.*, *212*(7), 572–582.

Milin, L., & Stanimarovic, S. (1950). Vitamins & pharmacology of pomegranate juice. *Medicinski Glasnik*, *4*(11-12), 259. PMID:14805886

Miller, E. R., Appel, L. J., Levander, O. A., & Levine, D. M. (1997). The effect of antioxidant vitamin supplementation on traditional cardiovascular risk factors. *Journal of Cardiovascular Risk*, *4*(1), 19–24. doi:10.1177/174182679700400104 PMID:9215516

Miller, G., Prakash, A., & Decker, E. (2002). *Whole-grain foods in health and disease*. St. Paul, MN: American Association of Cereal Chemists.

Mills, S., Ross, R. P., Hill, C., Fitzgerald, G. F., & Stanton, C. (2011). Mill intelligence: Mining milk for bioactive substances associated with human health. *International Dairy Journal*, *21*(6), 377–401. doi:10.1016/j.idairyj.2010.12.011

Milner, J. A., McDonald, S. S., Anderson, D. E., & Greenwald, P. (2001). Molecular targets for nutrients involved with cancer prevention. *Nutrition and Cancer*, *41*(1-2), 1–16. doi:10.1080/01635581.2001.9680606 PMID:12094610

Minamida, K., Ota, K., Nishimukai, M., Tanaka, M., Abe, A., Sone, T., & Asano, K. et al. (2008). *Asaccharobacter celatus* gen. nov., sp. nov., isolated from rat caecum. *International Journal of Systematic and Evolutionary Microbiology*, *58*(5), 1238–1240. doi:10.1099/ijs.0.64894-0 PMID:18450720

Ministry for food, agriculture, forestry and fisheries. (2011). *Main statistic information for food, agriculture, forestry and fisheries*. Author.

Mink, P. J., Scrafford, C. G., Barraj, L. M., Harnack, L., Hong, C. P., Nettleton, J. A., & Jacobs, D. R. Jr. (2007). Flavonoid intake and cardio vascular disease mortality: A prospective study in post-menopausal women. *The American Journal of Clinical Nutrition*, *85*, 895–909. PMID:17344514

Min, S., Harris, L., & Krochta, J. (2005). Antimicrobial effects of lactoferrin, lysozyme, and the lactoperoxidase system and edible whey protein films incorporating the lactoperoxidase system against Salmonella enterica and *Eschericchia coli* O157:H7. *Journal of Food Science*, *70*(7), 332–338. doi:10.1111/j.1365-2621.2005.tb11476.x

Miriyala, S., Panchatcharam, M., & Rengarajulu, P. (2007). Cardioprotective effects of curcumin. *Advances in Experimental Medicine and Biology*, *595*, 359–377. doi:10.1007/978-0-387-46401-5_16 PMID:17569220

Mishra, N. K., Chandini, D., Saijyothi, G., Divya, G., & Venkatalakshmi, I. (2014). Anti-inflammatory activity of Camellia sinensis by using cotton pellet granuloma in rat. *Pharma Science Monitor*, *5*(2), 108-17.

Mishra, A., Gopalakrishna, A. G., & Prabhakar, J. V. (1988). Factors affecting refining losses in rice (Oryza sativa L.) bran oil. *Journal of the American Oil Chemists' Society*, *65*(10), 1605–1609. doi:10.1007/BF02912563

Mitchell, B. S., Brooks, S. A., Leathem, A. J., & Schumacher, U. (1998). Do HPA and PHA-L have the same binding pattern in metastasizing human breast and colon cancers? *Cancer Letters*, *123*(1), 113–119. doi:10.1016/S0304-3835(97)00414-X PMID:9461027

Mitchell, J. H., Gardner, P. T., McPhail, D. B., Morrice, P. C., Collins, A. R., & Duthie, G. G. (1998). Antioxidant efficacy of phytoestrogens in chemical and biological model systems. *Archives of Biochemistry and Biophysics*, *360*(1), 142–148. doi:10.1006/abbi.1998.0951 PMID:9826439

Modriansky, M., & Gabrielova, E. (2009). Uncouple my heart: The benefits of inefficiency. *Journal of Bioenergetics and Biomembranes*, *41*(2), 133–136. doi:10.1007/s10863-009-9212-z PMID:19365715

Moghadasian, M. H., & Frohlich, J. J. (1999). Effects of dietary phytosterols on cholesterol metabolism & atherosclerosis: Clinical & experimental evidence. *The American Journal of Medicine*, *107*(6), 588–594. doi:10.1016/S0002-9343(99)00285-5 PMID:10625028

Moghaddam, G., Sharifzadeh, M., Hassanzadeh, G., Khanavi, M., Dolatshahi, F., Sadeghi, N., & Hajimahmoodi, M. et al. (2014). Anti-Ulcerative Potential of Punica granatum L. hydroalcoholic peel extract. *Tropical Journal of Pharmaceutical Research*, *13*(7), 1093–1097. doi:10.4314/tjpr.v13i7.12

Mohamed, S. (2014). Functional foods against metabolic syndrome (obesity, diabetes, hypertension and dyslipidemia) and cardiovascular disease. *Trends Fd Sci Tech.*, *35*(2), 114–128. doi:10.1016/j.tifs.2013.11.001

Mohan, M., Waghulde, H., & Kasture, S. (2010). Effect of pomegranate juice on Angiotensin II-induced hypertension in diabetic wistar rats. *Journal of Phytotherapy Research*, *24*(S2), 196–203. doi:10.1002/ptr.3090 PMID:20020514

Mokoena, M. P., Chelule, P. K., & Ggaleni, N. (2005). Reduction of fumonisin B1 and zearalenone by lactic acid bacteria in fermented maize meal. *Journal of Food Protection*, *68*, 2095–2099. PMID:16245712

Mokoena, M. P., Chelule, P. K., & Gqaleni, N. (2006). The toxicity and decreased concentration of aflatoxin B1 in natural lactic acid fermented maize meal. *Journal of Applied Microbiology*, *100*(4), 773–777. doi:10.1111/j.1365-2672.2006.02881.x PMID:16553732

Molassiotis, A., Fernadez-Ortega, P., Pud, D., Scott, J. A., Panteli, V., Margulies, A., & Patiraki, E. et al. (2005). Use of complementary and alternative medicine in cancer patients: A European survey. *Annals of Oncology*, *16*(4), 655–663. doi:10.1093/annonc/mdi110 PMID:15699021

Molla, M. D., Hidalgo-Mora, J. J., & Soteras, M. G. (2011). Phytotherapy as alternative to hormone replacement therapy. *Frontiers in Bioscience*, *3*(1), 191–204. doi:10.2741/s144 PMID:21196369

Mollard, R., Zykus, A., Luhovyy, B., Nunez, M., Wong, C., & Anderson, G. (2012). The acute effects of a pulse-containing meal on glycaemic responses and measures of satiety and satiation within and at a later meal. *The British Journal of Nutrition*, *108*(03), 509–517. doi:10.1017/S0007114511005836 PMID:22054112

Moller, M. E., Dahl, R., & Bockman, O. C. (1998). A possible role of the dietary fiber product, wheat bran, as a nitrite scavenger. *Food and Chemical Toxicology*, *26*(10), 841–845. doi:10.1016/0278-6915(88)90024-5 PMID:2851507

Monroy, A., Lithgow, G. J., & Alavez, S. (2013). Curcumin and neurodegenerative diseases- a review. *Int. Union Biochem. Mol. Biol.*, *39*(1), 122–132.

Montonen, J., Knekt, P., Jarvinen, R., Aromaa, A., & Reunanen, A. (2003). Whole grain and fiber intake and the incidence of type 2 diabetes. *The American Journal of Clinical Nutrition*, *77*(3), 622–629. PMID:12600852

Moon, K. A., Guallar, E., Umans, J. G., Devereux, R. B., Best, L. G., Francesconi, K. A., & Navas-Acien, A. et al. (2013). Association between exposure to low to moderate arsenic levels and incident cardiovascular disease: A prospective cohort study. *Annals of Internal Medicine*, *159*, 649–659. PMID:24061511

Moon, K., Guallar, E., & Navas-Acien, A. (2012). Arsenic exposure and cardiovascular disease: An updated systematic review. *Current Atherosclerosis Reports*, *14*(6), 542–555. doi:10.1007/s11883-012-0280-x PMID:22968315

Moon, Y. J., Wang, X., & Morris, M. E. (2006). Dietary flavonoids: Effects on xenobiotic and carcinogen metabolism. *Toxicology In Vitro*, *20*(2), 187–210. doi:10.1016/j.tiv.2005.06.048 PMID:16289744

Moreira, M. R., Ponce, A., Del Valle, C. E., & Roura, S. I. (2009). Edible coatings on fresh squash slices: Effect of film drying temperature on the nutritional and microbiological quality. *Journal of Food Processing and Preservation*, *33*, 226–236. doi:10.1111/j.1745-4549.2008.00295.x

Morgan, X. C., Segata, N., & Huttenhower, C. (2013). Biodiversity and functional genomics in the human microbiome. *Trends in Genetics*, *29*(1), 51–58. doi:10.1016/j.tig.2012.09.005 PMID:23140990

Morimitsu, Y., Kubota, K., Tashiro, T., Hashizume, E., Kamiya, T., & Osawa, T. (2002). Inhibitory effect of anthocyanins and colored rice on diabetic cataract formation in the rat lenses. *International Congress Series*, *1245*, 503–508. doi:10.1016/S0531-5131(02)00919-6

Morito, K., Hirose, T., Kinjo, J., Hirakawa, T., Okawa, M., Nohara, T., & Masamune, Y. et al. (2001). Interactions of phytoestrogens with estrogen receptors alpha and beta. *Biological & Pharmaceutical Bulletin*, *24*(4), 351–356. doi:10.1248/bpb.24.351 PMID:11305594

Morris, E. R., & Hill, A. D. (1996). Inositol phosphate content of selected dry beans, peas, and lentils, raw and cooked. *Journal of Food Composition and Analysis*, *9*(1), 2–12. doi:10.1006/jfca.1996.0002

Morris, M. C., Sacks, F., & Rosner, B. (1993). Does fish oil lower blood pressure? A meta-analysis of controlled trials. *Circulation*, *88*(2), 523–533. doi:10.1161/01.CIR.88.2.523 PMID:8339414

Mortensen, J. Z., Schmidt, E. B., Nielsen, A. H., & Dyerberg, J. (1983). The effect of N-6 and N-3 polyunsaturated fatty acids on hemostasis, blood lipids and blood pressure. *Thrombosis and Haemostasis*, *50*, 543–546. PMID:6636033

Morton, J. (1987). Pomegranate. In J. F. Morton (Ed.), Fruits of Warm Climates (pp. 352–355). Wallingford, UK: Cab-Direct Publishing.

Mosimann, A. L., Wilhelm-Filho, D., & Da Silva, E. L. (2006). Aqueous extract of *Ilex paraguariensis* attenuates the progression of atherosclerosis in cholesterol-fed rabbits. *BioFactors (Oxford, England)*, *26*(1), 59–70. doi:10.1002/biof.5520260106 PMID:16614483

Moslehishad, M., Ehsani, M. R., Salami, M., Mirdamadi, S., Ezzatpanah, H., Niasari, A. N., & Moosavi-Movahedi, A. A. (2013). The comparative assessment of ACE-inhibitory and antioxidant activities of peptide fractions obtained from fermented camel and bovine milk by *Lactobacillus rhamnosus* PTCC 1637. *International Dairy Journal*, *29*(2), 82–87. doi:10.1016/j.idairyj.2012.10.015

Moure, A., Domínguez, H., & Parajó, J. C. (2006). Antioxidant properties of ultrafiltration-recovered soy protein fractions from industrial effluents and their hydrolysates. *Process Biochemistry*, *41*(2), 447–456. doi:10.1016/j.procbio.2005.07.014

Mozzafera, P. (1997). Mate Drinking: Caffeine and Phenolic Acid Intake. *Food Chemistry*, *60*(1), 67–71. doi:10.1016/S0308-8146(96)00311-1

Mshandete, A. M., & Cuff, J. (2007). Proximate and nutrient composition of three types of indigenous edible wild mushrooms grown in Tanzania and their utilization prospects. *African Journal of Food Agriculture Nutrition and Development*, *7*(6), 1–16.

Muchuweti, M., Zenda, G., Ndhlala, A. R., & Kasiyamhuru, A. (2005). Sugars, organic acid and phenolic compounds in *Zizyphus mauritiana* fruit. *European Journal of Food Research and Technology.*, *221*(3-4), 570–574. doi:10.1007/s00217-005-1204-6

Mueller, M. S., Karhagomba, I. B., Hirt, H. M., & Wemakor, E. (2000). The potential of Artemisia annua L. as a locally produced remedy for malaria in the tropics: Agricultural, chemical and chemical aspects. *Journal of Ethnopharmacology*, *73*(3), 487–493. doi:10.1016/S0378-8741(00)00289-0 PMID:11091003

Mueller, M. S., Runyambo, N., Wagner, I., Bormann, S., Dietz, K., & Heide, L. (2004). Randomized controlled trial of a traditional preparation of Artemisia annua L. (Annual wormwood). *Trop Med Hyg*, *98*(5), 318–321. doi:10.1016/j.trstmh.2003.09.001 PMID:15109558

Muià, C., Mazzon, E., Di Paola, R., Genovese, T., Menegazzi, M., Caputi, A. P., & Cuzzocrea, S. et al. (2005). Green tea polyphenol extract attenuates ischemia/reperfusion injury of the gut. *Naunyn-Schmiedeberg's Archives of Pharmacology*, *371*(5), 364–374. doi:10.1007/s00210-005-1076-0 PMID:15997392

Mukkavilli, R., Gundala, S.R., Yang, C., Donthamsetty, S., Cantuaria, G., Jadhav, G.R., Vangala, S., Reid, M.D. & Aneja, R. (2014). Modulation of cytochrome P450 metabolism and transport across intestinal epithelial barrier by ginger biophenolics. *PLOS One, 9*(9), 1-12.

Muktar, H., & Ahmad, N. (2000). Tea polyphenols: Prevention pf cancer and optimizing health. *The American Journal of Clinical Nutrition*, *71*, 1698–1702.

Mukuddem-Petersen, J., Oosthuizen, W., & Jerling, J. C. (2005). A systematic review of the effects of nuts on blood lipid profiles in humans. *The Journal of Nutrition*, *135*, 2082–2089. PMID:16140880

Mulligan, A. A., Kuhnle, G. G., Lentjes, M. A., van Scheltinga, V., Powell, N. A., McTaggart, A., & Khaw, K. T. et al. (2013). Intakes and sources of isoflavones, lignans, enterolignans, coumestrol and soya-containing foods in the Norfolk arm of the European Prospective Investigation into Cancer and Nutrition (EPIC-Norfolk), from 7 d food diaries, using a newly updated database. *Public Health Nutrition*, *16*(08), 1454–1462. doi:10.1017/S1368980012003904 PMID:22939391

Mulvany, M. J. (2002). Small artery remodeling in hypertension. *Current Hypertension Reports*, *4*(1), 49–55. doi:10.1007/s11906-002-0053-y PMID:11790292

Murad, H. (2003). *U.S. Patent No. 6,630,163*. Washington, DC: U.S. Patent and Trademark Office.

Murray, M., Walchuk, C., Suh, M., & Jones, P. J. (2015). Green tea catechins and cardiovascular disease risk factors: Should a health claim be made by the United States Food and Drug Administration? *Trends in Food Science & Technology*, *41*(2), 188–197. doi:10.1016/j.tifs.2014.10.004

Mursu, J., Voutilainen, S., Nurmi, T., Tuomainen, T. P., Kurl, S., & Salonen, J. T. (2008). Flavonoid intake and the risk of ischaemic stroke and CVD mortality in middle-aged Finish men: The Kuopio Ischaemic Heat Disease Risk Factor Study. *The British Journal of Nutrition*, *100*(04), 890–895. doi:10.1017/S0007114508945694 PMID:18377681

Murti, K., & Paliwal, D. (2012). Exploration of preliminary phytochemical studies of seed of *Syzygium cumini*. *American Journal of Pharmacology and Toxicology.*, *7*(1), 12–14. doi:10.3844/ajptsp.2012.12.14

Muthayya, S., Hall, J., Bagriansky, J., Sugimoto, J., Gundry, D., Matthias, D., & Maberly, G. et al. (2012). Rice Fortification—an emerging opportunity to contribute to the elimination of vitamin and mineral deficiency worldwide. *Food and Nutrition Bulletin*, *33*(4), 296–307. doi:10.1177/156482651203300410 PMID:23424896

Muzzarelli, R. A. A. (1986). Filmogenic properties of chitin/chitosan. In R. A. A. Muzzarelli, C. Jeuniaux, & G. W. Gooday (Eds.), *Chitin in Nature and Technology* (pp. 389–396). New York: Plenum Press. doi:10.1007/978-1-4613-2167-5_48

Mwanri, A. W., Kogi-Makau, W., & Laswai, H. S. (2011). Nutrients and antinutrients composition of raw, cooked and sun- dried sweetpotato leaves. *African Journal of Food, Agriculture. Nutrition and Development*, *11*(5), 5142–5156.

Nabubuya, A., Muyonga, J. H., & Kabasa, J. D. (2010). Nutritional and hypocholesterolemic properties of *Termitomyces microcarpus* Mushrooms. *African Journal of Food, Agriculture, Nutrition and Development*, *10*(3), 2235–2257.

Nadeem, M., & Riaz, A. (2012). Cumin (*Cuminum cyminum*) as a potential source of antioxidants. *Pakistan Journal of Food Science*, *22*, 101–107.

Nagao, T., Hase, T., & Tokimitsu, I. (2007). A green tea extract high in catechins reduces body fat and cardiovascular risks in humans. *Obesity (Silver Spring, Md.)*, *15*(6), 1473–1483. doi:10.1038/oby.2007.176 PMID:17557985

Naidu, A. S. (2000). Lactoferrin, lactoperoxidase. In Natural food antimicrobial systems (pp. 17–132). New York: CRC Press.

Nakagawa, H., Hasumi, K., Woo, J. T., Nagai, K., & Wachi, M. (2004). Generation of hydrogen peroxide primarily contributes to the induction of Fe(II)-dependent apoptosis in Jurkat cells by (-)-epigallocatechin gallate. *Carcinogenesis*, *25*(9), 1567–1574. doi:10.1093/carcin/bgh168 PMID:15090467

Nakagawa, H., Wachi, M., Woo, J. T., Kato, M., Kasai, S., Takahashi, F., & Nagai, K. et al. (2002). Fenton reaction is primarily involved in a mechanism of (-)-epigallocatechin-3-gallate to induce osteoclastic cell death. *Biochemical and Biophysical Research Communications*, *292*(1), 94–101. doi:10.1006/bbrc.2002.6622 PMID:11890677

Nakatsu, C. H., Arsmstrong, A., Cavijo, A. P., Martin, B. R., Barnes, S., & Weaver, C. M. (2014). Fecal bacterial community changes associated with isoflavone metabolites in postmenopausal women after soy bar consumption. *PLoS ONE*, *9*, e108924. PMID:25271941

Nambiar, V. S., Dhaduk, J. J., Sareen, N., Shahu, T., & Desai, R. (2011). Potential functional implications of pearl millet (*Pennisetum glaucum*) in health and disease. *Journal of Applied Pharmaceutical Science*, *1*, 62–67.

Nam, S. H., Choi, S. P., Kang, M. Y., Kozukue, N., & Friedman, M. (2005). Antioxidative, antimutagenic, and anticarcinogenic activities of rice bran extracts in chemical and cell assays. *Journal of Agricultural and Food Chemistry*, *53*(3), 816–822. doi:10.1021/jf0490293 PMID:15686439

Nasir, M., & Sidhu, J. S. (2013). Chickpea, Lentil, Mung bean, Black gram, Pigeon Pea and India Vetch. In Pulses: Production, Processing and Nutritional Value. Wiley-Blackwell Publishing Co.

Nathan, C. (2006). Neutrophils and immunity: Challenges and opportunities. *Nature Reviews. Immunology*, *6*(3), 173–182. doi:10.1038/nri1785 PMID:16498448

National Center for Biotechnology Information. (2015a). *PubChem compound database; CID=65064*. Retrieved November 9, 2015 from https://pubchem.ncbi.nlm.nih.gov/compound/65064

National Center for Biotechnology Information. (2015b). *PubChem compound database; CID=72277*. Retrieved November 9, 2015 from https://pubchem.ncbi.nlm.nih.gov/compound/72277

National Center for Biotechnology Information. (2015c). *PubChem compound database; CID=107905*. Retrieved November 9, 2015 from https://pubchem.ncbi.nlm.nih.gov/compound/107905

National Center for Biotechnology Information. (2015d). *PubChem compound database; CID=182232*. Retrieved November 9, 2015 from https://pubchem.ncbi.nlm.nih.gov/compound/182232

National Center for Biotechnology Information. (2015e). *PubChem compound database; CID=114777*. Retrieved November 9, 2015 from https://pubchem.ncbi.nlm.nih.gov/compound/114777

National Center for Biotechnology Information. (2015f). *PubChem compound database; CID=22833650*. Retrieved November 9, 2015 from https://pubchem.ncbi.nlm.nih.gov/compound/22833650

National Center for Biotechnology Information. (2015g). *PubChem compound database; CID=5280343*. Retrieved November 2, 2015 from https://pubchem.ncbi.nlm.nih.gov/compound/5280343

National Center for Biotechnology Information. (2015h). *PubChem compound database; CID=5281672*. Retrieved November 2, 2015 from https://pubchem.ncbi.nlm.nih.gov/compound/5281672

National Center for Biotechnology Information. (2015i). *PubChem compound database; CID=5280863*. Retrieved November 2, 2015 from https://pubchem.ncbi.nlm.nih.gov/compound/5280863

National Center for Complementary and Integrative Health. (2015). *Complementary, alternative, or integrative health. What's in a name?* Retrieved November 9, 2015 from, https://nccih.nih.gov/sites/nccam.nih.gov/files/CAM_Basics_Whats_In_A_Name_03-26-2015.pdf

Naumann, E., Plat, J., Kester, A. M., & Mensink, R. P. (2008). The baseline serum lipoprotein profile is related to plant stanol induced changes in serum lipoprotein cholesterol and triacylglycerol concentrations. *Journal of the American College of Nutrition*, *27*(1), 117–126. doi:10.1080/07315724.2008.10719683 PMID:18460490

Naumann, E., van Rees, A. B., Onning, G., Oste, R., Wydra, M., & Mensink, R. P. (2006). Beta-Glucan incorporated into a fruit drink effectively lowers serum LDL-cholesterol concentrations. *The American Journal of Clinical Nutrition*, *83*, 601–605. PMID:16522906

Navarrate, A., Palacios-Espinosa, F., & Mata, R. (2011). Gastroprotective effect of Brickellia cavanillesii (Cav) B. L. Robinson (Asteraceae) in rats. *Planta Medica*, *77*, 52. doi:10.1055/s-0031-1273581 PMID:20560115

Navarro, V., Villarreal, M. L., Rojas, G., & Lozoya, X. (1996). Antimicrobial evaluation of some plants used in Mexican traditional medicine for the treatment of infectious diseases. *Journal of Ethnopharmacology*, *53*(3), 143–147. doi:10.1016/0378-8741(96)01429-8 PMID:8887021

Naveena, B. M., Sen, A. R., Kingsly, R. P., Singh, D. B., & Kondaiah, N. (2008). Antioxidant activity of pomegranate rind powder extract in cooked chicken patties. *International Journal of Food Science & Technology*, *43*(10), 1807–1812. doi:10.1111/j.1365-2621.2007.01708.x

Negi, P. S., Jayaprakasha, G. K., & Jena, B. S. (2003). Antioxidant and antimutagenic activities of pomegranate peel extracts. *Food Chemistry*, *80*(3), 393–397. doi:10.1016/S0308-8146(02)00279-0

Nesamvuni, C., Steyn, N. P., & Potgieter, M. J. (2001). Nutritional value of wild, leafy plants consumed by the Vhavenda. *South African Journal of Science*, *97*, 51–54.

Ness, A. R. (2001). Commentary: Beyond beta-carotene—antioxidants and cardiovascular disease. *International Journal of Epidemiology*, *30*(1), 143–144. doi:10.1093/ije/30.1.143 PMID:11171875

Ness, A. R., & Powles, J. W. (1997). Fruit and vegetables, and cardiovascular disease: A review. *International Journal of Epidemiology*, *26*(1), 1–13. doi:10.1093/ije/26.1.1 PMID:9126498

Ness, A. R., Powles, J. W., & Khaw, K. T. (1996). Vitamin C and cardiovascular disease: A systematic review. *Journal of Cardiovascular Risk*, *3*(6), 513–521. doi:10.1097/00043798-199612000-00006 PMID:9100087

Neumann, G., Noda, T., & Kawaoka, Y. (2009). Emergence and pandemic potential of swine-origin H1N1 influenza virus. *Nature*, *459*(7249), 931–939. doi:10.1038/nature08157 PMID:19525932

Nevin, K. G., & Rajamohan, T. (2006). Virgin coconut oil supplemented diet increases the antioxidant status in rats. *Food Chemistry*, *99*(2), 206–266. doi:10.1016/j.foodchem.2005.06.056

Nevin, K. G., & Rajamohan, T. (2014). Beneficial effects of virgin coconut oil on lipid parameters and i*n vitro* LDL oxidation. *Clinical Biochemistry*, *37*(9), 830–835. doi:10.1016/j.clinbiochem.2004.04.010 PMID:15329324

Newton, K. M., Reed, S. D., Uchiyama, S., Qu, C., Ueno, T., Iwashita, S., & Lampe, J. W. et al. (2015). A cross-sectional study of equol producer status and self-reported vasomotor symptoms. *Menopause (New York, N.Y.)*, *22*(5), 489–495. doi:10.1097/GME.0000000000000363 PMID:25380274

Nichenametla, S. N., Taruscio, T. G., Barney, D. L., & Exon, J. H. (2006). A review of the effects and mechanisms of polyphenolics in cancer. *Critical Reviews in Food Science and Nutrition*, *46*(2), 161–183. doi:10.1080/10408390591000541 PMID:16431408

Nielsen, I. L., & Williamson, G. (2007). Review of the factors affecting bioavailability of soy isoflavones in humans. *Nutrition and Cancer*, *57*(1), 1–10. doi:10.1080/01635580701267677 PMID:17516857

Nimni, M. E., Han, B., & Cordoba, F. (2007). Are we getting enough sulfur in our diet. *Nutrition and Metabolism (Lond)*, *4*, 24.

No, H. K., Meyers, S. P., Prinyawiwatkul, W., & Xu, Z. (2007). Applications of chitosan for improvement of quality and shelf life of Foods: A Review. *Journal of Food Science*, *72*(5), 87–100. doi:10.1111/j.1750-3841.2007.00383.x PMID:17995743

Noh, H. Y. (2014). *Effects of the processed sulfur supplementation on the growth performance and meat quality in pigs*. Konkuk University.

Noh, J. S., Choi, Y. H., & Song, Y. O. (2013). Beneficial effects of the active principle component of Korean cabbage kimchi via increasing nitric oxide production and suppressing inflammation in the aorta of aopE knockout mice. *The British Journal of Nutrition*, *109*(01), 17–24. doi:10.1017/S0007114512000633 PMID:22715945

Noh, K. A., Kim, D. H., Choi, N. S., & Kim, S. H. (1999). Isolation of fibrinolytic enzyme producing strains from kimchi. *Korean J. Food Sci. Technol*, *31*, 219–223.

Noncommunicable Diseases. (2015). *Fact sheet*. Retrieved from: www.who.int/mediacentre/factsheets/fs355/en/

Nongonierma, A. B., & Fitzgerald, R. J. (2015a). The scientific evidence for the role of milk protein-derived bioactive peptides in humans: A review. *J. Functional Foods*, *17*, 640–656. doi:10.1016/j.jff.2015.06.021

Nongonierma, A. B., & Fitzgerald, R. J. (2015b). Milk proteins as a source of tryptophan- containing bioactive peptides. *Food Function*, *6*(7), 2115–2127. doi:10.1039/C5FO00407A PMID:26027501

Normand, E. L., Ory, R. L., & Mod, R. R. (1981). Interactions of several bile acids with hemicelluloses from several varieties of rice. *Journal of Food Science*, *46*(4), 1159–1161. doi:10.1111/j.1365-2621.1981.tb03014.x

Normand, F. L., Ory, R. L., Mod, R. R., Saunders, R. M., & Gumbmann, M. R. (1984). Influence of rice hemicelluloses and α-cellulose on lipid and water content of rice faeces and on blood lipids. *Journal of Cereal Science*, *2*(1), 37–42. doi:10.1016/S0733-5210(84)80006-5

Normile, D. (2004). Yangtze seen as earliest rice site. *Science*, *275*(5298), 309. doi:10.1126/science.275.5298.309

Nuñez-Sánchez, M. A., García-Villalba, R., Monedero-Saiz, T., García-Talavera, N. V., Gómez-Sánchez, M. B., Sánchez-Álvarez, C., & Espín, J. C. et al. (2014). Targeted metabolic profiling of pomegranate polyphenols and urolithins in plasma, urine and colon tissues from colorectal cancer patients. *Molecular Nutrition & Food Research*, *58*(6), 1199–1211. PMID:24532260

Nwachukwu, I. D., Devassy, J. G., Aluko, R. E., & Jonesab, P. J. (2015). Cholesterol-lowering properties of oat β-glucan and the promotion of cardiovascular health: Did Health Canada make the right call? *Applied Physiology, Nutrition, and Metabolism*, *40*(6), 535–542. doi:10.1139/apnm-2014-0410 PMID:25933163

Nwauzoma, A. B., & Dawari, S. L. (2013). Study on the phytochemical properties and proximate analysis of *Piper Umbellatum* (LINN) from Nigeria. *American Journal of Research Communication*, *1*(7), 164–177.

Nyanhanda, T., Elaine, M. G., & Roger, D. H. (2014). Plant-derived foods for the attenuation of allergic airway inflammation. *Current Pharmaceutical Design*, *20*(6), 869–878. doi:10.2174/13816128113199990056 PMID:23701570

Nyau, V. (2014). Nutraceutical perspectives and utilization of common beans (*Phaseolus Vulgaris* L.): A review. *African Journal of Food Agriculture Nutrition and Development*, *14*, 9483–9496.

Nyyssonen, K., Parviainen, M. T., Salonen, R., Tuomilehto, J., & Salonen, J. T. (1997). Vitamin C deficiency and risk of myocardial infarction: Prospective population study of men from eastern Finland. *BMJ (Clinical Research Ed.), 314*(7081), 634–638. doi:10.1136/bmj.314.7081.634 PMID:9066474

O'Toole, T. E., Conklin, D. J., & Bhatnagar, A. (2008). Environmental risk factors for heart disease. *Reviews on Environmental Health, 23*, 167–202. PMID:19119685

Obodai, M., Ferreira, I. C. R. R., Fernandes, A., Barros, L., Mensah, D. L., Dzomeku, M., & Takli, R. et al. (2014). Evaluation of the chemical and antioxidant properties of wild and cultivated mushrooms in Ghana. *Molecules (Basel, Switzerland), 19*(12), 19532–19548. doi:10.3390/molecules191219532 PMID:25432007

Ochoa, T. J., & Cleary, T. G. (2009). Effect of lactoferrin on enteric pathogens. *Biochimie, 91*(1), 30–34. doi:10.1016/j.biochi.2008.04.006 PMID:18472012

Odhav, B., Beekrun, S., Akula, U., & Baijnath, H. (2007). Preliminary assessment of nutritional value of traditional leafy vegetables in KwaZulu-Natal, South Africa. *Journal of Food Composition and Analysis, 20*(5), 430–435. doi:10.1016/j.jfca.2006.04.015

Ogawa, M., Kumamaru, T., Satoh, H., Iwata, N., Omura, T., Kasai, Z., & Tanaka, K. (1987). Purification of protein body-I of rice seed and its polypeptide composition. *Plant & Cell Physiology, 28*, 1517–1527.

Ogunleye, A. A., Xue, F., & Michels, K. B. (2010). Green tea consumption and breast cancer risk or recurrence: A meta-analysis. *Breast Cancer Research and Treatment, 119*(2), 477–484. doi:10.1007/s10549-009-0415-0 PMID:19437116

Oh, Y. J., Hwang, I. J., & Leitzmann, C. (1993). Regular intake of kimchi prevent colon cancer. *Kimchi Sci Ind., 2*, 9.

Oki, T., Masuda, M., Kobayashi, M., Nishiba, Y., Furuta, S., Suda, I., & Sato, T. (2002). Polymeric procyanidins as radical-scavenging components in red-hulled rice. *Journal of Agricultural and Food Chemistry, 50*(26), 7524–7529. doi:10.1021/jf025841z PMID:12475265

Olaiya, C., & Adebisi, J. (2009). Phytoevaluation of the nutritional values of ten green leafy vegetables in South -Western Nigeria. *The Internet Journal of Nutrition and Wellness, 9*, 2.

Olivas, G. I., & Barbosa-Canovas, G. V. (2005). Edible coatings for fresh cut fruits. *Critical Reviews in Food Science and Nutrition, 45*(7-8), 657–670. doi:10.1080/10408690490911837 PMID:16371333

Olivas, G. I., Mattinson, D. S., & Barbosa-Canovas, G. V. (2007). Alginate coatings for preservation of minimally processed "Gala" apples. *Postharvest Biology and Technology, 45*(1), 89–96. doi:10.1016/j.postharvbio.2006.11.018

Olivas, G. I., Rodriguez, J. J., & Barbosa-Cánovas, G. V. (2003). Edible coatings composed of methylcellulose stearic acid, and additives to preserve quality of pear wedges. *Journal of Food Processing and Preservation, 27*(4), 299–320. doi:10.1111/j.1745-4549.2003.tb00519.x

Olumakaiye, M. F. (2011). Evaluation of nutrient contents of amaranth leaves prepared using different cooking methods. *Food and Nutrition Sciences, 2*(04), 249–252. doi:10.4236/fns.2011.24035

Ong, K. L., Cheung, B. M. Y., Man, Y. B., Lau, C. P., & Lam, K. S. L. (2007). Prevalence, awareness, treatment & control of hypertension among United States adults 1999–2004. *Hypertension, 49*(1), 69–75. doi:10.1161/01.HYP.0000252676.46043.18 PMID:17159087

Orech, F. O., Christensen, D. L., Larsen, T., Friis, H., Aagaard-Hansen, J., & Estambale, B. A. (2007). Mineral content of traditional leafy vegetables from western Kenya. *International Journal of Food Sciences and Nutrition, 58*(8), 595–602. doi:10.1080/09637480701350288 PMID:17852510

Organisation for Economic Co-operation and Development. (1999). *Consensus document on the biology of Oryza sativa (rice). Report No. ENV/JM/MONO(99)26.* OCED Environmental health and Safety Publications. Paris: Organisation for Economic Co-operation and Development.

Ortega, R. M., Palencia, A., & Lopez-Sobaler, A. M. (2006). Improvement of cholesterol levels and reduction of cardiovascular risk via the consumption of phytosterols. *The British Journal of Nutrition*, *96*(S1Suppl), 89S–93S. doi:10.1079/BJN20061708 PMID:16923260

Osabor, V. N., Ogar, D. A., Okafor, P. C., & Egbung, G. E. (2009). Profile of the African Bread Fruit (*Treculia africana*). *Pakistan Journal of Nutrition*, *8*(7), 1005–1008. doi:10.3923/pjn.2009.1005.1008

Oseni, T., Patel, R., Pyle, J., & Jordan, V. C. (2008). Selective estrogen receptor modulators and phytoestrogens. *Planta Medica*, *74*(13), 1656–1665. doi:10.1055/s-0028-1088304 PMID:18843590

Ostlund, R. E., Spilburg, C. A., & Stenson, W. F. (1999). Sitostanol administered in lecithin micelles potently reduces cholesterol absorption in humans. *The American Journal of Clinical Nutrition*, *70*, 826–831. PMID:10539742

Otieno, D. O., & Shah, N. P. (2007). Endogenous β-glucosidases and β-galactosidases activities from selected probiotic microorganisms and their role in isoflavone biotransformation in soymilk. *Journal of Applied Microbiology*, *103*(4), 910–917. doi:10.1111/j.1365-2672.2007.03438.x PMID:17897193

Otte, J., Shalaby, S. M. A., Zakora, M., & Neilsen, M. S. (2007). Fractionation and identification of ACE-inhibitory peptides from α-lactalbumin and β-casein produced by thermolysin-catalysed hydrolysis. *International Dairy Journal*, *17*(12), 1460–1472. doi:10.1016/j.idairyj.2007.04.008

Oulai, P. D., Zoue, L. T., Bedikou, M. E., Rose-Monde, M., & Niamke, L. S. (2014a). Impact of cooking on nutritive and antioxidant characteristics of leafy vegetables consumed in Northern Côte d'Ivoire. *International Journal of Plant. Animal and Environmental Sciences*, *4*, 576–583.

Oulai, P., Zoue, L., Megnanou, R., Doue, R., & Niamke, S. (2014b). Value of leafy vegetables consumed in Northern Côte D'ivoire. *European Scientific Journal*, *10*, 212–227.

Oyama, A., Ueno, T., Uchiyama, S., Aihara, T., Miyake, T., Kondo, S., & Matsunaga, K. (2012). The effects of natural S-equol supplementation on skin aging in postmenopausal women: A pilot randomized placebo-controlled trial. *Menopause (New York, N.Y.)*, *19*(2), 202–210. doi:10.1097/gme.0b013e318227427b PMID:21934634

Oyetayo, O. V. (2011). Medicinal Uses of Mushrooms in Nigeria: Towards Full and Sustainable Exploitation. *African Journal of Traditional, Complementary, and Alternative Medicines*, *8*(3), 267–274. doi:10.4314/ajtcam.v8i3.65289 PMID:22468005

Oyewole, O. B. (1997). Lactic fermented foods in Africa and their benefits. *Food Control*, *8*(5-6), 289–297. doi:10.1016/S0956-7135(97)00075-3

Pacheco-Palencia, L. A., Noratto, G., Hingorani, L., Talcott, S. T., & Mertens-Talcott, S. U. (2008). Protective effects of standardized pomegranate (*Punica granatum* L.) polyphenolic extract in ultraviolet-irradiated human skin fibroblasts. *Journal of Agricultural and Food Chemistry*, *56*(18), 8434–8441. doi:10.1021/jf8005307 PMID:18717570

Padayatty, S. J., Katz, A., Wang, Y., Eck, P., Kwon, O., Lee, J., & Levine, M. et al. (2003). Vitamin C as an antioxidant: Evaluation of its role in disease prevention. *Journal of the American College of Nutrition*, *22*(1), 18–35. doi:10.1080/07315724.2003.10719272 PMID:12569111

Padovani, R. M., Lima, D. M., Colugnati, F. A., & Rodriguez-Amaya, D. B. (2007). Comparison of proximate, mineral and vitamin composition of common Brazilian and US foods. *Journal of Food Composition and Analysis*, *20*(8), 733–738. doi:10.1016/j.jfca.2007.03.006

Pallauf, K., Rivas-Gonzalo, J. C., del Castillo, M. D., Cano, M. P., & de Pascual-Teresa, S. (2008). Characterization of the antioxidant composition of strawberry tree (*Arbutus unedo* L.) fruits. *Journal of Food Composition and Analysis*, *21*(4), 273–281. doi:10.1016/j.jfca.2007.11.006

Pan, D., Luo, Y., & Tanokura, M. (2005). Antihypertensive peptides from skimmed milk hydrolysate digested by cell-free extract of Lactobacillus helveticus JCM1004. *Food Chemistry*, *91*(1), 123–129. doi:10.1016/j.foodchem.2004.05.055

Pandey, K. B., & Rizvi, S. I. (2009). Plant polyphenols as dietary antioxidants in human health and disease. *Oxidative Medicine and Cellular Longevity*, *2*(5), 270–278. doi:10.4161/oxim.2.5.9498 PMID:20716914

Pang, G., Xie, J., Chen, Q., & Hu, Z. (2012). How functional foods play critical roles in human health. *Food Science and Human Wellness*, *1*(1), 26–60. doi:10.1016/j.fshw.2012.10.001

Pantack, E. T., Hsiao, C. B., & Garland, W. A. (1976). Stimulatory effect of vegetable on intestinal drug metabolism in the rat. *The Journal of Pharmacology and Experimental Therapeutics*, *198*, 277.

Pantsi, W. G., Bester, D. J., Esterhuyse, A. J., & Aboua, G. (2014). Dietary antioxidant properties of vegetable oils and nuts – the race against cardiovascular disease progression. In Antioxidant-antidiabetic agents and human health (pp. 209-238). InTech Publisher.

Pareek, S. (2013). Nutritional composition of jujube fruit. *Emirates Journal of Food and Agriculture.*, *25*(6), 463–470.

Pareek, S., Kitinoja, L., Kaushik, R. A., & Paliwal, R. (2009). Postharvest physiology and storage of *ber. Stew. Posthar. Rev.*, *5*(5), 1–10. doi:10.2212/spr.2009.5.5

Park, H. J., Chinnan, M. S., & Shewfelt, R. L. (1994). Edible corn-zein film coatings to extend storage life of tomatoes. *J. Food Process*, *18*(4), 317–331. doi:10.1111/j.1745-4549.1994.tb00255.x

Park, J. A., Tirupathi Pichiah, J. J., Yu, P. B., Oh, S. H., Daily, J. W. III, & Cha, Y. S. (2012). Anti-obesity effect of kimchi fermented with Weissella koreensis OK1-6 as starter in high-fat diet-induced obese C57BL/6J mice. *Journal of Applied Microbiology*, *113*(6), 1507–1516. doi:10.1111/jam.12017 PMID:22978326

Park, J. H., Ryu, M. S., Lee, Y. E., Song, G. S., & Ryu, K. S. (2003). A comparison of fattening performance, physic-chemical properties of breast meat, vaccine titers in cross bred meat type hybrid chicks fed sulfur. *Korean Journal of Poultry Science*, *30*, 211–217.

Park, K. Y. (1995). The nutritional evaluation, and antimutagenic and anticancer effects of kimchi. *J. Korean Soc. Food Nutr*, *24*, 169.

Park, K. Y., Jeong, J. K., Lee, Y. E., & Daily, J. W. III. (2014). Health benefits of kimchi (Korean fermented vegetables) as a probiotic food. *Journal of Medicinal Food*, *17*(1), 6–20. doi:10.1089/jmf.2013.3083 PMID:24456350

Park, S. H., Kyeong, M. S., Hqang, Y., Ryu, S. Y., Han, S. B., & Kim, Y. (2012). Inhibition of LPS binding to MD-2 co-receptor for suppressing TLR4-mediated expression of inflammatory cytokine by 1-dehydro-10-gingerdione from dietary ginger. *Biochemical and Biophysical Research Communications*, *419*(4), 735–740. doi:10.1016/j.bbrc.2012.02.091 PMID:22387540

Park, Y. W. (2009). Overview of bioactive components in milk and dairy products. In Y. W. Park (Ed.), *Bioactive Componentsin Milk and Dairy Products* (pp. 3–13). Blackwell Publishing. doi:10.1002/9780813821504.ch1

Parodi, P. W. (2009). Has the association between saturated fatty acids, serum cholesterol and coronary heart disease been over emphasized? *International Dairy Journal*, *19*(6-7), 345–361. doi:10.1016/j.idairyj.2009.01.001

Patel, M., & Naik, S. N. (2004). Gamma-oryzanol from rice bran oil – A review. *Journal of Scientific and Industrial Research*, *63*, 569–578.

Paterson, D. M. (2001). Oat antioxidants. *Journal of Cereal Science*, *33*(2), 115–129. doi:10.1006/jcrs.2000.0349

Pathak, L., Kanwal, A., & Agrawal, Y. (2015). Curcumin loaded self-assembled lipid-biopolymer nanoparticles for functional food applications. *J. Food Sci. Technol.*, *52*(10), 6143–6156. doi:10.1007/s13197-015-1742-2 PMID:26396362

Patil, S., & Jain, G. (2014). Holistic approach of *Trigonella foenum-graecum* in phytochemistry and pharmacology- A review. *Current Trends in Technology and Science*, *3*, 34–48.

Patra, J., Taylor, B., Irving, H., Roerecke, M., Baliunas, D., Mohapatra, S., & Rehm, J. (2010). Alcohol consumption and the risk of morbidity and mortality from different stroke types -a systematic review and meta-analysis. *BMC Public Health*, *10*(1), 258. doi:10.1186/1471-2458-10-258 PMID:20482788

Patrice, C., Laura, G. J., Jacqui, T., Kamlesh, K., & Melanie, D. J. (2010). Fruit and vegetable intake and incidence of type 2 diabetes mellitus: Systematic review and meta-analysis. *British Medical Journal*, *341*(4), c4229. doi:10.1136/bmj.c4229 PMID:20724400

Patrick, L. (2000). Beta-carotene: The controversy continues. *Alternative Medicine Review*, *5*(6), 530–545. PMID:11134976

Pawlowska, A. M., Leo, M. D., & Braca, A. (2006). Phenolics of *Arbutus unedo* L. (Ericaceae) fruits: Identification of anthocyanins and gallic acid derivatives. *Journal of Agricultural and Food Chemistry*, *54*(26), 10234–10238. doi:10.1021/jf062230o PMID:17177565

Pedersen, A., Sandström, B., & Amelsvoort, J. M. M. V. (1997). The effect of ingestion of inulin on blood lipids and gastrointestinal symptoms in healthy females. *The British Journal of Nutrition*, *78*(02), 215–222. doi:10.1079/BJN19970141 PMID:9301412

Pedreschi, R., & Cisneros-Zevallos, L. (2007). Phenolic profiles of Andean purple corn (*Zea mays* L.). *Food Chemistry*, *100*(3), 956–963. doi:10.1016/j.foodchem.2005.11.004

Peeters, P. H. M., Slimani, N., van der Schouw, Y. T., Grace, P. B., Navarro, C., Tjonneland, A., & Bingham, S. A. et al. (2007). Variations in plasma phytoestrogen concentrations in European adults. *The Journal of Nutrition*, *137*, 1294–1300. PMID:17449595

Pekkinen, J., Rosa, N. N., Savolainen, O. I., Keski-Rahkonen, P., Mykkanen, H., Poutanen, K., & Hanihineva, K. et al. (2014). Disintegration of wheat aleurone structure has an impact on the bioavailability of phenolic compounds and other phytochemicals as evidenced by altered urinary metabolic profile of diet-induced obese mice. *Nutrition and Metabolism*, *11*(1), 1–15. doi:10.1186/1743-7075-11-1 PMID:24383425

Pellegrini, A., Dettling, C., Thomas, U., & Hunziker, P. (2001). Isolation and characterization of four bactericidal domains in the bovine β-lactoglobulin. *Biochemicaet Biophysica Acta*, *1526*(2), 131–140. doi:10.1016/S0304-4165(01)00116-7 PMID:11325534

Pellegrini, N., Serafini, M., Salvatore, S., Del Rio, D., Bianchi, M., & Brighenti, F. (2006). Total antioxidant capacity of spices, dried fruits, nuts, pulses, cereals and sweets consumed in Italy assessed by three different in vitro assays. *Molecular Nutrition & Food Research*, *50*(11), 1030–1038. doi:10.1002/mnfr.200600067 PMID:17039458

Peltonen, K. D., El-Nezami, H. S., Salminen, S. J., & Ahokas, J. T. (2000). Binding of aflatoxin B1 by probiotic bacteria. *Journal of the Science of Food and Agriculture*, *80*(13), 1942–1945. doi:10.1002/1097-0010(200010)80:13<1942::AID-JSFA741>3.0.CO;2-7

Perabo, F. G., Von Löw, E. C., Ellinger, J., von Rücker, A., Müller, S. C., & Bastian, P. J. (2008). Soy isoflavone genistein in prevention and treatment of prostate cancer. *Prostate Cancer and Prostatic Diseases*, *11*(1), 6–12. doi:10.1038/sj.pcan.4501000 PMID:17923857

Pereira, D. I. A., & Gibson, G. R. (2002). Effects of consumption of probiotics and prebiotics on serum lipid levels in humans. *Critical Reviews in Biochemistry and Molecular Biology*, *37*(4), 259–281. doi:10.1080/10409230290771519 PMID:12236466

Pereira, M. A., O'Reilly, E., Augustsson, K., Fraser, G. E., Goldbourt, U., Heitmann, B. L., & Ascherio, A. et al. (2004). Dietary fiber and risk of coronary heart disease: A pooled analysis of cohort studies. *Archives of Internal Medicine*, *164*(4), 370–376. doi:10.1001/archinte.164.4.370 PMID:14980987

Perera, A., Meda, V., & Tyler, R. (2010). Resistant starch: A review of analytical protocols for determining resistant starch and of factors affecting the resistant starch content of foods. *Food Research International*, *43*(8), 1959–1974. doi:10.1016/j.foodres.2010.06.003

Perez-Jimenez, J., Neveu, V., Vos, F., & Scalbert, A. (2015). Identification of the 100 richest dietary sources of polyphenols: an application of the Phenol-Explorer database. *EJCN*. Retrieved from http://www.nature.com/ejcn/journal/v64/n3s/fig_tab/ejcn2010221t1.html

Pérez-Vásquez, A., García-Nolck, C., Linares, E., Bye, R., & Mata, R. (2014a). Antidiabetic activity and chemical composition of essential oil from Brickellia cavanillesii. *Planta Medica*, *80*(10), PD58. doi:10.1055/s-0034-1382479

Pérez-Vásquez, A., Hernadez-Arámburo, M., Linares, E., Bye, R., & Mata, R. (2014b). Validation of a HPLC-DAD method for chromenes markers in Brickellia cavanillesii. *Planta Medica*, *80*(10), PPL13. doi:10.1055/s-0034-1382649

Petchiammal, C., & Hopper, W. (2014). Antioxidant activity of proteins from fifteen varieties of legume seeds commonly consumed in India. *International Journal of Pharmacy and Pharmaceutical Sciences*, *6*, 476–479.

Peterson, J. J., Beecher, G. R., Bhagwat, S. A., Dwyer, J. T., Gebhardt, S. E., Haytowitz, D. B., & Holden, J. M. (2006). Flavanones in grapefruit, lemons, and limes: A compilation and review of the data from the analytical literature. *Journal of Food Composition and Analysis*, *19*, S74–S80. doi:10.1016/j.jfca.2005.12.009

Pietinen, P., Rimm, E. B., Korhonen, P., Hartman, A. M., Willett, W. C., Albanes, D., & Virtamo, J. et al. (1996). Intake of dietary fiber and risk of coronary heart disease in a cohort of Finnish men. The Alpha-Tocopherol, Beta-Carotene Cancer Prevention Study. *Circulation*, *94*(11), 2720–2727. doi:10.1161/01.CIR.94.11.2720 PMID:8941095

Pilšáková, L., Riečanský, I., & Jagla, F. (2010). The physiological actions of isoflavone phytoestrogens. *Physiological Research*, *59*, 651–664. PMID:20406033

Pilvi, T. K., Jauhiainen, T., Cheng, Z. J., Mervaala, E. M., Vapaatalo, H., & Korpela, R. (2006). Lupin protein attenuates the development of hypertension and normalises the vascular function of NaCl-loaded Goto- Kakizaki rats. *Journal of Physiology and Pharmacology*, *57*, 167–176. PMID:16845223

Pintó, X., Vilaseca, M. A., Balcells, S., Artuch, R., Corbella, E., Meco, J. F., & Grinberg, D. et al. (2005). A folat.e-rich diet is as effective as folic acid from supplements in decreasing plasma homocysteine concentrations In*terna.tional. Journal of Medical Science*, *2*(2), 58.

Pittler, M. H., & Ernst, E. (2004). Dietary supplements for body-weight reduction: A systematic review. *The American Journal of Clinical Nutrition*, *79*, 529–536. PMID:15051593

Pochapin, M. (2000). The effect of probiotics on *Clostridium difficile* diarrhea. *The American Journal of Gastroenterology*, *95*(1), S11–S13. doi:10.1016/S0002-9270(99)00809-6 PMID:10634221

Pogge, D., & Hansen, S. L. (2012). Effect of vitamin C on performance and antioxidant capacity of cattle fed varying concentrations of dietary sulfur. *Animal Industry Report*, *658*, 21.

Polunin, O., & Stainton, A. (1985). Pomegranate. In O. Polunin & A. Stainton (Eds.), Flowers of the Himalaya (pp. 532-534). New York: Oxford University Press.

Pool-Zobel, B., Veeriah, S., & Böhmer, F.D. (2005). Modulation of xenobiotic metabolising enzymes by anticarcinogens-focus on glutathione S-transferases and their role as targets of dietary chemoprevention in colorectal carcinogenesis. *Mutation Research/Fundamental and Molecular Mechanisms of Mutagenesis, 591*(1), 74-92.

Port'eres, R. (1976). African cereals: Eleusine, fonio, black fonio, teff, Brachiaria, Paspalum, Pennisetum, and African rice. In Origins of African Plant Domestication. Academic Press.

Port'eres, R. (1962). Berceauxagricolesprimairessur le continent africain. *Journal of African History*, *3*(02), 195–210. doi:10.1017/S0021853700003030

Possemiers, S., Bolca, S., Eeckhaut, E., Depypere, H., & Verstraete, W. (2007). Metabolism of isoflavones, lignans and prenylflavonoids by intestinal bacteria: Producer phenotyping and relation with intestinal community. *FEMS Microbiology Ecology*, *61*(2), 372–383. doi:10.1111/j.1574-6941.2007.00330.x PMID:17506823

Pradeep, B. V., Manojbabu, M. K., & Palaniswamy, M. (2008). Antibacterial activity of *Punica granatum* L. against gastro intestinal tract infection causing organisms. *Journal of Ethnobotanical Leaflets, 2008*(1), 143.

Prades, A., Dornier, M., Diop, N., & Pain, J.-P. (2012). Coconut water uses, composition and properties: A review. *Fruits*, *67*(2), 87–107. doi:10.1051/fruits/2012002

Prajapati, R. P., Kalariya, M., Parmar, S. K., & Sheth, N. R. (2010). Phytochemical and pharmacological review of *Lagenaria sicereria*. *J Ayurveda Integr Med*, *1*(4), 266–272. doi:10.4103/0975-9476.74431 PMID:21731373

Prakash-Maran, J., Priya, B., & Manikandan, S. (2014). Modeling and optimization of supercritical extraction of anthocyanin and phenolic compounds from *Syzygium cumini* fruit pulp. *Journal of Food Sciences and Technology.*, *51*(9), 1938–1946. doi:10.1007/s13197-013-1237-y PMID:25190849

Prasad, K. (2009). Flax seed and Cardiovascular Health. *Journal of Cardiovascular Pharmacology*, *54*(5), 369–377. doi:10.1097/FJC.0b013e3181af04e5 PMID:19568181

Probst, C., Bandyopadhyay, R., & Cotty, P. J. (2014). Diversity of aflatoxin-producing fungi and their impact on food safety in sub-Saharan Africa. *International Journal of Food Microbiology*, *174*, 113–122. doi:10.1016/j.ijfoodmicro.2013.12.010 PMID:24480188

Psaltopoulou, T., Naska, A., Orfanos, P., Trichopoulos, D., Mountokalakis, T., & Trichopoulou, A. (2004). Olive oil, the Mediterranean diet, and arterial blood pressure: The Greek European prospective investigation into cancer and nutrition (EPIC) study. *The American Journal of Clinical Nutrition*, *80*, 1012–1018. PMID:15447913

Pulido, R., Bravo, L., & Saura-Calixto, F. (2000). Antioxidant activity of dietary polyphenols as determined by a modified ferric reducing/antioxidant power assay. *Journal of Agricultural and Food Chemistry*, *48*(8), 3396–3402. doi:10.1021/jf9913458 PMID:10956123

Qin, J., Li, R., Raes, J., Arumugam, M., Burgdorf, K. S., Manichanh, C., & Wang, J. et al. (2010). A human gut microbial gene catalogue established by metagenomic sequencing. *Nature*, *464*(7285), 59–65. doi:10.1038/nature08821 PMID:20203603

Qiu, L. J., & Chang, R. Z. (2010). The origin and history of soybean. In G. Singh (Ed.), *The Soybean: Botany, Production and Uses*. Oxford, UK: CABI Publishing. doi:10.1079/9781845936440.0001

Qnais, E. Y., Elokda, A. S., Abu Ghalyun, Y. Y., & Abdulla, F. A. (2007). Antidiarrheal activity of the aqueous extract of *Punica granatum* (Pomegranate) peels. *Journal of Pharmaceutical Biology*, *45*(9), 715–720. doi:10.1080/13880200701575304

Quan, S., Tsuda, H., & Miyamoto, T. (2008). Angiotensin I-converting enzyme inhibitory peptides in skim milk fermented with Lactobacillus helveticus 130B4 from camel milk in Inner Mongolia, China. *Journal of the Science of Food and Agriculture*, *88*(15), 2688–2692. doi:10.1002/jsfa.3394

Queiroz-Monici, K. S., Costa, G. E., da Silva, N., Reis, S. M., & de Oliveira, A. C. (2005). Bifidogenic effect of dietary fiber and resistant starch from leguminous on the intestinal microbiota of rats. *Nutrition (Burbank, Los Angeles County, Calif.)*, *21*(5), 602–608. doi:10.1016/j.nut.2004.09.019 PMID:15850967

Quita, S. M., & Kurdi, A. F. L. (2010). Antigenotoxic and anticytotoxic effect of camel milk in mice treated with cisplatin. *Saudi Journal of Biological Sciences*, *17*(2), 159–166. doi:10.1016/j.sjbs.2010.02.010 PMID:23961073

Raghuram, T. C., Rao, U. B., & Rukmini, C. (1989). Studies on hypolipidemic effects of dietary rice bran oil in human subjects. *Nutrition Reports International*, *39*, 889–895.

Rahaiee, S., Moini, S., Hashemi, M., & Shojaosadati, S. A. (2015). Evaluation of antioxidant activities of bioactive compounds and various extracts obtained from saffron (*Crocus sativus* L.): A review. *Journal of Food Sciences and Technology.*, *52*(4), 1881–1888. doi:10.1007/s13197-013-1238-x PMID:25829569

Rahal, A., Kumar, A., Singh, V., Yadav, B., Tiwari, R., Chakraborty, S., & Dhama, K. (2014). Oxidative stress, prooxidants, and antioxidants: The interplay. *BioMed Research International*, *2014*, 1–19. doi:10.1155/2014/761264 PMID:24587990

Rahaman, S., Islam, R., Kamruzzaman, M., Alam, K., & Jamal, A.H.M. (2011). *Ocimum sanctum* L.: A review of phytochemical and pharmacological profile. *American Journal of Drug Discovery and Development*, 1-15.

Rahmouni, K., Correia, M. L. G., Haynes, W. G., & Mark, A. L. (2005). Obesity-associated hypertension – new insights into mechanisms. *Hypertension*, *45*(1), 9–14. doi:10.1161/01.HYP.0000151325.83008.b4 PMID:15583075

Raikos, V., & Dassios, T. (2014). Health-promoting properties of bioactive peptides derived from milk proteins in infant food: A review. *Dairy Sci. Technol.*, *94*(2), 91–101. doi:10.1007/s13594-013-0152-3 PMID:24511365

Raisz, L. G. (2005). Pathogenesis of osteoporosis: Concepts, conflicts, & prospects. *The Journal of Clinical Investigation*, *115*(12), 3318–3325. doi:10.1172/JCI27071 PMID:16322775

Rajagopalan, S., Kurz, S., Munzel, T., Tarpey, M., Freeman, B. A., Griendling, K. K., & Harrison, D. G. (1996). Angiotensin II-mediated hypertension in the rat increases vascular superoxide production via membrane NADH/NADPH oxidase activation. Contribution to alterations of vasomotor tone. *The Journal of Clinical Investigation*, *97*(8), 1916–1923. doi:10.1172/JCI118623 PMID:8621776

Ramadan, M. F. (2015). Nutritional value and applications of Nigella sativa essential oil: A mini review. *Journal of Essential Oil Research.*, *27*(4), 271–275. doi:10.1080/10412905.2015.1045564

Ramel, A., Alfredo Martinez, J., Kiely, M., Bandara, N. M., & Thorsdottir, I. (2010). Moderate consumption of fatty fish reduces diastolic blood pressure in overweight and obese European young adults during energy restriction. *Nutrition (Burbank, Los Angeles County, Calif.)*, *26*(2), 168–174. doi:10.1016/j.nut.2009.04.002 PMID:19487105

Ramshankar, V., & Krishnamurthy, A. (2014). Chemoprevention of oral cancer: Green tea experience. Journal of Natural Science. *Biologie Medicale*, *5*(1), 3–7.

Ramulu, P., & Udayasekhararao, P. (2006). Total insoluble and soluble dietary fiber contents of roots, tubers, vegetables, oilseeds, spices and condiments. *Journal of Food Sciences and Technology.*, *43*(4), 399–403.

Ranich, T., Bhathena, S. J., & Velasquez, M. T. (2001). Protective effect s of dietary phytoestrogens in chronic renal disease. *Journal of Renal Nutrition*, *11*(4), 183–193. doi:10.1016/S1051-2276(01)70036-2 PMID:11679998

Rao, A. V., & Rao, L. G. (2007). Carotenoids and human health. *Pharmacological Research*, *55*(3), 207–216. doi:10.1016/j.phrs.2007.01.012 PMID:17349800

Rao, B. S. N. (2003). Bioactive phytochemicals in Indian foods and their potential in health promotion and disease prevention. *Asia Pacific Journal of Clinical Nutrition*, *12*(1), 9–22. PMID:12737006

Rao, C. V., Newmark, H. L., & Reddy, B. S. (1998). Chemopreventive effect of squalene on colon cancer. *Carcinogenesis*, *19*(2), 287–290. doi:10.1093/carcin/19.2.287 PMID:9498278

Rather, M.A., Dar, B.A., Sofi, S.N., Bhat, B.A., & Qurishi, M.A. (2012). Foeniculum vulgare*: A comprehensive review of its traditional use, phytochemistry, pharmacology, and safety*. Doi: 10.1016/j.arabjc.2012.04.011

Ray, A., Dutta Gupta, S., & Ghosh, S. (2013). Isolation and characterization of potent bioactive fraction with antioxidant and UV absorbing activity from *Aloe vera berbadensis* Miller gel. *Journal of Plant Biochemistry and Biotechnology*, *22*(4), 483–487. doi:10.1007/s13562-012-0178-2

Raza, S., Graham, S. M., Allen, S. J., Sultana, S., Cuevas, L., & Hart, C. A. (1995). Lactobacillus GG promotes recovery from acute non-bloody diarrhea in Pakistan. *The Pediatric Infectious Disease Journal*, *14*(2), 107–111. doi:10.1097/00006454-199502000-00005 PMID:7746691

Reddy, K. S., & Katan, M. B. (2004). Diet, nutrition and the prevention of hypertension and cardiovascular diseases. *Public Health Nutrition*, *7*(1a), 167–186. doi:10.1079/PHN2003587 PMID:14972059

Reginatto, F. H., Athayde, M. L., Gosmann, G., & Schenkel, E. P. (1999). Methylxantines Accumulation in *Ilex* Species – Caffeine and Theobromine in Erva-Mate (*Ilex paraguariensis*) and Other *Ilex* Species. *Journal of the Brazilian Chemical Society*, *10*(6), 443–446. doi:10.1590/S0103-50531999000600004

Rehm, J., Baliunas, D., Borges, G. L. G., Graham, K., Irving, H. M., & Kehoe, T. (2010). The relation between different dimensions of alcohol consumption and burden of disease -An overview. *Addiction (Abingdon, England)*, *105*, 817–843. PMID:20331573

Reidah, I. M. (2013). *Characterization of phenolic compounds in highly-consumed vegetable matrices by using advanced analytical technique.* (Ph.D thesis). University of Granada.

Rein, D., Lotito, S., Holt, R. R., Keen, C. L., Schmitz, H. H., & Fraga, C. G. (2000). Epicatechin in human plasma:In vivo determination and effect of chocolate consumption on plasma oxidation status. *The Journal of Nutrition*, *130*, 2109S–2114S. PMID:10917931

Reinhart, K., Talati, R., White, C., & Coleman, C. I. (2009). The impact of garlic on lipid parameters: A systematic review and meta-analysis. *Nutrition Research Reviews*, *22*(01), 39–48. doi:10.1017/S0954422409350003 PMID:19555517

Reinisalo, M., Karlund, A., Koskela, A., Kaarniranta, K., & Karjalainen, R. O. (2015). Polyphenol stilbenes: Molecular mechanisms of defence against oxidative stress and aging-related diseases. *Oxidative Medicine and Cellular Longevity*, *2015*, 1–24. doi:10.1155/2015/340520 PMID:26180583

Rekha, C. R., & Vijayalakshmi, G. (2010). Bioconversion of isoflavone glycoside to aglycones, mineral bioavailability and vitamin B complex in fermented soymilk by probiotic bacteria and yeast. *Journal of Applied Microbiology*, *109*(4), 1198–1208. doi:10.1111/j.1365-2672.2010.04745.x PMID:20477889

Renaud, S., & de Lorgeril, M. (1992). Wine, alcohol, platelets, and the French paradox for coronary hearth disease. *Lancet*, *339*(8808), 1523–1526. doi:10.1016/0140-6736(92)91277-F PMID:1351198

Renz, H., Bradley, K., Saloga, J., Loader, J., Larsen, G. L., & Gelfand, E. W. (1993). T cells expressing specific V beta elements regulate immunoglobulin E production and airways responsiveness in vivo. *The Journal of Experimental Medicine*, *177*(4), 1175–1180. doi:10.1084/jem.177.4.1175 PMID:8459211

Ressureccion, A. V. A., Sales, J. M., Potrebko, I., Francisco, M. L. L. D., & Hitchcock, H. L. (2009). Peanuts: Bioactive food in a shell. *Food Technology*, *63*(12), 30–36.

Restuccia, D., & Spizzirri, U.G., Parisi, O.I., Cirillo, G., Curcio, M., Iemma, F., Puoci, F., … Picci, N. (2010). New EU regulation aspects and global market of active and intelligent packaging for food industry applications. *Food Control.*

Resurreccion, A. P., Juliano, B. O., & Tanaka, Y. (1979). Nutrient content and distribution in milling fractions of rice grain. *Journal of the Science of Food and Agriculture*, *30*(5), 475–481. doi:10.1002/jsfa.2740300506 PMID:470348

Reto, M., Figueria, M. E., Filipe, H. M., & Almedia, C. M. M. (2007). Chemical composition of green tea (Camellia sinensis) infusions commercialized in Portugal. *Plant Foods for Human Nutrition (Dordrecht, Netherlands)*, *62*(4), 139–144. doi:10.1007/s11130-007-0054-8 PMID:17899383

Reynolds, K., Chin, A., Lees, K. A., Nguyen, A., Bujnowski, D., He, J., & Rosell, M. S. (2006). A meta-analysis of the effect of soy protein supplementation on serum lipids. *The American Journal of Cardiology*, *98*(5), 633–640. doi:10.1016/j.amjcard.2006.03.042 PMID:16923451

Reynoso-Camacho, R., Ramos-Gomez, M., & Loarca-Pina, G. (2006). Bioactive components in common beans (Phaseolus vulgaris L.). In R. G. Guevara-Gonzalez & I. Torres-Pacheco (Eds.), Advances in Agricultural and Food Biotechnology (pp. 217–236). Academic Press.

Ricci-Cabello, I., Herrera, M. O., & Artacho, R. (2012). Possible role of milk derived bioactive peptides in the treatment and prevention of metabolic syndrome. *Nutrition Reviews*, *70*(4), 241–255. doi:10.1111/j.1753-4887.2011.00448.x PMID:22458697

Rice, A. L., West, K. P., & Black, R. (2004). Vitamin A deficiency. In Comparative quantification of health risks: Global and regional burden of disease attributable to selected major risk factors (vol. 1, pp. 212-256). World Health Organisation.

Rice, A. L., Sacco, L., Hyder, A., & Black, R. E. (2000). Malnutrition as an underlying cause of childhood deaths associated with infectious diseases in developing countries. *Bulletin of the World Health Organization*, *78*, 1207–1221. PMID:11100616

Richard, F. C., Goupy, P. M., & Nicolas, J. J. (1992). Cysteine as an inhibitor of enzymatic browning. 2. Kinetic studies. *Journal of Agricultural and Food Chemistry*, *40*(11), 2108–2114. doi:10.1021/jf00023a014

Ridlon, J. M., Kang, D. J., & Hylemon, P. B. (2006). Bile salt biotransformations by human intestinal bacteria. *Journal of Lipid Research*, *47*(2), 241–259. doi:10.1194/jlr.R500013-JLR200 PMID:16299351

Rimbach, G., Melchin, M., Moehring, J., & Wagner, A. E. (2009). Polyphenols from cocoa and vascular health-a critical review. *International Journal of Molecular Sciences*, *10*(10), 4290–4309. doi:10.3390/ijms10104290 PMID:20057946

Rimm, E. B., Katan, M. B., Ascherio, A., Stampfer, M. J., & Willett, W. C. (1996). Relation between intake of flavonoids and risk for coro-nary heart disease in male health professionals. *Annals of Internal Medicine*, *125*(5), 384–389. doi:10.7326/0003-4819-125-5-199609010-00005 PMID:8702089

Rimm, E. B., & Stampfer, M. J. (2000). Antioxidants for vascular disease. *The Medical Clinics of North America*, *84*(1), 239–249. doi:10.1016/S0025-7125(05)70216-9 PMID:10685137

Roberfroid, M. B. (2003). Introducing inulin-type fructans. *The British Journal of Nutrition*, *93*(S1), 13–26. doi:10.1079/BJN20041350 PMID:15877886

Robert, P., Gorena, T., Romero, N., Sepulveda, E., Chavez, J., & Saenz, C. (2010). Encapsulation of polyphenols and anthocyanins from pomegranate (Punica granatum) by spray drying. *International Journal of Food Science & Technology*, *45*(7), 1386–1394. doi:10.1111/j.1365-2621.2010.02270.x

Rocha, A., Wang, L., Penichet, M., & Martins-Green, M. (2012). Pomegranate juice & specific components inhibit cell & molecular processes critical for metastasis of breast cancer. *Breast Cancer Research and Treatment*, *136*(3), 647–658. doi:10.1007/s10549-012-2264-5 PMID:23065001

Rochfort, S., & Panozzo, J. (2007). Phytochemicals for health, the role of pulses. *Journal of Agricultural and Food Chemistry*, *55*(20), 7981–7994. doi:10.1021/jf071704w PMID:17784726

Rock, W., Rosenblat, M., Miller-Lotan, R., Levy, A. P., Elias, M., & Aviram, M. (2008). Consumption of wonderful variety pomegranate juice and extract by diabetic patients increases paraoxonase 1 association with high-density lipoprotein and stimulates its catalytic activities. *Journal of Agricultural and Food Chemistry*, *56*(18), 8704–8713. doi:10.1021/jf801756x PMID:18759451

Rodrigues, J., Assunção, M., Lukoyanov, N., Cardoso, A., Carvalho, F., & Andrade, J. P. (2013). Protective effects of a catechin-rich extract on the hippocampal formation and spatial memory in aging rats. *Behavioural Brain Research*, *246*, 94–102. doi:10.1016/j.bbr.2013.02.040 PMID:23473881

Rodrigues, K. A. F., Amorim, L. V., Dias, C. N., Moraes, D. F. C., Caneiro, S. M. P., & Carvalho, F. A. A. (2015). *Syzygium cumini* L. Skeels essential oil and its major constituent α–pinene exhibit anti-Leishmania activity through immunomodulation in vitro. *Journal of Ethnopharmacology*, *160*, 32–40. doi:10.1016/j.jep.2014.11.024 PMID:25460590

Rodríguez, C., Frias, J., Vidal-Valverde, C., & Hernández, A. (2008). Correlations between some nitrogen fractions, lysine, histidine, tyrosine, and ornithine contents during the germination of peas, beans, and lentils. *Food Chemistry*, *108*(1), 245–252. doi:10.1016/j.foodchem.2007.10.073

Rodriguez-Lopez, V., Moreno-Escobar, J. A., Avila-Torres, O., & Tlahuext, H. (2006). 6-Acetyl-5-hydroxy-2, 2-dimethyl-2H- Chromene. *Acta Crystallographica. Section E, Structure Reports Online*, *62*(9), 03616–03617. doi:10.1107/S1600536806028947

Roerecke, M., & Rehm, J. (2010). Irregular heavy drinking occasions and risk of ischemic heart disease: A systematic review and meta-analysis. *American Journal of Epidemiology*, *171*(6), 633–644. doi:10.1093/aje/kwp451 PMID:20142394

Roh, E., Kim, J. E., Kwon, J. Y., Park, J. S., Bode, A. M., Dong, Z., & Lee, K. W. (2015). Molecular Mechanisms of Green Tea Polyphenols with Protective Effects against Skin Photoaging.[Epub ahead of print]. *Critical Reviews in Food Science and Nutrition*, 00. doi:10.1080/10408398.2014.1003365 PMID:26114360

Rojas-Grau, M. A., Sobrino-Lopez, A., Tapia, M. S., & Martın-Belloso, O. (2006). Browning inhibition in fresh-cut 'Fuji' apple slices by natural anti-browning agents. *Journal of Food Science*, *71*(1), S59–S65. doi:10.1111/j.1365-2621.2006.tb12407.x

Rojas-Grau, M. A., Soliva-Fortuny, R., & Martin-Belloso, O. (2009). Edible coatings to incorporate active ingredients to fresh cut fruits: A review. *Trends in Food Science & Technology*, *20*(10), 438–447. doi:10.1016/j.tifs.2009.05.002

Rojas-Grau, M., Raybaudi-Massilia, R. M., Soliva-Fortuny, R. C., Avena-Bustillos, R. J., McHugh, T. H., & Martín-Belloso, O. (2007). Apple puree-alginate edible coating as carrier of antimicrobial agents to prolong shelf-life of fresh-cut apples. *Postharvest Biology and Technology*, *45*(2), 254–264. doi:10.1016/j.postharvbio.2007.01.017

Romanazzi, G., Nigro, F., Ippolito, A., Di Venere, D., & Salerno, M. (2002). Effects of pre- and postharvest chitosan treatments to control storage grey mold of table grapes. *Journal of Food Science*, *67*(5), 1862–1867. doi:10.1111/j.1365-2621.2002.tb08737.x

Rondini, E. A., & Bannink, M. R. (2012). Microarray analysis of genes differentially expressed by diet (black beans and soy flour) during azoxymethane-induced colon carcinogenesis in rats. *Journal of Nutrition and Metabolism*, *2012*, 1–17. doi:10.1155/2012/351796 PMID:22496968

Rooney, M. L. (1995). Active packaging in polymer films. In *Active Food Packaging* (pp. 74–110). Glasgow, UK: Blackie Academic & Professional. doi:10.1007/978-1-4615-2175-4_4

Rosa-Sibakov, N., Poutanen, K., & Micard, V. (2015). How does wheat grain, bran and aleurone structure impact their nutritional and technological properties? *Trends in Food Science & Technology*, *41*(2), 118–134. doi:10.1016/j.tifs.2014.10.003

Rosenblat, M., Hayek, T., & Aviram, M. (2006). Anti-oxidative effects of pomegranate juice (PJ) consumption by diabetic patients on serum and on macrophages. *Atherosclerosis*, *187*(2), 363–371. doi:10.1016/j.atherosclerosis.2005.09.006 PMID:16226266

Rosenfeldt, V., Michaelsen, K. F., Jakobsen, M., Larsen, C. N., Møller, P. L., Pedersen, P., & Pærregaard, A. et al. (2002). Effect of *Lactobacillus* strains in young children hospitalized with acute diarrhea. *The Pediatric Infectious Disease Journal*, *21*(5), 411–416. doi:10.1097/00006454-200205000-00012 PMID:12150178

Rosillo, M. A., Sánchez-Hidalgo, M., Cárdeno, A., Aparicio-Soto, M., Sánchez-Fidalgo, S., Villegas, I., & de la Lastra, C. A. (2012). Dietary supplementation of an ellagic acid-enriched pomegranate extract attenuates chronic colonic inflammation in rats. *Journal of Pharmacological Research*, *66*(3), 235–242. doi:10.1016/j.phrs.2012.05.006 PMID:22677088

Rowlands, D. J., Chapple, S., Siow, R. C., & Mann, G. E. (2011). Equol-stimulated mitochondrial reactive oxygen species activate endothelial nitric oxide synthase and redox signaling in endothelial cells: Roles for F-actin and GPR30. *Hypertension*, *57*(4), 833–840. doi:10.1161/HYPERTENSIONAHA.110.162198 PMID:21300668

Roy, F., Boye, J., & Simpson, B. (2010). Bioactive proteins and peptides in pulse crops: Pea, chickpea and lentil. *Food Research International*, *43*(2), 432–442. doi:10.1016/j.foodres.2009.09.002

Rozenn, N. L., Irena, B. K., Dariush, M., Lewis, H. K., Russell, P. T., & David, S. S. (2003). N-3 Polyunsaturated fatty acids, fatal ischemic heart disease, and nonfatal myocardial infarction in older adults: The Cardiovascular health study. *The American Journal of Clinical Nutrition*, *77*, 319–325. PMID:12540389

Rubio, C. A., & Befrits, R. (2008). Colorectal cancer in Crohn's disease — review of a 56-year experience in Karolinska Institute University Hospital. *Journal of Environmental Pathology, Toxicology and Oncology*, *27*(4), 257–266. doi:10.1615/JEnvironPatholToxicolOncol.v27.i4.20 PMID:19105531

Rubio, L. (2000). Physiological effects of legume storage proteins. *Nutrition Abstracts andReiew Series A. Human and Experimental*, *70*, 531–538.

Rueda, F. D. M. N. (2005). *Guava (*Psidium guajava *l.) fruit phytochemicals, antioxidant properties and overall quality as influenced by postharvest treatments*. (M.Sc Thesis). University of Florida.

Ruela de Sousa, R. R., Queiroz, K. C. S., Souza, A. C. S., Gurgueira, S. A., August, A. C., Miranda, M. A., & Aoyama, H. et al. (2007). Phosphoprotein levels, IMAPK activities and NFjB expression are affected by fisetin. *Journal of Enzyme Inhibition and Medicinal Chemistry*, *22*(4), 439–444. doi:10.1080/14756360601162063 PMID:17847710

Rüfer, C. E., Bub, A., Möseneder, J., Winterhalter, P., Stürtz, M., & Kulling, S. E. (2008). Pharmacokinetics of the soybean isoflavone daidzein in its aglycone and glucoside form: A randomized, double-blind, crossover study. *The American Journal of Clinical Nutrition*, *87*, 1314–1323. PMID:18469255

Rupp, H., & Maisch, B. (2003). Abdominal fat and sympathetic overactivity. *Herz*, *28*(8), 668–673. doi:10.1007/s00059-003-2517-5 PMID:14689100

Ryan, E. P. (2011). Bioactive food components and health properties of rice bran. *Journal of the American Veterinary Medical Association*, *238*(5), 593–600. doi:10.2460/javma.238.5.593 PMID:21355801

Ryan, E., Galvin, K., O'Connor, T., Maguire, A., & O'Brien, N. (2007). Phytosterol, squalene, tocopherol content and fatty acid profile of selected seeds, grains, and legumes. *Plant Foods for Human Nutrition (Dordrecht, Netherlands)*, *62*(3), 85–91. doi:10.1007/s11130-007-0046-8 PMID:17594521

Ryland, D., Vaisey-Genser, M., Arntfield, S. D., & Malcolmson, L. J. (2010). Development of a nutritious acceptable snack bar using micronized flaked lentils. *Food Research International*, *43*(2), 642–649. doi:10.1016/j.foodres.2009.07.032

Ryu, B.M., Ryu, S.H., Yang, Y.C., Lee, Y.S., Jeon, Y.S., & Moon, G.S. (2004). Morphological changes in the skin of hairless mouse fed various kimchi diet. *J. Korean Soc. Food Sci. Nutr*, *33*, 291-298.

Ryu, B. M. (2000). *Effect of kimchi on inhibition of skin aging of hairless mouse, (PhD. Disseration)*. Busan, Korea: Pusan National Univ.

Ryu, B. M., Ryu, S. H., Yang, Y. C., Lee, Y. S., Jeon, Y. S., & Moon, G. S. (2004). Morphological changes in the skin of hairless mouse fed various kimchi diet. *J Korean Soc Food Sci Nutr.*, *33*(9), 1469–1475. doi:10.3746/jkfn.2004.33.9.1469

Ryu, H. H., Kim, H. L., Chung, J. H., Lee, B. R., Kim, T. H., & Shin, B. C. (2010). Renoprotective effects of green tea extract on renin-angiotensin-aldosterone system in chronic cyclosporine-treated rats. *Nephrology, Dialysis, Transplantation*, *26*(4), 1188–1193. doi:10.1093/ndt/gfq616 PMID:20947539

Ryu, S. H., Jeon, Y. S., Kwon, M. J., Moon, J. W., Lee, Y. S., & Moon, G. S. (1997). Effect of kimchi ingaradients to reactive oxygen species in skin cell cytotoxicity. *J. korean Soc. Food Sci. Nutr.*, *26*(6), 998–1105.

Ryu, S. H., Jeon, Y. S., Kwon, M. J., Moon, J. W., Lee, Y. S., & Moon, G. S. (1997). Effect of kimchi ingredients to reactive oxygen species in skin cell cytotoxicity. *J. korean Soc. Food Sci. Nutr.*, *26*(5), 814–821.

Saavedra, J. (2000). Probiotics and infectious diarrhea. *The American Journal of Gastroenterology*, *95*(1), S16–S18. doi:10.1016/S0002-9270(99)00811-4 PMID:10634223

Sadat Ladjevardi, Z., Taghi-Gharibzahedi, S. M., & Mousavi, M. (2015). Development of a stable low-fat yogurt gel using functionality of psyllium (*Plantago ovata* Forsk) husk gum. *Carbohydrate Polymers*, *125*, 272–280. doi:10.1016/j.carbpol.2015.02.051 PMID:25857984

Sadler, M. (2003). Nutritional properties of edible fungi. *British Nutrition Foundation Nutrition Bulletin*, *28*(3), 305–308. doi:10.1046/j.1467-3010.2003.00354.x

Sah, B. N. P., Vasiljevic, T., McKechnie, S., & Donkor, O. N. (2014). Effect of probiotics on antioxidant and antimutagenic activities of crude peptide extract from yogurt. *Food Chemistry*, *156*, 264–270. doi:10.1016/j.foodchem.2014.01.105 PMID:24629967

Sainani, G. S., Desai, D. B., Gorhe, N. H., Natu, S. M., & Pise, D. V. (1979). Effects of dietary garlic on serum lipid prolic in Jain community. *The Indian Journal of Medical Research*, *69*, 776–779. PMID:511261

Salami, M., Moosavi-Movahedi, A. A., Ehsani, M. R., Yousefi, R., Haertlé, T., Chobert, J. M., & Niasari-Naslaji, A. et al. (2010). Improvement of the antimicrobial and antioxidant activities of camel and bovine whey proteins by limited proteolysis. *Journal of Agricultural and Food Chemistry*, *58*(6), 3297–3302. doi:10.1021/jf9033283 PMID:20175528

Salami, M., Moosavi-Movahedi, A. A., Moosavi-Movahedi, F., Ehsani, M. R., Yousefi, R., Farhadi, M., & Haertlé, T. et al. (2011). Biological activity of camel milk casein following enzymatic digestion. *The Journal of Dairy Research*, *78*(04), 471–478. doi:10.1017/S0022029911000628 PMID:21910944

Salariya, A. M. (2005). The effects of hydrothermal processing on antinutrients, protein and starch digestibility of food legumes. *International Journal of Food Science & Technology*, *40*(7), 695–700. doi:10.1111/j.1365-2621.2005.00978.x

Saldana, M. D., Zetzl, C., Mohamed, R. S., & Brunner, G. (2002). Extraction of Methylxantines from Guarana seeds, Mate leaves, and Cocoa Beans using Supercritical Carbon Dioxide and Ethanol. *Journal of Agricultural and Food Chemistry*, *50*(17), 4820–4826. doi:10.1021/jf020128v PMID:12166966

SaleemM.AdhamiV. M.SiddiquiI. A.MukhtarH. (2003) Tea

Saleem, M., Adhami, V. M., Siddiqui, I. A., & Mukhtar, H. (2003, September). Tea Beverage in Chemoprevention of Prostate Cancer: A Mini-Review. *Nutrition and Cancer*, *47*(1), 13–23. doi:10.1207/s15327914nc4701_2

Salgado, P. R., Lopez-Caballero, M. E., Gomez-Guillen, M. C., Mauri, A. N., & Montero, M. P. (2012). Exploration of the antioxidant and antimicrobial capacity of two sunflower protein concentrate films with naturally present phenolic compounds. *Food Hydrocolloids*, *29*(2), 374–381. doi:10.1016/j.foodhyd.2012.03.006

Salminen, S., Ouwehand, A. C., Benno, Y., & Lee, Y. K. (1999). Probiotics: How should they be defined? *Trends in Food Science & Technology*, *10*(3), 107–110. doi:10.1016/S0924-2244(99)00027-8

Sames, K., Schumacher, U., Halata, Z., Damme, E. V., Peumans, W., Asmus, B., & Moll, I. et al. (2001). Lectin. and proteoglycan histochemistry of Merkel cell carcinomas. *Experimental Dermatology*, *10*(2), 100–109. doi:10.1034/j.1600-0625.2001.010002100.x PMID:11260248

Samokhvalov, A. V., Irving, H. M., & Rehm, J. (2010). Alcohol as a risk factor for atrial fibrillation: A systematic review and meta-analysis. *European Journal of Cardiovascular Prevention and Rehabilitation*, *17*, 706–712. doi:10.1097/HJR.0b013e32833a1947 PMID:21461366

Samy, A. H., Omayma, A. R., & Mohammed, A. E. (2014). Protective Effect of Green Tea Extract on Cyclosporine A: Induced Nephrotoxicity in Rats. *The Journal of Biological Sciences*, *14*(4), 248–257. doi:10.3923/jbs.2014.248.257

Sánchez-Calvo, J. M., Rodríguez-Iglesias, M. A., Molinillo, J. M. G., & Macías, F. A. (2013). Soy isoflavones and their relationship with microflora: Beneficial effects on human Health in equol producers. *Phytochemistry Reviews*, *12*(4), 979–1000. doi:10.1007/s11101-013-9329-x

Sánchez-Muniz, F. J. (2012). Dietary fibre and cardiovascular health. *Nutricion Hospitalaria*, *27*(1), 31–45. PMID:22566302

Sandberg, A.-S. (2002). Bioavailability of minerals in legumes. *The British Journal of Nutrition*, *88*(S3), 281–285. doi:10.1079/BJN/2002718 PMID:12498628

Sangeethapriya, M., & Sidduraja, P. (2014). Health related functional characteristics and antioxidant potential of mucilage (dietary fiber) from Zizyphus mauritiana fruits. *Food Sci. Human Wellness*, *3*(2), 79–88. doi:10.1016/j.fshw.2014.05.003

Sang, S., Tian, S., Wang, H., Stark, R. E., Rosen, R. T., Yang, C. S., & Ho, C. T. (2003). Chemical studies of the antioxidant mechanism of tea catechins: Radical reaction products of epicatechin with peroxyl radicals. *Bioorganic & Medicinal Chemistry*, *11*(16), 3371–3378. doi:10.1016/S0968-0896(03)00367-5 PMID:12878131

Sankhari, J.M., Thounaojam, M.C., Jadeja, R. N., Devkar, R. V., Ramachandran, A. V. (2012). Anthocyanin-rich red cabbage (Brassica oleracea L.) extract attenuates cardiac and hepatic oxidative stress in rats fed an atherogenic diet. *Journal of Science and Food Agriculture*, *92*(8), 1688-1693.

Santhosha, S. G., Prakash, J., & Prabhavathi, S. N. (2013). Bioactive components of garlic and their physiological role in health maintenance: A review. *Food Biosci.*, *3*, 59–74. doi:10.1016/j.fbio.2013.07.001

Saranraj, P., Naidu, M. A., & Sivasakthivelan, P. (2013). Lactic acid bacteria and its antimicrobial properties: A review. *International Journal of Pharmaceutical & Biological Archives*, *4*(6), 1124–1133.

Sari, F., Turkmen, N., Polat, G., & Velioghi, Y. S. (2007). Total polyphenol, antioxidant and antibacterial activities of black mate tea. *Food Science and Technology Research*, *13*(3), 265–269. doi:10.3136/fstr.13.265

Sarkaki, A., Amani, R., Badavi, M., Moghaddam, A. Z., Aligholi, H., Safahani, M., & Haghighizadeh, M. H. (2008). Pre-treatment effect of different doses of soy isoflavones on spatial learning and memory in an ovariectomized animal model of Alzheimer's disease. *Pakistan Journal of Biological Sciences*, *11*, 1114–1119. doi:10.3923/pjbs.2008.1114.1119 PMID:18819549

Sarmadi, B. H., & Ismail, A. (2010). Antioxidative peptides from food proteins: A review. *Peptides*, *31*(10), 1949–1956. doi:10.1016/j.peptides.2010.06.020 PMID:20600423

Saroj, A., Pragadheesh, V. S., Palanivelu, , Yadav, A., Singh, S. C., Samad, A., & Chanotiya, C. S. et al. (2015). Antiphytopathogenic activity of *Syzygium cumini* essential oils, hydrocarbon fractions and its novel constituents. *Industrial Crops and Products*, *74*, 327–335. doi:10.1016/j.indcrop.2015.04.065

Sarrafzadegan, N., & Najafian, J. (1998). Prionties in cardiovascular prevention in Iran. *Iran Health Journal.*, *1*(Supp 1), 131.

Sarwar, M. T., Rahman, M. H., Raza, M. S., Rouf, S. M. A., & Rahman, M. N. (2014). Determination of Erucic acid content in traditional and commercial mustard oils of Bangladesh by gas- liquid chromatography. *Advances in Biochemistry*, *2*(1), 9–13. doi:10.11648/j.ab.20140201.12

SAS Institute. (2002). SAS User's Guide: Statistics. Cary, NC: SAS Institute Inc.

Satih, S., Chalabi, N., Rabiau, N., Bosviel, R., Fontana, L., Bignon, Y. J., & Bernard-Gallon, D. J. (2010). Gene expression profiling of breast cancer cell lines in response to soy isoflavones using a pangenomic microarray approach. *OMICS: A Journal of Integrative Biology*, *14*(3), 231–238. doi:10.1089/omi.2009.0124 PMID:20455703

Sato, T., & Miyata, G. (2000). The nutraceutical benefit, Part I: Green tea. *Nutrition (Burbank, Los Angeles County, Calif.)*, *16*(4), 315–317. doi:10.1016/S0899-9007(99)00301-9 PMID:10758375

Saura-Calixto, F., Serrano, J., & Perez-Jimemez, J. (2008). What constribution is beer to the intake of antioxidant in diet. In V. Preedy (Ed.), *Beer in health and disease prevention*. London: Academic Press.

Savolainen, O. I., Pekkinen, J., Katina, K., Poutanen, K., & Hanhineva, K. (2015). Glycosylated benzoxazinoids are degraded during fermentation of wheat bran. *Journal of Agricultural and Food Chemistry*, *65*(25), 5943–5949. doi:10.1021/acs.jafc.5b00879 PMID:26040909

Sawada, N., Iwasaki, M., Inoue, M., Takachi, R., Sasazuki, S., Yamaji, T., & Tsugane, S. et al. (2013). Dietary arsenic intake and subsequent risk of cancer: The Japan Public Health Center–based (JPHC) Prospective Study. *Cancer Causes & Control*, *24*(7), 1403–1415. doi:10.1007/s10552-013-0220-2 PMID:23666560

Sboui, A., Khorchani, T., Djegham, M., Agrebi, A., Elhatmi, H., & Belhadj, O. (2010). Anti-diabetic effect of camel milk in alloxan-induced diabetic dogs: A dose–response experiment. *Journal of Animal Physiology and Animal Nutrition*, *94*(4), 540–546. doi:10.1111/j.1439-0396.2009.00941.x PMID:19906135

Scalbert, A., Manach, C., Morand, C., Rémésy, C., & Jiménez, L. (2005). Dietary polyphenols and the prevention of diseases. *Critical Reviews in Food Science and Nutrition*, *45*(4), 287–306. doi:10.1080/1040869059096 PMID:16047496

Scalbert, A., & Williamson, G. (2000). Dietary intake and bioavailability of polyphenols. *The Journal of Nutrition*, *130*, 2073S–2085S. PMID:10917926

Scarafoni, A., Magni, C., & Duranti, M. (2007). Molecular nutraceutics as a mean to investigate the positive effects of legume seed proteins on human health. *Trends in Food Science & Technology*, *18*(9), 454–463. doi:10.1016/j.tifs.2007.04.002

Schaafsma, G., Meuling, W. J. A., van Dokkum, W., & Bouley, C. (1998). Effects of a milk product, fermented with Lactobacillus acidophilus and with fructo-oligosaccharides added, on blood lipids in male volunteers. *European Journal of Clinical Nutrition*, *52*(6), 436–440. doi:10.1038/sj.ejcn.1600583 PMID:9683397

Schell, M. A., Karmirantzou, M., Snel, B., Vilanova, D., Berger, B., Zwahlen, M. C., … Arigoni, F. (2002). The genome sequence of *Bifidobacterium longum* reflects its adaptation to the human gastrointestinal tract. *Proceedings of the Natural Academy of Science, USA 99*. doi:10.1073/pnas.212527599

Schiffrin, E. L. (2001). Effects of antihypertensive drugs on vascular remodeling: Do they predict outcome in response to antihypertensive therapy? *Current Opinion in Nephrology and Hypertension*, *10*(5), 617–624. doi:10.1097/00041552-200109000-00011 PMID:11496055

Schinella, G. R., Troiani, G., Davila, V., de Buschiazzo, P. M., & Tournier, H. A. (2000). Antioxidant Effects of an Aqueous Extract of *Ilex Paraguariensis*. *Biochemical and Biophysical Research Communications*, *269*(2), 357–360. doi:10.1006/bbrc.2000.2293 PMID:10708556

Schröder, C., Matthies, A., Engst, W., Blaut, M., & Braune, A. (2013). Identification and expression of genes involved in the conversion of daidzein and genistein by the equol-forming bacterium *Slackia isoflavoniconvertens*. *Applied and Environmental Microbiology*, *79*(11), 3494–3502. doi:10.1128/AEM.03693-12 PMID:23542626

Schubert, A., Zanin, F. F., Pereira, D. F., & Athayde, M. L. (2006). Variação anual de metilxantinas totais em amostras de *Ilex paraguariensis* St. Hill. (erva-mate) en Ijuí e Santa Maria, Estado do Rio Grande do Sul. *Quimica Nova*, *29*(6), 1233–1236. doi:10.1590/S0100-40422006000600016

Schubert, S. Y., Neeman, I., & Resnick, N. (2002). A novel mechanism for the inhibition of NF-κB activation in vascular endothelial cells by natural antioxidants. *The FASEB Journal*, *16*(14), 1931–1933. PMID:12368228

Schulze, M. B., Liu, S., Rimm, E. B., Manson, J. E., Willett, W. C., & Hu, F. B. (2004). Glycemic index, glycemic load,and dietary fiber intake and incidence of type 2 diabetes in younger and middle-aged women. *The American Journal of Clinical Nutrition*, *80*(2), 348–356. PMID:15277155

Schwen, R. J., Nguyen, L., & Jackson, R. L. (2012). Elucidation of the metabolic pathway of S-equol in rat, monkey and man. *Food and Chemical Toxicology*, *50*(6), 2074–2083. doi:10.1016/j.fct.2012.03.048 PMID:22449546

Sebti, I., Martial-Gros, A., Carnet-Pantiez, A., Grelier, S., & Coma, V. (2005). Chitosan polymer as bioactive coating and film against *Aspergillus niger* contamination. *Journal of Food Science*, *70*(2), 100–104. doi:10.1111/j.1365-2621.2005.tb07098.x

Seely, D., Mills, E. J., Wu, P., Verma, S., & Guyatt, G. H. (2005). The effects of green tea consumption on incidence of breast cancer and recurrence of breast cancer: A systematic review and meta-analysis. *Integrative Cancer Therapies*, *4*(2), 144–155. doi:10.1177/1534735405276420 PMID:15911927

Segura, J., & Ruilope, L. M. (2007). Obesity, Essential hypertension and rennin-angiotensin system. *Public Health Nutrition*, *10*(10A), 1151–1155. doi:10.1017/S136898000700064X PMID:17903324

Sehm, S. K., Magda, S. M., & Madiha, M. A. (2015). Effect of some plant oils and garlic on lipids of rats fed on high cholesterol diet. *International Food Research Journal*, *22*(3), 1307–1314.

Seibel, W., Sidhu, J. S., & Bruemmer, J. M. (1990). Composition of different whole wheat flours for performance in bread and *chapati*. Getreide Mehl u. *Brot.*, *44*(7), 208–210.

Seifu, E., Buys, E. M., & Donkin, E. F. (2005). Significance of the lactoperoxidase system in the dairy industry and its potential applications: A review. *Trends in Food Science & Technology*, *16*(4), 1–18. doi:10.1016/j.tifs.2004.11.002

Seki, T., & Hosono, T. (2015). Prevention of cardiovascular diseases by garlic-derived sulphur compounds. *Journal of Nutritional Science and Vitaminology*, *61*(Supplement), S83–S85. doi:10.3177/jnsv.61.S83 PMID:26598900

Selma, M. V., Espín, J. C., & Tomás-Barberán, F. A. (2009). Interaction between phenolics and gut microbiota: Role in human health. *Journal of Agricultural and Food Chemistry*, *57*(15), 6485–6501. doi:10.1021/jf902107d PMID:19580283

Selvaraj, V., Zakroczymski, M. A., Naaz, A., Mukai, M., Ju, Y. H., Doerge, D. R., & Cooke, P. S. et al. (2004). Estrogenicity of the isoflavone metabolite equol on reproductive and non-reproductive organs in mice. *Biology of Reproduction*, *71*(3), 966–972. doi:10.1095/biolreprod.104.029512 PMID:15151933

Sen, C. T. (2004). *Food Culture in India*. Greenwood Publishing Group.

Sengupta, A., Ghosh, S., & Das, S. (2004). Modulatory influence of garlic and tomato on cyclooxygenase-2 activity, cell proliferation and apoptosis during azoxymethane induced colon carcinogenesis in rat. *Cancer Letters*, *208*(2), 127–136. doi:10.1016/j.canlet.2003.11.024 PMID:15142670

Sengupta, R., & Bhattacharyya, D. K. (1996). Enzymatic extraction of mustard seed & rice bran. *Journal of the American Oil Chemists' Society*, *73*(6), 687–692. doi:10.1007/BF02517941

Sen, S., & Chakraborty, R. (2011). The role of antioxidants in human health. In A. Silvana & M. Hepel (Eds.), *Oxidative stress: Diagnostics, prevention, and therapy* (pp. 1–37). Washington, DC: American Chemical Society. doi:10.1021/bk-2011-1083.ch001

Sen, S., & Chakraborty, R. (2015). Antioxidant supplements: Friend or foe? In V. Rani & U. C. S. Yadav (Eds.), *Free radicals in human disease and health* (pp. 293–322). New Delhi: Springer Publication.

Sen, S., Chakraborty, R., Sridhar, C., Reddy, Y. S. R., & De, B. (2010). Free radicals, antioxidants, diseases and phytomedicines: Current status and future prospect. *International Journal of Pharmaceutical Sciences Review and Research*, *3*(1), 91–100.

Seo, B. J. (2012). *Antiviral effects of Leuconostoc mesenteroides YML003 isolated from Kimchi on pathogenic Avian influenza (H9N2) virus*. (Ph.D Thesis). Youngnam University, Daegu, Korea.

Seo, B. J., Rather, I. A., Kumar, V. J. R., Choi, U. H., Moon, M. R., Lim, J. H., & Park, Y. H. (2012). Evaluation of Leuconostoc mesenteroides YML003 as a probiotic against low-pathogenic avian influenza (H9N2) virus in chickens. *Journal of Applied Microbiology*, *113*(1), 163–171. doi:10.1111/j.1365-2672.2012.05326.x PMID:22548634

Servili, M., Sordini, B., Esposto, S., Urbani, S., Zeneziani, G., Maio, I. D., & Taticchi, A. et al. (2014). Biological activities of phenolic compounds of extra virgin olive oil. *Antioxidants*, *3*(1), 1–23. doi:10.3390/antiox3010001 PMID:26784660

Setchell, K. D. R., Brown, N. M., & Lydeking-Olsen, E. (2002). Clinical importance of the metabolite equol. A clue to the effectiviness of soy and its isoflavones. *The Journal of Nutrition*, *132*, 3577–3584. PMID:12468591

Setchell, K. D., Brown, N. M., Desai, P., Zimmer-Nechemias, L., Wolfe, B. E., Brashear, W. T., & Heubi, J. E. et al. (2001). Bioavailability of pure isoflavones in healthy humans and analysis of commercial soy isoflavone supplements. *The Journal of Nutrition*, *131*, 1362S–1375S. PMID:11285356

Setchell, K. D., & Clerici, C. (2010). Equol: History, chemistry, and formation. *The Journal of Nutrition*, *140*(7), 1355S–1362S. doi:10.3945/jn.109.119776 PMID:20519412

Setchell, K. D., Clerici, C., Lephart, E. D., Cole, S. J., Heenan, C., Castellani, D., & Heubi, J. E. et al. (2005). S-equol, a potent ligand for estrogen receptor beta, is the exclusive enantiomeric form of the soy isoflavone metabolite produced by human intestinal bacterial flora. *The American Journal of Clinical Nutrition*, *81*, 1072–1079. PMID:15883431

Setchell, K. D., & Cole, S. J. (2006). Method of defining equol-producer status and its frequency among vegetarians. *The Journal of Nutrition*, *136*, 2188–2193. PMID:16857839

Setchell, K. D., Faughnan, M. S., Avades, T., Zimmer-Nechemias, L., Brown, N. M., Wolfe, B. E., & Cassidy, A. et al. (2003). Comparing the pharmacokinetics of daidzein and genistein with the use of 13C-labeled tracers in premenopausal women. *The American Journal of Clinical Nutrition*, *77*, 411–419. PMID:12540402

Severino, J. F., Goodman, B. A., Kay, C. W., Stolze, K., Tunega, D., Reichenauer, T. G., & Pirker, K. F. (2009). Free radicals generated during oxidation of green tea polyphenols: Electron paramagnetic resonance spectroscopy combined with density functional theory calculations. *Free Radical Biology & Medicine*, *46*(8), 1076–1088. doi:10.1016/j.freeradbiomed.2009.01.004 PMID:19439236

Sezik, E., Yeşilada, E., Honda, G., Takaishi, Y., Takeda, Y., & Tanaka, T. (2001). Traditional medicine in Turkey X. Folk medicine in central Anatolia. *Journal of Ethnopharmacology*, *75*(2), 95–115. doi:10.1016/S0378-8741(00)00399-8 PMID:11297840

Shabo, Y., Barzel, R., Margoulis, M., & Yagil, R. (2005). Camel milk for food allergies in children. *Immunology and Allergies*, *7*, 796–798. PMID:16382703

Shahidi, F., & Chandrasekara, A. (2013). Millet grain phenolics and their role in disease risk reduction and promotion: A review. *Journal of Functional Foods*, *5*(2), 570–581. doi:10.1016/j.jff.2013.02.004

Shalash, M. R. (1984). The production and utilization of camel milk. In W. R. Cockrill (Ed.), *The Camelid: An all-purpose animal* (pp. 196–208). Uppsala, Sweden: Scandinavian Institute of African Studies.

Shams, H., Tahbaz, F., & Abadi, A. (2010). Effects of cooked lentils on glycemic control and blood lipids of patients with type 2 diabetes. *ARYA Atherosclerosis, 4*(1).

Shamsia, S. M. (2009). Nutritional and therapeutic properties of camel andhuman milks. *International Journal of Genetics and Molecular Biology*, *1*, 52-58.

Shane-McWhorter, L. (2007). Complimentary & alternative medicine (CAM) supplement use in people with diabetes: a clinician's guide. Alexandria, VA: American Diabetes Association (ADA).

Shantakumari, N., Eldeeb, R. A., Mabrouk Ibrahim, S. A., Sreedharan, J., & Otoum, S. (2014). Effect of PUFA on patients with hypertension: A hospital based study. *Indian Heart Journal, 66*(4), 408–414. doi:10.1016/j.ihj.2014.05.006 PMID:25173198

Sharp CQ, Kitchens KJ (1990). Using rice bran in yeast bread in a home baker. *Cereal Foods World, 35*, 1021-1024.

Shaw, D., Leon, C., Koley, S., & Murray, V. (1997). Traditional remedies and food supplements: A 5-year toxicology study (1991-1995). *Drug Safety, 17*(5), 342–356. doi:10.2165/00002018-199717050-00006 PMID:9391777

Shehata, M. S. M., & Soltan, S. S. A. (2013). Effects of bioactive component of kiwi fruit and avocado (fruit and seed) on hypercholesterolemic rats. *World Journal of Dairy & Food Sciences, 8*(1), 82–93.

Shei, L. C. (2008). *An Evaluation of Native West African Vegetables.* Paper presented at Conference on International Research on Food Security, Natural Resource Management and Rural Development, Tropentag, Germany.

Shema-Didi, L., Kristal, B., Sela, S., Geron, R., & Ore, L. (2014). Does pomegranate intake attenuate cardiovascular risk factors in hemodialysis patients. *The Journal of Nutrition, 13*(1), 18. doi:10.1186/1475-2891-13-18 PMID:24593225

Sheng, R., Gu, Z. L., Xie, M. L., Zhou, W. X., & Guo, C. Y. (2007). EGCG inhibits cardiomyocyte apoptosis in pressure overload-induced cardiac hypertrophy and protects cardiomyocytes from oxidative stress in rats. *Acta Pharmacologica Sinica, 28*(2), 191–201. doi:10.1111/j.1745-7254.2007.00495.x PMID:17241521

Shibuya, N. (1989). Comparative studies on the cell wall polymers obtained from different parts of rice grains. In N. G. Lewis & M. G. Paice (Eds.), *Plant cell wall polymers: biogenesis and biodegradation, Symp. No. 399* (pp. 333–344). Washington, DC: American Chemical Society. doi:10.1021/bk-1989-0399.ch024

Shimada, Y., Takahashi, M., Miyazawa, N., Abiru, Y., Uchiyama, S., & Hishigaki, H. (2012). Identification of a novel dihydrodaidzein racemase essential for biosynthesis of equol from daidzein in *Lactococcus* sp. strain 20-92. *Applied and Environmental Microbiology, 78*(14), 4902–4907. doi:10.1128/AEM.00410-12 PMID:22582059

Shimada, Y., Takahashi, M., Miyazawa, N., Ohtani, T., Abiru, Y., Uchiyama, S., & Hishigaki, H. (2011). Identification of two novel reductases involved in equol biosynthesis in *Lactococcus* strain 20-92. *Journal of Molecular Microbiology and Biotechnology, 2*(3-4), 160–172. doi:10.1159/000335049 PMID:22286043

Shimada, Y., Yasuda, S., Takahashi, M., Hayashi, T., Miyazawa, N., Sato, I., & Hishigaki, H. et al. (2010). Cloning and expression of a novel NADP(H)-dependent daidzein reductase, an enzyme involved in the metabolism of daidzein, from equol-producing *Lactococcus* strain 20-92. *Applied and Environmental Microbiology, 76*(17), 5892–5901. doi:10.1128/AEM.01101-10 PMID:20639368

Shim, Y. Y., Gui, B., Arnison, P. G., Wang, Y., & Reaney, M. J. T. (2015). Flaxseed (*Linum usitatissimum* L.) bioactive compounds and peptide nomenclature: A review. *Trends in Food Science & Technology, 38*(1), 5–20. doi:10.1016/j.tifs.2014.03.011

Shim, Y. Y., Gui, B., Wang, Y., & Reaney, M. J. T. (2015). Flaxseed (*Linum usitatissimum* L.) oil processing and selected products. *Trends in Food Science & Technology, 43*(2), 162–177. doi:10.1016/j.tifs.2015.03.001

Shin, J. S., Kim, M. A., & Lee, S. H. (2013). Comparison of physiological changes in broiler chicken fed with dietary processed sulfur. *Korean Journal of Food Preservation., 20*(2), 278–283. doi:10.11002/kjfp.2013.20.2.278

Shin, K. S., Chae, O. W., Park, I. C., Hong, S. K., & Choe, T. B. (1998). Antitumor effects of mice fed with cell lysate of *Lactobacillus plantarum* isolated from kimchi. *Korean J. Biotechnol. Bioeng., 13*, 357–363.

Shirai, K. (2004). Obesity as the core of the metabolic syndrome and the management of coronary heart disease. *Current Medical Research and Opinion, 20*(3), 295–304. doi:10.1185/030079903125003008 PMID:15025838

Shi, Y., Tian, F., Ru, Z., & Guo, L. (2011). Antioxidant activity of different fractions of wheat grains. *Advances in Biomedical Engineering*, *1-2*, 107–109.

Shohag, M. J. I., Wei, Y., & Yang, X. (2012). Changes of folate and other potential health- promoting phytochemicals in legume seeds as affected by germination. *Journal of Agricultural and Food Chemistry*, *60*(36), 9137–9143. doi:10.1021/jf302403t PMID:22906127

Shojaii, A., & Fard, M. A. (2012). Review of pharmacological properties and chemical constituents of *Pimpinella anisum*. *International Scholarly Research Network*, *2012*, 1–8. PMID:22848853

Shomaf, M., Takruri, H., & Faris, M. A. I. E. (2011). Lentils (Lens culinaris, L.) Attenuate Colonic Lesions and Neoplasms in Fischer 344 Rats. *Jordan Medical Journal*, *45*, 231–239.

Shori, A. B. (2013). Antioxidant activity and viability of lactic acid bacteria in soybean-yogurt made from cow and camel milk. *Journal of Taibahuniversity for Science*, *7*, 202-208.

Shrivastava, A. K., Singh, H. V., Raizada, A., & Singh, S. K. (2015). C-reactive protein, inflammation and coronary heart disease. *The Egyptian Heart Journal*, *67*(2), 89–97. doi:10.1016/j.ehj.2014.11.005

Shukla, M., Gupta, K., Rasheed, Z., Khan, K. A., & Haqqi, T. M. (2008). Consumption of hydrolyzable tannins-rich pomegranate extract suppresses inflammation & joint damage in rheumatoid arthritis. *The Journal of Nutrition*, *24*(7), 733–743. doi:10.1016/j.nut.2008.03.013 PMID:18490140

Shulman, G. I. (2004). Unraveling the cellular mechanisms of insulin resistance in humans: New insights from magnetic resonance spectroscopy. *Physiology (Bethesda, MD)*, *19*(4), 183–190. doi:10.1152/physiol.00007.2004 PMID:15304632

Siddhuraju, P., & Becker, K. (2007). The antioxidant and free radical scavenging activities of processed cowpea (*Vigna unguiculata* (L.) Walp.) seed extracts. *Food Chemistry*, *101*(1), 10–19. doi:10.1016/j.foodchem.2006.01.004

Siddiqui, N. S., & Patil, M. B. (2015). Assessment of antioxidant and cytotoxic activities of extracts of some *Zizyphus* species with identification of bioactive components. *European Journal of Medicinal Plants*, *8*(4), 202–213. doi:10.9734/EJMP/2015/17351

Sidhu, J. S. (2004). *Use of wheat bran and psyllium in breads and buns*. Final report, Project no. FB023C. Kuwait Institute for Scientific Research.

Sidhu, J. S. (1995). Wheat Usage in the Indian Subcontinent. In H. Faridi & J. M. Faubion (Eds.), *Wheat End Uses Around the World* (pp. 191–213). St. Paul, MN: American Association of Cereal Chemists.

Sidhu, J. S., Al-Hooti, S. N., & Al-Saqer, J. M. (1999). Effect of adding wheat bran and germ fractions on the chemical composition of high-fiber toast bread. *Food Chemistry*, *67*(4), 365–371. doi:10.1016/S0308-8146(99)00123-5

Sidhu, J. S., Al-Hooti, S. N., Al-Saqer, J. M., & Al-Othman, A. (2001). Studies on the development of pan bread using raw wheat germ. *Journal of Food Quality*, *24*(3), 235–247. doi:10.1111/j.1745-4557.2001.tb00605.x

Sidhu, J. S., Kabir, Y., & Huffman, F. G. (2007). Functional foods from cereal grains. *International Journal of Food Properties*, *10*(2), 201–230. doi:10.1080/10942910601045289

Sidhu, J. S., Seibel, W., Bruemmer, J. M., & Zwingelberg, H. (1989). Effect of whole wheat flour milling procedure and bran addition on bread quality. Getreide Mehl u. *Brot.*, *43*(12), 363–365.

Sidhu, J. S., & Zafar, T. A. (2012). Super fruits: Pomegranate, Wolfberry, Aronia, Acai, Noni and Amla. In N. K. Sinha, J. S. Sidhu, J. Barta, J. S. B. Wu, & M. P. Cano (Eds.), *Handbook of Fruits and Fruit Processing* (2nd ed.; pp. 653–679). New York: John Wiley & Sons Ltd., Publishers. doi:10.1002/9781118352533.ch35

Sierra, S., Lara-Villoslada, F., Olivares, M., Jiménez, J., Boza, J., & Xaus, J. (2005). Increased immune response in mice consuming rice bran oil. *European Journal of Nutrition*, *44*(8), 509–516. doi:10.1007/s00394-005-0554-y PMID:15719157

Sies, H. (1997). Oxidative stress: Oxidants and antioxidants. *Experimental Physiology*, *82*(2), 291–295. doi:10.1113/expphysiol.1997.sp004024 PMID:9129943

Sies, H., Stahl, W., & Sundquist, A. R. (1992). Antioxidant functions of vitamins. Vitamins E and C, beta-carotene, and other carotenoids. *Annals of the New York Academy of Sciences*, *669*(1), 7–20. doi:10.1111/j.1749-6632.1992.tb17085.x PMID:1444060

Silva, F. O., & Perrone, D. (2015). Characterization and stability of bioactive compounds from soybean meal. LWT-. *Food Science and Technology (Campinas.)*, *63*, 992–1000.

Silvia, A., Valencia-Chamorro, L., Palou, L., Miguel, A., Del R'Io, L., & Mari, A B. (2011). Antimicrobial Edible Films & Coatings for Fresh and Minimally Processed Fruits And Vegetables: A Review. *Critical Reviews in Food Science & Nutrition*, *51*, 872–900.

Simic, A., Manojlovic, D., Segan, D., & Todorovic, M. (2007). Electrochemical behavior and antioxidant and prooxidant activity of natural phenolics. *Molecules (Basel, Switzerland)*, *12*(10), 2327–2340. doi:10.3390/12102327 PMID:17978760

Simons, A. L., Renouf, M., Hendrich, S., & Murphy, P. A. (2005). Metabolism of glycitein (7;4'-dihydroxy-6-methoxy-isoflavone) by human gut microflora. *Journal of Agricultural and Food Chemistry*, *53*(22), 8519–8525. doi:10.1021/jf051546d PMID:16248547

Singh, M., Suman, S., & Shukla, Y. (2014). *New enlightenment of skin cancer chemoprevention through phytochemicals: in vitro & in vivo studies & the underlying mechanisms.* BioMed Research International.

Singh, A., & Quraishi, M. A. (2015). The extract of *Jamun* (*Syzygium cumini*) seed as green corrosion inhibitor for acid media. *Res. Chem. Intermed.*, *41*(5), 2901–2914. doi:10.1007/s11164-013-1398-3

Singh, B., Bajaj, M., Kaur, A., Sharma, S., & Sidhu, J. S. (1993). Studies on the development of high protein biscuits from composite flours. *Plant Foods for Human Nutrition (Dordrecht, Netherlands)*, *43*(2), 181–189. doi:10.1007/BF01087922 PMID:8475004

Singh, J., Upadhyay, A. K., Bahadur, A., Singh, B., Singh, K. P., & Rai, M. (2006). Antioxidant phytochemicals in cabbage (*Brassica oleracea* L. var. capitata). *Scientia Horticulturae*, *108*(3), 233–237. doi:10.1016/j.scienta.2006.01.017

Singh, M. B., Fotedar, R., & Lakshminarayana, J. (2008). Camel milk consumption pattern and its association with diabetes among Raika community of Jodhpur district of Rajasthan. *Ethno-Med*, *2*, 104–105.

Singh, R., De, S., & Belkheir, A. (2013). *Avena sativa* (Oat), a potential neutraceutical and therapeutic agent: An overview. *Critical Reviews in Food Science and Nutrition*, *53*(2), 126–244. doi:10.1080/10408398.2010.526725 PMID:23072529

Singh, S., & Immanuel, G. (2014). Extraction of antioxidants from fruit peels & its utilization in paneer. *Journal of Food Processing Technology*, *5*, 1–5.

Singletary, K. (2010). Ginger: An overview of health benefits. *Nutrition Today*, *45*(4), 171–183. doi:10.1097/NT.0b013e3181ed3543

Singletary, K. (2010). Turmeric: An overview of potential health benefits. *Nutrition Today*, *45*(5), 216–225. doi:10.1097/NT.0b013e3181f1d72c

Sinija, V. R., & Mishra, H. N. (2008). Green tea: Health benefit. *Journal of Nutritional & Environmental Medicine*, *17*(4), 232–242. doi:10.1080/13590840802518785

Sirtori, C. R., Galli, C., Anderson, J. W., Sirtori, E., & Arnoldi, A. (2009). Functional foods for dyslipidaemia and cardiovascular risk prevention. *Nutrition Research Reviews*, *22*(02), 244–261. doi:10.1017/S0954422409990187 PMID:20003590

Sirtori, C. R., & Lovati, M. R. (2001). Soy proteins and cardiovascular disease. *Current Atherosclerosis Reports*, *3*(1), 47–53. doi:10.1007/s11883-001-0010-2 PMID:11123848

Siruguri, V., & Bhat, R. V. (2015). Assessing intake of spices by pattern of spice use, frequency of consumption and portion size of spices consumed from routinely prepared dishes in southern India. *Nutrition Journal*, *14*(1), 7–15. doi:10.1186/1475-2891-14-7 PMID:25577292

Skeggs, L. T., Kahn, J. E., & Shumway, N. P. (1956). The preparation and function of the angiotensin-converting enzyme. *The Journal of Experimental Medicine*, *103*(3), 295–299. doi:10.1084/jem.103.3.295 PMID:13295487

Slavin, J. (2003). Why whole grains are protective: Biological mechanisms. *The Proceedings of the Nutrition Society*, *62*(1), 129–134. doi:10.1079/PNS2002221 PMID:12740067

Slavin, J. (2004). Whole grains and human health. *Nutrition Research Reviews*, *17*(01), 99–110. doi:10.1079/NRR200374 PMID:19079919

Sloan, F. A., & Gelband, H. (2007). *Cancer control opportunities in low-and middle-income countries*. National Academies Press.

Smith, F. I., & Eyzaguirre, P. (2007). African leafy vegetables: Their role in the World Health Organisation's global fruit and vegetable initiative. *African Journal of Food Agriculture Nutrition and Development*, *7*(3), 1–17.

Smith, S., Geeson, J., & Stow, J. (1987). Production of modified atmospheres in deciduous fruits by the use of films and coatings. *Horticulture Science*, *22*, 772–776.

Sofi, F., Cesari, F., Abbate, R., Gensini, G. F., & Casini, A. (2008). Adherence to Mediterranean diet and health status: Meta-analysis. *BMJ (Clinical Research Ed.)*, *337*(sep11 2), a1344. doi:10.1136/bmj.a1344 PMID:18786971

Sofi, F., Conti, A. A., Gori, A. M., Luisi, M. L. E., Casini, A., Abbate, R., & Gensini, G. F. (2007). Coffee consumption and risk of coronary heart disease: A meta-analysis. *Nutrition, Metabolism, and Cardiovascular Diseases*, *17*(3), 209–223. doi:10.1016/j.numecd.2006.07.013 PMID:17156982

Soneja, A., Drews, M., & Malinski, T. (2005). Role of nitric oxide, nitroxidative and oxidative stress in wound healing. *Pharmacological Reports*, *57*(Suppl), 108–119. PMID:16415491

Sones, K., Heaney, R. K., & Fenwick, G. R. (1984a). An estimate of the mean daily intake of glucosinolates from cruciferous vegetables in the UK. *Journal of the Science of Food and Agriculture*, *35*(6), 712–719. doi:10.1002/jsfa.2740350619

Song, Y. R. (2010). *Study on exopolysaccharides with antioxidant and antiaging activity produced by Bacillus sp. Strains isolated from Korea fermented food, Kimchi*. (M.S. Thesis). Chunbuk National University, Jeonju, Korea.

Song, R., Chen, C., Wang, L., Johnston, J., Kerr, B. J., Weber, T. E., & Shurson, G. C. (2013). High sulfur content in corn dried distillers grains with soluble protects against oxidized lipids by increasing sulfur-containing antioxidants in nursery pigs. *Journal of Animal Science*, *91*(6), 2715–2728. doi:10.2527/jas.2012-5350 PMID:23482577

Song, Y., He, K., Levitan, E. B., Manson, J. E., & Liu, S. (2006). Effects of oral magnesium supplementation on glycaemic control in Type 2 diabetes: Ameta-analysis of randomized double-blind controlled trials. *Diabetic Medicine*, *23*(10), 1050–1056. doi:10.1111/j.1464-5491.2006.01852.x PMID:16978367

Soris, T. P., Kala, K. B., Mohan, V. R., & Vadivel, V. (2010). The biochemical composition and nutritional potential of three varieties of *Vigna mungo* (L.) Hepper. *Advances in Bioresearch*, *1*, 6–16.

Sothornvit, R., & Krochta, J. M. (2000). Oxygen permeability and mechanical properties of films from hydrolyzed whey protein. *Journal of Agricultural and Food Chemistry*, *48*(9), 3913–3916. doi:10.1021/jf000161m PMID:10995290

Souli, A., Sebai, H., Rtibi, K., Chehimi, L., Sakly, M., Amri, M., & Marzouki, L. et al. (2015). Inhibitory effects of two varieties of tunisian pomegranate (*Punica granatum* L.) extracts on gastrointestinal transit in rat. *Journal of Medicinal Food*, *18*(9), 1007–1012. doi:10.1089/jmf.2014.0110 PMID:25775227

Sprent, J. I., Odee, D. W., & Dakora, F. D. (2009). Chemical composition of Marama bean (*Tylosema esculentum*) – A wild African bean with unexploited potential. *Journal of Experimental Botany*. doi:10.1093/jxb/erp342

Srinivasa Rao, K., Anand, S., & Venkateswarlu, P. (2010). Cadmium removal from aqueous solution using biosorbant *Syzygium cumini* leaf powder: Kinetic and equilibrium studies. *Korean Journal of Chemical Engineering*, *27*(5), 1547–1554. doi:10.1007/s11814-010-0243-2

Srinivasan, K. (2011). Traditional Indian Functional Foods. In J. Shi, C.-T. Ho, & F. Shahidi (Eds.), *Functional foods of the East* (pp. 51–84). Boca Raton, FL: CRC Press.

Srivastava, G., & Mehta, J. L. (2009). Currying the heart: Curcumin and cardioprotection. *Journal of Cardiovascular Pharmacology and Therapeutics*, *14*(1), 22–27. doi:10.1177/1074248408329608 PMID:19153099

Srivastava, R., Ahmed, H., Dixit, R. K., Dharamveer, , & Saraf, S. A. (2010). *Crocus sativus* L.: A comprehensive review. *Pharmacognosy Review*, *4*(8), 200–208. doi:10.4103/0973-7847.70919 PMID:22228962

Srivastava, S., & Chandra, D. (2013). Pharmacological potentials of *Syzygium cumini*: A review. *Journal of the Science of Food and Agriculture*, *93*(9), 2084–2093. doi:10.1002/jsfa.6111 PMID:23460190

Stadnik, J., & Keska, P. (2015). Meat and fermented meat products as a source of bioactive peptides. *Acta Sci. Pol. Technol. Aliment.*, *14*(3), 181–190. doi:10.17306/J.AFS.2015.3.19

Stahl, W., & Sies, H. (2003). Antioxidant activity of carotenoids. *Molecular Aspects of Medicine*, *24*(6), 345–351. doi:10.1016/S0098-2997(03)00030-X PMID:14585305

Stamoulis, K.G., Pingali, P., & Shetty, P. (2004). Emerging challenges for food and nutrition policy in developing countries. *e-Journal of Agricultural and Development Economics*, *1*(2), 154–167.

Stangeland, T., Remberg, S. F., & Lye, K. A. (2009). Total antioxidant activity in 35 Ugandan fruits and vegetables. *Food Chemistry*, *113*(1), 85–91. doi:10.1016/j.foodchem.2008.07.026

Stanley W., Jacob, M. D., Ronald M., Lawrence, M.D. & Zucker, M. (1998). *The Miracle of MSM*. The Berkley Publishing Group.

Stark, A. H., & Madar, Z. (2002). Olive oil as a functional food: Epidemiology and nutritional approaches. *Nutrition Reviews*, *60*(6), 170–176. doi:10.1301/002966402320243250 PMID:12078915

Steensma, A., Noteborn, H. P., & Kuiper, H. A. (2004). Comparison of Caco-2, IEC-18 and HCEC cell lines as a model for intestinal absorption of genistein, daidzein and their glycosides. *Environmental Toxicology and Pharmacology*, *16*(3), 131–139. doi:10.1016/j.etap.2003.11.008 PMID:21782699

Steer, T., Johnson, I. T., Gee, J. M., & Gibson, G. R. (2003). Metabolism of the soyabean isoflavone glycoside genistin in vitro by the human gut bacteria and the effect of prebiotics. *The British Journal of Nutrition*, *90*(03), 635–642. doi:10.1079/BJN2003949 PMID:13129470

Stein, F. L. P., Schimidt, B., & Furlong, E. B. (2005). Vascular Responses to Extractable Fractions of *Ilex paraguariensis* in Rats Fed Standard and High Cholesterol Diets. *Biological Research for Nursing*, *7*(2), 146–156. doi:10.1177/1099800405280521 PMID:16267376

Steinmetz, K. A., & Potter, J. D. (1991). Vegetables, fruit, and cancer. I. Epidemiology. *Cancer Causes & Control*, *2*(5), 325–357. doi:10.1007/BF00051672 PMID:1834240

Steinmetz, K. A., & Potter, J. D. (1991). Vegetables, fruit, and cancer. II. Mechanisms. *Cancer Causes & Control*, *2*(6), 427–442. doi:10.1007/BF00054304 PMID:1764568

Stenberg, M., Marko-Varga, G., & Oste, R. (2002). Enantio separation of D- and L-amino acids by a coupled system consisting of an ion-exchange column and a chiral column and determination of D-aspartic acid and d-glutamic acid in soy products. *Food Chemistry*, *79*(4), 507–512. doi:10.1016/S0308-8146(02)00215-7

Stephen, A. M., Dahl, W. J., Sieber, G. M., van Blaricom, J. A., & Morgan, D. R. (1995). Effect of green lentils on colonic function, nitrogen balance, and serum lipids in healthy human subjects. *The American Journal of Clinical Nutrition*, *62*(6), 1261–1267. PMID:7491890

Stephens, N. G., Parsons, A., Schofield, P. M., Kelly, F., Cheeseman, K., & Mitchinson, M. J. (1996). Randomised controlled trial of Vitamin E in patients with coronary disease: Cambridge Heart Antioxidant Study (CHAOS). *Lancet*, *347*(9004), 781–786. doi:10.1016/S0140-6736(96)90866-1 PMID:8622332

Stevenson, D. E., & Hurst, R. D. (2007). Polyphenolic phytochemicals – just antioxidants or much more? *Cellular and Molecular Life Sciences*, *64*(22), 2900–2916. doi:10.1007/s00018-007-7237-1 PMID:17726576

Steyn, N. P., Mann, J., Bennett, P. H., Temple, N., Zimmet, P., Tuomilehto, J., & Louheranta, A. et al. (2004). Diet, nutrition and the prevention of type 2 diabetes. *Public Health Nutrition*, *7*(1a), 147–165. doi:10.1079/PHN2003586 PMID:14972058

Steyn, N. P., Olivier, J., Wirter, P., Burger, S., & Nesamvuni, C. (2001). A survey of wild, green, leafy vegetables and their potential in combating micronutrient deficiencies in rural populations. *South African Journal of Science*, *97*, 276–278.

Stoltzfus, R., Mullany, L., & Black, R. E. (2004). Iron deficiency Anaemia. In Comparative quantification of health risks: Global and regional burden of disease attributable to selected major risk factors (vol. 1, pp. 163-209). World Health Organisation.

Stone, A., Massey, A., Theobald, M., Styslinger, M., Kane, D., Kandy, D., . . . Davert, E. (2011). *Africa's indigenous crops.* Retrieved April 20, 2015 from http://www.worldwatch.org/system/files/NtP-Africa%27s-Indigenous-Crops.pdf

Stopforth, J. D., Skandamis, P. N., Davidson, P. M., & Sofos, J. N. (2005a). Naturally ocurring compounds: Animal sources. In Antimicrobials in Food (pp. 453–505). Boca Raton, FL: CRC Press.

Stopforth, J. D., Sofos, J. N., & Busta, F. F. (2005b). Sorbic acid and sorbates. In Antimicrobials in Food (pp. 49–90). Boca Raton, FL: CRC Press.

Stowe, C. B. (2011). The effects of pomegranate juice consumption on blood pressure & cardiovascular health. *Complementary Therapies in Clinical Practice*, *17*(2), 113–115. doi:10.1016/j.ctcp.2010.09.004 PMID:21457902

Street, D. A., Comstock, G. W., Salkeld, R. M., Schuep, W., & Klag, M. J. (1994). Serum antioxidants and myocar-dial infarction. Are low levels of carotenoids and α-tocopherol risk factors for myocardial infarction? *Circulation*, *90*(3), 1154–1161. doi:10.1161/01.CIR.90.3.1154 PMID:8087925

Subash, S., Braidy, N., Essa, M. M., Zayana, A. B., Ragini, V., Al-Adawi, S., & Guillemin, G. J. et al. (2015). Long-term (15 mo) dietary supplementation with pomegranates from Oman attenuates cognitive & behavioral deficits in a transgenic mice model of Alzheimer's disease. *The Journal of Nutrition*, *31*(1), 223–229. doi:10.1016/j.nut.2014.06.004 PMID:25441596

Subash, S., Essa, M. M., Al-Asmi, A., Al-Adawi, S., Vaishnav, R., Braidy, N., & Guillemin, G. J. (2014). Pomegranate from Oman alleviates the brain oxidative damage in transgenic mouse model of Alzheimer's disease. *Journal of Traditional & Complementary Medicine*, *4*(4), 232. doi:10.4103/2225-4110.139107 PMID:25379464

Subhash, G. P., Virbhadrappa, S. R., & Vasanth, O. K. (2010). *Spinacia oleracea* Linn: A pharmacognostic and pharmacological overview. *International Journal of Research in Ayurveda & Pharmacy*, *1*, 78–84.

Su, D., Zhang, R., Hou, F., Zhang, M., Guo, J., Huang, F., & Wei, Z. et al. (2014). Comparison of the free and bound phenolic profiles and cellular antioxidant activities of litchi pulp extracts from different solvents. *BMC Complementary and Alternative Medicine*, *14*(1), 9. doi:10.1186/1472-6882-14-9 PMID:24405977

Sugimoto, T., Tanaka, K., & Kasai, Z. (1986). Molecular species in the protein body II (PB-II) of developing rice endosperm. *Agricultural and Biological Chemistry*, *50*, 3031–3035.

Sugiyama, Y., Masumori, N., Fukuta, F., Yoneta, A., Hida, T., Yamashita, T., & Tsukamoto, T. et al. (2013). Influence of isoflavone intake and equol-producing intestinal flora on prostate cancer risk. *Asian Pacific Journal of Cancer Prevention*, *14*(1), 1–4. doi:10.7314/APJCP.2013.14.1.1 PMID:23534704

Sugiyama, Y., Nagata, Y., Fukuta, F., Takayanagi, A., Masumori, N., Tsukamoto, T., & Mori, M. et al. (2014). Counts of *Slackia* sp. strain NATTS in intestinal flora are correlated to serum concentrations of equol both in prostate cancer cases and controls in Japanese men. *Asian Pacific Journal of Cancer Prevention*, *15*(6), 2693–2697. doi:10.7314/APJCP.2014.15.6.2693 PMID:24761887

Suleria, H. A. R., Butt, M. S., Anjum, F. M., Saeed, F., & Khalid, N. (2015). Onion: Nature protection against physiological threats. *Critical Reviews in Food Science and Nutrition*, *55*(1), 50–66. doi:10.1080/10408398.2011.646364 PMID:24915405

Sumner, M. D., Elliott-Eller, M., Weidner, G., Daubenmier, J. J., Chew, M. H., Marlin, R., & Ornish, D. et al. (2005). Effects of pomegranate juice consumption on myocardial perfusion in patients with coronary heart disease. *The American Journal of Cardiology*, *96*(6), 810–814. doi:10.1016/j.amjcard.2005.05.026 PMID:16169367

Sumpio, B. E., Cordova, A. C., Berke-Schlessel, D. W., Qin, F., & Chen, Q. H. (2006). Green tea, the 'Asian paradox,' and cardiovascular disease. *Journal of the American College of Surgeons*, *202*(5), 813–825. doi:10.1016/j.jamcollsurg.2006.01.018 PMID:16648021

Sundram, K. (2015). *Palm oil: Chemistry and nutrition updates*. Retreated from: www.americanpalmoil.com/pdf/DR%20 Sundram.pdf

Suru, S. M., & Ugwu, C. E. (2015). Comparative assessment of onion and garlic extracts on endogenous hepatic and renal antioxidant status in rat. *Journal of Basic and Clinical Physiology and Pharmacology*, *26*(4), 347–354. doi:10.1515/jbcpp-2014-0088 PMID:25536663

Swami, S. B., Thakor, N. S. J., Patil, M. M., & Haldankar, P. M. (2012). Jamun (*Syzygium cumini* L.): A review of its food and medicinal uses. *Food and Nutrition Sciences*, *3*(08), 1100–1117. doi:10.4236/fns.2012.38146

Swayne, D. E., & Suarez, D. L. (2000). Highly pathogenic avian influenza. *Rev Sci Tech Off Inter Epiz*, *19*(2), 463–482. doi:10.20506/rst.19.2.1230 PMID:10935274

Taddei, S., Ghiadoni, L., Virdis, A., Versari, D., & Salvetti, A. (2003). Mechanisms of endothelial dysfunction: Clinical significance and preventive non-pharmacological therapeutic strategies. *Current Pharmaceutical Design*, *9*(29), 2385–2402. doi:10.2174/1381612033453866 PMID:14529554

Taira, H., Nakagahra, M., & Nagamine, T. (1988). Fatty acid composition of indica, sinica, japonica, and japonica groups of nonglutinous brown rice. *Journal of Agricultural and Food Chemistry*, *36*(1), 45–47. doi:10.1021/jf00079a011

Taira, H., Taira, H., & Fujii, K. (1979). Influence of cropping season on lipid content and fatty acid composition of lowland nonglutinous brown rice. *Nihon Sakumotsu Gakkai Kiji*, *48*(3), 371–377. doi:10.1626/jcs.48.371

Tai, T. Y., Tsai, K. S., Tu, S. T., Wu, J. S., Chang, C. I., Chen, C. L., & Wu, C. H. et al. (2012). The effect of soy isoflavone on bone mineral density in postmenopausal Taiwanese women with bone loss: A 2-year randomized double-blind placebo-controlled study. *Osteoporosis International*, *23*(5), 1571–1580. doi:10.1007/s00198-011-1750-7 PMID:21901480

Takeda, A. T. (2004). Triterpenes and Triperpenoidal Glycosides from the Fruits of *Ilex Paraguariensis* (Mate). *Journal of the Brazilian Chemical Society*, *15*(2), 205–211. doi:10.1590/S0103-50532004000200008

Takeda, Y., Hizukuri, S., & Juliano, B. O. (1987). Structures of rice amylopectin with low and high affinities for iodine. *Carbohydrate Research*, *168*(1), 79–88. doi:10.1016/0008-6215(87)80008-3

Taku, K., Melby, M. K., Kurzer, M. S., Mizuno, S., Watanabe, S., & Ishimi, Y. (2010). Effects of soy isoflavone supplements on bone turnover markers in menopausal women: Systematic review and meta-analysis of randomized controlled trials. *Bone*, *47*(2), 413–423. doi:10.1016/j.bone.2010.05.001 PMID:20452475

Taku, K., Melby, M. K., Nishi, N., Omori, T., & Kurzer, M. S. (2011). Soy isoflavones for osteoporosis: An evidence-based approach. *Maturitas*, *70*(4), 333–338. doi:10.1016/j.maturitas.2011.09.001 PMID:21958941

Taku, K., Umegaki, K., Ishimi, Y., & Watanabe, S. (2008). Effects of extracted soy isoflavones alone on blood total and LDL cholesterol: Meta-analysis of randomized controlled trials. *Journal of Therapeutics and Clinical Risk Management*, *4*, 1097–1103. PMID:19209289

Talalay, P. (1989). Mechanisms of induction of enzymes that protect against chemical carcinogenesis. *Advances in Enzyme Regulation*, *28*, 237–250. doi:10.1016/0065-2571(89)90074-5 PMID:2696344

Talathoti, G. K., Satyanarayana, S. V., & King, P. (2014). Equilibrium and thermodynamic studies of methylene blue biosorption from aqueous solution using *Syzygium cumini* L. J. *Enviorn. Res. Develop.*, *8*(4), 964–973.

Tanaka, K., Ogawa, M., & Kasai, Z. (1977). The rice scutellum. II. A comparison of scutellar and aleurone electron-dense particles by transmission electron microscopy including energy-dispersive X-ray analysis. *Cereal Chemistry*, *54*, 684–689.

Tanaka, K., Sugimoto, T., Ogawa, M., & Kasai, Z. (1980). Isolation and characterization of two types of protein bodies in the rice endosperm. *Agricultural and Biological Chemistry*, *44*, 1633–1639.

Tanaka, K., Yoshida, T., Asada, K., & Kasai, Z. (1973). Subcellular particles isolated from aleurone layer of rice seeds. *Archives of Biochemistry and Biophysics*, *155*(1), 136–143. doi:10.1016/S0003-9861(73)80016-5 PMID:4712443

Tanaka, T., Kohno, H., Murakami, M., Shimada, R., Kagami, S., Sumida, T., & Ogawa, H. et al. (2000). Suppres.sion of azoxymethane-induced colon carcinogenesis in male F344 rats by mandarin juices rich in β-cryptoxanthin and hesperidin Interna.tional. *Journal of Cancer*, *88*(1), 146–150.

Tanaka, T., Kohno, H., Shimada, R., Kagami, S., Yamaguchi, F., Kataoka, S., & Ohigashi, H. et al. (2000). Prevention of colonic aberrant crypt foci by dietary feeding of garcinol in male F344 rats. *Carcinogenesis*, *21*(6), 1183–1189. doi:10.1093/carcin/21.6.1183 PMID:10837008

Tanaka, Y., Resurrecci6n, A. P., Juliano, B. O., & Bechtel, D. B. (1978). Properties of whole and undigested fraction of protein bodies of milled rice. *Agricultural and Biological Chemistry*, *42*, 2015–2023.

Tandaon, V. R., Verma, S., Singh, J. B., & Mahajan, A. (2005). Antioxidants and cardiovascular health. *Drug Review*, *7*(2), 61–64.

Tang, N., Wu, Y., Zhou, B., Wang, B., & Yu, R. (2009). Green tea, black tea consumption and risk of lung cancer: A meta-analysis. *Lung Cancer (Amsterdam, Netherlands)*, *65*(3), 274–283. doi:10.1016/j.lungcan.2008.12.002 PMID:19128856

Taniya, A. J., Kabir, Y., & Hoque, M. M. (2015). *Occurrence of emerging food borne pathogens in common fast foods and inactivation of pathogens with essential oil.* (Unpublished M. Phil Dissertation). University of Dhaka, Bangladesh.

Tan, P. L., Peh, K. K., Gan, C. Y., & Liong, M. T. (2014). Bioactive dairy ingredients for food and non-food applications. *Acta Alimentaria*, *43*(1), 113–123. doi:10.1556/AAlim.43.2014.1.12

Tanveer, A., Farooq, U., Akram, K., Hayat, Z., Shafi, A., Nazar, H., & Ahmad, Z. (2015). Pomegranate extracts: A natural preventive measure against spoilage & pathogenic microorganisms. *Food Reviews International*, *31*(1), 29–51. doi:10.1080/87559129.2014.961074

Tapia, M., Rojas-Grau, M., Rodriguez, F., Ramirez, J., Carmona, A., & Martin-Belloso, O. (2007). Alginate- and gellan-based edible films for probiotic coatings on fresh-cut fruits. *Journal of Food Science*, *72*(4), 190–196. doi:10.1111/j.1750-3841.2007.00318.x PMID:17995771

Tapsell, L.C. (2006). Health benefits of herbs and spices: The past, the present, the future. *Medical Journal of Australia, 185*(4 suppl), S2-S4.

Tapsell, L. C., Hemphill, I., Cobiac, L., Patch, C. S., Sullivan, D. R., Fenech, M., & Inge, K. E. et al. (2006). Health benefits of herbs and spices: The past, the present, the future. *The Medical Journal of Australia*, *185*, 4–24. PMID:17022438

Taruvinga, A., & Nengovhela, R. (2015). *Consumer perceptions and consumption dynamics of African leafy vegetables(ALVs): Evidence from Feni communal area, Eastern Cape Province, South Africa.* Paper presented at the 5th International Conference on Biomedical Engineering and Technology, Seoul, Korea. Doi doi:10.773/IPCBEE.2015.V81.16

Taubert, D., Roesen, R., Lehmann, C., Jung, N., & Schoming, E. (2007). Effects of low habitual cocoa intake on blood pressure and bioactive nitric oxide: A randomized controlled trial. *JAMMA*, *298*(1), 49–60. doi:10.1001/jama.298.1.49 PMID:17609490

Taylor, B., Irving, H. M., Baliunas, D., Roerecke, M., Patra, J., Mohapatra, S., & Rehm, J. (2009). Alcohol and hypertension: Gender differences in dose-response relationships determined through systematic review and meta-analysis. *Addiction (Abingdon, England)*, *104*(12), 1981–1990. doi:10.1111/j.1360-0443.2009.02694.x PMID:19804464

Taylor, J. R. N., Belton, P. S., Beta, T., & Duodu, C. K. (2014). Increasing the utilization of sorghum, millets and pseudocereals: Developments in science of their phenolic phytochemicals, biofortification and protein functionality. *Cereal Science*, *59*(3), 257–275. doi:10.1016/j.jcs.2013.10.009

Taylor, S. L. (1986). Immunological and allergic properties of cows' milk proteins in humans. *Journal of Food Protection*, *49*, 239–250.

Teeguarden, R. (2007). *The pro-oxidant/antioxidant dance of life. dragon time — summer 2007.* Retrieved from http://www.bluetoad.com/article/The+Pro-OxidantAntioxidant+Dance+of+Life/10364/0/article.html

Teklehaymanot, T., Giday, M., Medhin, G., & Mekonnen, Y. (2007). Knowledge and use of medicinal plants by people around DebreLibanos monastery in Ethiopia. *Journal of Ethnopharmacology*, *111*(2), 271–283. doi:10.1016/j.jep.2006.11.019 PMID:17187950

Teng, P. S., Kropff, M. J., Ten Berge, H. F. M., Dent, J. B., Lansigan, F. P., & Van Laar, H. H. (1997). Approaches at the Farm and Regional Levels. Los Ba˜nos: International Rice Research Institute.

Terra, X., Montagut, G., Bustos, M., Llopiz, N., Ardevol, A., Blade, C., & Blay, M. et al. (2009). Grape-seed procyanidins prevent low-grade inflammation by modulating cytokine expression in rats fed a high-fat diet. *The Journal of Nutritional Biochemistry*, *20*(3), 210–218. doi:10.1016/j.jnutbio.2008.02.005 PMID:18602813

Tharanathan, R., & Mahadevamma, S. (2003). Grain legumes—a boon to human nutrition. *Trends in Food Science & Technology*, *14*(12), 507–518. doi:10.1016/j.tifs.2003.07.002

Thavarajah, D., Ruszkowski, J., & Vandenberg, A. (2008). High potential for selenium biofortification of lentils (*Lens culinaris* L.). *Journal of Agricultural and Food Chemistry*, *56*(22), 10747–10753. doi:10.1021/jf802307h PMID:18954072

Thavarajah, P., Sarker, A., Materne, M., Vandemark, G., Shrestha, R., Idrissi, O., & Vandenburg, A. et al. (2011). A globa.l survey of effects of genotype and environment on selenium concentration in lentils (*Lens culinaris* L): Impli. cations for nutritional fortification strategies. *Food Chemistry*, *125*(1), 72–76. doi:10.1016/j.foodchem.2010.08.038

Tho, H., Oshima, K., Suzuki, T., Hattori, M., & Morita, H. (2013). Complete genome sequence of the equol-producing bacterium *Adlerkreutzia equolifaciens* DSM 19450. *Genome Announcements*, *1*, e00742. PMID:24051320

Thomas, L. V., & Delves-Broughton, J. (2005). Nisin. In P. M. Davidson, J. N. Sofos, & A. L. Branen (Eds.), *Antimicrobials in Food* (pp. 237–274). Boca Raton, FL: CRC Press.

Thompson, L. U. (1994). Antioxidants and hormone-mediated health benefits of whole grains. *Critical Reviews in Food Science and Nutrition*, *34*(5&6), 473–497. doi:10.1080/10408399409527676 PMID:7811379

Thompson, L. U., Boucher, B. A., Liu, Z., Cotterchio, M., & Kreiger, N. (2006). Phytoestrogen content of foods consumed in Canada, including isoflavones, lignans, and coumestan. *Nutrition and Cancer*, *54*(2), 184–201. doi:10.1207/s15327914nc5402_5 PMID:16898863

Tijerina-Saenz, A., Innis, S. M., & Kitts, D. D. (2009). Antioxidant capacity of human milk and its association with vitamins A and E and fatty acid composition. *Acta Paediatrica (Oslo, Norway)*, *98*(11), 1793–1798. doi:10.1111/j.1651-2227.2009.01437.x PMID:19807706

Tiwari, U., & Cummins, E. (2013). Fruits and vegetables. In B. K. Tiwari, N. P. Brunton, & C. S. Brennan (Eds.), *Handbook of plant food phytochemicals: Sources, stability and extraction* (pp. 107–137). Oxford, UK: John Wiley & Sons Ltd. doi:10.1002/9781118464717.ch5

Topo, E., Soricelli, A., D'Aniello, A., Ronsini, S., & D'Aniello, G. (2009). The role and molecular mechanism of D-aspartic acid in the release and synthesis of LH and testosterone in humans and rats. *Reproductive Biology and Endocrinology*, *7*(1), 120–131. doi:10.1186/1477-7827-7-120 PMID:19860889

Totelin, L. (2015). When foods become remedies in ancient Greece: The curious case of garlic and other substances. *Journal of Ethnopharmacology*, *167*, 30–37. doi:10.1016/j.jep.2014.08.018 PMID:25173971

Tousen, Y., Abe, F., Ishida, T., Uehara, M., & Ishimi, Y. (2011). Resistant starch promotes equol production and inhibits tibial bone loss in ovariectomized mice treated with daidzein. *Metabolism: Clinical and Experimental*, *60*(10), 1425–1432. doi:10.1016/j.metabol.2011.02.009 PMID:21550090

Trachootham, D., Lu, W., Ogasawara, M. A., Valle, N. R., & Huang, P. (2008). Redox regulation of cell survival. *Antioxidants & Redox Signalling*, *10*(8), 13430–1374. doi:10.1089/ars.2007.1957 PMID:18522489

Tresserra-Rimbau, A., Medina-Remon, A., Estruch, R., & Lamuela-Raventos, R. M. (2014). Coffee polyphenol and high cardiovascular risk parameters. In V. Preedy (Ed.), *Coffee in health and disease prevention* (p. 388). London: Academic Press.

Trio, P. Z., Sixiang, Y., He, X., He, J., Sakao, K., & Hou, D. X. (2014). Chemopreventive functions and molecular mechanisms of garlic organosulfur compounds. *Food Functions*, *5*(5), 833–844. doi:10.1039/c3fo60479a PMID:24664286

Trock, B., Lanza, E., & Greenwald, P. (1990). Dietary fiber, vegetables, and colon cancer: Critical review and meta-analyses of the epidemiologic evidence. *Journal of the National Cancer Institute*, *82*(8), 650–661. doi:10.1093/jnci/82.8.650 PMID:2157027

Troszyńska, A., Amarowicz, R., Lamparski, G., Wołejszo, A., & Baryłko-Pikielna, N. (2006). Investigation of astringency of extracts obtained from selected tannins-rich legume seeds. *Food Quality and Preference*, *17*(1), 31–35. doi:10.1016/j.foodqual.2005.04.006

Troszynska, A., & Ciska, E. (2002). Phenolic compounds of seed coats of white and coloured varieties of pea (*Pisum sativum* L.) and their total antioxidant activity. *Czech Journal Food Science*, *20*, 15–22.

Tsangalis, D., Ashton, J. F., McGill, A. E. J., & Shah, N. P. (2002). Enzymic transformation of isoflavone phytoestrogens in soy milk by β-glucosidase producing bifidobacteria. *Journal of Food Science*, *67*(8), 3104–3113. doi:10.1111/j.1365-2621.2002.tb08866.x

Tsao, A. S., Liu, D., Martin, J., Tang, X. M., Lee, J. J., El-Naggar, A. K., & Papadimitrakopoulou, V. et al. (2009). Phase II randomized, placebo-controlled trial of green tea extract in patients with high-risk oral premalignant lesions. *Cancer Prevention Research (Philadelphia, Pa.)*, *2*(11), 931–941. doi:10.1158/1940-6207.CAPR-09-0121 PMID:19892663

Tsao, R. (2010). Chemistry and biochemistry of dietary polyphenols. *Nutrients*, *2*(12), 1231–1246. doi:10.3390/nu2121231 PMID:22254006

Tsen, S. Y., Siew, J., Lau, E. K. L., Afiqah bte Roslee, F., Chan, H. M., & Loke, W. M. (2014). Cow's milk as a dietary source of equol and phenolic antioxidants: Differential distribution in the milk aqueous and lipid fractions. *Dairy Sci. Technol.*, *94*(6), 625–632. doi:10.1007/s13594-014-0183-4

Tsuji, H., Moriyama, K., Nomoto, K., & Akaza, H. (2012). Identification of an enzyme system for daidzein-to-equol conversion in *Slackia* sp. strain NATTS. *Applied and Environmental Microbiology*, *78*(4), 1228–1236. doi:10.1128/AEM.06779-11 PMID:22179235

Tsuji, H., Moriyama, K., Nomoto, K., Miyanaga, N., & Akaza, H. (2010). Isolation and characterization of the equol-producing bacterium *Slackia* sp. strain NATTS. *Archives of Microbiology*, *192*(4), 279–287. doi:10.1007/s00203-010-0546-z PMID:20237913

Tucker, K. L., Selhub, J., Wilson, P. W., & Rosenberg, I. H. (1996). Dietary intake pattern relates to plasma folate and homocysteine concentrations in the Framingham Heart Study. *The Journal of Nutrition*, *126*(12), 3025. PMID:9001370

Tucker, L. A., & Thomas, K. S. (2009). Increasing total dietary fiber intake reduces risk of weight and fat gain in women. *The Journal of Nutrition*, *139*(3), 576–581. doi:10.3945/jn.108.096685 PMID:19158230

Tumwet, T. N., Mwangi, A. M., Kogi-makau, W., & Kang, E. K. (2013). Effect of different cooking methods on the nutritional value of some African indigenous leafy vegetables in Kenya. In *Proceedings of African Crop Science Conference* (vol. 11, pp 441 - 443). Kampala, Uganda: ACSJ.

Tzulker, R., Glazer, I., Bar-Ilan, I., Holl, D., Aviram, M., & Amir, R. (2007). Antioxidant activity, polyphenol content & related compounds in different fruit juices & homogenates prepared from 29 different pomegranate accessions. *Journal of Agricultural and Food Chemistry*, *55*(23), 9559–9570. doi:10.1021/jf071413n PMID:17914875

Uchiyama, S., Ueno, T., & Suzuki, T. (2007). Identification of a newly isolated equol-producing lactic acid bacterium from the human feces. *Journal of Intestinal Microbiology*, *21*, 217–220. doi:10.11209/jim.21.217

Ueland, P. M., Refsum, H., Beresford, S. A., & Vollset, S. E. (2000). The controversy over homocysteine and cardiovascular risk. *The American Journal of Clinical Nutrition*, *72*(2), 324–332. PMID:10919921

Umeta, M., West, C. E., & Fufa, H. (2005). Content of zinc, iron, calcium and their absorption inhibitors in foods commonly consumed in Ethiopia. *Journal of Food Composition and Analysis*, *18*(8), 803–817. doi:10.1016/j.jfca.2004.09.008

United States Department of Agriculture (USDA). (2011). *National Nutrient Database for standard reference release 28*. Retrieved from http://ndb.nal.usda.gov/

Urashima, T., Kitaoka, M., Asakuma, S., & Messer, M. (2009). Milk oligosaccharides. In Advanced Dairy Chemistry. Lactose, Water, Salts and Minor Constituents (pp. 295-349). New York, NY: Springer Science Business Media.

Urashima, T., Murata, S., & Nakamura, T. (1997). Structural determination of monosialyltrisaccharides obtained from caprine colostrum. *Comparative Biochemistry and Physiology*, *116B*(4), 431–435. doi:10.1016/S0305-0491(96)00269-6 PMID:9149396

Urchin Tea. (2012, December 11). *The Oldest Tea Tree on the Earth*. Retrieved from http://teaurchin.blogspot.com/2012/12/the-worlds-oldest-tea-tree.html

Urgert, R., van Vliet, T., Zock, P. L., & Katan, M. B. (2000). Heavy coffee consumption and plasma homocysteine: A randomized controlled trial in healthy volunteers. *The American Journal of Clinical Nutrition*, *72*, 1107–1110. PMID:11063436

USDA. (2010). *USDA Database for the Oxygen Radical Absorbance Capacity (ORAC) of Selected Foods, Release2*. Retrieved from www.ars.usda.gov/SP2UserFiles/Place/12354500/Data/ORAC/ORAC_R2.pdf

USDA. (2010). *USDA National Nutrient Database for Standard Reference, Release 23*. Retrieved from http://www.ars.usda.gov/research/publications/publications.htm?seq_no_115=243584

Uusiku, N. P., Olefose, A., Duodu, K. G., Bester, M. J., & Faber, M. (2010). Nutritional value of leafy vegetables of sub-Saharan Africa and the potential contribution to human health: A review. *Journal of Food Composition and Analysis*, *23*(6), 499–509. doi:10.1016/j.jfca.2010.05.002

Uusitalo, U., Pietinen, P., & Puska, P. (2002). *Dietary transition in developing countries: Challenges for chronic disease prevention*. Retrieved April 20, 2015 from http://whqlibdoc.who.int/publications/9241590416.pdf

Valcic, S., Burr, J. A., Timmermann, B. N., & Liebler, D. C. (2000). Antioxidant chemistry of green tea catechins. New oxidation products of (-)-epigallocatechin gallate and (-)-epigallocatechin from their reactions with peroxyl radicals. *Chemical Research in Toxicology*, *13*(9), 801–810. doi:10.1021/tx000080k PMID:10995252

Valero, M., & Frances, E. (2006). Synergistic bactericidal effect of carvacrol, cinnamaldehyde or thymol and refrigeration to inhibit Bacillus cereus in carrot broth. *Food Microbiology*, *23*(1), 68–73. doi:10.1016/j.fm.2005.01.016 PMID:16942988

Vali, S. R., Ju, Y., Kaimal, T. N. B., & Chern, Y. (2005). A process for the preparation of food grade rice bran wax & determination of its composition. *Journal of the American Oil Chemists' Society*, *82*(1), 57–64. doi:10.1007/s11746-005-1043-z

Valko, M., Leibfritz, D., Moncol, J., Cronin, M. T. D., Mazur, M., & Telser, J. (2007). Free radicals and antioxidants in normal physiological functions and human disease. *The International Journal of Biochemistry & Cell Biology*, *39*(1), 44–84. doi:10.1016/j.biocel.2006.07.001 PMID:16978905

van Dam, R. M., Hu, F. B., Rosenberg, L., Krishnan, S., & Palmer, J. R. (2006). Dietary calcium and magnesium, major food sources, and risk of type 2 diabetes in U.S. black women. *Diabetes Care*, *29*(10), 2238–2243. doi:10.2337/dc06-1014 PMID:17003299

Van der Klaauw, A. A., & Farooqi, I. S. (2015). The hunger genes: Pathways to obesity. *Cell*, *161*(1), 119–132. doi:10.1016/j.cell.2015.03.008 PMID:25815990

van der Schouw, Y. T., de Kleijn, M. J., Peeters, P. H., & Grobbee, D. E. (2000). Phyto-oestro-gens and cardiovascular disease risk. *Nutrition, Metabolism, and Cardiovascular Diseases*, *10*, 154–167. PMID:11006924

van Huis, A. (2003). Insects as food in sub-Saharan Africa. *Insect Science and Its Application*, *23*, 163–185.

Van Weerdn, E. J., & Schutte, J. B. (1976). Relation between methionine and inorganic sulphate in broiler rations. *Poultry Science*, *55*(4), 1476–1748. doi:10.3382/ps.0551476 PMID:951375

VanEtten, C. H., Daxenbickler, M. E., Tookey, H. L., Kwolek, W. F., Williams, P. H., & Yoder, O. C. (1980). Glucosinolates: Potential toxicants in cabbage cultivars. *Journal of the American Society for Horticultural Science*, *105*, 710–714.

Vankar, P. S. (2008). Effectiveness of antioxidant properties of fresh and dry rhizomes of Curcuma longa (Long and Short varieties) with dry turmeric spice. *Int. J. Food Engg.*, *4*(8), 1–30.

Varraso, R., Kabrhel, C., Goldhaber, S. Z., Rimm, E. B., & Camargo, C. A. Jr. (2012). Prospective study of diet and venous thromboembolism in US women and men. *American Journal of Epidemiology*, *175*(2), 114–126. doi:10.1093/aje/kwr377 PMID:22180874

Vaspreet, J., Dornez, E., Ende, W. V., Delcour, J. A., & Courtin, C. M. (2015). Cereal grain fructans: Structure, variability and potential health effects. *Trends in Food Science & Technology*, *43*(1), 32–42. doi:10.1016/j.tifs.2015.01.006

Veer, P.V., Jansen, M.C.J.F., Klerk, M., & Kok, F.J. (1999). Fruits and vegetables in the prevention of cancer and cardiovascular disease. *Public Health Nutrition*, *3*(1), 103–107. PMID:10786730

Vehoeven, D. T., Goldbohn, R. A., van Poppel, G., Verhagen, H., & van den Brandt, P. A. (1996). Epidemiological studies on brassica vegetables and cancer risk. *Cancer Epidemiology, Biomarkers & Prevention*, *5*, 733–748. PMID:8877066

Veigas, J. M., Shrivasthava, R., & Neelwarne, B. (2008). Efficient amelioration of carbon tetrachloride induced toxicity in isolated rat hepatocytes by *Syzygium cumini* Skeels extract. *Toxicology In Vitro*, *22*(6), 1440–1446. doi:10.1016/j.tiv.2008.04.015 PMID:18538978

Velie, E. M., Schairer, C., Flood, A., He, J. P., Khattree, R., & Schatzkin, A. (2005). Empirically derived dietary patterns and risk of postmenopausal breast cancer in a large cohort study. *The American Journal of Clinical Nutrition*, *82*, 1308–1319. PMID:16332665

Venkateswarlu, S., Natesh Kumar, B., Prasad, C. H., Venkateswarlu, P., & Jyothi, N. V. V. (2014). Bio-inspired green synthesis of Fe3O4 spherical magnetic nanoparticles using *Syzygium cumini* seed extract. *Physica B, Condensed Matter*, *449*, 67–71. doi:10.1016/j.physb.2014.04.031

Venn, B., & Mann, J. (2004). Cereal grains, legumes and diabetes. *European Journal of Clinical Nutrition*, *58*(11), 1443–1461. doi:10.1038/sj.ejcn.1601995 PMID:15162131

Venter, C. S., & van Eyssen, E. (2011). More legumes for better overall health. *South African Journal of Clinical Nutritional*, *14*(suppl), S32–S38.

Verghese, M., Rao, D., Chawan, C., Walker, L., & Shackelford, L. (2006). Anticarcinogenic effect of phytic acid (IP 6): Apoptosis as a possible mechanism of action. *LWT-Food Science and Technology*, *39*(10), 1093–1098. doi:10.1016/j.lwt.2005.07.012

Vermeiren, L., Devlieghere, F., Beest, M., de Kruijf, N., & Debevere, J. (1999). Developments in the active packaging of foods. *Trends in Food Science & Technology*, *10*(3), 77–86. doi:10.1016/S0924-2244(99)00032-1

Vernarelli, J. A., & Lambert, J. D. (2012). Tea consumption is inversely associated with weight status, and other markers for metabolic syndrome in US adults. *European Journal of Nutrition*, *52*(3), 1039–1048. doi:10.1007/s00394-012-0410-9 PMID:22777108

Vertuani, S., Angusti, A., & Manfredini, S. (2004). The antioxidants and pro-antioxidants network: An overview. *Current Pharmaceutical Design*, *10*(14), 1677–1694. doi:10.2174/1381612043384655 PMID:15134565

Vidal, A., Fallarero, A., Peña, B. R., Medina, M. E., Gra, B., Rivera, F., & Vuorela, P. M. et al. (2003). Studies on the toxicity of *Punica granatum* L.(Punicaceae) whole fruit extracts. *Journal of Ethnopharmacology*, *89*, 295–300. PMID:14611895

Vidal-Valverde, C., Frias, J., Sierra, I., Blazquez, I., Lambein, F., & Kuo, Y. H. (2002). New functional legume foods by germination: Effect on the nutritive value of beans, lentils and peas. *European Food Research and Technology*, *215*(6), 472–477. doi:10.1007/s00217-002-0602-2

Vieira, A. J. S. C., Telo, J. P., Pereira, H. F., Patrocínio, P. F., & Dias, R. M. B. (1999). Antioxi-dant effect of naturally occurring xanthines on the oxidative damage of DNA bases. *The Journal of Chemical Physics*, *96*, 116–123.

Vijaykumar, M. V., Pandey, V., Mishra, G. C., & Bhat, M. K. (2010). Hypolipidemic effect of fenugreek seeds is mediated through inhibition of fat accumulation and upregulation of LDL receptor. *Obesity (Silver Spring, Md.)*, *18*(4), 667–674. doi:10.1038/oby.2009.337 PMID:19851306

Vila-Donat, P., Caprioli, G., Maggi, F., Ricciutelli, M., Torregiani, E., Vittori, S., & Sagratini, G. (2015). Effective clean-up and ultra-high-performance liquid chromatography-tandem mass spectrophotometry for isoflavone determination in legumes. *Food Chemistry*, *174*, 487–494. doi:10.1016/j.foodchem.2014.11.047 PMID:25529710

Villareal, C. P., & Juliano, B. O. (1989). b. Comparative level of waxy gene product of endosperm starch granules of different rice ecotypes. *Starch*, *41*(10), 369–371. doi:10.1002/star.19890411002

Villarreal G. M. A., Estrada, S. S., Guadarrama, A. B. A., & Molina, R. V. (2014). Antidiabetic and antihypertensive effect of Brickellia cavanillesii. *Planta Med, 80*, P2B3. Doi: 10.1055/s-0034-1394880

Villegas, R., Liu, S., Gao, Y. T., Yang, G., Li, H., Zheng, W., & Shu, X. O. (2007). Prospective study of dietary carbohydrates, glycemic index, glycemic load, and incidence of type 2 diabetes mellitus in middleaged Chinese women. *Archives of Internal Medicine*, *167*(21), 2310–2316. doi:10.1001/archinte.167.21.2310 PMID:18039989

Vinas, R., & Smith, E. E. (2013). Preliminary evaluation of Prodigiosia herbal tea in cytotoxicity and Glut 2 expression of HepG2 cells. *Toxicological and Environmental Chemistry*, *90*(4), 669–678. doi:10.1080/02772248.2013.801977

Vinskofski, S. (2015). Medicinal herbal tea: infusions and decoctions. *Learning and Yearning*. Retrieved October 23, 2015 from http://learningandyearning.com/infusions-and-decoctions

Vinson, J. A., Jang, J., Dabbagh, Y. A., Serry, M. M., & Cai, S. (1995). Plant Polyphenols Exhibit Lipoprotein-Bound Antioxidant Activity using an *in vitro* Oxidation Model for Heart Disease. *Journal of Agricultural and Food Chemistry*, *43*(11), 2798–2799. doi:10.1021/jf00059a004

Virtanen, T., Pihlanto, A., Akkanen, S., & Korhonen, H. (2007). Development of antioxidant activity in milk whey during fermentation with lactic acid bacteria. *Journal of Applied Microbiology*, *102*(1), 106–115. doi:10.1111/j.1365-2672.2006.03072.x PMID:17184325

Visioli, F., & Hagen, T. M. (2007). Nutritional strategies for healthy cardiovascular aging: Focus on micronutrients. *Pharmacological Research*, *55*(3), 199–206. doi:10.1016/j.phrs.2007.01.008 PMID:17317208

Vitrac, X., Moni, J. P., Vercauteren, J., Deffieux, G., & Merillon, J. M. (2002). Direct liquid chromatography analysis of resveratrol derivatives and flavanonols in wines with absorbance and fluorescence detection. *Analytica Chimica Acta*, *458*(1), 103–110. doi:10.1016/S0003-2670(01)01498-2

Vlachojannis, C., Zimmermann, B. F., & Chrubasik-Hausmann, S. (2015). Efficacy & safety of pomegranate medicinal products for cancer. *Journal of Evidence-Based Complementary & Alternative Medicine. Article ID*, *258598*. doi:10.1155/2015/258598

von Acker, S. A., de Groot, M. J., van der Berg, D. J., Tromp, M. N., Donne-Op den Keider, G., van der Vijgh, W. J., & Bast, A. (1996). A Quantum Chemical Explanation of the Antioxidant Activity of Flavonoids. *Chemical Research in Toxicology*, *9*(8), 1305–1312. doi:10.1021/tx9600964 PMID:8951233

von Schacky, C. (2004). Omega-3 fatty acids and cardiovascular disease. *Current Opinion in Clinical Nutrition and Metabolic Care*, *7*(2), 131–136. doi:10.1097/00075197-200403000-00005 PMID:15075702

Vorarat, S., Managit, C., Iamthanakul, L., Soparat, W., & Kamkaen, N. (2010). Examination of antioxidant activity and development of rice bran oil and gamma-oryzanol microemulsion. *Journal of Health Research*, *24*(2), 67–72.

Vorster, I. H. L., van Rensburg, W. J., van Zijl, J. J. B., & Venter, S. L. (2007). The importance of traditional leafy vegetables in South Africa. *African Journal of Food, Agriculture. Nutrition and Development*, *7*, 49–54.

Vucenik, I., & Shamsuddin, A. M. (2006). Protection against cancer by dietary IP6 and inositol. *Nutrition and Cancer*, *55*(2), 109–125. doi:10.1207/s15327914nc5502_1 PMID:17044765

Wada, K., Nakamura, K., Tamai, Y., Tsuji, M., Kawachi, T., Hori, A., & Nagata, C. et al. (2013). Soy isoflavone intake and breast cancer risk in Japan: From the Takayama study. *International Journal of Cancer*, *133*, 952–960. PMID:23389819

Wada, Y., & Lonnerdal, B. (2014). Bioactive peptides derived from human milk proteins- mechanism of action. *The Journal of Nutritional Biochemistry*, *25*(5), 503–514. doi:10.1016/j.jnutbio.2013.10.012 PMID:24411973

Wagacha, J. M., & Muthomi, J. W. (2008). Mycotoxin problem in Africa: Current status, implications to food safety and health and possible management strategies. *International Journal of Food Microbiology*, *124*(1), 1–12. doi:10.1016/j.ijfoodmicro.2008.01.008 PMID:18258326

Wahlqvist, M. L. (2013). Antioxidant relevance to human health. *Asia Pacific Journal of Clinical Nutrition*, *22*(2), 117–176. PMID:23635359

Wallace, T. C. (2011). Anthocyanins in Cardiovascular Disease. *Advances in Nutrition*, *2*(1), 1–7. doi:10.3945/an.110.000042 PMID:22211184

Wallis, I. R. (1999). Dietary supplements of methionine increase breast meat yield and decrease abdominal fat in growing broiler chickens. *Australian Journal of Experimental Agriculture*, *39*(2), 131–141. doi:10.1071/EA98130

Walstra, P., Wouters, J. T. M., & Geurts, T. J. (2008). Milk for liquid consumption. In Dairy Science and Technology (pp. 421-444). CRC, Taylor & Francis.

Wang, C., Harris, W., Chung, M., Lichtenstein, A. H., Balk, E. M., Kupelnick, B., & Lau, J. et al. (2006). n-3 Fatty acids from fish or fish-oil supplements, but not a-linolenic acid, benefit cardiovascular disease outcomes in primary- and secondary-prevention studies: A systematic review. *The American Journal of Clinical Nutrition*, *84*, 5–17. PMID:16825676

Wang, D., Wang, L., Zhu, F., Zhu, J., Chen, X. D., Zou, L., & Li, L. et al. (2008). *In vitro and in vivo* studies on the antioxidant activities of the aqueous extracts of Douchi (A traditional Chinese slat fermented soybean food). *Food Chemistry*, *17*(4), 1421–1428. doi:10.1016/j.foodchem.2007.09.072

Wang, H. P., Yang, J., Qin, L. Q., & Yang, X. J. (2015). Effect of Garlic on Blood Pressure: A Meta-Analysis. *Journal of Clinical Hypertension*, *17*(3), 223–231. doi:10.1111/jch.12473 PMID:25557383

Wang, H., Ng, T., Ooi, V. E., & Liu, W. (2000). Effects of lectins with different carbohydrate-binding specificities on hepatoma, choriocarcinoma, melanoma and osteosarcoma cell lines. *The International Journal of Biochemistry & Cell Biology*, *32*(3), 365–372. doi:10.1016/S1357-2725(99)00130-2 PMID:10716633

Wang, R., Ding, Y., Liu, R., Xiang, L., & Du, L. (2010). Pomegranate: Constituents, bioactivities and pharmacokinetics. *Fruits. Vegetable and Cereal Science and Biotechnology*, *4*(2), 77–87.

Wang, T., Hicks, K. B., & Moreau, R. (2002). Antioxidant activity of phytosterols, oryzanol & other phytosterol conjugates. *Journal of the American Oil Chemists' Society*, *79*(12), 1201–1206. doi:10.1007/s11746-002-0628-x

Wang, X. L., Hur, H. G., Lee, J. H., Kim, K. T., & Kim, S. I. (2005). Enantioselective synthesis of S-equol from dihydrodaidzein by a newly isolated anaerobic human intestinal bacterium. *Applied and Environmental Microbiology*, *71*(1), 214–219. doi:10.1128/AEM.71.1.214-219.2005 PMID:15640190

Wang, X. L., Kim, H. J., Kang, S. I., Kim, S. I., & Hur, H. G. (2007). Production of phytoestrogen S-equol from daidzein in mixed culture of two anaerobic bacteria. *Archives of Microbiology*, *187*(2), 155–160. doi:10.1007/s00203-006-0183-8 PMID:17109177

Wareing, P. W., Westby, A., Gibbs, J. A., Allotey, L. T., & Halm, M. (2001). Consumer preferences and fungal and mycotoxin contamination of dried cassava products from Ghana. *International Journal of Food Science & Technology*, *36*(1), 1–10. doi:10.1046/j.1365-2621.2001.00419.x

Warner, K., Vick, B., Kleingartner, L., Isaak, R., & Doroff, K. (2015). *Compositions of sunflower, nusun (mid-oleic sunflower) and high-oleic sunflower oils*. Retreated from: https://www.sunflowernsa.com/uploads/resources/51/warner_.pdf

Warshafsky, S., Kramer, R. S., & Sivak, S. L. (1993). Effect of garlic on total serum cholesterol: A meta-analysis. *Annals of Internal Medicine*, *119*(7_Part_1), 599–605. doi:10.7326/0003-4819-119-7_Part_1-199310010-00009 PMID:8363171

Waterman, E., & Lockwood, B. (2007). Active components and clinical applications of olive oil. *Alternative Medicine Review*, *12*, 331–342. PMID:18069902

Wei, C. C., Yu, C. W., Yen, P. L., Lin, H. Y., Chang, S. T., Hsu, F. L., & Liao, V. H. (2014). Antioxidant activity, delayed aging, and reduced amyloid-β toxicity of methanol extracts of tea seed pomace from Camellia tenuifolia. *Journal of Agricultural and Food Chemistry*, *62*(44), 10701–10707. doi:10.1021/jf503192x PMID:25295856

Weickert, M. O., Mohlig, M., Schofl, C., Arafat, A. M., Otto, B., Viehoff, H., & Pfeiffer, A. F. (2006). Cereal. fiber improves whole-body insulin sensitivity in overweight and obese women. *Diabetes Care*, *29*(4), 775–780. doi:10.2337/diacare.29.04.06.dc05-2374 PMID:16567814

Wei, P., Liu, M., Chen, Y., & Chen, D.-D. (2012). Systematic review of soy isoflavone supplements on osteoporosis in women. *Asian Pacific Journal of Tropical Medicine*, *5*(3), 243–248. doi:10.1016/S1995-7645(12)60033-9 PMID:22305793

Wei, Q.-K., Chen, T.-R., & Chen, J.-T. (2007). Using *Lactobacillus* and *Bifidobacterium* to produce the isoflavone aglycones in fermented soymilk. *International Journal of Food Microbiology, 117*(1), 120–124. doi:10.1016/j.ijfoodmicro.2007.02.024 PMID:17477997

Weisburger, J. H. (1999). Mechanisms of action of antioxidants as exemplified in vegetables, tomatoes and tea. *Food and Chemical Toxicology, 37*(9-10), 943–948. doi:10.1016/S0278-6915(99)00086-1 PMID:10541449

Wei, X. J., Wu, J., Ni, Y. D., Lu, L. Z., & Zhao, R. Q. (2011). Antioxidant effect of a phytoestrogen equol on cultured muscle cells of embryonic broilers. *In Vitro Cellular & Developmental Biology. Animal, 47*(10), 735–741. doi:10.1007/s11626-011-9464-x PMID:22083625

Wells, J. H. (1993). Utilization of rice bran & oil in human diets. *Louisiana Agriculture, 36*, 4–8.

Were, B. A., Okware, A. O., Gudu, S., Welander, M., & Carlsson, A. S. (2006). Seed oil content and fatty acid composition in East African sesame (*Sesamum indicum L.*) accessions evaluated over 3 years. *Field Crops Research, 97*(2-3), 254–260. doi:10.1016/j.fcr.2005.10.009

Weststrate, J. A., Poppel, G. V., & Verschuren, P. M. (2002). Functional foods, trends and future. *The British Journal of Nutrition, 88*(S2), S233–S235. doi:10.1079/BJN2002688 PMID:12495465

WHO. (2004). *Iodine status worldwide: WHO Global Database on Iodine Deficiency*. Retrieved July 15, 2015, from http://www.who.int/nutrition/publications/micronutrients/iodine_deficiency/9241592001/en/

WHO. (2008). *Worldwide prevalence of anaemia 1993–2005: WHO global database on anaemia*. Retrieved July 15, 2015 from http://www.who.int/vmnis/anaemia/prevalence/en/

WHO. (2009). *Global prevalence of vitamin A deficiency in populations at risk 1995–2005. WHO Global Database on Vitamin A Deficiency*. Retrieved July 15, 2015 from http://www.who.int/vmnis/database/vitamina/x/en/

WHO. (2012). *Estimated incidence, mortality and prevalence worldwide in 2012*. Retrieved May 23, 2015, from http://globocan.iarc.fr/Pages/fact_sheets_cancer.aspx

Wikimedia Commons. (2007). *Chemical structure of glucosinolates*. Retrieved from https://commons.wikimedia.org/wiki/File:Glucosinolates.png

Wilcox, J. N., & Blumenthal, B. F. (1995). Thrombotic mechanisms in atherosclerosis: Po-tential impact of soy proteins. *The Journal of Nutrition, 125*, 631S–638S. PMID:7884545

Wilcox, M. L., Burton, S., Oyweka, R., Namyalo, R., Challand, S., & Lindsey, K. (2011). Evaluation and pharmacovigilance of projects promoting cultivation and local use of Artemisia annua for malaria. *Malaria Journal, 10*(84), 1–6. PMID:21214892

Wild, S., Roglic, G., Green, A., Sicree, R., & King, H. (2004). Global prevalence of diabetes: Estimates for the year 2000 and projections for 2030. *Diabetes Care, 27*(5), 1047–1053. doi:10.2337/diacare.27.5.1047 PMID:15111519

Williams, J. H., Phillips, T. D., Jolly, P. E., Stiles, J. K., Jolly, C. M., & Aggarwal, D. (2004). Human aflatoxicosis in developing countries: A review of toxicology, exposure, potential health consequences, and interventions. *The American Journal of Clinical Nutrition, 80*, 1106–1122. PMID:15531656

Winham, D. M., & Hutchins, A. M. (2007). Baked bean consumption reduces serum cholesterol in hypercholesterolemic adults. *Nutrition Research (New York, N.Y.), 27*(7), 380–386. doi:10.1016/j.nutres.2007.04.017

Winter, J. (2005). The phytosterol phenomenon. *Func Food Nutraceutic.*, 24–30.

Wiseman, H., Casey, K., Bowey, E. A., Duffy, R., Davies, M., Rowland, I. R., & Clarke, D. B. et al. (2004). Influence of 10 wk of soy consumption on plasma concentrations and excretion of isoflavonoids and on gut microflora metabolism in healthy adults. *The American Journal of Clinical Nutrition*, *80*, 692–699. PMID:15321810

Witte, V. C., Krause, G. F., & Bailey, M. E. (1970). A new extraction method for determining 2-thiobarbituric acid values of pork and beef during storage. *Journal of Food Science*, *35*(5), 582–585. doi:10.1111/j.1365-2621.1970.tb04815.x

Wolever, T. M., Katzman-Relle, L., Jenkins, A. L., Vuksan, V., Josse, R. G., & Jenkins, D. J. (1994). Glycaemic index of 102 complex carbohydrate foods in patients with diabetes. *Nutrition Research (New York, N.Y.)*, *14*(5), 651–669. doi:10.1016/S0271-5317(05)80201-5

Wolfram, S., Weber, T., Grenacher, B., & Scharrer, E. (1995). A Na(+)-dependent mechanism is involved in mucosal uptake of cinnamic acid across the jejunal brush border in rats. *The Journal of Nutrition*, *125*(5), 1300–1308. PMID:7738690

Women's Health Initiative. (2010). *Findings from the WHI Postmenopausal Hormone Therapy Trials*. Retrieved from: http://www.nhlbi.nih.gov/whi/

Womeni, H. M., Linder, M., Tiencheu, B., Mbiapo, F. T., Villeneuve, P., Fanni, J., & Parmentier, M. (2009). Oils of insects and larvae consumed in Africa: Potential sources of polyunsaturated fatty acids. *Oilseeds and Fats Crops Lipids*, *16*, 230–235.

Won, T.J., Kim, B.J., Lim, Y.T., Song, D.S., & Oh, E.S., Lee Do, I., & Hwang, K.W. (2011). Modulation of Th1/Th2 balance by Lactobacillus strains isolated kimchi via stimulation of macrophage cell line J774A.1 in vitro. *Journal of Food Science*, *76*, H55–H61. PMID:21535768

World Health Organization (W.H.O.). (2009). *Cardiovascular diseases (CVDs). Fact sheet N° 317*. Available at: http://www.who.int/mediacentre/factsheets/fs317/en/ index.html

World Health Organization (WHO). (2003). *Traditional Medicine*. Retrieved November 9, 2015 from, http://www.who.int/mediacentre/factsheets/2003/fs134/en/

World Health Organization (WHO). (2008). *The global burden of diseases: 2004 update*. Retrieved from www.who.int/healthinfo/global_burden_disease/GBD_report_2004updat

World Health Organization (WHO). (n.d.) Fact Sheet. Retrieved from: www.who.int/mediacentre/factsheets/fs355/en/)

World Health Organization. (2014). *The top ten causes of death. Fact sheet no. 310*. Retrieved October 23, 2015 from http://www.who.int/mediacentre/factsheets/fs310/en/

World Health Organization. (2015). *Guidelines for the treatment of malaria* (3rd ed.). Retrieved November, 7 2015 from http://apps.who.int/iris/bitstream/10665/162441/1/9789241549127_eng.pdf?ua=1

Wu, C., Gao, Q., Kjelgren, R. K., Guo, X., & Wang, M. (2013). Yields, phenolic profiles and antioxidant activities of *Ziziphus jujube* mill. in response to different fertilization treatments. *Molecules (Basel, Switzerland)*, *18*(10), 12029–12040. doi:10.3390/molecules181012029 PMID:24084012

Wu, J., Ho, S. C., Zhou, C., Ling, W. H., Chen, W. Q., Wang, C. L., & Chen, Y. M. (2009). Coffee consumption and risk of coronary heart diseases: A meta-analysis of 21 prospective cohort studies. *International Journal of Cardiology*, *137*(3), 216–225. doi:10.1016/j.ijcard.2008.06.051 PMID:18707777

Wu, N., Fu, K., Fu, Y., Zu, Y., Chang, F., Chen, Y., & Gu, C. et al. (2009). Antioxidant activities of extracts and main components of pigeonpea [*Cajanus cajan* (L.) Millsp.] leaves. *Molecules (Basel, Switzerland)*, *14*(3), 1032–1043. doi:10.3390/molecules14031032 PMID:19305357

Xia, M., Ling, W., Zhu, H., Wang, Q., Ma, J., Hou, M., & Ye, Q. et al. (2007). Anthocyanin prevents CD40-activated proinflammatory signaling in endothelial cells by regulating cholesterol distribution. *Arteriosclerosis, Thrombosis, and Vascular Biology*, *27*(3), 519–524. doi:10.1161/01.ATV.0000254672.04573.2d PMID:17158355

Xiaoming, C., Ying, F., Hong, Z., & Zhiyonga, C. (2010). Review of the nutritive value of edible insects. In *Proceedings of a workshop on Asia-Pacific resources and their potential for development* (pp 85-92), Bangkok, Thailand: Food and Agriculture Organisation.

Xie, Z., Fan, J., Charlebois, D., Roussel, D., Dube, C., Charles, M. T., & Khanizadeh, S. (2014). Agronomic characteristics and phytochemical profiles of advanced june-bearing strawberry lines for the northern Candian climate. *Agricultural and Food Science*, *23*, 38–47.

Xu, B. J., Han, L. K., Zheng, Y. N., Lee, J. H., & Sung, C. K. (2005). In vitro inhibitory effect of triterpenoidal saponins from Platycodi Radix on pancreatic lipase. *Archives of Pharmacal Research*, *28*(2), 180–185. doi:10.1007/BF02977712 PMID:15789748

Xu, B., & Chang, S. (2007). A comparative study on phenolic profiles and antioxidant activities of legumes as affected by extraction solvents. *Journal of Food Science*, *72*(2), S159–S166. doi:10.1111/j.1750-3841.2006.00260.x PMID:17995858

Xu, B., & Chang, S. K. (2008). Effect of soaking, boiling, and steaming on total phenolic contentand antioxidant activities of cool season food legumes. *Food Chemistry*, *110*(1), 1–13. doi:10.1016/j.foodchem.2008.01.045 PMID:26050159

Xu, B., & Chang, S. K. (2010). Phenolic substance characterization and chemical and cell-based antioxidant activities of 11 lentils grown in the Northern United States. *Journal of Agricultural and Food Chemistry*, *58*(3), 1509–1517. doi:10.1021/jf903532y PMID:20058926

Xu, B., & Chang, S. K. C. (2012). Comparative study on anti-proliferation properties and cellular antioxidant activities of commonly consumed food legumes against nine human cancer cell lines. *Food Chemistry*, *134*(3), 1287–1296. doi:10.1016/j.foodchem.2012.02.212 PMID:25005945

Xu, B., Yuan, S., & Chang, S. (2007). Comparative analyses of phenolic composition, antioxidant capacity, and color of cool season legumes and other selected food legumes. *Journal of Food Science*, *72*(2), S167–S177. doi:10.1111/j.1750-3841.2006.00261.x PMID:17995859

Xu, K. Z. Y., Zhu, C., Kim, M. S., Yamahara, J., & Li, Y. (2009). Pomegranate flower ameliorates fatty liver in an animal model of type 2 diabetes & obesity. *Journal of Ethnopharmacology*, *123*(2), 280–287. doi:10.1016/j.jep.2009.03.035 PMID:19429373

Xu, L., Du, B., & Xu, B. (2015). A systematic, comparative study on the beneficial health components and antioxidant activities of commercially fermented soy products marketed in China. *Food Chemistry*, *174*, 202–213. doi:10.1016/j.foodchem.2014.11.014 PMID:25529671

Xu, Y., Zhang, J. J., Xiong, L., Zhang, L., Sun, D., & Liu, H. (2010). Green tea polyphenols inhibit cognitive impairment induced by chronic cerebral hypoperfusion via modulating oxidative stress. *The Journal of Nutritional Biochemistry*, *21*(8), 741–748. doi:10.1016/j.jnutbio.2009.05.002 PMID:19615878

Yadav, D., Yadav, S. K., Khar, R. K., Mujeeb, M., & Akhtar, M. (2013). Turmeric (*Curcuma longa* L.): A promising spice for phytochemical and pharmacological activities. *International Journal of Green Pharmacy*, *7*(2), 82–89. doi:10.4103/0973-8258.116375

Yadav, R., & Kaushik, R. (2011). A study of phytochemical constituents and pharmacological actions of *Trigonella foenum-graecum*: A review. *International Journal of Pharmacy & Technology*, *3*, 1022–1028.

Yagil, R. (1987). Camel milk - A review. *Farm Animals*, *2*, 81–99.

Yamakuchi, M., Bao, C., Ferlito, M., & Lowenstein, C. J. (2008). Epigallocatechin gallate inhibits endothelial exocytosis. *Biological Chemistry*, *389*(7), 935–941. doi:10.1515/BC.2008.095 PMID:18627310

Yamamoto, T., Hsu, S., Lewis, J., Wataha, J., Dickinson, D., Singh, B., & Schuster, G. et al. (2003). Green tea polyphenol causes differential oxidative environments in tumor versus normal epithelial cells. *The Journal of Pharmacology and Experimental Therapeutics*, *307*(1), 230–236. doi:10.1124/jpet.103.054676 PMID:12954803

Yamamoto, Y., & Gaynor, R. (2001). Therapeutic potential of inhibition of NF-kB pathway in the treatment of inflammation and cancer. *The Journal of Clinical Investigation*, *107*(2), 135–142. doi:10.1172/JCI11914 PMID:11160126

Yamori, Y. (2006). Food factors for aterosclerosis prevention: Asian perspective derived from analyses of worldwide dietary biomarkers. *Experimental and Clinical Cardiology*, *11*, 94–98. PMID:18651042

Yanagihara, K., Takigahira, M., Mihara, K., Kubo, T., Morimoto, C., Morita, Y., & Seyama, T. et al. (2013). Inhibitory effects of isoflavones on tumor growth and cachexia in newly established cachectic mouse models carrying human stomach cancers. *Nutrition and Cancer*, *65*(4), 578–589. doi:10.1080/01635581.2013.776089 PMID:23659450

Yang, C. S., & Landau, J. M. (2000). Effects of tea consumption on nutrition and health. *The Journal of Nutrition*, *130*, 2409–2412. PMID:11015465

Yang, G. Y., Liao, J., Li, C., Chung, J., Yurkow, E. J., Ho, C. T., & Yang, C. S. (2000). Effect of black and green tea polyphenols on c-jun phosphorylation and H(2)O(2) production in transformed and non-transformed human bronchial cell lines: Possible mechanisms of cell growth inhibition and apoptosis induction. *Carcinogenesis*, *21*(11), 2035–2039. doi:10.1093/carcin/21.11.2035 PMID:11062165

Yasuhiko, T., & Fumio, I. (1988). Recent technical advances in rice bran oil processing (II About refining process). Transactions of the Kokushikan Univ. *Faculty of Engineering*, *21*, 118–124.

Yawadio, R., Tanimori, S., & Morita, N. (2007). Identification of phenolic compounds isolated from pigmented rices and their aldose reductase inhibitory activities. *Food Chemistry*, *101*(4), 1616–1625. doi:10.1016/j.foodchem.2006.04.016

Yener, F. Y. G., Korel, F., & Yemenicioglu, A. (2009). Antimicrobial activity of lactoperoxidase system into crosslinked alginate films. *Journal of Food Science*, *74*(2), 73–79. doi:10.1111/j.1750-3841.2009.01057.x PMID:19323761

Yen, G. C., & Wei, Q. K. (1993). Myrosinase activity and total glucosinolate content of cruciferous vegetables, and some properties of cabbage myrosinase in Taiwan. *Journal of the Science of Food and Agriculture*, *61*(4), 471–475. doi:10.1002/jsfa.2740610415

Ying, H., Jiang, H., Liu, H., Chen, F., & Du, Q. (2014). Ethyl acetate-n-butanol gradient solvent system for high-speed countercurrent chromatography to screen bioactive substances in okra. *J. Chromatog.*, *1359*, 117–123. doi:10.1016/j.chroma.2014.07.029 PMID:25069743

Yokoyama, S., Oshima, K., Nomura, I., Hattori, M., & Suzuki, T. (2011). Complete genomic sequence of the equol-producing bacterium *Eggerthella* sp. strain YY7918, isolated from adult human intestine. *Journal of Bacteriology*, *193*(19), 5570–5571. doi:10.1128/JB.05626-11 PMID:21914883

Yokoyama, S., & Suzuki, T. (2008). Isolation and characterization of a novel equol-producing bacterium from human feces. *Bioscience, Biotechnology, and Biochemistry*, *72*(10), 2660–2666. doi:10.1271/bbb.80329 PMID:18838805

Yoon, S. H., & Rhee, J. S. (1982). Composition of waxes from crude rice bran oil. *Journal of the American Oil Chemists' Society*, *59*(12), 561–563. doi:10.1007/BF02636324

Yordi, E. G., Pérez, E. M., Matos, M. J., & Villares, E. U. (2012). Antioxidant and pro-oxidant effects of polyphenolic compounds and structure-activity relationship evidence. In Nutrition, well-being and health (pp. 2-48). InTech Publisher.

You, W. C., Zhang, L., Gail, M. H., Ma, J. L., Chang, Y. S., Blot, W. J., & Xu, G. W. et al. (1998). Fraumeni JF Jr. *Helicobacter pylori* infection, garlic intake and precancerous lesions in a Chinese population at low risk of gastic cancer. *International Journal of Epidemiology*, *27*(6), 941–944. doi:10.1093/ije/27.6.941 PMID:10024185

Yuan, J.-P., Wang, J.-H., & Liu, X. (2007). Metabolism of dietary soy isoflavones to equol by human intestinal microbiota. Implications for health. *Molecular Nutrition & Food Research*, *51*(7), 765–781. doi:10.1002/mnfr.200600262 PMID:17579894

Yuan, Y. V., & Kitts, D. D. (1997). Endogenous antioxidants: role of antioxidant enzyme in biological systems. In F. Shahidi (Ed.), *Natural antioxidants- Chemistry, health effects, and applications* (pp. 258–270). Champaign, IL: Amer Oil Chemists Society.

Yu, D., Shu, X. O., Li, H., Xiang, Y. B., Yang, G., Gao, Y. T., & Zhang, X. (2013). Dietary carbohydrates, refined grains, glycemic load, and risk of coronary heart disease in Chinese adults. *American Journal of Epidemiology*, *178*(10), 1542–1549. doi:10.1093/aje/kwt178 PMID:24008907

Yu, E. J. (2004). *The cytotoxic, antioxidative, and antihypertensive activities in Dolsanleaf mustard and its kimchi. (Ph.D)*. Yosu, Korea: Yosu National University.

Yue, P., & Waring, S. (1998). Resistant starch in food applications. *Cereal Foods World*, *43*, 90–695.

Yu, J., Ahmedna, M., & Goktepe, I. (2005). Effects of processing methods and extraction solvents on concentration and antioxidant activity of peanut skin phenolics. *Food Chemistry*, *90*(1-2), 199–206. doi:10.1016/j.foodchem.2004.03.048

Yu, M. H., Im, H. G., Im, N. K., Hwang, E. Y., Choi, J. H., Lee, E. J., & Seo, H. J. et al. (2009). Anti-hypertensive activities of Lactobacillus isolated from Kimchi. *Korean J. Food Sci. Technol.*, *41*(4), 428–434.

Yun, Y. R., Kim, H. J., & Song, Y. O. (2014). Kimchi methanol extract and the kimchi active compound, 3'-(4'-hydroxyl-3',5'-dimethoxyphenyl)propionic acid, downregulate CD36 in THP-1 macrophages timulated by oxLDL. *Journal of Medicinal Food*, *8*(8), 886–893. doi:10.1089/jmf.2013.2943 PMID:25010893

Yu, S. Y., Lee, Y. J., Kim, J. D., Kang, S. N., Lee, S. K., Jang, J. Y., & Lee, O. H. et al. (2013). Phenolic composition, antioxidant activity and anti-adipogenic effect of hot water extract from safflower (*Carthamus tinctorius* L.) seed. *Nutrients*, *5*(12), 4894–4907. doi:10.3390/nu5124894 PMID:24288028

Yusuf, S., Dagenais, G., Pogue, J., & Sleight, P. (2000). Vitamin E supplementation and cardiovascular events in high-risk patients. The Heart Outcomes Prevention Evaluation Study Investigators. *The New England Journal of Medicine*, *345*, 154–160. PMID:10639540

Yusuf, S., Hawken, S., Ounpuu, S., Dans, T., Avezum, A., Lanas, F., & Lisheng, L. et al. (2004). Effect of potentially modifiable risk factors associated with myocardial infarction in 52 countries (the INTERHEART study): Case-control study. *Lancet*, *364*(9438), 937–952. doi:10.1016/S0140-6736(04)17018-9 PMID:15364185

Yu, Z. T., Yao, W., & Zhu, W. Y. (2008). Isolation and identification of equol-producing bacterial strains from cultures of pig faeces. *FEMS Microbiology Letters*, *282*(1), 73–80. doi:10.1111/j.1574-6968.2008.01108.x PMID:18328079

Zamora-Ros, R., Knaze, V., Luján-Barroso, L., Kuhnle, G. G., Mulligan, A. A., Touillaud, M., & González, C. A. (2012, August). Dietary intakes and food sources of phytoestrogens in the European Prospective Investigation into Cancer and Nutrition (EPIC) 24-hour dietary recall cohort. *European Journal of Clinical Nutrition*, *66*(8), 932–941. doi:10.1038/ejcn.2012.36 PMID:22510793

Zand, J., Rountree, R., Rountree, B., & Walton, R. (2003). *Smart medicine for a healthier child: A practical A-to-Z to natural and conventional treatments for infants and children*. New York: Pengium.

Zawistowski, J. (2014). Regulation of Functional Foods in Selected Asian Countries in the Pacific Rim. In Nutraceutical and Functional Food Regulations in the United States and Around the World (2nd ed.). Food Science and Technology. doi:doi:10.1016/B978-0-12-405870-5.00024-4 doi:10.1016/B978-0-12-405870-5.00024-4

Zeng, Y., Chen, H., Ni, T., Ruan, R., Feng, L., Nie, C., & …, Vaupel, J.W. (2015). GxE interactions between FOXO genotypes and drinking tea are significantly associated with prevention of cognitive decline in advanced age in China. *The Journals of Gerontology. Series A, Biological Sciences and Medical Sciences*, *70*(4), 426–433. doi:10.1093/gerona/glu060 PMID:24895270

Zhang, B., Deng, Z., Ramdath, D. D., Tang, Y., Chen, P. X., Liu, R., & Tsao, R. et al. (2015). Phenoli.c profiles of 20 Canadian lentil cultivars and their contribution to antioxidant activity and inhibitory effects on α-glucosidase and pancreatic lipase. *Food Chemistry*, *172*, 862–872. doi:10.1016/j.foodchem.2014.09.144 PMID:25442631

Zhang, H., Jiang, L., Ye, S., Ye, Y., & Ren, F. (2010). Systematic evaluation of antioxidant capacities of the ethanolic extract of different tissues of jujube (*Zizyphus jujube* Mill.) from China. *Food and Chemical Toxicology*, *48*(6), 1461–1465. doi:10.1016/j.fct.2010.03.011 PMID:20230870

Zhang, H., Kong, B., Xiong, Y. L., & Sun, X. (2009). Antimicrobial activities of spice extracts against pathogenic and spoilage bacteria in modified atmosphere packaged fresh pork and vacuum packaged ham slices stored at 4°C. *Meat Science*, *8*(4), 686–692. doi:10.1016/j.meatsci.2008.11.011 PMID:20416570

Zhang, H., Spitz, M. R., Tomlinson, G. E., Schabath, M. B., Minna, J. D., & Wu, X. (2002). Modification of lung cancer susceptibility by green tea extract as measured by the comet assay. *Cancer Detection and Prevention*, *26*(6), 411–418. doi:10.1016/S0361-090X(02)00127-7 PMID:12507225

Zhang, J., Ge, Y., Han, F., Li, B., Yan, S., Sun, J., & Wang, L. (2014). Isoflavone content of soybean cultivars from maturity group 0 to VI grown in Northern and Southern China. *Journal of the American Oil Chemists' Society*, *91*(6), 1019–1028. doi:10.1007/s11746-014-2440-3 PMID:24882872

Zhang, L. L., & Lin, Y. M. (2009). Antioxidant tannins from *Syzygium cumini* fruit. *African Journal of Biotechnology*, *8*, 2301–2309.

Zhang, M., Guo, B., Zhang, R., Chi, J., We, Z., Xu, Z., & Tang, X. (2006). Separation, purification and identification of antioxidant compositions in black rice. *Agricultural Sciences in China*, *5*(6), 431440. doi:10.1016/S1671-2927(06)60073-4

Zhang, R. F., Zhang, F. X., Zhang, M. W., Wei, Z. C., Yang, C. Y., Zhang, Y., & Chi, J. W. et al. (2011). Phenolic composition and antioxidant activity in seed coats of 60 Chinese black soybean (*Glycine max* L. Merr.) varieties. *Journal of Agricultural and Food Chemistry*, *59*(11), 593–544. doi:10.1021/jf201593n PMID:21548651

Zhang, R., Zhang, X., Wu, K., Wu, H., Sun, Q., Hu, F. B., & Giovannucci, E. L. (2016). Rice consumption and cancer incidence in US men and women. *International Journal of Cancer*, *138*(3), 555–564. doi:10.1002/ijc.29704 PMID:26219234

Zhang, X. D., Zhao, X. Y., Zhang, M., Liang, Y., Xu, X. H., D'Arcy, C., & Holman, J. (2008). A case-control study on green tea consumption and the risk of adult leukemia. *Zhonghua Liu Xing Bing Xue Za Zhi*, *29*(3), 290–293. PMID:18788532

Zhao, H., Zhang, H., & Yang, S. (2014). Phenolic compounds and its antioxidant activities in ethanolicextracts from seven cultivars of Chinese jujube. *Food Science and Human Wellness*, *3*(3-4), 183–190. doi:10.1016/j.fshw.2014.12.005

Zhao, S. P., Liu, L., Cheng, Y. C., Shishehbor, M. H., Liu, M. H., Peng, D. Q., & Li, Y. L. (2004). Xuezhikang, an extract of cholestin, protects endothelial function through antiinflammatory and lipid-lowering mechanisms in patients with coronary heart disease. *Circulation, 110*(8), 915–920. doi:10.1161/01.CIR.0000139985.81163.CE PMID:15313947

Zhao, X., Yuan, Z., Fang, Y., Yin, Y., & Feng, L. (2013). Characterization and evaluation of major anthocyanins in pomegranate (*Punica granatum* L.) peel of different cultivars and their development phases. *European Food Research and Technology*, *236*(1), 109–117. doi:10.1007/s00217-012-1869-6

Zhao, Z., & Moghadasian, M. H. (2008). Chemistry, natural sources, dietary intake and pharmacokinetic properties of ferulic acid: A review. *Food Chemistry*, *109*(4), 691–702. doi:10.1016/j.foodchem.2008.02.039 PMID:26049981

Zheng, W., Hou, Y., Su, Y., & Yao, W. (2014). Lactulose promotes equol production and changes the microbial community *in vitro* of daidzein by fecal inocula of sows. *Anaerobe*, *25*, 47–52. doi:10.1016/j.anaerobe.2013.11.011 PMID:24315807

Zhou, K., Su, L., & Yu, L. (2004). Phytochemicals and antioxidant properties in wheat bran. *Journal of Agricultural and Food Chemistry*, *52*(20), 6108–6114. doi:10.1021/jf049214g PMID:15453674

Zhou, Z., Robards, K., Helliwell, S., & Blanchard, C. (2004). The distribution of phenolic acids in rice. *Food Chemistry*, *87*(3), 401–406. doi:10.1016/j.foodchem.2003.12.015

Zhu, J., Vinas, R., & Smith, E. E. (2008). In vitro evaluation of human liver cancer cells and the potential cytotoxicity of Tecoma stans (Bignoniaceae) and Brickellia cavanillesii (Asteraceae) both single and in combination. *Toxicological and Environmental Chemistry*, *90*(4), 801–808. doi:10.1080/02772240701740387

Zhu, Y., Soroka, D., & Sang, S. (2015). Oxyphytosterols as active ingredients in wheat bran suppress human colon cancer cell growth: Identification, chemical synthesis, and biological evaluation. *Journal of Agricultural and Food Chemistry*, *63*(8), 2264–2276. doi:10.1021/jf506361r PMID:25658220

Zielinski, H. (2002). Low molecular weight antioxidants in the cereal grains- a review. *Polish J. Food Nutr. Sci.*, *11/51*(1), 3–9.

Zilic, S., Basic, Z., Sukalovic, V. H. T., Makasimovic, V., Jankovic, M., & Filipovic, M. (2014). Can the sprouting process applied to wheat improve the contents of vitamins and phenolic compounds and antioxidant capacity of the flour? *International Journal of Food Science & Technology*, *49*(4), 1040–1047. doi:10.1111/ijfs.12397

Ziouzenkova, O., Gieseg, S. P., Ramos, P., & Esterbauer, H. (1996). Factors affecting resistance of low density lipoproteins to oxidation. *Lipids*, *31*(1Suppl), 71–76. doi:10.1007/BF02637054 PMID:8729097

Zorov, D. B., Bannikova, S. Y., Belousov, V. V., Vyssokikh, M. Y., Zorova, L. D., Isaev, N. K., & Plotnikov, E. Y. et al. (2005). Reactive oxygen and nitrogen species: Friends or foes? *Biochemistry (Moscow)*, *70*(2), 215–221. doi:10.1007/s10541-005-0103-6 PMID:15807661

Zou, Y., Chang, S. K. C., Gu, Y., & Qian, S. Y. (2011). Antioxidant activity and phenolic compositions of lentil (*Lens culinaris* var. Morton) extract and its fractions. *Journal of Agricultural and Food Chemistry*, *59*(6), 2268–2276. doi:10.1021/jf104640k PMID:21332205

Zozio, S., Servent, A., Hiol, A., Mbeguie, D., Cosmidis, L., Lucien, J. M., & Pallet, D. (2015). Processed Z. *Mauritiana* Lamk in the formula of high nutritional value cake. *J. Food. Process. Technol.* http:// dx.dio.org/10.4172/2157-7110.1000444

About the Contributors

Omar Alhaj is an assistant Professor of Dairy Biotechnology at King Saud University, Kingdom of Saudi Arabia. His Ph.D. and MSc. were awarded from Wales University, United Kingdom. He served as assistant professor and industry consultant at a number of institutions. He has been awarded a number of research project grants in his field. He authored a number of manuscripts and books, and he served as reviewer for several peer reviewed journals and has a number of international research collaborations worldwide. He teaches various courses and supervises a number of MSc. students. His professional interests include bovine and camel milk protein chemistry, enzymology and bioactivity of isolated casein peptides as cholesterol reducer, ACE-inhibitor, antioxidant, anticancer and antimicrobial activity. He has worked on the effect of probiotic bacteria on peptides and amino acids profiles from milk proteins; moreover, he has been studying probiotics growth and survival in different sources of milk. Recently, he served as internal accreditation auditor and assessor for King Saud University.

Susana Delgado is affiliated to IPLA, a dairy-oriented research institute belonging to CSIC, the Spanish largest public research institution. She is part of the Functional Dairy Cultures (FDC) research team and works on several aspects of dairy and human gastrointestinal microbiology. These studies aim to select appropriate microorganisms to be used for, or added to, fermented dairy products. Current research of FDC focuses on the identification and characterization of isoflavone-activating and metabolizing bacteria from the human gut.

Etetor Roland Eshiet is a graduate of Texas Tech University's, The Institute of Environmental and Human Health (TIEHH) and the Department of Environmental Toxicology doctoral program. He possesses a Bachelor of Science (Hons) degree in Applied Chemistry, and a Masters' degree in Petroleum Chemistry & Petrochemicals. He has obtained certifications, with distinction, in Data Management for Clinical Research (DMCR) and Design and Interpretation of Clinical Trials (DICT) from the Department of Biomedical Informatics, Vanderbilt University and Bloomberg School of Public Health, John Hopkins University respectively. He is a literary consultant, a Healthcare Information Technology (HIT) consultant and the Co-Founder/Managing Partner of SEEED (Sustainable Energy Environmental and Educational Development), an international consulting organization with points of contacts (poc) in Europe and West-Africa. Dr. Eshiet has publications in highly reputable peer-reviewed scientific journals, and is working in tandem with a team of other experts to publish a book. He is a member of the board of directors of EL-THOMP College of Technology, Nigeria.

Han Eung-Soo, PhD, is Lead Researcher, Research and Development Division, New Production Process and Fermentation, at the World Institute of Kimchi, Korea.

Ana Belén Flórez is affiliated to IPLA, a dairy-oriented research institute belonging to CSIC, the Spanish largest public research institution. She is part of the Functional Dairy Cultures (FDC) research team and works on several aspects of dairy and human gastrointestinal microbiology. These studies aim to select appropriate microorganisms to be used for, or added to, fermented dairy products. Current research of FDC focuses on the identification and characterization of isoflavone-activating and metabolizing bacteria from the human gut.

Lucía Guadamuro is affiliated to IPLA, a dairy-oriented research institute belonging to CSIC, the Spanish largest public research institution. She is part of the Functional Dairy Cultures (FDC) research team and works on several aspects of dairy and human gastrointestinal microbiology. These studies aim to select appropriate microorganisms to be used for, or added to, fermented dairy products. Current research of FDC focuses on the identification and characterization of isoflavone-activating and metabolizing bacteria from the human gut.

Md. Zakir Hossain Howlader joined as a lecturer in the Department of Biochemistry at the University of Dhaka in 1995 after completion of M.Sc. in 1993. For Ph.D. research, he was awarded Japanese Government Scholarship (Monbukagakusho) and joined in the Laboratory of Nutrition under faculty of Agriculture in Tohoku University, Japan. After completion of Ph.D., he returned to the Department of Biochemistry. From 2008, he was working as a Professor in the same Department. From September 2009 to March 2011, he worked as a Postdoctoral Research Fellow in the Lab of Physiological Functions of Foods in Kyoto University, Japan. He is working in Nutritional and Clinical Biochemistry, specially Rice Glycemic Index, Rice Nutrition, and Rice bran.

Tariq Ismail is working as Assistant Professor of Food Sciences in Institute of Food Science & Nutrition, Bahauddin Zakariya University, Multan - Pakistan. He did his master in Food Science & Technology while his doctoral research is in the domain of Nutraceuticals and Functional Foods. To date, he has authored several quality publications on biomolecules and their disease preventive and curative properties particularly focusing on the chemopreventive properties of natural micro and macromolecules in inflammatory disorders, cardiovascular diseases, various types of cancer, diabetes and infectious diseases. His studies focus on exploration and utilization of fruits and vegetables for the production of novel foods bearing functional and nutraceutical properties.

Kim Hyun Ju, PhD, is Senior Researcher, Research and Development Division, Industrial Technology Research Group, at the World Institute of Kimchi, Korea.

Marena Manley was born in 1961 and grew up in the Northern Cape, South Africa. She obtained her BSc in Food Science degree at Stellenbosch University and subsequently her Honours and MSc degrees at the University of Pretoria. She received her PhD (Food Science) in 1995 from the University of Plymouth, UK. After 18 months in industry, she joined Stellenbosch University in 1997 as a lecturer where she is currently appointed as Professor. Her research interests involve the application of near-infrared (NIR) spectroscopy, NIR hyperspectral imaging and lately also X-ray micro-computed tomography to study whole grain endosperm texture and other cereal defects. More recently she also studies antioxidants of cereal grain as well as the effect of heat processing on phenolics of cereals.

Baltasar Mayo is affiliated to IPLA, a dairy-oriented research institute belonging to CSIC, the Spanish largest public research institution. He is part of the Functional Dairy Cultures (FDC) research team and works on several aspects of dairy and human gastrointestinal microbiology. These studies aim to select appropriate microorganisms to be used for, or added to, fermented dairy products. Current research of FDC focuses on the identification and characterization of isoflavone-activating and metabolizing bacteria from the human gut.

John Muyonga is a Professor of Food Science at Makerere University, where he has worked since 1997. He holds a B.Sc. in Food Science from Makerere University, an M.S. in Food Science from Cornell University and a PhD from University of Pretoria. Prof. Muyonga has served as Dean School of Food Technology, Nutrition and Bioengineering at Makerere University since 2011. Prof Muyonga's research covers aspects of food protein chemistry, characterisation of nutraceutical components from foods materials, food lipids and the effect of processing on nutritional and functional properties of foods. He has studied the effect of different traditional processing conditions for beans, millet, grain amaranth and cooking bananas on nutritional and rheological properties. Prof is widely published, with over 1300 citations in widely indexed journals. He has won multiple research and consultancy contracts. Prof Muyonga is passionate about linking research to development.

Sophie Nansereko holds a BSc. In Food Science and Technology and a MSc. in Applied Human Nutrition from Makerere University. Her research covered aspects of post-harvest handling of groundnuts, as well as application of HACCP along the groundnut value chain. She has over seven years' experience in community food, health and nutrition projects, including working with the Ministry of Health and NGOs. Her professional interests involve developing and implementing innovative interventions aimed at improving the health, nutrition and food security of vulnerable communities.

Judith Kanensi Okoth is a lecturer at Jomo Kenyatta University of Agriculture and Technology (JKUAT), in Kenya where she has worked since 2006. She received her PhD in Foods, Nutrition and Dietetics in 2014 from Kenyatta University in Kenya. She obtained her BSc and Msc degrees in Food Science and Technology at JKUAT. Her career interest involves improving the lives of Kenyans especially the vulnerable groups through research backed development of affordable nutrient dense food products and positive contribution to Government policies on food and nutrition.

Santosh Jain Passi received her Ph.D. in Food and Nutrition from the University of Delhi. She is a Public Health Nutrition Consultant (independent), as well as Former Director, Institute of Home Economics (University of Delhi), Hauz Khas Enclave, New Delhi, Associate and Honorary Consultant (Nutrition and Extension), Nutrition Foundation of India, Qutab Institutional Area, New Delhi Honorary Professor - Public Health Nutrition, Amity University, NOIDA (UP) Head - Public Health Nutrition Division, LSTech Ventures Pvt. Ltd, Udyog Vihar, Gurugram, Honorary Consultant, VTC & Community Health and Nutrition Research and Training Centre, NDSE-I, New Delhi and Ex-Public Health and Nutrition Expert cum Course Coordinator (MoHFW). She has been teaching for nearly 43 years - courses in Foods, Nutrition, Public Nutrition, Dietetics and Research Method. She has a number of papers/ articles published in the field of Foods and Nutrition in various journals, newspapers, periodicals etc.; she has edited the reports of seminars/workshops and have more than 80 abstracts published in various proceedings/ abstract booklets of conferences. She has participated and presented papers in various international, national, Conferences/ Seminars/Symposia; and chaired various scientific sessions.

Saikat Sen is working as Associate Professor, Department of Pharmacy, Assam down town University, Guwahati, India. He gained his Master Degreed (M. Pharm in Pharmacology) from College of Pharmacy, SRIPMS, Coimbatore in 2008 and Ph.D in Pharmaceutical Sciences from JNT University Anantapur, Andhra Pradesh (2014). He has authored two books and contributed different peer reviewed edited books published by American Chemical Society (USA), Springer Publishers and Stadium Press LLC. Nearly 50 research and review articles in reputed national/international journals was added to his credit, presented several scientific papers, attended a number of national and international conferences and delivered invitee lecture in an international forum. Dr. Sen is working as Editorial Board/Advisory Board Member and reviewer of several international and national journals. He also received monetary reward from J For Res in collaboration of Govt. of China to continue his research in herbal medicine. He is member of different professional bodies around the world and involve enthusiastically in scientific research on traditional/folk medicinal system and to develop active research culture.

Jiwan S. Sidhu has a B.Sc. Agri. & A.H., PAU, Ludhiana, India, M.Sc. Food Technology, IFTTC, CFTRI, Mysore, India, Ph.D. Grain Science, Kansas State University, USA, and a PG Diploma in Business Mgt., PAU Ludhiana, India. He has about 45 years of teaching and research experience. He is currently Professor of Food Science, College of Life Sciences, KU, since Sept 19, 2004, and Director of Masters' Program since Sept. 2012. He has published 94 research papers in peer-reviewed journals, 25 book chapters in USA books, and 53 general papers.

Ernest E. Smith is an Associate Professor in the Department of Environmental Toxicology and The Institute of Environmental and Human Health, at Texas Tech University. He received his undergraduate degree in Agricultural Sciences, with a major in animal science from Prairie View A&M University, Prairie View, Texas, and his Ph.D. in Food Science and Technology - Toxicology from Texas A&M University. His teaching and research interests include reproductive and developmental effects of environmental contaminants, as well as the development and understanding of biomarkers of the endocrine systems in developing offspring and adults. He is the author of several peer-reviewed publications and has been awarded several research grants from federal, state, and private sources to investigate various aspects of developmental biology and toxicology. Currently, his research group is focused on characterizing membrane transport proteins and the mechanisms of herbal extracts in the control of glucose transport and metabolism.

Ilona Steenkamp obtained a BSc Food Science degree at the University of Stellenbosch in 2008, after which she completed her MSc degree in 2010, also at Stellenbosch University. Thereafter she was involved in research focusing on the sensory characterisation of rooibos and honeybush teas. She was also appointed as temporary lecturer for cereal science and food chemistry and analysis, and has since been acting in a consulting capacity for the Stellenbosch Food Science Department.

Tasleem A. Zafar, currently employed as an Associate Professor at Kuwait University, earned her Ph.D. degree in the area of Foods and Nutrition at Purdue University, West Lafayette, Indianan, USA. She obtained a substantial research experience as Postdoctoral fellow and as Research Associate at Purdue University, USA and University of Toronto, Canada before she joined the Department of Food Science and Nutrition, College of life Sciences, Kuwait University in 2005. Her primary research interests focus on to develop a good breakthrough for the epidemic ailment of obesity and diabetes through food. Exploring individual micronutrient capacities, for example, calcium, magnesium, and vitamin D, as well as through manipulation of the energy components of the diet such as dietary r resistant starch may help in enhancement of the insulin sensitizing effects and the satiety power of meals. Furthermore, mineral metabolism and bone health status are also her compassion. Dr. Zafar has published more than 20 original research articles in peer-reviewed journals and contributed chapters to four scholarly books on Fruits, Vegetables and Functional Foods, published by Wiley-Blackwell Publishing Co., New York, USA and by IGI Global (formerly Idea Group Inc.), USA. She is an honorary editor of the Pakistan Journal of Home-Economics (PJHE) and has served as an honorary reviewer for Journal Medicinal Foods, Journal of Applied Physiology, Nutrition and Metabolism, Journal of Food Science and Technology and British Journal of Nutrition.

Index

P

R

S

T

U

V

W

Y

www.ingramcontent.com/pod-product-compliance
Lightning Source LLC
LaVergne TN
LVHW080621300926
849162LV00005B/1227